D0053746

TIME TO HEAL

Time to Heal

*American Medical Education
from the Turn of the Century
to the Era of Managed Care*

Kenneth M. Ludmerer

OXFORD
UNIVERSITY PRESS
1999

OXFORD
UNIVERSITY PRESS

Oxford   New York
Athens   Auckland   Bangkok   Bogotá   Buenos Aires
Calcutta   Cape Town   Chennai   Dar es Salaam   Delhi
Florence   Hong Kong   Istanbul   Karachi   Kuala Lumpur
Madrid   Melbourne   Mexico City   Mumbai   Nairobi   Paris
São Paulo   Singapore   Taipei   Tokyo   Toronto   Warsaw

and associated companies in
Berlin   Ibadan

Copyright © 1999 by Oxford University Press, Inc.

Published by Oxford University Press, Inc.
198 Madison Avenue, New York, New York 10016

Oxford is a registered trademark of Oxford University Press, Inc.

All rights reserved. No part of this publication may be
reproduced, stored in a retrieval system, or transmitted,
in any form or by any means, electronic, mechanical,
photocopying, recording, or otherwise, without the
prior permission of Oxford University Press.

Library of Congress Cataloging-in-Publication Data
Ludmerer, Kenneth M.
Time to Heal : American medical education from the turn of the
century to the era of managed care / Kenneth M. Ludmerer.
p. cm.   Includes bibliographical references and index.
ISBN 0-19-511837-5
1. Medical education—United States—
History—20th century.   I. Title.
II. Title : American medical education from the
turn of the century to the era of managed care.
[DNLM : 1. Education, Medical—history—United States.
2. History of Medicine, 20th Cent.—United States.
W 18 L945t 1999]
R745.L843   1999   610'.71'1730904—dc21
DNLM/DLC for Library of Congress   98-55496

1 3 5 7 9 8 6 4 2

Printed in the United States of America
on acid-free paper

For Loren

Contents

Preface

THIS BOOK WAS WRITTEN with two objectives in mind. The first was to provide a comprehensive interpretive history of American medical education from the beginning of the twentieth century through the present. The second was to alert readers to changes the marketplace has exerted on the way doctors learn and practice medicine in the current era of "managed care." Thus, the story relates to the larger practice of medicine and to many current anxieties about health care in America among patients, health care professionals, and the public.

It would have been impossible for me to have conceptualized this book without the experience of having written an earlier book on medical education, *Learning to Heal: The Development of American Medical Education* (Basic Books, 1985), which examined the creation of the country's system of medical education from the Civil War through World War I. In this sense, work for the present volume began in 1976. However, the need for another book became apparent to me in the late 1980s as the managed care movement began to spread rapidly. Many medical schools and teaching hospitals were no longer receiving enough clinical income to allow their educational and research programs to be fully supported. More subtle but more important, the learning environment for medical students and house officers was eroding, and professional values in medical practice were being marginalized. The origins of these dilemmas preceded the 1980s and could not be explained just by a hostile marketplace. Rather, they arose in part from actions (or inactions) within academic medicine itself during the second half of the century. This book represents an effort to help understand these events.

The most important sources for this book were unpublished records from medical schools, hospitals, faculty members, administrators, students, and various private and public organizations. These sources provided rich detail obtainable in no other fashion. During my research, I visited a representative sample of approximately one-quarter of the country's academic medical centers. If certain institutions are represented more frequently in the text, it is usually because their archival holdings were more extensive. In general, records became particularly voluminous for the period after 1965, illustrating one of the daunting problems of researching contemporary history. (For example, the minutes and agenda items of the Executive Council of the Association of American Medical Colleges from 1932 to 1956 were contained in one storage box; the records from 1957 to 1991 required 42 boxes.) The notes to the book are purposely long for the benefit of interested readers. However, the book may be read without returning to the notes, and no one need be distracted by them.

At the beginning of the project it quickly became apparent that the evolution of medical education in America could not be fully understood without being placed in a broad social and cultural context. Thus, I also read extensively in social, cultural, and educational history and medical sociology. The notes serve as a guide to the secondary literature to which I owe so much. It did not lessen my interest in the subject to discover that the history of medical schools and teaching hospitals was in fact a prism of many of the social, cultural, and political forces transforming American society as a whole during the twentieth century.

This book has been crafted so that chapters and sections may be read individually without having to read what precedes or follows. However, the chapters are tightly interrelated, and I hope that readers will find that the narrative is more than the sum of the parts. Every measure has been taken to assure accuracy. Given the rapid-fire changes of the current health care environment, it would be surprising if certain details discussed in Chapters 17 and 18 did not become outdated during the time it took to publish the book—perhaps a new merger between teaching hospitals or medical schools, or a previously announced merger falling apart. However, such epiphenomena will not alter the nature of the transforming forces, the challenges and opportunities American medical education faces for the twenty-first century, or the choices that we as a society will have to make about our health care system in the future. Thus, readers should find the analysis provided in the last two chapters to be salient, even if the landscape should appear slightly different in the near future.

Throughout the narrative I have endeavored to be objective and balanced so that the book might be useful to those of divergent viewpoints about how American medical education and practice should proceed. Those looking to divine the future by reading these pages will be disappointed. The past did not occur in an inevitable or predictable fashion; neither will the future. However, the past bears powerfully on the present in American medicine. Thus, it is my hope that this historical analysis will help illuminate the current dilemmas we face and provide guidance as we make choices about the future of our health care system.

The title of the book conveys a dual meaning. An overarching theme of the book is the importance of time to every aspect of good medicine. Sufficient time is required to learn to heal, to teach how to heal, to practice the art of healing, and to discover new ways to heal. During the current managed care era, time is being squeezed out of each of these activities, which is perhaps the most alarming transformation of all those occurring in American medicine at the present moment. In addition, though both the profession and public at large have recently experienced profound angst about medical education and practice, a historical understanding of the creation of these dilemmas suggests ways out of the predicament. Thus, it is also time to use this knowledge to begin healing our ailing systems of medical education and practice while they are still superb—and salvageable.

Acknowledgments

A T THE END OF A LONG JOURNEY, it is a great pleasure to thank the many persons whose encouragement, advice, and support were so instrumental along the way. While writing this book, I have been unusually fortunate in the assistance I have received from friends and colleagues. Their generous contributions have immeasurably enriched the final product.

Research for the book involved years of travel to scholarly repositories throughout the country, and I am indebted to the many archivists and librarians who aided and encouraged me during this demanding and seemingly endless stage of the project. The notes will serve as an index to the dozens of staffs that so graciously provided assistance. I am especially grateful to Adele Lerner, who at the start of the project guided me through the linear mile of records at the New York Hospital–Cornell Medical Center, and to Susan Crawford, Mark Frisse, and Paul Anderson of the Washington University Medical School Library. I would also like to thank the Rockefeller Archive Center and American Philosophical Society for grants-in-aid that facilitated some of the early travel.

Much of the research, particularly for the most recent decades, was conducted in the offices of medical school deans and hospital presidents, where I was typically the first scholar ever to examine the materials. I was surprised—and inspired—by the willingness of medical school and hospital officials to make their most confidential records open to my inspection. So free was my access to the materials that I was often the one to lock up the office at night. Such willingness among medical educators to allow themselves to be scrutinized, despite knowing that not all that would be found would be flattering, served as a remarkable indication of their commitment to meeting the current challenges in health care decisively and constructively.

During both the research and writing, I benefited from the support and suggestions of many friends and colleagues, who were always available for conversations and musings. I would especially like to thank Garland Allen, Paul Beeson, Henry Berger, Iver Bernstein, Morton Bogdonoff, Gerald Dunne, Mary Ann Dzuback, I. Jerome Flance, Donald Fleming, Renée Fox, Mark Frisse, Thomas Gallagher, Daniel Goodenberger, Jack Hexter, Harry Jonas, Michael Karl, David Kipnis, David Konig, Joseph Losos, Gerald Perkoff, Henry Schwartz, Monte Throdahl, Peter Tuteur, Richard Walter, and Carl Wellman. I have been touched and inspired by these and other individuals in ways they probably do not even realize. I also learned much from serving on a task force on medical education sponsored by the Acadia Institute during a formative stage of the project.

A number of colleagues generously took the time to read all or parts of an earlier version of the book. I would like to thank Paul Beeson, Iver Bernstein, Gert Brieger, Roger Bulger, Mary Ann Dzuback, Donald Fleming, Renée Fox, Mark Frisse, Thomas Gallagher, Daniel Goodenberger, Hugh Hawkins, Diane Katzman, Joseph Kett, David Kipnis, Gerald Perkoff, Linda Sage, Rosemary Stevens, Monte Throdahl, and Michael Whitcomb for their helpful and insightful comments. I am equally grateful to the scholars who participated in a conference in March 1997 to discuss an earlier version of Part III of the book, as well as to the Milbank Memorial Fund for arranging the meeting. I would also like to thank Marietta Magnus for the faithful secretarial and computer assistance she provided and Jeffrey House of Oxford University Press for his constructive suggestions, sage advice, and steady encouragement.

To a few persons I would like to express my special appreciation. Daniel Fox was a source of encouragement and ideas throughout the project. His suggestions on how to strengthen the preliminary manuscript were invaluable, and he became a friend of the book in the broadest possible ways. Ralph Morrow was a continual source of encouragement, advice, and wisdom. Throughout the project we talked regularly, and he offered many helpful suggestions on the preliminary manuscript. In addition, whenever I was stuck, he was available, which was fortunate for me since he was someone whose judgment I particularly trusted. Jordan, Lindsey, and Cissy Ludmerer enriched the book by their presence. Loren Ludmerer was a fountainhead of ideas, guidance, and encouragement, and her many insightful comments and suggestions improved the book enormously. In addition, she contributed to the project in many diverse and important ways that only authors can fully understand.

The most difficult part of the project involved the decision to carry the story through the present and to write a book that spoke to many of the large anxieties of today's health care world. Had the narrative ended with Chapter 16, the book would have been ready for publication two or three years earlier. In this context, I am extremely grateful to the Washington University Department of Medicine for providing an unusually supportive environment that allowed me to undertake a large project where success was not guaranteed. I am also indebted to a number of private foundations for the indispensable financial support they provided: the Henry J. Kaiser Family Foundation, the American Medical Association Foundation, the Charles E. Culpeper Foundation, the Spencer Foundation, and especially, the Josiah Macy, Jr. Foundation. These organizations accepted the notion that it would be important to have a study that examined and analyzed medical education from a broad point of view. My hope is that they will feel that their trust has been justified.

Introduction

IT IS HARDLY AN ACCIDENT that the twentieth century has been called "the health century." Americans have been blessed with a soaring life expectancy, declining infant mortality, control of the infectious and nutritional diseases that have ravaged the human race throughout recorded history, and important advances against modern-day killers like cancer, coronary artery disease, and stroke. Technological marvels such as computer-guided scanners and organ transplantation have astonished and amazed the public, as have remarkable breakthroughs in genetic medicine and biotechnology. It is difficult to know which seems more like science fiction: the recent cloning of a sheep (and the prospect of cloning human beings), or the World Health Organization's expansive definition of health as the presence of physical, mental, socioeconomic, and spiritual well-being, not the absence of sickness.

No factor has been more important to the achievements of medical practice in the United States than the country's medical schools and teaching hospitals (or academic health centers, as the joint institutions are typically called). Their importance lay in the education of the nation's doctors, generation of new medical knowledge, introduction and evaluation of innovative clinical practices, and provision of the most sophisticated medical care available. During most of the twentieth century, an admiring public obligingly catered to their needs, and the institutions accordingly prospered. Nevertheless, academic health centers also grew insular, and at century's end the public was withdrawing much of its traditional support of them. As the millennium approached, medical schools and teaching hospitals were in jeopardy, with disturbing implications for the future quality of medical care in America. It is this paradox of academic health centers—that they were so successful, so central to the nation's health, and ultimately so threatened—that is the central concern of the story told in the following pages.

❦ . ❦ . ❦

This book is intended to provide a synthetic history of American medical education from the turn of the twentieth century through the present. A major focus is the four years of medical school—the period of undergraduate medical education. However, the book explores many other topics, such as premedical training, admissions, residency and specialty education (graduate medical education), the institutions of medical training, and the complex interactions between academic health centers and the society they were created to serve. The story includes such issues as the financing of medical education, the expansion of medical research, the creation of new medical schools, the problems encountered by minority and women students, the changing relationship between teaching and research, the difficulty of retaining the art of medicine in a technological age, the erosion of medical education's traditional patient base, the growing tension between egalitarian and educational ideals, and the complex relationships between medical schools and teaching hospitals, medical schools and universities, and academic health centers and their surrounding neighborhoods.

This history is very much a study of people, not just institutions. A primary objective is to recapture the experience of students, house officers, faculty, administrators, and patients and to describe how their day-to-day lives in the medical world have evolved over the course of a century. Similarly, the book examines the relationships among these various groups, such as how faculty have established authority over students and house officers, how those in training have prodded their instructors to remain intellectually honest, how learners have coped with the sometimes brutal training conditions, and the ways in which the relationships between students and patients have changed. The book also examines certain unseemly events in the history of medical education, such as admission quotas and the ongoing tensions between "town" (community physicians) and "gown" (medical faculties).

Traditionally, most writings in the history of medicine have emphasized either the intellectual development of medicine (the "internalist" approach) or the social, economic, and political context of medicine (the "externalist" approach). This book is characterized by the attempt to incorporate both perspectives. Important to this discussion are the changes in medical education and practice that have resulted from the internal development of medicine, particularly the increasing reductionism (molecular level of analysis) of medical knowledge. However, the book also interprets medical education in its external context: higher education in America, the evolving health care delivery system, and the major cultural trends of the twentieth century.

A strong sociological perspective also pervades the book. A striking observation is that the power of medical education is limited, particularly regarding its ability to produce doctors who are caring, socially responsible, and capable of behaving as patient advocates in all practice environments. Indeed, much of the behavior of physicians reflects influences from outside the medical school, such as the character and values of those who choose to enter medicine, the cultural climate of the time, and the particular rewards and incentives offered by medical practice. It is important to recognize that the caliber of doctors we have represents a negotiation between medical education and society. Our physicians reflect the type of people and society we are, not just the efforts of academic health centers. It would not be an exaggeration to say that as a nation we ultimately get the type of doctors we deserve.

In view of the many similarities among medical schools, it is possible to speak in these pages of American medical education as a whole. All schools must conform to uniform standards to receive accreditation, all teach the same corpus of knowledge, and graduates of all schools are entitled to practice anywhere in the United States. However, it is equally important to recognize the striking diversity that exists among medical schools. Some are private, others public. Most utilize major teaching hospitals for their clinical work, but many new schools use smaller community hospitals. The level of research activities varies markedly from one school to another, as does the commitment to special missions, such as the production of primary care practitioners or the education of racial minorities. No school is without its distinctive local traditions. This dual perspective of commonality and individuality is important to understanding American medical schools fully, even if it is not possible in this book to provide an account of each school.

It is sometimes tempting to interpret the evolution of American medical education as the response of medical schools and teaching hospitals to powerful external forces: the Depression, World War II, the National Institutes of Health, private medical insurance, Medicare and Medicaid, and the managed care movement. This view is only partially correct, for individuals also mattered. This fact goes a long way toward explaining the relative professional ascent of some schools and relative decline of others. It would be a great error to view the history of American medical education as devoid of people or personalities.

Precisely because individuals were important, American medical education did not develop in a predictable or inevitable fashion. At every point choices were made—some with good results, others with less salutary consequences. If American medical schools and teaching hospitals were in a precarious position at the end of the century, it was not because anyone desired to do them harm but because poor decisions were made or unforeseen consequences occurred. Nevertheless, for those who wish to do so, opportunities to influence medical education in a more constructive direction are still present. The lesson of history is that the future is not predetermined and that individuals can make a difference.

❦ · ❦ · ❦

In view of the book's broad scope, it may be useful to identify the major themes.

By World War I, the modern medical school and teaching hospital in the United States had been created, and the first revolution in American medical education (often called the "Flexnerian" revolution, after Abraham Flexner, the author of an influential report on medical education in 1910) was complete. This revolution called for medical schools to be university-based, for faculty to be engaged in original research, and for students to participate in "active" learning through laboratory study and real clinical work. The origins of the revolution dated to the mid-nineteenth century, when a revolution occurred regarding how medicine should be taught. Subsequently, this intellectual revolution begot a social and economic revolution that allowed the new educational ideas to be implemented. During the revolution an implicit social contract was established. Society would provide the necessary financial, political, and moral support of medical education and research. In exchange, medical faculties would remember that they existed to serve, and the measure of their success would be the quality of their academic work and their success at ensuring that medical practice in America was conducted according to high, professionally determined standards.

From the beginning, the modern American medical school had a tripartite mission: education, research, and patient care. However, the relative importance of these activities varied with time. From World War I to World War II, the educational mission was paramount. Teaching was the end in itself, and patient care was pursued only insofar as it was needed to facilitate teaching. Faculties prided themselves on providing an educational environment that focused on the needs of learners, a group that expanded during this time to include interns and residents as well as medical students.

As medical faculties taught, they also engaged in research. By the 1930s the United States had become the foremost nation in medical research in the world. After World War II, however, research replaced teaching as the dominant activity of most medical faculties. This resulted primarily from the expansion of the National Institutes of Health. By 1965, federal grants and contracts typically accounted for 60 percent or more of the budgets of research-intensive medical schools. However, all medical schools shared in the wealth, and at virtually every school, the research enterprise grew to a size that before the war would have been considered unimaginable.

As the period from World War I to World War II was the educational era, and that from World War II to 1965 the research era, the period after

1965 was the clinical era. Since the 1940s, with the spread of private medical insurance in the United States, medical faculties had increasingly engaged in the private practice of medicine. However, after the passage of Medicare and Medicaid in 1965, the amount of faculty practice began to soar, as millions of "ward" (charity) patients became paying patients overnight. Within 15 years, the size of the clinical enterprise eclipsed that of the academic enterprise at virtually every school, and faculties typically generated 50 percent or more of their income from private practice. Clinical revenue allowed an extraordinary expansion of faculty sizes and salaries, particularly in the clinical departments.

During each of these three eras, medical schools experienced enormous growth. In 1910, a leading medical school might have had a budget of $100,000. By 1940, that budget typically had grown to $1,000,000; by 1965, to $20,000,000; and by 1990, to $200,000,000 or more. At most schools, growth was unplanned and by accretion, with new programs piling on top of existing ones. By the 1980s, medical schools were no longer cohesive organizations. Education, research, and patient care, once interrelated activities held in some sort of balance, had each been magnified to the point that they could no longer be readily balanced with each other.

As medical schools grew, a number of conspicuous changes occurred. The education of medical students, once the central mission of medical schools (and their one unique activity), was no more than a by-product of what contemporary academic health centers were doing in the 1980s. Throughout the century, medical schools had been situated in part in the university and in part in the health care delivery system. Now, the medical school's ties to the university had significantly weakened, while its involvement in the health care delivery system had correspondingly grown. During the course of the century, academic health centers had evolved primarily in a faculty-driven fashion, as opposed to a style that concentrated on the needs of learners or the wishes of society for medical schools to help improve the health care delivery system.

Though education by the 1980s was rarely a high institutional priority, the quality of medical education obtainable in the United States remained superb. This was because all medical learning was ultimately self-learning. Throughout the century, the high quality of American medical education depended far less on the formal curriculum than it did on attracting motivated, capable students and providing them unfettered opportunities to learn. Essential to this learning environment were good laboratories and libraries, an ample and diverse supply of patients, and stimulating teachers and colleagues. Most important of all was the fact that medical education was conducted in settings where learners were provided sufficient time with patients so that patients could be studied and understood.

In the 1980s and 1990s, with the spread of the managed care movement, the supportive environment for academic health centers rapidly began to change. Managed care (a generic term encompassing a variety of new approaches to financing and delivering medical care) arose as an attempt to correct serious, long-standing problems in the health care delivery system. Soon, however, many problems with managed care also became apparent, among which were its deleterious effects on academic health centers. Managed care organizations insisted on paying the lowest possible price for medical care. In this new environment, academic health centers, which had higher costs than community hospitals because of education, research, charity care, and certain highly specialized clinical services, suddenly found their financial viability threatened.

Specific responses of academic health centers to this situation varied, but the general thrust was to expand their clinical enterprises still further so that they might make up in volume what they were losing in price. More patients could be seen if faculties treated patients more quickly—by decreasing the length of stay and increasing the turnover of inpatients, or by brief, rapid-fire office visits for outpatients. Medical school and teaching hospital officials, who once measured their success by the physicians they educated and the new knowledge they produced, now increasingly focused on their institution's profitability and market share, with scant discussion of what was happening to education and research.

By the late 1990s, it was clear that the competitive, market-driven response of most faculties was generally successful in terms of maintaining or even increasing clinical income. However, in the process, the quality of academic work at most schools began to suffer. At many schools, clinical teachers and investigators were forced to spend more and more time seeing patients, sometimes to the near abandonment of their educational responsibilities. More insidious and more serious, the increasing speed with which patients were treated wreaked havoc on the learning environment of academic health centers, whose quintessential feature had always been that it had allowed students and house officers enough time with patients for educational objectives to be met. Equally disturbing were the potential long-term effects of educating the nation's doctors in a commercial atmosphere where the good visit was a short visit, where patients were "consumers," and where institutional officials spoke more often of the financial balance sheet than of service and the relief of suffering. Such an environment did little to validate the altruism and idealism that students typically brought with them to the study of medicine.

Ironically, in the 1990s it became apparent that what was good for medical schools and medical faculties was not necessarily good for medical education. Schools could remain financially strong and continue to pay their faculty high salaries if the professors spent more time in patient care and less in teaching and research. Similarly, medical schools and teaching hospitals could do well financially if patients were admitted and discharged so quickly that learners could no longer profit from their contact with them. At the end of the decade, faculty practice had many strong advocates among medical educators, as did medical research. However, education had surprisingly few defenders or champions. It was by far the most endangered part of the medical school's traditional mission.

Thus, as the millennium approached, a second revolutionary period in American medical education had begun—one characterized by the dismantling of the infrastructure of medical education that had served the country well for most of the twentieth century. The learning environment at academic health centers was eroding, faculty research was decreasing, and faculty incomes, as at the proprietary schools of the nineteenth century, depended mainly on the private practice of medicine rather than on teaching and research. The social contract between society and medical education had been bilaterally broken. Society was no longer providing academic health centers sufficient financial or political support. In turn, medical faculties had grown inwardly focused. They seemed unwilling to make sacrifices to protect education, and they appeared similarly unwilling to fulfill their traditional responsibility of standing up for high standards of care.

Since medical education and medical practice were inextricably linked, these events carried disturbing implications for the American public. It was difficult to imagine the quality of care remaining high in the United States if the quality of medical education was eroding and if clinical research was tapering off. Similarly, it did not bode well for the quality of care if medical faculties were unwilling to execute their traditional responsibility of defining and maintaining the standards of practice. In the 1990s this was a matter of no small concern, for many serious questions had been raised in the popular media about the quality of care under managed care. It was also not clear that medical schools were effectively instilling among physicians their fiduciary duty to patients. There was increasing talk in the 1990s of doctors serving the needs of populations, health care systems, and organizations; surprisingly little was heard from medical educators about the need for doctors to remain their patients' friend, counselor, and advocate.

As the twenty-first century approached, medical schools still ranked among the crown jewels of the country's educational system, and the quality of medical practice in America remained high. More disturbing than the actual damage inflicted was the projection of recent trends. The most important immediate challenge medical education faced was to adapt to its rapidly changing environment without compromising its core value of service to society or its core mission of education, research, and determining the standards of care. Fortunately for the American public, the second revolution was just beginning. That meant there was still time for individuals within and without the profession to influence events so that both society and medical education might be better served.

PART I

Fulfilling the Social Contract

Medical Education as a Public Trust and the Capture of Public Confidence

1

Creating the System

ONE COULD SCARCELY BLAME American medical educators in the 1920s if they appeared smug. Observing the condition of medical training in the United States and abroad, they noted with undisguised pleasure that American medical education was nowhere to be surpassed. In the course of the preceding half century American medical education had evolved from the worst in industrialized civilization to the very best. To many, this transformation was "the marvel of the educational world."[1]

Among those who proudly surveyed the condition of American medical education was Abraham Flexner. No one name has ever been more closely identified with medical education than Flexner's.[2] Once an obscure headmaster of a private high school in Louisville, he gained prominence in 1910 by writing a famous muckraking report for the Carnegie Foundation for the Advancement of Teaching, *Medical Education in the United States and Canada*, frequently termed the "Flexner report."[3] This report, which castigated American medical schools for their commercialism and deplorably low standards, launched Flexner into national prominence as arbiter of educational reform and earned him another job—secretary of John D. Rockefeller's huge foundation, the General Education Board. As a foundation officer, dispensing tens of millions of Rockefeller dollars to selected medical schools, he embarked upon the upgrading of standards as a personal crusade. Dogmatic, rigid, and acerbic, though incredibly charming and ingratiating when he chose to be, Flexner readily acknowledged his tendency "to butt in" to the affairs of medical schools.[4] Thus, it was with considerable pleasure in 1930 that he reflected upon what had been accomplished in American medical education. "Positive and immense progress has . . . been made." Anyone who knew conditions early in the century would be "amazed" at the change.[5]

Such enthusiasm was understandable, for American medical education had undergone a startling transformation.[6] At the close of the Civil

War, it did not take much hard work to become a doctor in America. Entrance requirements to medical school were nonexistent, other than the ability to pay the fees. Courses were superficial and brief. The typical path to a medical degree consisted of two 16-week terms of lectures, the second term repeating the material of the first. Instruction was almost wholly didactic, consisting of lectures and textbook reading. Laboratory work in the scientific subjects and student participation in patient care in the clinical courses were not to be found. Medical school faculties were tiny, typically numbering seven or eight. The instructors owned the schools and operated them for profit—hence the term "proprietary schools" to denote them. A school might conduct business on the second floor above a corner drug store, and it was unheard of for a school to have laboratories, pursue research, or possess a genuine affiliation with a university or hospital. American students not satisfied with the casual education offered in this country had to go to Europe for more comprehensive and thorough instruction in the medical sciences and clinical specialties.

By the 1920s a revolution had occurred, one that is often called the Flexnerian revolution. Entrance requirements had been established, the course of instruction had been expanded to four years of nine-month terms, and the scientific components of the curriculum had been greatly strengthened. Didactic teaching had been deemphasized, and in its place the laboratory and clinical clerkship provided the core of the learning experience. The proprietary school had been replaced by the university medical school, replete with new laboratories and facilities, a burgeoning army of full-time instructors, a commitment to research, a proliferation of new hospital facilities and affiliations, and a bureaucratic administrative structure. The quality of American medical education now surpassed that provided by European schools. That this was so could be seen in the results of licensing examinations. In the 1920s over 60 percent of graduates of European medical schools, whether European or native born, failed to pass the New York state licensing examination, compared with a failure rate of 14 percent among graduates of United States schools.[7]

The creation of America's system of medical education was a long, arduous process that began in the mid-nineteenth century amid the birth of experimental medicine on the Continent and the migration of American medical graduates to France and Germany to acquire the latest scientific knowledge and, more important, an understanding of scientific methodology and technique. In the early 1870s, the first lasting reforms occurred as Harvard, Pennsylvania, and Michigan extended their course of study to three years, added new scientific subjects to the curriculum, required laboratory work of each student, and began hiring full-time medical scientists to the faculty. In the late 1870s, the plans for the new Johns Hopkins Medical School were announced, though for financial reasons the opening was delayed until 1893. When the school finally did open, it immediately became the model by which all other medical schools were measured, much as the Johns Hopkins University in 1876 had become the model for the modern research university. A college degree was required for admission, a four-year curriculum with nine-month terms was adopted, classes were small, students were frequently examined, the laboratory and the clerkship were the primary teaching devices, and a brilliant full-time faculty made medical research as well as medical education part of its mission. In the 1880s and 1890s, schools across the country started to emulate the pioneering schools, and a campaign to reform American medical education began. By the turn of the century, the university medical school had become the acknowledged ideal, and proprietary schools were already closing for want of students.

Nevertheless, much work remained to be done, mainly because schools lacked the financial resources and clinical facilities to execute their new ideas of how to teach medicine. It was at that point that Abraham Flexner joined the staff of the Carnegie Foundation. Contrary to a widespread myth, Flexner made no intellectual contribution to the discussion of how physicians should be taught. The ideas he popularized to the public in his report were those that had developed within medical faculties during the 1870s and 1880s. Still, his report proved indispensable to the reform movement. It made the reform of medical education a cause célèbre, transforming what previously had largely been a private matter within the profession into a broad social movement similar to other reform movements of progressive era America. The public responded by opening its pocketbook, and in the decade that followed the report the money and clinical facilities that had long eluded medical schools at last became available. In addition, an outraged public, scandalized by Flexner's acerbic depiction of the proprietary schools still in existence, brought a sudden end to the proprietary era through the enactment of state licensing laws, which mandated that medical schools operated for profit would no longer be accredited.

Why should the Flexner report have exuded such indignation and moral outrage? The answer lies in the fact that in the early twentieth century it made a difference to the public how its doctors were trained. The condition of medical practice had improved immeasurably since the Civil War, when doctors routinely performed such noxious treatments as bleeding, purging, and blistering—long after these so-called "heroic" treatments had been shown to be ineffective by the French clinical school. Nevertheless, at the turn of the century medical practice did not consistently reflect the state of medical knowledge, particularly when the practices of older doctors and doctors trained at the weaker medical schools were considered. It was estimated that a patient in 1900 stood only a fifty-fifty chance of benefiting from an encounter with a random physician.[8] In 1912, one recent graduate of Harvard Medical School starting a practice in Nebraska was stunned to learn that his microscope was the only one in that section of the country—a full 30 years after the enunciation of the germ theory of disease and the creation of the science of bacteriology.[9]

Medical schools, Flexner argued, were public trusts. Now that scientific medicine was offering genuinely effective treatments, it was unconscionable to allow any physician to receive an inferior training.[10]

The relationship between medical knowledge and medical practice is complex and has varied over place and time. Nevertheless, in early twentieth-century America, medical practice clearly lagged behind medical knowledge. The revolution in medical education was necessitated by the fact that medical schools were not consistently translating the existing body of scientific knowledge into medical practice. The gap between what was known and what was taught was unacceptably wide. The social mission of the Flexnerian revolution was to ensure, in a democratic society, that the best possible scientific training be made available to every person studying medicine. The revolution succeeded brilliantly in bringing this about. As a result, the quality of medical education began to determine the quality of available medical care. Improvements in medical education were now translated into an elevation in the level of practice; the ordinary citizen at last could be confident in the care he would receive from any licensed physician. This was the meaning of the Flexnerian revolution.

❦ · ❦ · ❦

As may be inferred from the above discussion, the creation of America's system of medical education occurred in two overlapping stages. It began as a revolution in ideas concerning the purpose and methods of medical education. After the Civil War, medical educators began rejecting traditional notions that medical education should inculcate facts through rote memorization. Rather, the new objective of medical education was to produce problem-solvers and critical thinkers who knew how to find out and evaluate information for themselves. To do so, medical educators deemphasized traditional didactic teaching methods—lectures and textbooks—and began speaking of the importance of self-education and learning by doing. Through laboratories and clinical clerkships, students were to be active participants in their learning, not passive observers as before. A generation before John Dewey, medical educators were espousing the ideas of what later came to be called "progressive education."

Learning by doing greatly increased the demands on medical schools, for the new teaching methods were extremely costly to implement. Thus, an intellectual revolution gave rise to an institutional revolution. The proprietary medical school was abandoned, and the university medical school was created. Funds were raised, new laboratories and facilities were built, clinical facilities were acquired, and full-time faculty with research interests were hired. Medical schools, which had existed as autonomous institutions during the proprietary era, became closely affiliated with universities and teaching hospitals. After the opening of the Johns Hopkins Medical School in 1893, the intellectual revolution in medical education was complete. Subsequent developments in the reform movement were concerned primarily with creating a new institutional structure for medical education that would allow the desired educational methods to be carried out.

As America's new system of medical education emerged, the focus of reformers was on "undergraduate medical education" (the education of medical students in medical school) and not on "graduate medical education" (the formal training that physicians receive after graduation from medical school, such as internship, residency, and fellowship). At the turn of the century, graduation from medical school was considered sufficient preparation for practice. Few doctors were taking internships; even fewer, residencies or specialty training. However, by the 1920s the reorganized medical school had the capacity to meet new responsibilities that might arise as scientific and social circumstances changed. Thus, the modern medical school not only accommodated the needs of undergraduate medical education early in the twentieth century but residency and specialty training soon thereafter and a much larger program of research and patient care after World War II.

It is important to recognize that the revolution in medical education came from within the medical profession. As William Welch, the legendary first dean of the Johns Hopkins Medical School, put it, "The advancement and development of medicine in itself required an improvement in the methods of teaching medicine."[11] Of course, the new system would not have been created without the financial help of foundations, philanthropists, ordinary citizens, and state and local governments. However, the idea that students should learn by doing and the conviction that research belongs in medical schools sprang from the evolution of medical science itself. Leaders of academic medicine energetically disseminated this idea to the profession and public and helped raise the funds to bring those ideas to institutional reality. In this sense, the revolution in medical education represented an outstanding example of what recent writers on organizational behavior have called "proactive" thinking.[12] Medical educators defined their vision of an ideal system of medical education—one that was in the best interests of both the medical profession and society—and then devised a strategy to create that system. In doing so they demonstrated considerable entrepreneurial skill and an uncanny ability to remain focused on long-term goals.

Though the new system was brilliantly successful, its creation did not come without costs or problems. To members of the working class, denied a career in medicine because of the more rigid entrance requirements of the modern medical school, the passing of the proprietary school may not have seemed such a good thing. Private practitioners, relegated to peripheral teaching roles by the upstart and sometimes supercilious full-time academicians, harbored more than a few grudges and resentments. Rural communities, popular sites for graduates of proprietary schools to locate, found themselves attracting fewer new doctors. And reflective individuals began to ask thorny questions about medical education. What is the role of education in determining physician behavior? What should be the role of the medical school in improving the health care system of the country? These and other troubling issues tended to arouse little passion in the early twentieth century, so great was the infatuation with what medical education had achieved. Nevertheless, in the decades that followed, these dilemmas were to prove persistent—for medical education, and for the American educational system in general.

Progressive Medical Education

The complex story of the creation of America's system of medical education involved many important elements. Scientific advance, technological achievement, and individual and collective professional ambition played indispensable roles. So did a host of important social factors, such as the rationalization of America's school system, the rise of the modern university, the country's economic growth, the development of a tradition of philanthropy, the reform impulse of the progressive era, and the new responsibilities that local, state, and federal government began to assume for the regulation of society's affairs.

Nevertheless, at the heart of the transformation of American medical education was a revolution in ideas concerning how medicine should be taught. Traditional teaching devices—the lecture and textbook—diminished in importance. Instead, emphasis was placed on laboratory work in the scientific subjects and hospital work with real responsibility for patient care in the clinical years, in the hope that students would develop the power of critical reasoning, the capacity to generalize, and the ability to find out and evaluate information for themselves. In the American medical school, as in the American college, the days when students' sole task was to memorize the innumerable details of the lectures or textbooks had passed.

The revolution in educational philosophy arose from the rapid growth of medical knowledge in the nineteenth century. In the first half of the century, the French clinical school conducted its pathbreaking work. The science of pathology was created, techniques of physical examination were developed, statistical methods were for the first time applied to clinical investigations, and the hospital became the center of medical teaching and research. The French empiricists, believing only what their senses told them, discredited the traditional notion that disease results from imbalanced "humors" in the body; instead, they showed that disease is a localized phenomenon that can be anatomically detected in specific organs. The pace of discovery accelerated in midcentury, as the experimental era in medical research began. The enunciation of the theory of the cell, the creation of modern physiology, the articulation of the cellular theory of disease, the rise of experimental pathology—all demonstrated the explanatory power of experimental medicine and the importance to medical thought of the basic medical sciences. Excitement over fundamental research increased still further in the 1870s and early 1880s, with the articulation of the germ theory of disease, the isolation and identification of the specific microorganisms that cause tuberculosis and many other dreaded diseases, and the birth of the science of bacteriology. New drugs—for example, aspirin and chloral hydrate—began to appear, and surgery underwent an astonishing development after antiseptic techniques came into general employ.[13]

With these discoveries, a major epistemological shift occurred. It became clear that experimental methods could be applied to the study of disease and therapeutics, not just the healthy condition. For the first time, the causes of disease were being explained in fundamental terms, and from basic science new treatments were being developed. Scientific knowledge no longer represented a curiosity, irrelevant to the concerns of ordinary doctors. Rather, such knowledge began to reshape and direct clinical practice. Moreover, through experimental research, the process of discovery had been normalized. Much remained to be learned, but laboratory research offered the promise that more knowledge and treatments would soon be forthcoming.

How should medical schools cope with the onslaught of new information? This was the challenge medical educators faced as they contemplated the ever-growing tide of discovery and the exponential rise in the number of books and journals. "The time has gone by when one mind can encompass all which has been ascertained in the medical sciences,"[14] Welch wrote in 1886. Moreover, they had to contend with the even more daunting realization that knowledge is not fixed. They recognized that knowledge not only grows but evolves—a metaphor that was not lost on them in the wake of the theory of evolution. No one could take solace in what he thought he knew, for today's "truths" might readily be disproved by new research. "Your new text books will be antiquated in five years,"[15] John Shaw Billings, a pioneering medical educator, warned the graduating medical school class of the University of Pennsylvania.

To medical educators, there was but one viable approach to managing the information explosion: to redesign medical education so that it should have a procedural rather than a substantive emphasis. Instead of enforcing the memorization of established facts and dogmas, medical education should teach students how to acquire and evaluate information themselves. In developing sound habits of thought, students must learn that knowledge derived from personal observation and experience was to be trusted far more than the dictates of any authority. Since there was simply too much to learn, and what was "known" would undoubtedly change, students first and foremost must be able to understand biological principles and formulate sound judgments. In addition, physicians needed to be able to remain up-to-date throughout a professional career—something they could reasonably hope to accomplish only if they had mastered the methods of self-education.

In the early twentieth century, the idea that students should learn by doing was not confined to medical education alone. Throughout the educational system—the elementary school, the high school, the college—educators were speaking of the importance of active learning and an experiential approach to acquiring knowledge. The challenge to education at every level was the same: to foster the ability to acquire information for oneself, so that old habits or ideas might be cast aside for the new as conditions or circumstances changed. A catechistic view of knowledge was no more suitable for the ordinary citizen struggling to cope with the many changes in day-to-day life than it was for the average physician struggling to keep abreast of evolving medical ideas. Accordingly, in education at every level, many leaders were arguing that the main goal should be the promotion of problem-solving, self-learning, and critical thinking. This concept of education, complex in its origin, was popularly known as "progressive education" and most closely associated with the ideas of John Dewey.[16] Abraham Flexner espoused these educational principles as fervidly as Dewey himself, and his writings on medical education constituted primers on progressive education. "Though medicine can be learned," Flexner wrote in 1925, "it cannot be taught."[17] "Active participation—doing things—is therefore the fundamental note of medical teaching."[18]

The applicability of these concepts to medical education remains strong today, and every generation of medical educators since the 1870s has expressed its belief in them. Yet, it is not easy to teach students how to think critically, particularly in a discipline so laden with important facts as medicine. The history of twentieth-century medical education is one of striving to attain these ideals rather than one of actual realization. Nevertheless, these concepts have persisted as the goals of medical education, even if progressive education has faded as the underlying inspiration of common school education. This reflects the great intellectual demands that progressive education places on both teachers and students: it takes very talented instructors to inspire students to think for themselves and motivated and gifted students to do so. Progressive education has traditionally been considered a representation of the democratic spirit in education, but, ironically, it survived in institutional form in the United States largely at a level of instruction targeted for the elite.

Fund-Raising

In progressive medical education students were expected to learn more than they were taught. However, the new approach placed great demands on the schools as well. Much more money was needed, for medical education had become both labor and capital intensive. Many more instructors were required to provide the close supervision, personalized instruction, and unhurried discussions with students that progressive medical education demanded. New land had to be purchased, buildings and classrooms constructed, laboratories equipped, clinics established, and higher operating expenses provided. As medical schools began to define research as part of their mission, more money still was needed. The sums required greatly exceeded that which a school could expect from tuition fees.

Before 1910, money for medical education remained in extremely short supply. One of the fundamental challenges medical schools faced was acquiring the funds to implement the desired educational changes. In 1891, the total endowments for American medical schools amounted to only $500,000, in contrast to $18,000,000 for theological schools.[19] For the next 20 years, despite some success at raising money, the lack of funds continued to undermine most efforts to improve medical education.

In the years immediately following the Flexner report, the financial troubles of medical education were finally alleviated. Medical schools received huge amounts of money that in the aggregate amounted to hundreds of millions of dollars. The most visible force was the large national foundations, especially the General Education Board and Carnegie Corporation. The General Education Board alone contributed $61 million by 1928 and, by restricting the use of its money to endowments, helped make innovations at those schools self-sustaining. However, foundation support was far from essential for a medical school to succeed. Schools also received generous support from private philanthropists, ordinary citizens, and state and local governments. By the 1920s medical education was on a solid financial footing, and the acquisition of this money made possible the implementation of many long-desired educational goals.[20] Equally important, since state legislatures and philanthropic foundations were permanent institutions whose concern for medical education persisted, a means for the continued support of medical education and research had been established.

By World War I, medical education and research might have seemed obvious targets of support, so impressive had been the development of medical science over the preceding generation. Of great importance to those who would provide financial aid to medical schools, more and more discoveries carried practical benefits. The germ theory of disease allowed a rational approach to be taken in public health and helped lead to the use of antiseptic techniques in the operating room. The specific causes of numerous infectious diseases were identified. Hormones and vitamins were discovered and specific treatments developed—for example, thyroid extract for myxedema. Immunology blossomed, as effective antitoxins were discovered against tetanus and diphtheria and vaccines developed against rabies, typhoid, and bubonic plague. Great excitement arose over the use of new diagnostic techniques: electrocardiograms; X-rays; and chemical, hematologic, and serologic tests of blood and urine. The popular press filled with paeans to modern medicine. In 1924 one such work, entitled *Fifty Years of Medical Progress*, spoke of the preceding half century as "the golden age of medical progress." The "general advance has been so enormous that one cannot fail to be struck with amazement."[21]

Adding to the enthusiasm, medicine seemed to possess the method—experimental laboratory research—by which even greater conquest of disease would be forthcoming. What mattered most, both to doctors and the public, was that the major discoveries of medicine had not occurred by chance but by the use of systematic experimentation and the application of fundamental principles of biology and chemistry. Experimental research, boasted one prominent medical scientist, provided "a powerful agent for extending knowledge."[22] In 50 years, predicted another, "science will have practically eliminated all forms of disease."[23] Such faith in scientific method was part of a widespread reverence for science in progressive era America.

The excitement over scientific medicine was instrumental to the success schools now enjoyed in fund-raising. However, the acquisition of funds was a complex process, and donors gave to medical schools for a variety of reasons. The growing ability of medicine to intervene in the natural history of disease appealed to the period's prevailing notions of "scientific philanthropy," which valued most highly those endeavors that sought to alter the causes of problems rather than simply to palliate surface conditions.[24] Altruism, the death of a family member, the lack of heirs, an egocentric desire to see one's name immortalized on a building or laboratory, the desire for power, the quest for social legitimization—all these motives influenced one benefactor or another. Donors, large and small, had agendas of their own, choosing to support some schools or projects over others. No benefactor had a more sharply defined agenda than Abraham Flexner, who as secretary of the General Education Board would consider for support only schools that had adopted his version of the "full-time plan"—the appointment to clinical departments of salaried instructors who derived no income from seeing patients. Some writers have argued that medical philanthropy served the needs of the corporate class by directing the attention of workers to health rather than to the underlying inequities of a capitalistic society, thereby dissipating potential social unrest.[25] Money was power, and contributors to medical education knew that.

Nevertheless, raising money was not easy. Many reluctant benefactors or legislatures had to be wooed. The president of Cornell University complained to the president of Columbia of the great work involved in persuading the very rich of New York City to give money to medical schools. "Our multi-millionaires will naturally not give money till they have definite knowledge about the nature and character of the institution which is to receive it."[26] Few with money would give to medical schools on demand; they had to be presented with sound justifications and a specific plan. This created the opportunity and necessity for leaders of medical education to truly lead.

Medical educators responded to the challenge. From the earliest days of the reform movement they campaigned zealously to arouse public interest in medical science. Increasingly, their efforts bore fruit, now that medicine was rapidly rising in "cultural authority."[27] Individuals such as Victor Vaughan (Michigan), Henry Bowditch (Harvard), John Collins Warren (Harvard), L. Emmett Holt (Physicians and Surgeons), William Pepper (Pennsylvania), and Christian Holmes (Cincinnati) gained fame as exceptional fund-raisers. They made notable contributions not only to the intellectual growth of their disciplines but also to the development of their respective medical schools.

No one was more renowned for his entrepreneurial gifts than William Welch, the professor of pathology and dean of the Johns Hopkins Medical School. His judgment, insight, and force of personality gained him the ready ear of lawmakers, philanthropists, foundation officials, university presidents, and U.S. presidents. He contributed to the development not only of Johns Hopkins but of academic medicine generally in the United States. For example, he established the country's first medical research journal and first school of public health, he helped establish the first "full-time plan" for clinical faculty, and he helped organize the Rockefeller Institute for Medical Research. Gifted with extraordinary executive ability and administrative skill, he could have been a captain of industry had he so chosen, and his influence in helping build a system of medical education in the United States was comparable to the work of banker J. P. Morgan in creating a system of vertically integrated corporations in American business.[28]

If medical educators acted with zeal, it was because they had much at stake. Since American physicians had begun traveling to German universities for postgraduate medical study, they had returned to the United States with a new ideal: that of being able to spend their full time in teaching and research, just like their German professors had been doing. At the beginning of the reform era no full-time medical school positions existed in the United States, and throughout the nineteenth century the lack of opportunities for research was the great frustration of those aspiring to careers in academic medicine. Leaders of medical education therefore had a dual interest: upgrading the quality of education, and developing academic medicine as a viable career in the United States. Raising funds for the modern medical school was a professional life-or-death mission for them.[29]

The drive to establish academic medicine as a secure career in the United States was similar to events in other emerging scholarly disciplines in late nineteenth-century America. In virtually every academic subject, from physics to philosophy, scholars were engaged in the same struggle to "professionalize" their fields—that is, to establish academic departments, professional societies, and scholarly journals and to seek the funds to support research and train advanced students. The effort of physicians to establish academic medicine as a secure career represented but one of the innumerable ways in which the evolution of medical education in the United States was connected with the development of the educational system in general and higher education in particular.

The creation of medicine's endowment involved a complex interplay between donors and medical entrepreneurs, with each group acting for reasons of its own, and each group leaving an indelible imprint on the shape that American medical education ultimately assumed. Underlying the dialectic between benefactors and recipients was the fact that experimental medicine was working. For academic medicine—and for the medical profession in general—this was to be both a blessing and a curse. With each success of medical research, popular expectations for further medical "conquests" rose, and leaders of academic medicine did little to try to contain the soaring expectations. Yet, the higher the expectations, the greater the potential disappointment if the results of the investment were less than anticipated. In the ever-rising expectations for scientific medicine were seeds of disillusionment that could erupt at any time if medicine did not perform as expected.

Medicine and the University

In the mid-nineteenth century, the university may have seemed an unlikely home for medical education since the antebellum college was scarcely a place where higher learning was vigorously pursued. As universities began assuming their modern form after the Civil War—assuming responsibility for the production, not just the transmission, of knowledge—they became much more interested in medical education.[30] Universities with affiliated medical schools began to take control of those schools; many without medical schools either created their own or established real relationships with existing schools. A cadre of visionary university presidents—James B. Angell of Michigan; Seth Low and Nicholas Murray Butler of Columbia; Daniel Coit Gilman of Johns Hopkins; Benjamin Wheeler of California; William Rainey Harper of Chicago; Charles Van Hise of Wisconsin; George Vincent of Minnesota; Robert Brookings of Washington University; Samuel McCormick of Pittsburgh; and Arthur Hadley of Yale—took command of building their medical schools as they did their law, divinity, engineering, education, and graduate schools. The reform coalition that created the modern American medical school was led not only by medical school professors and deans but also by eminent university presidents, who saw that control of medical schools would help validate the university's claim to hegemony in all matters of higher education and professional training.

Perhaps no university president was more closely identified with the creation of the modern medical school than Charles Eliot of Harvard University. In 1869, when Eliot, a young chemist and Boston Brahmin, assumed the presidency of the university, the medical school was a typical proprietary school, described in one account as "a money-making institution, not much better than a diploma mill."[31] To Eliot, it was imperative that medicine be taught in a rigorous, scientific fashion—and that proper educational techniques, emphasizing empirical observations and the questioning of traditional authority, be brought to bear in every department and school of the university. Immediately upon assuming the presidency, Eliot took the unprecedented step of assuming the chair at a meeting of the medical faculty. Overcoming the stiff opposition of several senior faculty members, the redoubtable Eliot, with the aid of younger faculty members who supported him, imposed upon the school the new system of instruction that took effect in 1871. Over the next 40 years, Eliot sat in the chair at virtually every meeting of the medical school faculty, guiding the school from one improvement to another. No other episode better illustrated the modern university's desire to take medical education under its wing.[32]

Initially, the idea of moving medical education into the universities engendered considerable resistance among physicians, especially the physician-owners of proprietary schools, who were reluctant to turn over their businesses to someone else. In addition, the university was not an inevitable location for medical research. In some European countries, independent research institutes rather than universities were the major home of medical research. Nevertheless, as medical faculties increasingly came under the influence of the German university model, they saw that there was much to gain by being a professional school of a university. Affiliations with universities made sense because of their commitment to advanced teaching, research, and the legitimization of the pursuit of scholarship as a career. In addition, universities infused money and intellectual vigor into their medical schools and helped ensure that the schools would develop along genuine academic lines. Soon, medical faculties committed to reform began to regard the university as their greatest friend and protector.

Not surprisingly, as the medical school moved into the university, it changed. Its mission was now educational, not profit-making as in the proprietary era. As one manifestation of this change, schools began to limit class size to ensure that every student have the opportunity for practical instruction and personalized supervision. The dean of the Cornell University Medical College remarked, "We do not desire such huge numbers [of students] as we cannot handle more than about a hundred in a single class and give practical teaching, as we are doing at present."[33] Similarly, the faculty at Physicians and Surgeons voted to limit its class size to 100 to allow for "personal contact with the individual student."[34] Gone were the days when medical schools engaged in ruthless competition to maximize enrollments and profits.

In addition, movement into the university facilitated the emergence of academic medicine as a separate career from medical practice. In the late nineteenth century, medical schools began making full-time academic appointments in the basic science disciplines, and during World War I, in the clinical departments as well. The entry of medical education into the university gave a rationale to this process. Repeatedly, academic physicians were likened not to practitioners but to university professors in other disciplines since all devoted their energies to advanced teaching and research. In Flexner's words, "The professor of medicine is primarily a student of problems and a trainer of men," which made the medical professor no different from "the professor . . . of law, of economics, of all subjects whatsoever."[35] For this reason, many preferred the use of the term "university system" to "full-time system."

To the joy of medical educators, the new identity of medical education as a university discipline carried a profound payoff: the task of raising funds became much easier. Donors of all types found the idea of contributing to a university department much more palatable than that of contributing to the private business of a group of doctors. Of the hundreds of millions of dollars raised for medical education in the creative period, proprietary schools received almost none. As Welch observed, "The only type of school which can expect to receive support from the public must be a university medical school."[36] A university affiliation in itself did not guarantee success at raising money, but without an affiliation, a school stood virtually no chance at all.

Even at its inception, the American university was a diverse place, with many functions to perform and constituencies to serve. Yet, ideals of research and advanced teaching remained at its core. This was why Abraham Flexner—and university leaders in general—felt that the graduate school of arts and sciences, together with the medical school and law school, represented "the heart of a university."[37] Even if many medical schools were located apart from their parent university, medical schools had clearly become university enterprises, for they had adopted university values.

As medical schools moved into the university, they also moved into the country's educational system. Medical educators, like teachers everywhere, were concerned with the process of learning. All educators needed to understand how to organize the educational environment to maximize learning, and they struggled with similar issues: what subjects to teach, how to order subjects in relation to each other, how many subjects to teach at one time, how much time to give to formal lectures and how much to laboratory work or independent study, and how best to examine and evaluate students. Henry Pritchett, the president of the Carnegie Foundation for the Advancement of Teaching, repeatedly said that "medical education is an educational rather than a professional problem."[38] Medical education could not be properly discussed or understood apart from general education.

As the modern university and medical school were being created, their fate became irrevocably bound with that of the broader educational system. The university could flourish only as long as the underlying elementary and secondary schools produced enough qualified students to take full advantage of university opportunities. Similarly, scientific medical education could thrive only if the university produced enough premedical students who had taken the necessary preparatory courses. Only after 1900 did demanding entrance requirements become commonplace. Time was needed for attendance at the elementary schools, secondary schools, and colleges to grow large enough to allow enforceable entrance requirements to be introduced.[39] Medical schools thus became situated at the pinnacle of the country's educational pyramid: elementary and high schools at the bottom, open to all; universities above, open to some; and medical schools, together with other graduate and professional schools, at the very top, accessible only to those who had earned their way there academically. A once fluid educational system had become structured and rigid, and a division of labor ensued. Lower tiers served egalitarian purposes by offering educational opportunity for the masses; the higher levels carried out a more purely educational mission by providing advanced instruction to the academically elite who had gained their position through merit.[40] America's system of medical education, in the end, became an integral part of the country's educational system as a whole.

The Emergence of the Teaching Hospital

Medical education occupied an unusual place in higher education. Through the case workup, it was linked to the health care delivery system, not just to the university. To execute their mission, medical schools needed hospital facilities as well as university affiliations. Yet, whereas universities quickly became eager to affiliate with medical schools, hospitals did not. Throughout the late nineteenth century and even into the twentieth, hospitals were decidedly chilly toward allowing anything more than nominal educational activities to be conducted inside their doors. To persuade hospital trustees to permit their institutions to be used for genuine educational and investigative purposes, rather than merely to provide care for the sick, was one of the most difficult and frustrating challenges medical educators faced in creating a new system of training doctors.

The need for hospital facilities arose in part from the intellectual requirements of progressive medical education. Students were expected to be active learners throughout their medical training, not just in the scientific work of the first two years of the curriculum. The desired teaching device was the clinical clerkship, whereby students, under supervision, were given actual responsibility for the management of hospitalized patients. They would take admitting histories from patients, perform complete physical examinations, order or perform appropriate laboratory tests, initiate a course of treatment, follow their patients' daily progress, write the notes in the chart, order further studies or alter therapy as needed, and report regularly on events to senior staff physicians. Emphasis was placed on the intensive and thorough study of a limited number of patients rather than on having superficial contact with many, in order to train the clerks in proper methods and techniques. "Competent practitioners of medicine can be trained in but one way," stated Arthur Dean Bevan, chairman of the Council on Medical Education of the American Medical Association, "and that is in the hospital and in the dispensary, which are the clinical laboratories in which the students must study."[41] In the view of informed observers, the responsibility given clinical clerks exerted a remarkable effect in transforming them from students into doctors.

In the late nineteenth century there were solid educational reasons why medical schools needed hospital affiliations. By the turn of the century a research imperative had emerged as well. Clinical science was maturing as a learned discipline, and faculty in the clinical departments required hospitalized patients and clinical laboratories to conduct their scholarly investigations of disease and therapeutics. As Flexner put it, "The hospital should be the laboratory of the clinical teacher, and the conditions essential to the physiologist are equally material to the teaching and research of the internist."[42] For the modern medical school to do its work, it needed to control strong teaching hospitals deeply rooted in university medicine.

American hospitals had always cooperated in medical education, and after the Civil War their activities in that area noticeably increased. As the demands of medical education became greater, and as the American hospital underwent its transformation from a sleepy domicile for the deserving poor into a large, bustling institution where scientific medical care was actively delivered, the hospital's involvement in medical education grew. Hospital amphitheaters were used for clinical lectures, outpatient clinics were used for demonstrative teaching, and groups of students were brought into the wards for an hour or two a day, a few days a week, to practice physical diagnosis and hear interesting patients discussed. But there hospitals drew the line. Trustees and administrators guarded their prerogatives jealously. They saw their mission as patient care, not medical education and research. They vigorously protected their independence and their patients from any disruptions and inconveniences that might arise from having students set loose on the wards. Hospitals condoned clinical education—as long as that education involved passive learning and tight control of student activity. When it came to permitting the clerkship and encouraging clinical research, one hospital after another repeatedly refused to help. As a result, in the judgment of virtually every university and medical school leader of the period, the greatest single deficiency of medical education in the early 1900s was the conduct of work in the clinical departments.[43]

The model of clinical instruction to which all schools aspired was that of the Johns Hopkins Medical School. When the school opened in 1893, it had the good fortune of having a large, modern, well-equipped hospital of its own, which had been provided for in Johns Hopkins's will along with the medical school and university. The medical school made all staff appointments to the hospital, clinical research was not only permitted but encouraged, and the clinical clerkship immediately became the standard vehicle of instruction in all the major clinical departments. But no other medical school was so fortunate. A few schools, such as Michigan and Pennsylvania, also owned their own hospitals, and at such schools the clerkship and clinical research showed some signs of life. However, no school at this time, except for Johns Hopkins, owned a hospital large enough and sufficiently well financed to allow the clerkship to be available to all students in all rotations. Other schools, without hospitals of their own, were wholly dependent on the grace of affiliated hospitals to permit instruction and research, and here medical schools received one rebuff after another when they attempted to persuade hospitals to do so.

By the early 1900s, many hospitals began to consider taking a more active partnership in teaching and research. The success of the Johns Hopkins Hospital had been an inspiration, as that institution had achieved international eminence by combining a hospital's traditional humanitarian activities with educational and research excellence. The modern hospital had emerged, with its emphasis on providing the most up-to-date scientific care.[44] Now that medical practice was changing so rapidly, the modern hospital became much more receptive to developing closer relations with the leaders of medical research—the academic physicians. Medical schools and medical students had both improved in quality over the preceding four decades, thereby commanding greater respect from hospitals. School and hospital officials recognized that financial benefits could accrue to their respective institutions if they were to divide certain expenses and achieve economies of scale—an attractive selling point in a society infatuated with the cult of "efficiency." And medical educators lobbied incessantly, in public and private, for new affiliations with hospitals. Medical entrepreneurs recognized that the control of teaching hospitals was as central to the development of the clinical disciplines as endowments and laboratory facilities were to the proper conduct of the scientific departments.

Most important, a new consensus, accepted by medical educators and hospital officials alike, held that education and research improved the care of patients in a hospital. In this view, the presence of armies of students and faculty ensured that every detail of the moment-to-moment care of patients would receive prompt attention. The continuous presence of students served as an intellectual prod to the faculty, stimulating thorough study and discussion of patients. With so many examiners, there was little chance that significant symptoms or signs would escape notice or that possible therapeutic measures would be overlooked. And the presence of bedside clinical investigation led to a more careful study of patients, which benefited not only the immediate patient but also other patients, should something new be discovered. The intellectual excitement of teaching hospitals attracted the most accomplished physicians to the staff. It soon became apparent that the most up-to-date information on the management of diseases was to be found in university hospitals, where the search for the cause, mechanisms, and cure of human afflictions was actively being pursued.

Francis W. Peabody helped ease any remaining doubts about the desirability of a more active educational and scientific role for hospitals. Peabody, a New England aristocrat and professor of medicine at Harvard Medical School, was one of the most brilliant clinical investigators of the early twentieth century, having served as the first resident physician of the Hospital of the Rockefeller Institute in New York, the first resident physician of the Peter Bent Brigham Hospital in Boston, and the first director of the Thorndike Memorial Laboratory at the Boston City Hospital. For all his academic accomplishments, he was also a compassionate and humane physician, whose presence had an uplifting effect on the medical profession that rivaled that of the legendary Johns Hopkins professor of medicine, William Osler. Peabody's famous essay, "The Care of the Patient," became the classic text for students and physicians seeking to practice humane medicine. ("The secret of the care of the patient," he wrote, in words that have been immortalized, "is in caring for the patient."[45]) In Peabody, the concept of the teaching hospital had a vigorous advocate. When he spoke, hospital officials listened, for the man whose name was synonomous with caring could hardly be dismissed as a brash academic upstart. "There are few influences that exert as elevating an effect on the standard of professional work in a hospital as the presence in it of medical teaching," he wrote in 1923. "This is so true that the phrase 'teaching hospital' is almost synonymous with a good hospital."[46] Largely owing to his persuasion, the Boston City Hospital, after years of refusal, finally agreed to become a teaching hospital of the modern type, and trustees of other institutions heard his words as well.[47]

In response to these various developments, after 1910 the situation of clinical teaching rapidly changed. In the ensuing 15 years, hospitals across the country, prodded by aggressive medical faculties, reconsidered their role in teaching and research, and the modern teaching hospital was created, with the Johns Hopkins Hospital the model. Mergers in St. Louis between the Washington University School of Medicine and Barnes and St. Louis Children's Hospitals, in New York between the College of Physicians and Surgeons and Presbyterian Hospital, and in Boston between Harvard Medical School and the Peter Bent Brigham Hospital catalyzed the process. From there, subsequent affiliations between medical schools and hospitals occurred with rapidity. In many instances, particularly in the case of private medical schools, meaningful affiliations were established with existing nonprofit (voluntary) or municipal hospitals. In other instances, especially in the case of state medical schools, funds appropriated by the state legislatures were used to construct modern teaching hospitals that were owned and operated by the fortunate medical school.[48] By the 1920s, the historic antagonism between hospitals and medical education had finally been broken.

Not every medical school succeeded at finding a teaching hospital, and failure to do so was as harsh a blow to a school's survival as the inability to raise sufficient funds. Both a sizeable budget and control of a modern teaching hospital were necessary for accreditation under the new state licensing laws that appeared during World War I. Many honorable schools, for lack of suitable clinical facilities, either closed their doors or merged with other schools. Schools in relatively unpopulated parts of the country were at a particular disadvantage, for the greatest number and variety of patients were found in the large hospitals of metropolitan areas. With the creation of the teaching hospital, medical education, once found as often in the country as in the city, became primarily an urban activity.

As the teaching hospital emerged, tensions and disagreements with medical schools did not disappear. Nevertheless, a new era had clearly begun. Both medical schools and teaching hospitals became convinced that they were indispensable to each other's welfare and that the pursuit of education and research contributed to good patient care. Teaching hospitals, which were proud institutions seeking international recognition, quickly learned that without educational and investigative elements they would be no different from community hospitals. They now accepted their new academic responsibilities enthusiastically. Similarly, medical schools recognized that they could not do good work without having control of strong teaching hospitals. Accordingly, the perpetual and relentless quest for clinical facilities was to be a constant in their behavior throughout much of the twentieth century.

However, in one of the great ironies of American medical education, the new view that a harmony existed among education, research, and patient care was never proven, only assumed. Lurking beneath the repeated assertions of the interdependence of these functions was a troubling reality: the medical school's primary commitment was to education and research; the hospital's, to patient care. Could a hospital ever be a real part of a university if its primary obligations were to patient care? Could a medical school remain true to university values if its activities in patient care became too demanding? So successful and impressive were the new unions between medical schools and teaching hospitals that for much of the twentieth century these questions went virtually unasked. But the equilibrium between educational and service responsibilities was potentially unstable—a stark reality that would haunt both medical schools and teaching hospitals in a later era.

Establishing the Social Contract

By the 1920s, the revolution in American medical education had been completed. The modern medical school, with its huge physical plants, sophisticated laboratory facilities, growing number of full-time faculty, and unswerving research mission—not to mention its new affiliations with universities and teaching hospitals—bore no more resemblance to the proprietary school than the twentieth-century factory did to the craftsman's workshop. The transformation occurred by design, not by accident. From the 1870s onward, medical school and university leaders had defined their ideal vision of medical education and worked to help create the social and economic support necessary to fulfill that vision. Though the public ultimately supported the reforms and provided the economic means by which the changes could be made, the initiative for reform came from within the medical profession—or, that is, from the leaders of academic medicine who developed a new vision, and the university leaders who aided and supported them in their work.

An overview can barely suggest the complexity of the movement or the frustrations, failures, and mistakes that occurred along the way. Had the task of institution-building been easy, it would not have taken half a century to accomplish, nor would so many medical educators have been disappointed with one or another detail of the new system. Success was never inevitable or guaranteed. Nevertheless, the singular feature of the creative period was the ability of academic leaders to persevere. They thought in terms of the long-term; they expressed a vision and, as a group, never gave up in their quest to persuade others to support that vision.

Central to the success of the new system of medical education was that it served the needs of both the academic physicians who inspired it and the public that supported it. An implicit social contract emerged: medical schools would produce the type of doctor society needed, and in return society would provide the schools the resources they required to conduct education and research on a high plane. The American public clearly began fulfilling its end of the social contract. They provided medical schools with generous levels of public support, and individual patients came to be used in education and research to a degree that would have flabbergasted most nineteenth-century hospital officials. The public gladly invested in medical education and research so that the health of future generations might be better than its own.

In turn, the system of medical education served the needs of society. Most directly, the high quality of the product of the transformed medical school allowed the public to be much more confident in the capability of the average physician. As one medical school dean wrote, the meaning of the Flexnerian revolution was "that if medicine was to be taught at all it was to be taught well."[49] Moreover, medical schools were continually improving medical practice through their success at discovering new knowledge and translating that knowledge into everyday medical care. The new state licensing laws, which drove inferior schools out of business, were also interpreted by the public as a manifestation of the profession's social responsibility. In the words of one medical official, "The movement to place the practice of medicine under legal control has met with quite universal approval in this country. . . . This [licensing] is not for the purpose of protecting physicians but for the purpose of protecting the people against the unqualified, ignorant and dishonest practitioners."[50] As medical schools went about their work, they were often explicitly conscious of being a public trust. Thus, President Nicholas Murray Butler of Columbia University advised his medical faculty always to "keep in mind that we are a public service institution and see that you do not fail to help the public."[51]

Scientific medical education and research also came to be seen as an aid to the nation's industrial competitiveness—a perception not unimportant to a pragmatic, business-minded country. For instance, the conquest of hookworm was important to the economic development of the South and the attraction of Northern capital to that region.[52] The completion of the Panama Canal was less a tribute to American engineering excellence than to American medical research. Without the elimination of yellow fever, it is doubtful that construction could have been completed, as the French discovered in their unsuccessful attempt to build a canal.[53] Frederick T. Gates, the chief financial and philanthropic advisor to John D. Rockefeller, justified the idea of creating the Rockefeller Institute for Medical Research by noting, "Pasteur's inquiries on anthrax and on the diseases of fermentation had saved the French nation a sum in excess of the entire cost of the Franco-German war."[54] Many others justified the support of medical research with dollar calculations. For much of the twentieth century, investment in medical education, research, and practice would continue to be perceived as an economic good for the country.

Academic physicians, and the medical profession more broadly, fulfilled their end of the social contract in a variety of other ways as well. Medical educators not only supported but also helped lead the public health movement, and individuals such as William Welch, William Osler, Victor Vaughan, and L. Emmett Holt were as important to that movement as they were to the development of medical education. Prominent medical educators also fought against quackery, fraud, and patent medicines and actively participated in the campaign that led to the country's first pure food and drug legislation. Medical schools gained much notice for the patriotism they exhibited during World War I. Many schools contributed notably to the war effort—operating their medical school and teaching hospitals at home with a skeleton staff; sending some of their most prominent faculty to Europe to establish and run hospital bases abroad.[55] Distinguished researchers such as Harvard physiologist Walter Cannon put aside their own investigations to pursue projects that served wartime needs—in Cannon's case, developing new methods of cardiopulmonary resuscitation.[56] Though complaints of greedy doctors were not uncommon, statistically the average physician after World War I could expect to earn between one and one-half to two times the income of the average worker, and it was at this time that the profession ended fee-splitting.[57] Henry Pritchett, who explicitly described the practice of medicine as a public trust, counselled youths that they should enter medicine out of a desire to be of public service, for the medical profession was not financially prosperous and those entering it should not expect to be able to become wealthy from the practice of medicine.[58] At this time, medical educators and the profession at large supported a variety of liberal reforms, not the least of which was compulsory health insurance.[59] Activities of physicians in general, as well as those of medical schools in particular, gave the public confidence that medicine was fulfilling its end of the social contract.

The new system of medical education fitted remarkably well with the conditions of medical practice of the early twentieth century. In an era dominated by infectious and nutritional diseases, the accomplishments of scientific medicine were astonishing—and achieved at relatively low cost. The predominance of acute diseases made the hospital a logical center of medical care should a serious illness or surgical emergency strike. Requirements for ongoing office care were much less in an era when chronic diseases and conditions associated with aging were not as frequent. The relatively modest level of hospital costs led to few complaints about underwriting the expense of clinical education through hospital charges. Moreover, the long duration of hospital stays (average stay in 1900, two to three weeks), lack of life-sustaining technologic equipment, and strong reliance on bedside observations in managing patients resulted in an outstanding opportunity for students. They could follow the natural history of disease, learn principles of therapy, develop personal relationships with patients and families, and make real contributions to patient care. The educational system was well suited to medical practice of the era and provided students a nearly ideal introduction to the life of a physician.

The success of the new system should not obscure the fact that not everyone was happy with it. Owners of proprietary schools and private practitioners displaced in authority at honorable medical schools were scarcely enamored with the triumph of the university medical schools. Nor were women, racial and religious minorities, immigrants, and economically or culturally disadvantaged youths, who found entrance to medical school much more difficult than before. Many medical educators expressed concern about the rigidity of the new system, worrying that too much standardization might cause a school to lose the ability to make a legitimate exception or experiment along a new educational pathway. Rural areas perhaps lost the most. Well supplied with physicians during the proprietary era, they now began to find themselves at a competitive disadvantage for graduates of the university medical schools. Whether the growing maldistribution of physicians represented a response to educational policy or to social and economic incentives beyond a medical school's ability to control was actively debated—a debate that would reverberate among medical educators and policy-makers throughout the twentieth century.

In addition, the new system fostered a narrowing of medical schools' interests to issues of technical concern. From the beginning, the focus of the modern medical school was on disease organically defined, not on the system of health care or on society's health more generally. Nowhere could this be better seen than in the attitude of Johns Hopkins, the model for all modern schools. Even there, in a university so sympathetic to education in public health, preventive medicine was never satisfactorily incorporated into undergraduate or graduate medical education. Preventive issues received little attention in the curriculum, and their teaching was considered a responsibility primarily of the faculty of the school of public health, not of the school of medicine.[60] The school exhibited scarcely more interest in economic issues than in disease prevention. The Committee on the Costs of Medical Care asked it to undertake work in this area, but the faculty coolly declined.[61] No school better illustrated the achievements of scientific medicine, or the narrowness of the vision that scientific medical education initially assumed, than Johns Hopkins.

Nevertheless, despite lingering concerns, few contrary voices were raised after the new system had been created, so immediately discernible were its achievements. America was embarking on a love affair with scientific medicine, whatever its imperfections, that was to last for most of the twentieth century. The greatest achievement of the new system, in the minds of many, was that it was never meant to be immutable. Flexner himself wrote in 1910: "This solution deals only with the present and near future,—a generation, at most. In the course of the next thirty years needs will develop of which we here take no account."[62] The flexibility and freedom to change—indeed, the mandate to do so—was part of the system's mission from the very beginning. Contrary to popular myth, the system was always intended to evolve.

2

The American Medical School
Between the World Wars

O N THE SURFACE, there may have appeared to be less diversity of
purpose within the medical school than among other parts of the
educational system. Lower branches of the educational system had
responsibilities that did not apply to medical schools: the custodial function, the assimilative function, and the vocational function. Even the
social advancement function—such an important raison d'être for public
education—was less important to medical education since virtually all
physicians were assured a privileged place in society. Further differentiation—where medical graduates did specialty training, or whether they
took specialty training at all—was less important as a sign of social position than the mere fact of being a doctor.

There was also more cohesiveness between students and faculty in
medical schools than in the undergraduate branches of the university
system. Though most college students shared their professors' upper-
middle-class backgrounds, relatively few shared their instructors' scholarly interests, love of books, or quest for a contemplative life. College for
many students was a place for play—a stopping point in a life journey
motivated by worldly concerns and material values. The serious scholarly efforts of the instructors were often viewed by students in a jocular
fashion. Medical students, by contrast, were a serious lot—a self-chosen
group who shared their professors' interests in ideas, abstractions,
knowledge, and professional values. The academic experience meant
much the same thing to them as to their teachers.

Thus, medical schools after World War I went about their work with
little disagreement that their primary purpose was academic. External
demands on medical schools to provide clinical services to large populations of patients or to reform an ailing health care system were minimal at
this time. Nevertheless, beneath medical schools' seemingly circumscribed mission lay a multiplicity of roles: education, research, and

patient care. Before World War II these diverse roles were considered mutually dependent, much as a three-legged stool requires each of its legs. Few at the time could imagine how tensions among them would grow as medical research became increasingly sophisticated and as medical schools became more tightly involved with the country's medical care system.

Typically regarded as a quiet time in American medical education, the interwar period was in fact highly dynamic. Medical research advanced and medical schools grew in size, wealth, and complexity. The values associated with the Flexnerian revolution became generalized—particularly the commitment of medical schools to research. If American medical schools after World War II were to grow so large as to dwarf pre–World War II medical schools, that was because a solid institutional infrastructure was already in place that could effectively utilize the massive infusion of federal and private funds.

What drove this incipient juggernaut? If any one force predominated, that was the desire of medical scholars, like scholars throughout the university, to engage in research. During this period research was modest in scale, and faculties remained highly committed to teaching. Yet, medical research evolved from an activity designed to enhance teaching to one that by World War II had taken on a life of its own. The fact that investigators were helping solve the pressing medical problems of the time— acute diseases—seemed to validate the notion that research was in the interest of the public as well as medical scientists. Left unanswered, however, was the question of how the public would be served by a faculty-driven, laboratory-focused definition of the medical school in other intellectual and social circumstances. This question would be put to the test in the second half of the twentieth century, when the challenges of chronic diseases and a diseased medical care system began to make themselves apparent.

Education

If most post–World War I medical schools had any one function they professed to be of greatest importance, that activity was education—the training of medical students and house officers to be physicians. In the words of Arthur Dean Bevan, professor of surgery at Rush Medical College and chairman of the Council on Medical Education of the American Medical Association, "The duty of a medical school and its first function is to train competent practitioners of medicine."[1] Such sentiments were expressed throughout the era by local schools like Kansas and Nebraska, national schools like Chicago and Yale, and special mission schools like Woman's Medical College of Pennsylvania.

Medical schools had always been in business to produce doctors. Indeed, nineteenth-century medical schools had focused solely upon teaching. What was notable about American medical schools between the world wars, however, was the degree to which teaching remained their primary mission, even as they adopted new responsibilities of research and patient care. To most faculty members of the era—even many of the most productive scientific investigators—the teaching of medical students came first.

The measures of medical faculties' commitment to education were many. Faculties were small; of necessity a great amount of their time was consumed by teaching. At Michigan, the average faculty member devoted about 60 percent of his time to teaching or to preparation for teaching.[2] At most schools, with fewer research programs than Michigan, an even greater percentage of the faculty's time went into teaching. Educational expenses consumed the dominant portion of medical school budgets, even at the most prominent research schools. For instance, of the total expenditures of the Cornell University Medical College in 1933, $449,170 was spent for teaching, compared with $88,510 for research and $112,234 for everything else.[3] At Johns Hopkins, teaching was considered so integral to all the school's activities that the school paid no faculty salaries specifically for research. It was expected that any instructor wishing to do research would find the opportunity to do so.[4]

Teaching was taken seriously by everyone. Even the most senior faculty members were routinely present in student laboratories and clinics, and they knew the students well. In the preclinical departments, such behavior was typified by George Corner of the University of Rochester, one of the country's premier anatomists. Corner proudly recalled how he once won five cents from students in the histology laboratory who had bet that he could not properly identify certain salivary gland specimens. None of Corner's students was spared the opportunity for such daily personal interactions with the professor. Like so many senior preclinical scientists of the period, Corner also accepted university duties with good humor. Thus he served on the medical school admissions committee, chaired the library committee, organized a history of medicine club, advised the dean on administrative and financial matters, taught in the anatomy and histology laboratories, and counseled students and faculty—all as he pursued his pioneering work that led to the discovery of the hormone progesterone.[5]

In the clinical departments, faculty members were also heavily involved in teaching. Even departmental chairmen made daily rounds, conducted medical histories, performed physical examinations, made diagnostic and therapeutic decisions, and discussed cases—all under the watchful eyes of physicians in training. Among the most famous was Soma Weiss, physician-in-chief of the Peter Bent Brigham Hospital and Hersey Professor of the Theory and Practice of Physics at Harvard Medical School. An outstanding clinical investigator and charismatic department chairman, Weiss took a keen interest in students and house officers, stimulating them with his warm personality and deep concern for their intellectual development and personal well-being. Weiss was always roaming the wards. When he was not performing consultations, he was visiting his own patients. He loved being called in from home for consultation at night. Even in the wee hours, he would bring enthusiasm and fresh insight to a case and discuss every detail with the house officers and students. He would often end such trips with an impromptu visit to the emergency room to see what clinical treasures might have come in and what teaching "pearls" he might impart.[6]

Corner and Weiss exemplified the dedication, work habits, and values that many preclinical and clinical faculty members of the period brought to their teaching. Individuals such as these left an indelible imprint on their students, and many who studied medicine during the era have remembered it nostalgically. To students between the wars, many professors were larger than life. David E. Rogers, the former president of the Robert Wood Johnson Foundation, has said of this period: "It was still a time for heroes; heroes, who often shaped the values and aspirations of young people."[7]

Though few instructors became legends, known by name to medical students and physicians everywhere, faculty members in medical schools across the land labored quietly and unpretentiously, dedicated to medicine and committed to their students. In both the preclinical and clinical subjects, they not only provided personalized instruction but maintained their presence over sustained periods of time, thereby allowing relationships to be established with students. Especially in the clinical departments, medical professors routinely served as role models—even for the vast majority of students for whom they may not have personally served as mentors. Few students of the era were not in some way touched by their professors.

In educating physicians, medical schools were perceived as a public trust. Their mission was to train skilled practitioners of medicine, and the health of the nation was considered to be dependent on the quantity and quality of physicians produced. How might the country's high maternal mortality rate be lowered, one professor of obstetrics asked?—only by greater support of the teaching of obstetrics.[8] More generally, how might the health of the nation best be guaranteed? According to a faculty committee of the Johns Hopkins School of Medicine, only in one way: by preserving excellence in medical education.[9]

Even before World War II, some observers recognized that there was more to assuring the country's health than simply having well trained doctors. In 1932 the dean of the College of Physicians and Surgeons of Columbia University declared that medicine was "as much a social as it is a biological science" and proceeded to describe some of "the broad problems of medical economics" that needed to be addressed if the health needs of the community were to be maximally served.[10] Nevertheless, to almost all at this time, the training of doctors had become the cornerstone to assuring the nation's health. An influential midcentury report felt that it was "useless" to consider such issues as access or cost without reference to "the central need of having a sufficient number of trained physicians capable of providing a type of medical care that can justify elaborate plans for distributing and paying for it."[11] Such assumptions about the centrality of medical education to the nation's health, though never proven and certainly challenged in a later period, were nonetheless highly plausible during an era of acute diseases. Such assumptions also squared neatly with traditional American optimism that scientific and technological "progress" contained the key to the solution of social problems.[12] If anyone had doubts that the nation's health depended on the quality of medical education, those doubts were seldom expressed.

Research

The forerunner of the modern American medical school had a strictly demarcated task: education. Its immediate constituency was its students; its purpose was to teach. However, the modern American medical school had been created primarily for medical scholars by medical scholars. Accordingly, research was one of its major activities. Even if teaching occupied most of its time, it was research that allowed the medical school to be a genuine part of the university.

The "professionalization" of American medical research, to use the argot of historians and sociologists of science, had been underway long before World War I. Indeed, as sociologist Joseph Ben-David has demonstrated, the development of American medical research occurred so dramatically that by 1920 the United States already led the world in new medical discoveries (*see Figure 1*).[13] However, after World War I no other activity of the American medical school grew more rapidly than research. Medical research developed from a poorly supported enterprise conducted at relatively few schools to an established activity that by World War II was pursued at almost all schools. Most medical research (the term "biomedical" was not yet used) was done at a relatively small number of elite medical schools located primarily on the East Coast or in the Great Lakes region—just as American scholarship of the period was concentrated in approximately 20 universities in those parts of the country.[14] (Some of the leading medical journals of the era bore their names: the *Bulletin of the Johns Hopkins Hospital*, the *Yale Journal of Biology and Medicine*, the *Journal of the Mount Sinai Hospital*.) However, the amount and quality of research grew significantly even at the majority of schools with smaller research programs, and it was the unusual school that did not aspire to do more in this area.

Especially impressive was the development of research within the ten or 15 schools that were setting the standards. For example, between 1912 and 1935 Harvard Medical School increased its total expenditures from $300,000 to $1,200,000, with the increase going almost entirely toward research. By 1953, a year that reflected the early impact of federal grants, the school was spending over $2,000,000 a year on research—a 100-fold

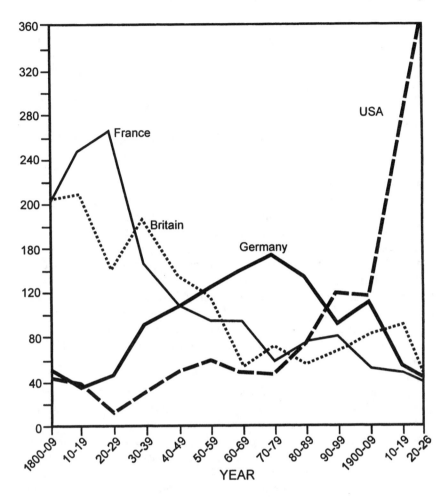

Figure 1 *Changes in the relative share of medical discoveries in selected countries, 1800–1926*

increase over the $21,000 it spent in 1910.[15] This investment in medical research reaped dividends, as judged by the respect given to American medical research worldwide. Between 1925 and 1950, 12 Americans received or shared the Nobel Prize in physiology or medicine—nearly twice as many as that from the second most successful country, Great Britain, with seven prizes.

It was between the wars that many of the characteristics of modern medical research became apparent. The outpouring of scholarship, both in the preclinical and clinical disciplines, was immense. By 1934 there were approximately 33,000 scientific periodicals, with a high proportion relating directly or indirectly to medicine.[16] At the same time a distinct trend toward multiauthorship and shorter papers was occurring.[17]

Department chairmen and deans struggled to keep abreast of research emanating even from within their own faculties. In 1940 the chairman of surgery at Cornell spoke with astonishment of the 145 publications his faculty had produced the preceding academic year. The dean of the school pointed out that the annual departmental reports submitted to him "comprise some 125 closely typewritten pages, mainly describing research activities."[18]

During this period other important indications of the growing maturity of American medical research became apparent. As one sign of the increasing intellectual sophistication of medical research, faculty positions in the preclinical departments increasingly became the province of Ph.D. investigators, not physician-scientists as before World War I. As medical research became more fundamental, medical schools began acquiring the characteristics of graduate schools. Indeed, many schools established programs leading to graduate degrees (Sc.D.s, M.A.s, and Ph.D.s) in preclinical subjects like biochemistry, physiology, and bacteriology.[19] Medical schools also began providing more research opportunities in the preclinical sciences to "research fellows"—physicians who had completed their medical training and were now seeking further scientific background in preparation for academic careers. Probably the school with the largest number of research fellows was Harvard Medical School, which in the 1939–40 academic year had 87 fellows in the preclinical departments.[20]

The period between the wars was a prosperous time for medical scholarship. In the preclinical disciplines an outpouring of knowledge occurred in every field. In biochemistry, the period witnessed profound advances in the understanding of carbohydrate metabolism, the processes of energy exchange within cells, and the structure and function of proteins and macromolecules. Classical physiology matured, providing a sophisticated understanding of how human organs function. Pharmacology, the least developed of all the preclinical subjects prior to World War I, was increasingly able to explain the chemical and physiological actions of drugs on tissues. Research in the field became experimentally based in the style of organic chemistry and physiology rather than in the earlier descriptive style of nineteenth-century "materia medica."

Similar advances occurred in the study of the causes and mechanisms of disease. As new classes of disease-producing microbial organisms— fungi, viruses, and parasites—were discovered, "bacteriology" was transformed into "microbiology." Pathology, the study of diseased organs and tissues, continued its evolution from an observational to an experimental science. Patient-oriented research by clinicians also flourished. In keeping with traditional observational studies in the field, new diseases were identified and their natural histories clarified. In addition, clinical research began to evolve into an experimental discipline, as clinical investigators increasingly utilized the laboratory to answer questions posed by observations on patients. The result was an explosion in the

Table 1   A comparison between the more important specific therapeutic
remedies available in 1913 and in 1943

1913	*1943*	
Salvarsan	Arsenicals	Vitamin A
Quinine	Liver extract	Vitamin B, thiamin,
Vermifuges	Heparin	niacin, riboflavin, etc.
Thyroid extract	Epinephrine	Vitamin C
Digitalis	Insulin	Vitamin D
Emetine	Thyroxin	Vitamin E
	Parathyroid extract	Vitamin K
	Adrenal cortex extract	Dihydrotachysterol
	Estrogenic hormones	Antitoxin
	Progesterone	Immune sera
	Androgenic hormones	Prostigmine
	Anterior pituitary	Thiouracil
	Pitressin	Sulfonamides
	Pitocin	Tyrothricin
	Placental hormones	Penicillin

understanding of the chemical and physiological mechanisms of disease—the so-called "pathophysiology" of disease.[21]

Most important to doctors—and the public—the period between the
wars witnessed striking therapeutic advances. The evolution of
endocrinology resulted in the discovery of new hormones, some of which
were in regular clinical use by World War II. The discovery of insulin had
come from medical research in the 1920s; so had the use of liver extract to
treat pernicious anemia. Surgery became more daring, and new operative
subspecialties like neurosurgery, urology, and orthopedic surgery rapidly
developed. The 1920s and 1930s witnessed the rise of nutritional science
and the discovery of a host of vitamins—developments of enormous
importance to both preventive and curative medicine. The 1920s and
1930s came to be labelled the era of the "vitamin hunters."[22] By the early
1940s, the antibiotic age had begun, and both sulfonamide drugs and
penicillin were in use. Not to be overlooked, after World War I the pharmaceutical industry matured, and during the 1920s and 1930s it developed many new drugs that quickly found their way into medical practice
for specific treatments or for the amelioration of symptoms.[23] The physician-in-chief of the Peter Bent Brigham Hospital proudly described the
great expansion of medicine's therapeutic war chest that had occurred
between World War I and World War II (*see Table 1*).[24]

Though such developments may seem humble to a later era accustomed to high-technology wizardry, a continuous onslaught of new pharmaceuticals, and one new sophisticated molecular discovery after

another, the power of medical science from the perspective of the time was awe-inspiring. By 1944, in response to both preventive and curative medicine, gross mortality in the United States had fallen 40 percent from 1900, and life expectancy had increased from 47 years in 1900 to over 60 years.[25] The pestilential diseases that had ravaged the human race throughout history had been controlled, and chronic and degenerative diseases—the ironic consequence of living longer—had become the primary cause of mortality and morbidity. In 1940 Ernest P. Boas described chronic diseases as the modern "plague," now that infectious and nutritional diseases had finally been controlled.[26]

America's ascent to world leadership in medical research occurred as part of a broader process involving all of American science. By World War I, American science had gone far toward achieving independence and intellectual respectability, but the war hastened that process by the enforced isolation of American science from European science. Science made spectacular contributions to the war effort, which elevated its prestige and fueled further private funding.[27] University opportunities for research and graduate study grew accordingly. By the mid-1930s America had established world leadership not only in medical research but also in genetics, physics, and astronomy. In the 1930s, in the throes of the Depression, universities were spending at least $50 million a year on research. Industry, cognizant of the utilitarian value of science, was spending two to four times that amount.[28] By World War II, the United States was the foremost center for scientific research in the world.

❦ · ❦ · ❦

Four characteristics of American medical research during the interwar period are especially important to understanding the twentieth-century history of American medical education. The first pertains to research in the preclinical departments. At this time the intellectual orientation of these fields was toward the clinical departments, not the university— toward an understanding of disease mechanisms and treatments, not fundamental biology and chemistry, even as biological and chemical techniques were increasingly utilized in their work. Preclinical faculty were studying problems essential to the development of medicine as a practical science; they were custodians of the knowledge and subject matter that were "relevant" to students and practitioners of medicine, even if that relevance often became apparent only at some point later in a physician's training. For this reason they were commonly viewed as the "handmaidens" of the clinical disciplines.

Scientific knowledge is always in transition, and the period between the wars witnessed considerable maturation of the preclinical sciences. Biochemistry is a case in point. Shortly before World War I, Jacques Loeb—fictionalized as Max Gottlieb, the idealization of the pure medical scientist, in Sinclair Lewis's *Arrowsmith*—advanced a mechanistic conception of life and predicted that life processes would ultimately be reduced to chemical and physical explanations. By 1944, Oswald T. Avery, Colin M. Macleod, and Maclyn McCarty had shown that DNA is the "transforming principle" of pneumococcus—that is, that the genetic endowment of each strain of pneumococcal bacteria resided in the DNA molecule. Recent historical studies have shown in detail how the coming of age of molecular biology in the 1950s owed much to the development of biochemistry in the 1930s and 1940s.[29] The transformation of biochemistry into a branch of general biology was especially apparent in England and Germany, where its location in universities rather than medical schools contributed to an earlier determination that the field should establish its scientific independence and end its servitude to medicine— the clearest example yet described of how institutional structure can influence the intellectual content and self-perception of a discipline.[30]

Nevertheless, before World War II preclinical scientists, especially in the United States, remained focused primarily on problems of direct medical significance. The use of the term "preclinical" to describe the departments of the first two years of medical school represented no accident of nomenclature but a specific reference to the role that teaching and research in these departments played during this period. A cursory glance at preclinical research illustrates this point. Otto Folin, an outstanding biochemist, established his reputation by developing analytic methods to determine the chemical constitutents of blood, urine, and body tissues.[31] Walter Cannon, Harvard's distinguished physiologist, was continually interested in the translation of his research into practical applications. Until his retirement in 1942, he carried the title of "consulting physiologist" to the Peter Bent Brigham Hospital, a reflection of his efforts to help link the work of Harvard's Department of Physiology with the activities of the clinic.[32] Even the greatest preclinical scientists would routinely look to medicine for questions to ask in their research. When considering a new project, Vincent du Vigneaud, who won a Nobel Prize for his work on vasopressin, regularly asked his physician friends if they thought it was likely to be important.[33] Collaborative projects among preclinical scientists and clinicians were common. One of the most important collaborations, which began in the 1920s and lasted for over three decades, occurred between physiologist Homer W. Smith and members of the department of medicine at the New York University School of Medicine—a collaboration that gave birth to the discipline of nephrology.[34]

The orientation of the preclinical sciences toward medicine had many causes, but it primarily reflected the fact that the smallest unit of study was the cell. "Cells in biology," Alfred E. Cohn of the Rockefeller Institute for Medical Research wrote in 1928, "are to be regarded as the analogues of atoms in physics."[35] Most work in the preclinical sciences involved higher levels of biological organization—tissues, organs, and whole organisms. As a result, borders between subjects were considered firm and inviolable. Biochemistry was biochemistry; physiology was physiology; pathology, pathology; and microbiology, microbiology—each subject taught by a separate department and defined as sharply and discretely by its intellectual content as college undergraduate subjects like mathematics, history, and classics. These fields were "more or less watertight compartments,"[36] a medical school curriculum committee said of them in 1930. Upon completing a course, students had a definite sense of "finishing" the subject matter, however misleading that sense might have been.

The second characteristic pertains to research in the clinical departments, or "clinical research" for purposes of this discussion. The essential feature of clinical research at this time was that it involved the study of patients. The majority of clinical research consisted of descriptions of various diseases and the development of new tests and procedures. The primary sources of data were meticulous bedside observations of patients, retrospective review of hospital charts, and the use of the clinical diagnostic laboratories of the hospital. Henry Dolger, a prominent clinical investigator at the Mount Sinai Hospital of New York, recalled how he went about conducting his studies demonstrating that diabetics who live long enough often develop vascular complications. "When I made observations about the eyes in diabetes, I made them myself. I took the records of 200 patients. I analyzed them and studied them at night. I left my home, my kids, and I'd be in the record room from 8:00 until 11:00. When I got home, I'd sit down and would write until 3:00 in the morning. That's the way it was done."[37]

The importance of patients in clinical research was seen in the emphasis that was placed on maintaining thorough clinical records. Henry A. Christian, chief of medicine of the Peter Bent Brigham Hospital, considered the creation of a set of complete, typed hospital records of all patients at the hospital to be the institution's "greatest single achievement."[38] If this type of clinical research could be said to make particular use of any one underlying preclinical science, that science was pathology, for it was the autopsy examination that allowed the appearance of tissues and organs to be correlated with the clinical symptoms and physical findings observed while the patient was alive. Christian himself exemplified this approach to clinical investigation. A careful bedside observer with a thorough background in pathology, he was quick to see clinical entities that were peculiar or discrete, and in this way he described certain syndromes that now bear his name, such as Hand-Schüler-Christian disease.

After World War I, clinical research entered a second, more mature phase. It came to be appreciated that experimental methods applied to the study of disease and therapeutics, not just to the preclinical disciplines. Though observational studies and record-room research continued, the most exciting work increasingly involved the search to explain the physiological mechanisms of disease. Clinical investigators, armed with new knowledge about metabolic pathways, fluid and electrolyte homeostasis, acid-base balance, immunology, and other laboratory subjects, began applying experimental methods to unraveling the mechanisms of human disease.

However, in an observation whose importance can scarcely be exaggerated, the work of the physiologically oriented clinical investigator remained just as focused on patients as that of the traditional clinical researcher. What was new was that science, to use the phrase of A. McGehee Harvey, was brought to the bedside.[39] The questions asked arose from observations of patients; clinical investigators went to their laboratories—almost invariably located in hospital rather than medical school buildings—to search for solutions; answers found helped explain the pathophysiology of disease and often led to diagnostic procedures or therapeutic interventions. Thus, Robert F. Loeb and Dana W. Atchley of Columbia, troubled by the fact that 50 percent of diabetics in ketoacidosis would die despite the administration of insulin, used new biochemical and physiological techniques to study fluid and electrolyte metabolism in these patients. The result was a rational form of treatment with intravenous fluid and electrolyte infusions that, together with insulin administration, markedly reduced the mortality of this condition.[40]

The third characteristic of medical research between the wars was the relatively short distance from the standard student courses to the forefront of medical research. In every department, a congruence existed between the required teaching of the medical school courses and the specific research problems faculty were pursuing when not teaching. This observation helps explain the continued enthusiasm for student teaching that was regularly found. Faculty members experienced the joy and excitement of teaching medical students the knowledge, techniques, and problems they were encountering in their own original work. Instructors regularly noted with pleasure the facility with which medical students were mastering difficult research techniques as part of the standard laboratory instruction.[41] For students also, being close to the forefront of knowledge was beneficial, for it allowed them to see the faculty in their natural habitats. In the preclinical laboratories, students learned to appreciate the day-to-day life of an experimental scientist. In the clinical subjects, students would regularly encounter their professors at the bedside examining patients or in the hospital record room reviewing charts, as the patient-focused nature of clinical research kept professors continually in view.

The fourth important characteristic of medical research before World War II was the high authority it commanded without complex methods to demonstrate the "statistical significance" of an observation. "Numerical" methods in medical research had long been in use, but they were notable for their mathematical simplicity. A rigorous discipline of "biostatistics" to help structure studies, eliminate investigator and participant bias, control for multiple interacting factors, and determine levels of statistical significance had not yet emerged. It is notable that Koch's postulates (the criteria for demonstrating a microbial cause of a disease) did not contain the concept of a control and that the first randomized controlled trial of a therapeutic substance (the use of the antibiotic streptomycin to treat tuberculosis) was conducted only after World War II.

The ability of medical researchers to speak authoritatively with modest statistical documentation resulted from the intellectual nature of the major problems that confronted them: acute diseases. Here, the time frame was compressed and the results were often measured by life or death. Complex statistics were not necessary to demonstrate that a bacterium caused an acute infection or that sulfonamides and penicillin allowed patients with acute meningitis to live who otherwise would have died within hours or days. The recoveries of critically ill patients were so dramatic that what happened could not be missed. It required the challenge of a different type of scientific problem—chronic diseases—to stimulate the development of biostatistics after World War II.[42] Though medical knowledge and the capacity of medical practice to diagnose and treat disease were to grow to extraordinary heights in the second half of the twentieth century, the authority of medicine would never again be so clear or unchallenged as it was in the early and middle decades of the century when it was dealing primarily with acute diseases.

❧ · ❧ · ❧

By virtue of successfully confronting many acute diseases, medical research (and by extension, medical practice) came to enjoy an exalted position in the public eye. The public's infatuation with medicine was reflected in popular culture—a string of movies with titles such as "Men in White," "The White Parade," and "The Magic Bullet." Medical schools were deemed worthy of continued financial support by state and local governments, philanthropists, and foundations. The contrast that Richard Shryock drew between American physicians' exalted status in 1946 and their position of ignominy 100 years before was startling.[43]

Reinforcing the public's adulation of medical research was the attitude of the researchers themselves: their view that medical research was a calling, their conspicuous disdain for commercialism, and their lack of interest in personal financial reward, provided that their laboratory and department were well supported. Medical scientists were hardly without ego or ambition. However, they sought nonmonetary rewards: approval and recognition from their peers and, for a lucky few, from society. The currency of academic medicine was not dollars but publications, appointments, titles, memberships, and awards.

There was no better indication of the antipathy of medical schools toward commercialism than their attitude toward patents. In their view, the objective of medical research was to promote the public welfare, not to enable individuals or institutions to profit financially from inventions or discoveries. Most medical schools would not hold patents or accept royalties from patents that arose from university work. At the University of Rochester, for instance, neither George Corner nor the school's dean gave any thought to patenting Corner's discovery of the hormone progesterone. It was their position that no medical discovery should be commercially restricted, even for the benefit of a university.[44]

Although there were a few exceptions to this pattern,[45] this was the policy at the two most important schools, Johns Hopkins and Harvard. At Hopkins, the dean declared that "universities (and particularly medical schools) do not belong in business. . . . any commercialization of the institutions will in the long run do the institutions great harm. Universities being supported by philanthropy and by State grants should not sell themselves in any way."[46] Neither the school nor individual faculty members owned patents, and the school refused royalties from patents growing out of medical school research.[47] Harvard Medical School went further. Not only were patents by faculty members prohibited, but the school offered to provide legal advice to faculty members who desired help to prevent others from patenting their discoveries or inventions.[48] When Harvard Medical School dedicated its patent on liver extract for the treatment of pernicious anemia to the public, it engaged in a "venomous discourse" with the "burned up" Eli Lilly Company, which had invested more than $1,000,000 in the work. Lilly wanted "a special 'in'," but the school refused "in the belief that Harvard professors worked for the public interest."[49] In research, as well as in education, American medical schools acted as a public trust.

Patient Care

The third responsibility of the modern medical school was patient care. Faculty provided consultations for private practitioners and supervised the interns and residents in treating the indigent patients of teaching hospitals. Patient care was essential for faculty to maintain their clinical and teaching skills and to obtain material for research. Faculty practice was also important for good education, for it allowed students to be exposed to exemplary clinicians and the highest quality medical practice.

Who were the outstanding clinicians and clinical teachers? As clinical research matured after World War I, this was not a trivial question. Clinical research, like all research, required large amounts of undistracted time. Furthermore, as clinical research entered its analytic stage, additional competency in the preclinical disciplines, not just clinical medicine, had to be acquired and maintained. With the field becoming so demanding, some feared that investigators might lose touch with clinical medicine, becoming sterile practitioners and ineffective clinical teachers. Such were the concerns of William Osler, probably the most influential American internist ever. In 1912 he objected to the proposition that the clinical departments of the Johns Hopkins Medical School should be placed on a full-time (university) basis because full-time clinicians might become "clinical prigs." A full-time system, he warned, might be "a very good thing for science, but a bad thing for the profession."[50]

Nevertheless, clinical investigators had hardly given up contact with patients. As noted earlier, clinical research of the era required investigators to spend considerable time at the bedside. Soon it became apparent that no one knew more about patient care than the clinical scientists, who were continually studying patients, diseases, and treatments. They began to serve regularly as clinical consultants—not just for cases of rare diseases in specialties but for difficult diagnostic and therapeutic cases of any kind. The view emerged that patient care, education, and research were inseparably linked and that the most up-to-date and thorough clinicians were those actively engaged in research. "Triple threats"—those who excelled in patient care, teaching, and research—could and did exist.[51]

In a nontechnological era in which patient care depended mainly on bedside skill and clinical acumen, no one could extract more information from patients or use clinical information more wisely than these master clinicians. Arthur L. Bloomfield, who became chairman of the Department of Medicine at the Stanford Medical School in 1926, was one such individual. He regularly made morning rounds at the bedside with students and house officers, demonstrating diagnostic virtuosity and exceptional clinical acumen. One former student recalled how with Bloomfield, "instruments were there for use rather than show; we six students watched the way a medical professor actually performed an examination." Bloomfield was "The Professor," and his clinical judgments were the final word.[52] Another clinical virtuoso and "triple threat" was David P. Barr, chairman of the Department of Medicine at Washington University and later Cornell and a pioneer in the development of physiologically oriented clinical research. An inveterate showman, Barr delighted in teaching students physical examination. His demonstrations of the technique of percussion were legendary. According to David E. Rogers, "One of his favorite stunts was to have a student hide a 50-cent piece deep within a loaf of bread. With meticulous precision, his pen beneath his teeth, he would percuss out its location, marking it carefully on the crust. Then he would have another student section the loaf to show its accuracy."[53]

Clinical excellence was not confined to full-time clinical faculty. Innumerable private practitioners possessed formidable clinical and teaching skills and provided medical schools invaluable services as "voluntary" clinical faculty members. In addition, during this period the line between academic medicine and private practice blurred. It was not uncommon for private practitioners to make important contributions to clinical research, particularly in the area of descriptive clinical studies. Nevertheless, the intellectual underpinnings of medicine were such that research, education, and patient care were considered interrelated. Many clinical investigators carried a commanding presence as practitioners. Even Osler later recanted and agreed that research would enhance a physician's clinical skills.[54]

Though clinical faculty took their patient care duties seriously, they did not try to expand their consulting practices. Patient care was undertaken only insofar as it was necessary to advance the schools' academic mission of education and research. At Johns Hopkins, for instance, surgical chairmen from William Halsted to Alfred Blalock would try to go to the laboratory every day and chide other members of the department who did not. Blalock was unimpressed if one of his staff had a heavy operating schedule. He would scold a busy operator, telling him that laboratory work was possible with one operation a day but not three.[55]

To clinical professors, their university identity came first. They considered themselves students of problems and trainers of future generations of physicians. Patient care, beyond that necessary to remain clinically, scientifically, and educationally alive, only diverted them from their primary mission. Medical faculties regularly acted on this belief. For example, at Johns Hopkins fees from private patients in 1929 amounted to $10,000 for the departments of medicine, pediatrics, surgery, and obstetrics combined—hardly evidence that the full-time staff was being diverted into patient care for the financial gain of themselves, the school, or the hospital.[56]

Although the volume of patients seen by faculties was relatively small, it would be incorrect to conclude that medical schools or their teaching hospitals were unimportant to the delivery of medical services in the United States. The new knowledge, practices, and technologies they generated, the doctors they trained, the consultations they provided to practitioners in need of help—these activities were essential to the operation of the American medical care system, even if the volume of services delivered directly by medical schools was intentionally limited. Through consultations, education, and research, medical schools were in business to service, maintain, and upgrade the delivery system—but not to be the delivery system.

Faculty Culture

Compared with the pre-Flexnerian period, medical schools of the 1920s were large and organizationally complex. They also had become part of a national system of medical education in which schools shared standardized definitions, values, and operating procedures. In the newly rationalized system of medical education, college graduates with the proper credentials could be admitted to any medical school in the country. Medical schools offered a standardized curriculum that allowed their graduates to apply for internships or enter practice in every state. Faculty administrative procedures also became very similar. Witness, for instance, the standardization of academic titles, a process that was completed by the 1930s.[57]

For all their emerging complexity, medical schools remained informal, congenial places. Schools were not so large or bureaucratic as to encroach

on faculty members' scholarly leisure, close associations, or intimate discussions with colleagues. To Arnold Rich, a distinguished Johns Hopkins
pathologist who later bemoaned the intrusion of the federal government
in medical research after World War II and steadfastly refused to apply
for federal grants, the interwar period was still a time in which faculty
could enjoy "the element of repose, the quiet pursuit of knowledge, the
friendship of books, the pleasures of conversations, and the advantages
of solitude."[58] Kenneth Blackfan, physician-in-chief of Boston Children's
Hospital from 1923 to 1941, considered his colleagues and himself "com-
rades in the enjoyable adventure against disease."[59] Rich and Blackfan
were far from alone in viewing the pre–World War II period in this fashion, for that era was a unique time when American medicine had come of
age yet had not been affected by the size, competitiveness, and financial
stakes of post–World War II medical research.

Faculty life during this period has been described as a period of
"threadbare gentility."[60] The term "threadbare" referred to the meager
academic salaries, particularly at the junior level. Of course, faculty
salaries varied considerably from school to school. In the 1930s, a full professor in a preclinical department at Harvard could make up to $13,000,
whereas a professor of similar rank at the University of Mississippi, the
University of South Dakota, and Creighton would make no more than
$3,600.[61] (The range of salaries at 66 medical schools in 1939 is shown in
Table 2.[62]) Clinical professors could usually supplement their university
salaries with fees from private consultations, which typically gave them a
20 to 50 percent premium compared with faculty of similar rank and
seniority in preclinical departments. Even so, there was still a large discrepancy between an academic income and what a successful practitioner could make, and a conspicuous proportion of full-time clinical
professors were individuals of independent means.

Financial deprivations were particularly severe at the lower academic
ranks. For instance, junior faculty at Georgetown were "entirely too
engrossed with the vicissitudes of life and financial matters"[63] to be able
to concentrate on their work. The prospect of low pay influenced some
contemplating academic positions to choose other careers. In 1920 a
highly regarded young embryologist declined a junior position in
anatomy at Johns Hopkins because he could not live on $1,000 a year. He
apologized to the dean for having to mention "these trivial personal
things" but explained that "I have no independent income" and wish to
live "in moderate comfort" and "pay off some of my indebtedness."[64]
Academic medicine was clearly a calling. Faculty members were paid in
part through the opportunity to do research and receive academic recognition, not through salary alone.

If the financial rewards of academic medicine were less than in a later
period, the emotional rewards were arguably greater and the quality of
life richer. Many commentators have claimed that medical research was
more satisfying and more fun.[65] This had to do with the smaller size and

Table 2   Range of salaries paid in the basic science departments of schools ranking highest and lowest in salary scales

Full-time Faculty	Ten Highest	Ten Lowest
Professor	$12,000–$16,000	$2,249–$4,455
Associate Professor	$6,000–$10,000	$2,062–$3,500
Assistant Professor	$4,500–$8,000	$1,980–$2,550
Instructor	$3,000–$6,000	$1,050–$1,800
Assistant	$2,000–$3,600	$637–$1,200

greater collegiality of academic departments and the relative technological simplicity of medical research. A medical school before World War II that had a few dozen full-time faculty members was large. Departmental barriers were minimal and easily surmounted, administrative regulations were few, schools operated with a flexibility and absence of bureaucracy that has long been forgotten, and investigators were spared the time and worry of applying for federal grants. Research in both preclinical and clinical departments was supported by small foundation grants, legislative appropriations, or a school's own resources. Equipment was sparse, so faculty members regularly borrowed from one another. Laboratory equipment and supplies used for teaching were often used for research as well. Paul Beeson recalls how world-class scientists like Oswald Avery and René Dubos at the Rockefeller Institute in the early 1940s had "cubbyhole" offices and worked by themselves without technicians.[66] The tradeoff for working in a modest research environment was that faculty members did not have to bring in their salaries from outside sources. Research grants during this period were expressly for the actual expenses of research, not for the faculty member's time.

The small size of medical schools, the clinical orientation of the scientific departments, and the commitment of clinical faculty to establishing clinical research as an academic discipline resulted in an unusual harmony and cooperation within most pre–World War II medical schools. This was manifested by routine collaboration among departments in teaching and research, regular interdepartmental luncheons and conferences, and schoolwide journal groups and research clubs—which would often meet at night or on Saturdays. A sense was present that the medical school was a family, with the various parts working together for the larger whole. Senior faculty would look out for junior faculty, as at the Peter Bent Brigham Hospital, where the chief of internal medicine went to great lengths to ensure that the younger instructors received proper credit of authorship for their investigative work.[67] Clinical departments would look out for preclinical departments, often using surplus income from patient fees to help support them.

The pre–World War II medical school was characterized by an extraordinary commingling of social and scientific life. A tone of aristocratic collegiality permeated medical education. At the University of Southern California, the Executive Faculty held their regular meetings at the exclusive California Club; at New York University, the Advisory Committee of the medical faculty met in similar posh surroundings at several private clubs; at Mount Sinai, the journal club met every Friday night at the Harmonie Club.[68] The conviviality of the club extended to numerous professional societies of academicians. Thus, there was the Clinical Society of Genito-Urinary Surgeons, the American Gynecological Club, the American Clinical and Climatological Association, the Cosmopolitan Club, and the Peripatetic Club—all known for good fellowship as well as for clinical and scientific leadership. No club was more renowned than the Interurban Clinical Club, whose central importance in the development of clinical science can scarcely be exaggerated, yet which was equally well known for its elegant black-tie dinners and the camaraderie among its elected members.[69]

Medical school life was all-consuming. Where did the professional end and the personal begin? At the University of Southern California, faculty wives regularly hosted teas for medical students (as well as for each other); at Cornell, students entertained the faculty and their scientific guests, such as the American Association of Anatomists.[70] Discussion groups would be well attended at night; lecture halls and conference rooms would be overflowing on Saturdays. Though more will be said of students, house officers, and voluntary faculty, they, too, were part of the medical school family. This was best personified by house officers, who lived in the hospital, did not marry, and were always on duty. To them the medical school and teaching hospital literally were the family.

Ruling the roost of the pre–World War II medical school were the senior faculty members, particularly the department chairmen. Whether in the laboratory or at the bedside, they influenced lives and careers and exemplified high professional values. Though many famous professors served their fields nationally, they travelled relatively little, particularly when they had teaching or patient-care responsibilities. Their impact was a personal one, whether guiding a first-year student through an anatomical dissection or a surgical resident through a new operation. Their authority was unquestioned. In the clinical departments, the power of the chairmen derived not just from the administrative powers of the office but from the fact that they were the consummate clinical authorities. "The academic physicians were the best, and medical students respected these men just as medieval monks had respected their abbots."[71]

Junior faculty assisted ably in the operation of the medical school, but theirs was a more insecure life. Aside from the problem of low pay, they had to endure the paucity of opportunities for promotion. Most medical schools followed a strict pyramid system of faculty appointments, which meant that there could be no more than one full professor in a department. The rank of associate professor was often reserved for individuals qualified for a full professorship awaiting such an appointment. Faculty sizes grew substantially at this time, but the bulk of the growth occurred in the lower academic ranks. At Harvard Medical School, for instance, the ratio of junior faculty to full professors grew from 5.4 to 1 in 1920 to 15 to 1 in 1940.[72]

Also part of the family were the voluntary (part-time) faculty—private practitioners who donated their time to medical teaching in exchange for academic titles and admitting privileges to the teaching hospital. Voluntary faculty were universally present at private medical schools, and they played important roles at some state schools as well. In the aggregate a school's voluntary faculty would provide thousands of hours of teaching each year at no cost to the school. Voluntary faculty occasionally chafed at their subordinate role in medical school governance, and at some schools they tended to receive the less prestigious teaching assignments. However, at most schools the esprit de corps between the part-time and full-time staffs remained strong, and private faculty were generally considered members of the family.

Part of the harmony of the pre–World War II medical school resulted from the cohesiveness of its purpose: education, research, and patient care intertwined. The interdependence of these activities was illustrated by the career of Harvard hematologist George R. Minot. It was from careful observations of his patients—spending countless hours listening to their stories, extracting their dietary histories, and thinking "ever more about food"—that he began his pioneering inquiries that ultimately led to the discovery that liver feedings could cure pernicious anemia, a previously fatal disease. He shared the Nobel Prize for this discovery in 1934. Yet, even as he found great joy poring for hours at a time at blood smears under a microscope, he would continually remind students that "studying his [a patient's] blood does not study the patient," and throughout his career he remained an outstanding clinical teacher and bedside doctor. He continued to see private patients until his retirement, and he warned about letting research interfere with one's view of medicine as a whole. To this Nobel laureate it was "essential that every doctor, regardless of his field of interest, should keep his hands on patients."[73]

Another quality of American medical schools of this period was their adherence to high standards of intellectual honesty. George W. Corner of the University of Rochester, for instance, delayed publication of the discovery of progesterone until he could perform each step of the chemical isolation himself. He was not content that his colleague, the gifted chemist Willard Allen, had already done the experiments.[74] It was customary in this period for chairmen in all departments to read every paper emanating from their staffs. In such a climate, scientific fraud was a non-issue.[75] Generosity in publication was frequently extended to students. Thus, physiologist Walter Cannon of Harvard, like his mentor Henry Bowditch and Bowditch's mentor, Carl Ludwig, would omit his name from the papers of students working in his laboratory—even if he had been extensively involved in the project. Cannon, as did other intellectual descendents of Ludwig, adopted the German physiologist's attitude that there could be no better way to encourage students' interest in research than to allow them to see their names in print.[76]

The ultimate manifestation of the pre–World War II medical school's sense of family was the willingness of all to expose their errors. The most important clinical conference was the mortality conference, where pathologists and clinicians, usually in a room overflowing with full-time staff, voluntary faculty, house officers, and students, would discuss the clinical presentation and autopsy findings of a patient who had died. Almost always, something was to be learned—a diagnostic insight, a scientific observation, or a lesson on how to avoid an error in the future. House officers competed zealously with each other to secure the highest percentage of autopsies on their patients who died, and hospitals similarly competed, for a high autopsy rate was considered the mark of a great teaching hospital. Another vehicle to discuss failure or mistakes was the published case report. Thus, when an early dean of Cornell surgically removed the kidney of an unusual patient who had been born with only one kidney, rather than hide his mistake, he published an account of it so that others might be warned against committing the same mistake.[77]

Every year medical faculty would be renewed during their annual scientific meetings. This was true of every discipline, but it was especially true of clinical scientists, who would gather each spring for their most important meetings (the Association of American Physicians, the American Society for Clinical Investigation, and the American Federation for Clinical Research) in Atlantic City. To medical educators the term "Atlantic City" connoted not the city in New Jersey but the intellectual and personal cohesiveness of academic medicine and clinical science. For several days the best, brightest, and most aspiring clinical investigators would present papers, engage in intense discussions, and stay up to all hours probing the meaning of the latest reports. The boardwalk of Atlantic City witnessed a continual promenade of clinical scientists, young and old, engrossed in conversation. The tacky hotels and restaurants were sites of some of the most important discussions in American medicine. The presentations of the young workers received the most intense scrutiny, and jobs were often offered to investigators completing residencies or fellowships. For all who participated, the meetings were a reminder that the family of academic medicine was a national one.

The metaphorical family of the medical school also had its outcasts. Medical faculties, like most university faculties, were overwhelmingly white, male, and Christian. Individuals who were not often endured great indignities, provided they could obtain faculty positions at all. African-Americans encountered the greatest obstacles. Except for the two black medical schools, Howard and Meharry, professorships for black doctors were virtually nonexistent, and even junior appointments were extremely rare and difficult to obtain. Perhaps the most remarkable story of an African-American medical scientist was that of Vivien Thomas, a dignified and self-effacing high school graduate from Nashville who ultimately was made a member of the medical faculty and awarded an honorary doctorate by the Johns Hopkins University in recognition of his pioneering investigations in cardiovascular surgery and for his role in training young surgeons. With no formal education beyond high school, Thomas was instructed in laboratory techniques by Alfred Blalock and Joseph W. Beard and served as Blalock's principal laboratory technician at Vanderbilt and Johns Hopkins. Thomas became an extraordinary operative technician and a superb designer of chemical and physiological experiments. It was Blalock's name that was immortalized in the Blalock-Taussig "blue baby" operation, but it was Thomas who perfected the surgical techniques for this pioneering operation in the laboratory and who guided Blalock through the first successful use of the operation on a human baby at Johns Hopkins in 1945.[78]

Women medical faculty encountered similar, if less severe, obstacles that mirrored challenges they faced in receiving opportunities to do original work throughout American higher education.[79] Faculty appointments were given to women much more readily than to African-Americans, but recognition and advancement came very slowly. The brilliant anatomist, Florence Rena Sabin, was passed over for the department chairmanship at the University of Illinois College of Medicine because she was a woman.[80] Alice Hamilton, the founder of the field of occupational medicine and a person considered by her dean as "greatly superior to any man"[81] in the field, was privately (though not publicly) frustrated at being Harvard's only woman faculty member and at the school's refusal to offer her anything more than a succession of temporary appointments. She retired in 1935 as an assistant professor, highly honored outside her institution but not within.[82] Salaries for women faculty were usually lower than those for men of comparable rank and seniority, and if medical schools granted leaves of absence for pregnancy at all, it was usually without pay. For the first half of the century, apparently the only medical school in the nation that would appoint a woman dean was Woman's Medical College of Pennsylvania.[83]

Jews encountered the most organized discrimination in academic medicine, a reflection of the high number of qualified Jewish aspirants for professorships and the intense nativist sentiment that pervaded America after World War I. Medical faculties, like faculties throughout the university, established formal or informal quotas for Jews, particularly to senior positions. Throughout the archival records of medical schools of this period, when the issue of faculty appointments came up, comments continually appeared regarding a candidate's Jewishness. Thus, historian of medicine Charles Singer was described as "a very aggressive, persistent, commercial Jew"; pathologist Arnold Rich as "a

very brilliant Jew."[84] Solicited for suggestions for a new anatomy chairman at the University of California at San Francisco, one medical dean
replied that some of the best younger candidates were Jews, but "I shall
not mention them until I hear that additional suggestions [regarding
them] would be welcome."[85]

Many Jews succeeded in having brilliant careers in academic medicine, but prejudice was always a thin layer away. Brothers Abraham and
Simon Flexner—highly assimilated German Jews who steadfastly
retained their idealistic belief in America as a land of fairness and opportunity—bristled at occasional incidents of anti-Semitism they encountered.[86] Jewish faculty at Yale fared worse than at most medical schools,
despite the presence from 1920 to 1935 of a Jewish dean, Milton C. Winternitz. Winternitz has been described as "almost a caricature of the
American Jew trying to become part of gentile society" who "rejected
Jews, Judaism, and Jewish associations in his drive for achievement."[87]
Jewish faculty at Yale knew they had to be much better than their gentile
counterparts to succeed, and it was an unwritten rule at the school that
Jews would not be promoted above the rank of associate professor.[88]

The above discussion suggests that the pre–World War II medical
school, like so many families, harbored considerable conflict, not just
good feeling. Usually tensions lay below the surface. However, in some
instances conflict visibly erupted. A common occasion would be the
appointment of a new department chairman or clinical chief. Many who
had dutifully served the previous chairman suddenly found themselves
unappreciated and displaced. Thus, the department of surgery of Cornell
was disrupted when the intensely academic George Heuer, who had little
use for the practitioner-consultant type of surgeon who had previously
staffed the department, was appointed chairman. Upon taking over,
Heuer found that he did not have the clean slate he had been promised.
The former chairman, who was made to feel miserable, did not cooperate
with Heuer. The result was "two professors of surgery at absolute logger-
heads—neither one willing to cooperate with the other, and each
extremely resentful of the other."[89]

There was never any guarantee that faculty would get along. In the
hierarchical medical school, junior faculty were vulnerable to dressing-
downs, often without cause. At Johns Hopkins a senior surgeon, William
F. Rienhoff Jr., suggested a project on pancreatitis to a junior colleague.
The young investigator was unable to get an appointment with Rienhoff
to discuss the results of the work despite months of trying. Thinking
Rienhoff had lost interest in the project, he showed a draft of the paper to
another person. Upon learning this, an irate Rienhoff immediately sum-
moned him and delivered a severe scolding. Such idiosyncratic behavior,
which was not considered unusual for Rienhoff, contributed to his being
passed over for department chairman.[90]

One special area of conflict concerned salary. Instructors did not enter
academic medicine with high income expectations, but even the most

dedicated faculty often chafed at perceived inequities in compensation. At school after school, preclinical faculty resented the higher salaries received by their counterparts in the clinical departments. To preclinical instructors, arguments that medical schools needed to respond to market forces, or that a clinical professor's job was more taxing because of the additional demands of patient care, were nonpersuasive. They felt that all university professors should be paid on the same scale.

Even within the same or similar departments, dissension frequently occurred over inequalities of pay. At Harvard Medical School, Dean Edsall often discussed with President Lowell his difficulties at quelling unrest among the leading scientists of the faculty over the issue of salary. Harvard, like all schools, had a salary range for each academic rank. In the preclinical departments in 1930, the scale was as follows: assistants, $1,200 to $3,800; instructors, $1,800 to $4,000; assistant professors, $3,500 to $6,500; associate professors, $5,000 to $12,000; professors, $7,000 to $13,000. Thus, an associate professor might earn more than a full professor. Knowledge among the faculty that a wide salary range existed frequently led to unrest, jealousy, and at times outspoken dissension. One usually noncomplaining professor of international renown complained bitterly to Edsall when he discovered that a former pupil, now a member of the teaching staff, was receiving a distinctly higher salary than his.[91]

Considerable conflict was also apparent in the governance of the medical school, as manifested by the evolving power relationships among and within various departments. During World War I, anatomy was the strongest preclinical department and pharmacology the weakest. By World War II, biochemistry had become the strongest preclinical department, and the chair of anatomy had become the most difficult position for most medical schools to fill. In the clinical fields, the situation was more stable. Internal medicine and surgery were the dominant departments intellectually and politically. Because of its strong foundation on clinical science, internal medicine was generally considered the backbone of the medical school. "Minor" fields—radiology, neurology, dermatology—had not yet achieved departmental status, though they frequently clamored to be so recognized. For now, internal medicine and surgery held their fields together and staved off fragmentation and subspecialization. Thus, they could command the most medical school resources, dominate the operations of the school, and control the curriculum.

The greatest conflict in medical schools of this period—one that was to resonate in medical schools throughout the twentieth century—was the tension between teaching and research. That teaching and research invigorated each other was widely appreciated. However, there was also an intrinsic conflict between the two: they each competed for a faculty member's limited time. Even Abraham Flexner on one occasion acknowledged that teaching and research "encroach on a common fund of time and energy" and hence are "more or less antagonistic."[92]

What is notable about American medical schools before World War II was the importance that almost all schools began placing on research. A school's reputation for scholarship became the primary measure of its standing in comparison with other schools. Accordingly, in academic medicine, like other university disciplines, published papers became the new currency, and most schools used publications rather than teaching excellence as the chief criterion for promotion.[93] Many schools complained loudly about the intrusion of teaching on the faculty's opportunities for research. The main justification for not increasing the size of medical school classes (which remained unchanged from World War I to World War II, despite a several-fold increase in the number of faculty) was to protect research time. In the race to succeed, there was considerable inflation in the number of publications and devaluation of the quality. "In the stampede of scientific literature the quantity of it conceals much good work, and the ordinary quality of it degrades the standard of medical research and its written record,"[94] an officer of the Rockefeller Foundation wrote in 1941.

An emphasis on research was found not just at elite institutions but at almost all medical schools. For instance, Hahnemann and the University of Arkansas, schools with distinct teaching missions, hoped to develop a much stronger presence in research. Their faculty frequently expressed the importance of research to a medical school.[95] Howard, continually struggling to remain solvent, also encouraged its faculty to spend as much time as possible doing research. Some teachers at the school believed that Howard had actually developed an "over emphasis in attempting to make the College of Medicine a research institution rather than a school."[96] The majority of schools lacked the resources to compete with the research elite, but they often dreamed of doing so.

Perhaps the most telling indication of the importance of research to medical faculty lay in the primal drive to propagate. Though medical schools produced mainly practitioners—the career choice made by at least 95 percent of graduates before World War II[97]—the greatest ambition of faculty was to produce people like themselves—future researchers, preferably in their own field. Faculty pride and a school's prestige were tightly enmeshed with the number of medical scholars they produced. Students picked up quickly on this aspect of faculty culture. How, besides good grades, could a student best compete for a "competitive" residency after graduation? The answer, universally known among medical students, was clear: to profess an interest in an academic career.

The above discussion is not to suggest that teaching suffered because of the pre–World War II medical school's attention to research but that good teaching often occurred by happenstance rather than design. A senior professor at one prominent school pointed out that "teaching as a whole has improved" at his institution. However, "The importance attached to it by many staff members appears to have waned appreciably."[98] In the American medical school, as the American university, a faculty-determined definition of institutional mission prevailed. Accomplishment was measured primarily by research productivity rather than by excellence in teaching, caring for patients, or addressing the broader health needs of society. In this environment the massive postwar infusion of federal funds created the research behemoths of the present, both in the medical school and the "multiversity."

Diversity and Development

Medical schools in America were a heterogeneous lot. The variation among medical schools was less than among colleges and universities, which were far greater in number and charged with nonacademic functions not attached to medical schools. However, the diversity in facilities, personnel, resources, quality, and mission among medical schools was notable. Each school (and there were 76 in 1929, 77 after the University of Southern California reopened in 1933) had a unique personality and history, reflective of its own traditions and circumstances.

No city better illustrated the diversity of American medical education than Philadelphia. In addition to an osteopathic school, there were five medical schools: Pennsylvania, a typical research-oriented school; Jefferson, a clinically oriented school; Hahnemann, a former homeopathic school; Woman's Medical College of Pennsylvania; and Temple, which had been founded in 1901 as a night school to allow economically impoverished groups the opportunity to enter medicine, and which remained committed to the education of the economically disadvantaged and victims of discrimination. Similar contrasts could be found in several other cities as well.

The reputations of medical schools fell along a spectrum. At the top was an aristocracy of 12 to 15 schools, mainly private and located in the East. These schools, exemplified by Harvard and Johns Hopkins, were the most prominent centers of medical research. They had the largest number of full-time faculty, the best facilities, and the largest endowments and budgets. Most schools were in the respectable middle: solid institutions known for excellent teaching, but where research was conducted on a smaller scale. Most state medical schools were of this type, as were many private schools, such as Jefferson, Emory, Northwestern, St. Louis University, the University of Southern California, and Stanford. At the lower end were approximately 20 schools that were continually on and off probation with the accrediting agencies (the Council on Medical Education and Hospitals of the American Medical Association and the Association of American Medical Colleges). These schools struggled with little money, inadequate laboratory and clinical facilities, and few full-time instructors. They engaged in little research and frequently would admit students who had not satisfied published admission requirements. Among these were many Southern schools, two-year schools like North Dakota and South Dakota, independent (nonuniversity affiliated) schools like the Long Island College of Medicine and Hahnemann, and underfunded schools such as Creighton, Meharry, Ohio State, Buffalo, and Wayne University.

Schools varied in mission as well as reputation. Those of the aristocracy had a national constituency. They attracted students from around the country, and their graduates dispersed nationally. These schools conducted the largest amount of research and trained the majority of medical scientists. Most schools were local institutions. They served a specific region or state and defined their primary mission as the production of practicing doctors rather than medical scientists. A few leading state schools, such as Michigan and Minnesota, experienced conflicting objectives. As public schools, they felt a strong responsibility to the state—educating practitioners who would practice there; providing consultative and charity medical care to state residents. Yet as strong university medical schools, they experienced the same desire to achieve excellence in research and advanced teaching as the elite private schools. Noble in purpose, feeble in pocketbook, were the special mission schools—Woman's Medical College of Pennsylvania for women, and Howard and Meharry for African-Americans. During this period Woman's Medical College was less central to the education of women than Meharry and Howard were for African-Americans. Woman's enrolled approximately 10 percent of women medical students in the United States, compared with Meharry and Howard, which together enrolled 87 percent of the country's black medical students.[99] This was a reflection of the more restrictive medical and societal barriers that faced African-Americans.

Though schools on the whole were much stronger than before World War I, those on the lower tiers were still problematic. For instance, Hahnemann assigned out-of-date textbooks in the biochemistry course, and lectures on the subject did not reflect current concepts. Students had to study collateral reading to pass licensing examinations, and they were not given credit on school examinations for answers that were scientifically correct but that differed from the obsolete point of view presented in the course.[100] At Georgetown, junior and senior students had few opportunities to study hospitalized patients. A Georgetown regent complained in 1929 that the school had "no right" to take their tuition until teaching improved.[101] Few schools encountered such severe obstacles as Howard, which was engaged in an incessant struggle to make ends meet financially. Unlike some private schools that could raise tuition, Howard had to keep its tuition low because so many of its students were impoverished.[102] Rivaling Howard for poverty was Meharry, which not only was unable to provide competitive salaries to faculty but also was unable to build up resources to provide retirement annuities for its staff.[103]

Nevertheless, the overall quality of American medical schools had become unmistakably excellent. A medical dean noted in 1924 that, with a few exceptions, the course of study was so similar at medical schools "that it makes little difference which school a student attends."[104] Even the weakest schools of this period were far stronger and more respectable than most medical schools of the proprietary era. This was seen in the behavior of the accrediting agencies, which in the 1920s shifted their focus from eliminating substandard medical schools to eliminating substandard medical education. They would place weaker schools on probation and offer constructive suggestions for improvement, rather than swiftly disaccredit a school, as they had done to so many proprietary schools before World War I.[105]

The period between the world wars witnessed considerable growth at American medical schools. The greatest growth occurred during the 1920s, as academic medicine's first great bull market occurred. Fueled by postwar prosperity and generous philanthropic and state support, medical schools enjoyed a golden age. Schools expanded, new faculty positions were created, academic salaries rose, and the volume of research increased. This was an especially prosperous time for clinical departments, which received the greatest attention of deans and fund-raisers. By the decade's end, clinical departments often surpassed the preclinical departments in size and funding. To many medical schools, growth became an imperative. As a Harvard official put it, "The [medical] institution which ceases to grow almost inevitably stagnates and begins to decay."[106] The imperative to grow was not confined to medical schools. It was also a defining characteristic of research universities of the period.[107]

The 1930s were a period of retrenchment for medical schools, as for many organizations and institutions seeking to remain afloat during the Depression. At major and minor schools alike, operations were curtailed, hiring and promotion freezes instituted, and salaries cut.[108] Nevertheless, even the Depression could not curtail the development of medical schools. Contributions from foundations and wealthy individuals continued unabated, and medicine in the 1930s was the most generously supported area of university research.[109] By 1940, many American medical schools were operating with budgets ten times greater than those of a generation before. At the time of the Flexner report, $100,000 was considered the necessary annual budget to run an "ideal" medical school—a level of income enjoyed by very few schools. By 1939, many leading schools had annual budgets surpassing $1,000,000, and the median expenditure of American medical schools had risen to $244,350.[110]

Significantly, most of the new funds were earmarked for research. Faculty sizes grew, physical plants expanded, and departmental budgets increased—even as the number of medical students remained unchanged. This was especially true of the elite research schools. An important study of medical education in 1932 observed that the increasing wealth of medical schools was often not being used for education. "The large expenditures of some medical schools should not be regarded as the standard for all because medical students can be well trained in schools which have modest budgets."[111]

As before World War I, funds for growth came from state and local governments, foundations, individual donors, tuition, and endowment income. New sources of support became available as well, particularly research grants from pharmaceutical houses and other industrial concerns. The broad-based nature of private support was evidenced by the success of Harvard Medical School, which rose to national leadership without receiving a major grant from the once dominant General Education Board.

Medical schools continued to be aided financially by their parent universities. This was especially important for less wealthy schools, which depended on their parent universities for substantial portions of their budget and for help with fund-raising. However, the ability of medical schools to generate research grants, clinical income, and large gifts led to an unprecedented degree of autonomy from the rest of the university. This was especially so at the elite research schools. At Washington University, the inability of the university chancellor, George R. Throop, to gain control of the medical school's finances led to a deep rift between him and the medical school dean, Philip Shaffer. The university's board sided with Shaffer, which helped bring about Throop's resignation.[112]

As medical schools grew, they competed vigorously with one another. No school was immune to raids on its faculty for notable medical scientists, who would be wooed by other institutions with promises of higher salaries, academic promotions, and greater opportunities for research. Dean David Edsall of Harvard frequently voiced his worry about the "striking offers" to Harvard professors and planned strategies on how "to hold our men."[113] Schools that might not be able to compete with the elite would compete with others on the same level. Thus, Meharry and Howard would try to outbid each other when making faculty appointments.[114] Local competition was fierce in cities with several medical schools and teaching hospitals, such as Boston, New York, Philadelphia, and Chicago. In New Orleans, Tulane and Louisiana State University competed vigorously for control of Charity Hospital. In the early 1930s, when Tulane controlled the hospital, up to 36 Tulane graduates but few Louisiana State graduates would receive internships at Charity each year. When Louisiana State University gained control, the number of new interns from Tulane immediately fell to 9, and 42 graduates of Louisiana State University received appointments instead.[115]

As medical schools grew larger and more complex, so did their administrative structures. Governance, once simple and informal, became increasingly challenging and formalized. Someone was needed to lead the recruitment for new faculty, mediate intrafaculty disputes, raise funds, foster relationships with foundations, philanthropists, and government agencies, manage financial affairs, serve as a liaison with the university and hospital, supervise the physical facilities, and oversee the educational programs. Those tasks fell to the dean.

Before World War I the deanship was a part-time, often honorific position. Administration was simple; virtually no school even had a comprehensive system of cost accounting. After the war the administrative responsibilities of the deanship grew significantly, as did the underlying administrative infrastructure of secretaries, clerks, messengers, typewriters, telephones, records, and filing systems. By 1939, full-time deans had become more common, the office of the dean began to encompass various assistant deanships, and medical school committees began to proliferate.[116] The execution of the dean's duties was now a devouring task. This fact came to the dismay of many deans who had accepted their positions mistakenly thinking they could keep their hand in teaching or research. Even David Edsall of Harvard—the greatest administrative animal among medical school deans of the period—repeatedly complained of the toll the deanship was taking on his scientific work and his health, and on several occasions he even considered resigning.[117]

For all their growth, medical schools before World War II were still small enterprises relative to the behemoths they would later become. Their financial needs were modest and funding sources broad-based. This fact, coupled with the lack of regulation of the country's medical system, allowed them a high degree of autonomy. Medical school leaders went about the business of managing their schools remarkably free to pursue their own agendas. As always, medical schools remained dependent on the good will of society for support. However, the period between the wars was one in which medical schools were able to achieve a remarkably high degree of control over their own destiny.

The Rise of Harvard Medical School

As World War II began, it appeared that Johns Hopkins would retain its position as the country's leading medical school for the foreseeable future. Hopkins was among the schools selected by the General Education Board to receive endowments to create full-time clinical departments, and the school received funds from the Rockefeller Foundation in 1916 to establish the country's first school of public health. As late as 1926 an eminent member of the faculty of rival Harvard Medical School spoke enviously of the prominence of Johns Hopkins in American medicine.[118]

However, by the end of World War I Johns Hopkins was no longer so dominant. Compared with Harvard, Johns Hopkins was handicapped by a smaller faculty, a more modest budget, and a series of mediocre appointments to key faculty positions. Moreover, Johns Hopkins did not have a large body of alumni from either the medical school or the university to draw upon for support. As the war ended, the school did not seem so robust as before. No one doubted its continued excellence, but other schools were rapidly catching up.[119]

In the early 1900s Harvard was still a regional school, with 93 percent of its students coming from New England.[120] In the immediate post-Flexnerian period no school underwent so rapid or dramatic a transformation. A new era began with the appointment of A. Lawrence Lowell as university president in 1909 and David L. Edsall as dean of the school in 1918. Soon Harvard surpassed Johns Hopkins as the nation's archetypical medical school—a position it retained, despite stiff competition, for the rest of the twentieth century.[121]

Lowell and Edsall worked closely with each other to transform Harvard into a national school. Lowell, a strong-willed, self-righteous, somewhat humorless Boston Brahmin with an unusually broad outlook on education, took medical school affairs seriously—advising his dean on matters of curriculum, personnel, and finances. Like his predecessor, President Charles Eliot, Lowell even attended meetings of the medical faculty. However, unlike Eliot, whose personality and presence dominated the medical school, Lowell was more removed. He counseled Edsall on various matters but made clear that the final decision belonged to the dean.[122] Accordingly, the postwar development of the school was much more a result of the vision and energy of Edsall, who acted with great independence. Lowell himself acknowledged Edsall's singular influence in developing the school.[123]

Immediately on assuming the deanship, Edsall, a trained laboratory worker who had become a pioneering clinical investigator at the University of Pennsylvania and the Massachusetts General Hospital, undertook the school's revitalization. He made the cultivation of research his primary focus as dean. Under this outstanding fund-raiser, persuasive recruiter, and wise administrator, the school thrived. From 1918 to 1930, the budget of the school grew from approximately $200,000 to nearly $800,000 per year, and the number of faculty with major research responsibilities more than doubled to 179.[124] New facilities for research were built and older facilities repaired and updated. Investigation in both the preclinical and clinical disciplines flourished, and a thriving program of graduate study in the basic medical sciences was nurtured as well.

By the time Edsall retired as dean in 1935, Harvard Medical School had become the nation's most prestigious, largely because of its unparalleled laboratory and clinical resources and its phenomenal record of accomplishment in medical research. A regional school no longer, nearly 70 percent of its student body came from outside New England, attracted by the presence of so many distinguished teachers and investigators on the faculty.[125] Based on many criteria—the degree of competitiveness for admission, student performance on standardized tests and licensing examinations, the amount of research support, the size of the budget and endowment, success at producing medical researchers and teachers, and faculty honors and awards—Harvard Medical School had become the leading school, the grudging reluctance of several institutions close behind to concede the lead notwithstanding.

As Harvard rose to national prominence, a major issue was thrown into sharp relief: Was the medical school's mission research or education? Lowell worried that the school was producing too few physicians. The class size was limited to 125 students, a number that had not changed since 1900 despite rising numbers of outstanding applicants and a large growth in the faculty and facilities.[126] To Lowell a medical school was a public instrument meant to help furnish the country with an adequate supply of well-trained physicians. He was disturbed that more and more of the school's resources were pouring into research without a concomitant increase of medical teaching.

Lowell was not bashful about discussing this point with Edsall. He told the dean on one occasion that providing medical education to all suitable applicants was "our duty to the community."[127] Neither was Eliot, who remained active in Harvard affairs even after retiring from the presidency and who agreed with Lowell. Eliot told Edsall that the school's failure to enlarge the student body represented "a shocking abandonment of the right conception of the function of a good medical school toward the public welfare."[128]

Edsall and the medical faculty readily brushed the criticisms of the two presidents aside. In their minds they already had enough students. They felt that any more would interfere with research. In no uncertain terms Edsall said to Lowell: "I am quite sure that most of the important men in the School would be intensely disappointed and much disturbed if the number [of medical students] were larger than at present. . . . I do not see how we can push them further than that [the amount of teaching they are already doing] without making it very difficult and trying for them."[129]

For the rest of his presidency, Lowell tried unsuccessfully to persuade Edsall to reconsider the issue of class size and institutional mission. Lowell continually stated his belief, privately and publicly, that the number of medical students was too small relative to the size of the physical plant and faculty. However, he could not convince Edsall to increase enrollment. When Lowell retired in 1933, the size of the entering class was still 125, unchanged from the turn of the century. Lowell and Edsall were good friends who usually saw eye-to-eye, and their long relationship had proven extremely fruitful for the medical school. The issue of the number of students, Lowell told Edsall on his retirement from the presidency, was "the only point on which we have ever seriously disagreed."[130]

In the battle between Edsall and Lowell, some of the main directions and ironies of twentieth-century medical education were laid bare. That Edsall "won" was indicative of the growing autonomy of medical schools from their parent universities. After World War I, the ability of medical schools to raise funds on their own gave them a new independence from the universities that had nurtured them during the creative period. Of course, no other medical school was as wealthy as Harvard. Many still depended heavily on their parent universities for financial aid, and some never stopped doing so. On the whole, however, medical schools became the richest and most self-sufficient branch of the university, and many began to operate with an administrative autonomy that would have flabbergasted the creators of the system.

In the confrontation between Lowell and Edsall, the mission of Harvard Medical School was sharply debated. Lowell believed that the school had an obligation to produce more doctors; Edsall believed equally strongly that the school's first duty was research. With Edsall's victory over Lowell, the vision of the medical school turned inward. A faculty-oriented priority (research) triumphed over a society-oriented priority (education and the immediate provision of doctors). What happened at Harvard was characteristic of what was happening at leading medical schools across the country. Schools were developing more to serve the intellectual interests of the faculty than to meet the needs of students and society at large.

The above observations, of course, are hardly meant to suggest that research that explains, mitigates, or cures disease is not a public service. The importance to the public of medical research between the wars, which resulted in the discovery of cures for many nutritional and infectious diseases, can scarcely be exaggerated. Such work provided tangible solutions to problems that had been ravaging the human race since the dawn of history. Yet, the congruence between the intellectual interests of medical scientists and the health needs of society was fortuitous. How might medical research be popularly perceived, it could be asked, if the results were not so immediate and dramatic, or if the medical schools were felt not to be addressing the greatest health needs of society? Herein lay the fundamental ambiguity of American medical schools: their social role as a public trust, versus the faculties' desire to pursue their scientific curiosity. Torn between their intellectual interests and the recognition that to gain patronage they must produce useful knowledge, medical schools' tension was intrinsic to the nature of all scientific research, as scientists since the time of Francis Bacon could attest.

3

Undergraduate
Medical Education

IF KNOWLEDGEABLE PHYSICIANS agreed on one principle, it was that
medical education was a lifelong process. The education of a physician
began long before medical school, since a student's success at learning
medicine depended heavily on the aptitude, characteristics, and educational background that person brought to medical school in the first
place. The four years of medical school—"undergraduate medical education," as it came to be called—were focused on principles and fundamentals. Specialized training was reserved for after the completion of medical
school. All practicing physicians, general practitioners and specialists
alike, needed to remain up-to-date, whether through continuing medical
education courses or informal conferences, discussions, and readings.
From this perspective, the education of a physician was viewed as a continuum, not as a succession of isolated experiences.

Though a medical education was never complete, medical schools
between the wars came close to producing a finished product. This was
because most physicians at that time entered general practice. Accordingly, before World War II undergraduate medical education remained
the primary focus of medical faculties. The Association of American
Medical Colleges in 1935 declared that its "primary and sole interest is in
the medical student from the time he enters medical school until he
graduates."[1]

Traditionally, writers have examined undergraduate medical education mainly in terms of courses and curriculum. However, formal medical instruction represented only one of many important forces that
shaped physicians. Another significant influence was the "hidden curriculum"—the implicit messages continually conveyed, the education
that occurred by example rather than by word, and the imprinting of attitudes and values that regularly occurred. In addition, medical students
themselves had much to say about how they learned medicine. Far from

being passive flotsam in the educational ocean, they had an important impact on the environment of medical schools.

In their work, medical educators faced many general educational challenges that were not unique to medicine. The central pedagogic issues of medical education—the search for a core curriculum and the tension between theoretical and practical knowledge—were similar to those that instructors and administrators faced throughout higher education. In addition, medical educators wrestled with the same dilemma concerning mission that educators everywhere faced: the role of education in influencing attitudes and behavior. For the entire twentieth century these challenges were to resonate throughout medical education—and the educational system as a whole.

Admissions

To even a casual observer, it was clear that medical education could not proceed out of synchrony with the rest of the country's educational system. Medical schools were dependent on earlier levels of education for producing a large enough pool of well-prepared students. Early in the century, when the number of applicants with college backgrounds was small, this was readily apparent. At all but the most competitive schools, admission was open to anyone with a high school degree. Accordingly, attrition was exceedingly high, for those without college preparation usually dropped out or failed.

After the Flexner report, admissions standards to medical school rose rapidly. This was made possible by the extraordinary growth in the number of academically prepared applicants. From 1890 to 1930, a period in which the population of the United States roughly doubled, the number of students enrolled in secondary schools increased from 357,813 to 4,799,867. During the same period, the number of students enrolled in colleges and universities increased from approximately 122,000 to 1,085,799.[2] World War I represented an especially important takeoff point. After the war, a college education for the first time became integral to success for those seeking wealth or social prestige in America.[3] One result was a much higher number of academically qualified students applying to medical school.

By World War I, medical schools for the first time could fill their classes with well-prepared students. In 1915, roughly half the schools required a minimum of one year of college, the other half two years. By 1937, more than half of the schools required at least three years of college. Ninety-two percent of all students admitted to medical school that year had taken at least three years of college, and over half had obtained a baccalaureate degree.[4] Incoming medical students in the 1930s were viewed as "not only the most competent group of students ever admitted to our medical schools, but by and large the best group of students in training for any profession throughout the country."[5]

Through the 1920s almost all qualified applicants were accepted. However, in the late 1920s competition for medical school became much keener as the number of qualified applicants began to greatly exceed the available positions. In 1929–30 only 48 percent of the nation's 13,569 applicants were accepted.[6] Throughout the 1930s those figures remained approximately the same. Rejected applicants who still wished to become doctors had little choice but to go abroad to study. In the 1930s a considerable number did so, particularly Jewish students from the state of New York.[7]

Medical educators recognized that the decision to study medicine had something to do with personal characteristics, cultural values, and the perceived attractiveness of medicine as a career, though no one could *precisely* explain medicine's growing popularity as a career or how premedical students might have differed from undergraduates who pursued other fields.[8] Nevertheless, this was of little worry to medical schools, which now rejoiced at being able to conduct medical education on a far higher plane. Students entered medical school already knowing the alphabet of science, which allowed the four years of medical school to be preserved for purely medical subjects. Academic failure became much less common. By the 1930s the national attrition rate had fallen to 15 percent, most of which occurred during the first year of study.[9] At elite schools that were highly competitive for admission, attrition rates were much lower still.

What course of study should students preparing for medicine undertake? This troublesome issue perplexed medical school and university officials alike. Everyone agreed that in an era of scientific medicine, a college education alone did not suffice. Rather, specific courses were required so that students could begin medical study without having to take remedial work. These consisted of biology or zoology, inorganic chemistry, organic chemistry, and physics. Most medical schools required or recommended courses in English, mathematics, and a foreign language as well.[10]

Beyond these requirements, there was great confusion concerning the best preparation for medical school. Officially, medical school officials espoused the importance of a broad general education, not a narrow scientific training. However, faculties frequently sent the opposite message. This dilemma was illustrated at the University of Michigan. The medical school dean met repeatedly with premedical students to tell them "that the purpose of their preparation was to give them a broad general education."[11] Yet, the majority of individual faculty at the school believed that "science courses are still paramount for medical students."[12] James B. Conant, A. Lawrence Lowell's successor as president of Harvard University, summarized the dilemma in 1939: "I realize that many deans, professors and members of the medical profession protest that what they all desire is a man with a liberal education, not a man with four years loaded with premedical sciences. The trouble is very few people believe this group of distinguished witnesses. Least of all the students."[13] Accordingly, the overwhelming majority of applicants applied to medical school having majored in a scientific subject.

Though medical schools sought qualified students, most were not eager to increase the number admitted. Medical deans knew precisely how many students the school's dissection facilities, student laboratories, and hospital wards could accommodate. The situation at the College of Physicians and Surgeons of Columbia University was typical. In 1918, to ensure that all students "can be adequately taught and trained," the school reduced the size of the first-year class by one-half. The faculty found this experience "infinitely more satisfactory" than trying to teach larger numbers of students as before.[14] In emphasizing educational quality, medical schools were thought to be acting in a socially responsible fashion. Virtually no one in the 1920s and 1930s, inside or outside the profession, thought the country was suffering from too few physicians.

Medical educators and admissions officers debated endlessly how to select the finest candidates from the growing applicant pool: whether to rely on grades, courses taken, letters of recommendation, or the personal interview. Virtually all admissions committees valued that elusive quality of "character," though no one knew exactly how to define or measure it. To help make their deliberations more "scientific," some admissions committees began using the results of the Medical Aptitude Test, a standardized "objective" test introduced by medical educators and educational psychologists at George Washington University in the late 1920s and recommended for general use by the Association of American Medical Colleges in 1931. However, no instrument of measurement, alone or in conjunction with others, could allow them to determine with confidence which applicants would make the best practitioners or medical scientists. The Medical Aptitude Test could accurately predict which students would achieve academic success during the formal course work of medical school, but not future success at practicing medicine.[15]

Distinct patterns could be observed in the practices of admissions committees. Certain undergraduate colleges were favored. Harvard Medical School, for instance, preferred students from established universities like Harvard, Yale, Princeton, and Stanford and prestigious colleges like Amherst and Williams. The chance for admission from these institutions was one in three or four, compared with one in seven or eight for students from less prestigious schools.[16] Some schools favored children or grandchildren of alumni or applicants personally known to a faculty member or someone whose advice was considered reliable.[17] Most schools frowned upon older applicants, no matter how qualified and how meritorious their reasons for seeking to enter medicine.[18] Preference was also given to those who could pay—in part because schools wanted the tuition fees, and in part because schools generally believed that students who had to work their way through would not do well academically.[19] Attention was also given to the geographic origin of students—especially by public schools seeking to fulfill their mandate to educate state residents, and elite private schools seeking a nationally diverse student body.

Some students stood at a distinct disadvantage in the admissions process. One group was African-Americans. The problems of educating blacks were hardly unique to medicine, but discrimination and inequality were as severe in medical schools as anywhere in the educational system. Through World War II, with the exception of Meharry and Howard, African-Americans attended medical school in very small numbers. Many schools, whether Southern institutions like the Medical College of Georgia or Northern schools like Harvard, had never admitted a black medical student.[20] Some schools, such as the University of Michigan, were more receptive to admitting African-Americans, but school officials remained wary of admitting too many because of high dropout rates—an observation they did not know whether to attribute to poor academic preparedness or the lack of money.[21] Blatant racism was sometimes found. Many faculty at the College of Physicians and Surgeons of Columbia University felt that African-Americans were mentally inferior to Caucasians, and the school would admit only the most unusually superior applicants of the race.[22] Many schools received very few applications from qualified blacks. However, as one advocacy group for African-Americans observed, the fact of discrimination at many medical schools was well known. Many blacks were reluctant to apply to schools other than Meharry or Howard because they were convinced they would be rejected. In their view, all that would happen would be that they would lose the nonrefundable application fees.[23]

Women also encountered obstacles in pursuing careers in medicine, though less severe than those faced by African-Americans.[24] When Woman's Medical College of Pennsylvania was organized in 1850, coeducation in medical schools did not exist. Over the next century, most medical schools eliminated their formal barriers to coeducation, so that by 1946 all but two medical schools were open to women. Nevertheless, American culture before World War II, with its persistent Victorian stereotypes of "proper" female roles and its deep-rooted hesitation at even allowing women to vote, hardly provided encouragement for women to enter medicine. Moreover, many schools that did admit women still had a *numerus clausus*. At Michigan, for example, there was a female quota of 10 percent of the entering class; at Physicians and Surgeons, of 20 students per class.[25] Many medical educators argued that a medical education would be "wasted" on women who might forsake their career for a family. Some midcentury studies documented educators' claim that women physicians spent less time at their careers than men—though these studies also concluded that women had made a substantial contribution to the nation's health.[26]

In the highly charged nativist climate of the 1920s that saw the enactment of immigration restriction legislation, vitriolic prejudices existed against the admission of Catholics, Italians, Jews, and other ethnic or religious minorities. By virtue of their success in climbing the educational and social ladder, the most rigid, formalized quotas were faced by Jews. Between 1880 and 1925, the Jewish population in the United States increased from 200,000 to over 4,000,000, and Jewish youths sought admission to college and medical school in high numbers. Medical schools, in the words of an official of Harvard Medical School, felt "overwhelmed by the number of Jewish lads who are applying for admission."[27] The fact that most Jewish applicants were Eastern European Jews rather than German Jews as before was not lost on medical school admissions committees as frightened of the "new" immigration as the rest of American society. In the early 1920s a backlash began. The first manifestation was the creation of quotas at many elite private colleges. Soon quotas appeared in medical schools and other areas of professional and graduate training.[28] By the late 1930s and early 1940s, rigid quotas were found throughout medical education. In the early 1940s, 3 out of every 4 non-Jewish students were accepted, in contrast to 1 out of 13 Jewish students.[29]

Discrimination against Jews was most intense in New York, where the number of Jewish applicants was the highest. At the College of Physicians and Surgeons, the enrollment of Jewish students between 1920 and 1940 dropped from 47 percent of the class to 6 percent; at Cornell during the same period, from 40 percent to 5 percent. At the City College of New York, a magnet to outstanding but poor Jewish students, the percentage of applicants accepted to medical school declined from 58.4 percent in 1925 to 20 percent in 1941 and fell still further after America's entry into World War II.[30] Quotas appeared in surprising places. Woman's Medical College of Pennsylvania, hardly unfamiliar with discrimination, itself discriminated against Jews.[31] The schools without Jewish quotas, such as New York University and Tufts, often came under pressure to conform with prevailing patterns of discrimination.[32]

Medical school officials always publicly denied the existence of Jewish quotas or anti-Jewish prejudice. However, school records revealed otherwise. References to an individual's having the typical traits of an "eastside New York Jew" abounded in documents and correspondence.[33] Questions regularly appeared on application forms concerning candidates' race, religion, and birthplace, and, at some schools, whether candidates had ever changed their names. Since the state of New York had an especially high number of Jewish applicants, followed by the New England states, schools could use the goal of a geographically diverse student body as a disguise for anti-Semitism. Similarly, a school's insistence on accepting students of only the proper "character" for medicine could also be used for weeding out Jews and other "undesirables."[34]

Poor students were also at a distinct disadvantage in becoming physicians—not because they were denied admission, but because of indirect barriers relating to high tuition and the scarcity of scholarship aid. By the late 1920s, the median medical school tuition had reached approximately $250 per year, and books, fees, and living expenses had to be paid for as well.[35] During the Depression, this level of expenditure was out of reach to students from many working-class families—even those willing to work part-time while in school. Few schools had much scholarship money. Accordingly, the sociological composition of medical student bodies shifted toward the affluent.[36]

Medical schools were deeply troubled by the lack of scholarships. Faculty were known to contribute personally to loan or scholarship funds,[37] and most schools tried hard to raise money for financial aid. However, these efforts were usually unsuccessful. The heart of the problem was the ambiguity regarding whether the private practice of medicine was a public service or a business. One generous contributor to the University of Southern California wondered how far the public should go "in paying for an individual's higher education, especially when that higher education is used mainly for his personal livelihood."[38] Confusion regarding whether medical practice was a private business or public service was to haunt efforts to acquire funds for scholarships throughout the twentieth century.

Ultimately, the sociological composition of the student body shifted toward individuals of means. Such an observation would not be surprising to recent critics of the American educational system who have argued that true equality in education depends on socioeconomic equality.[39] From the first stages of education, children from economically disadvantaged families faced obstacles much more frequently than children from wealthier families—substandard local schools and a social environment that worked against maximum learning. Working-class students who succeeded in high school were still at an educational disadvantage. If they could afford college at all, they were often unable to pay the expenses of a more prestigious one. If they did enroll at an elite college, time spent working their way through school frequently occurred at the cost of their studies or of their participation in the social and cultural life of college, the latter to acquire personal contacts useful later in life. These observations are not meant to deny that for many the educational system did work as an instrument of social mobility, but rather, that the dilemmas of medical education were those of the American educational system as a whole.

Training for Uncertainty

In medical school, the specific work of becoming a doctor began. The goal of medical school was to equip students with the fundamentals of medical science to prepare them for medical practice. Instruction in fundamental concepts, scientific reasoning, and critical thinking would hopefully provide students the intellectual tools for a lifetime of professional study and practice. Principles of progressive medical education, articulated in the 1870s, dominated the discourse on medical education in the interwar years, as they were to do throughout the twentieth century.

The medical curriculum in the United States was arranged logically—that is, the course work was constructed so that each subject was based on courses that preceded and prepared for those that followed. The first two years contained the preclinical disciplines in a rationally arranged order: anatomy, biochemistry, physiology, pathology, bacteriology, pharmacology, pathophysiology, and an introduction to history-taking and physical examination. The last two years provided instruction in the various clinical subjects. Most of the time was devoted to the "major" fields of surgery, internal medicine, obstetrics and gynecology, pediatrics, and psychiatry. Lesser amounts of time were spent in specialized areas like urology, neurology, ophthalmology, anesthesiology, and orthopedics. The course of study was designed to familiarize students with the structure, function, and behavior of the human organism in health and disease, to acquaint them with the causes, physiological disturbances, and natural history of the various diseases, to provide an introduction to principles of therapeutics and surgery, and to present the environmental and social influences that affect health, illness, and recovery. Instruction emphasized active learning through laboratories, clerkships, and small-group discussions so that students might learn how to acquire information and solve problems.[40]

The structure of the medical curriculum had been established in the late nineteenth century. The content of the curriculum, however, was highly dynamic, reflecting the evolution of medical science and the changing pattern of diseases encountered in medical practice. Thus, during the interwar period the hours devoted to anatomy fell, while those given to biochemistry rose. Individual courses also evolved. In pharmacology, for instance, emphasis shifted from the identification of drugs and compounding of prescriptions to the study of the physiological effects of drugs and principles of drug therapy. Clinical courses began devoting more time to vascular and degenerative diseases, as those illnesses became more prevalent in the 1920s and 1930s.

Though the curriculum assumed a similar appearance at all medical schools, details varied considerably. In 1940, the number of hours of physiology ranged from 180 to 336; bacteriology, from 90 to 326.[41] These differences reflected the varying scientific strength and political influence of different departments at different schools. During the first two years, the majority of schools taught the preclinical subjects in some form of a block system: anatomy before physiology, pathology before pharmacology. Yet, some provided concurrent instruction. Similarly, in the clinical clerkships there were notable variations in the amount of patient material, degree of responsibility given to students, and allocation of time between inpatient and outpatient work.

In constructing a curriculum, medical instructors were concerned with creating a rich educational environment. They incessantly debated details: topics to include in the lectures, the proper distribution of time between didactic and practical work, the number and types of laboratory experiments, the proper number of students to assign to each cadaver or laboratory bench, the most desirable ratio of instructors to students, the best way to bridge the gap between the laboratory and clinical courses, when and how to introduce students to patients, and how to achieve the best balance between the study of rare diseases that might have heuristic value and that of common illnesses routinely seen in everyday practice. Evaluation procedures received especially lengthy discussion. Should there be many examinations or a few comprehensive ones? written or oral? essay, multiple choice, or practical? letter or numerical grades? Medical educators derived ideas on these matters from their own insights into medical education as well as from each other. Any school contemplating a major reform would first survey what other schools had done.

No curricular issue was more important than broad questions concerning the proper content of medical education. As specialization became more prevalent after World War I, educators wondered whether one curriculum could serve the needs of all students—future psychiatrists and surgeons, aspiring general practitioners, and future medical scientists. What represented the core knowledge and skills that every physician should be expected to have? Similarly, there was much debate about how theoretical a medical education should be. Everyone recognized that progress in medical care derived from the profession's scientific underpinnings, but the great majority of graduates became practitioners, not medical scientists. To what degree should medical education emphasize scientific principles, and to what degree should it provide practical instruction of immediate clinical applicability? This search to define the core knowledge necessary to the general education of physicians mirrored a similar search in higher education to define the core components of general education that all liberal arts students should receive. And the controversy in medical schools over theoretical versus practical goals mirrored an analogous debate in universities over liberal culture versus utility. These debates were to envelop both medical and university educators for the rest of the twentieth century.[42]

The greatest deficiency of medical education was its lack of an efficient excretory system. As medical knowledge continued to grow, the curriculum's reflective response was to attempt to accommodate that knowledge. However, the curriculum quickly became bloated. Lectures too easily substituted for independent learning; too little time remained for thinking, self-development, and personal initiative. The typical medical course, 32 weeks per year during World War I, grew to 36 weeks by World War II, and many students studied during the summers as well.[43] Some felt that a fifth year of medical school should be required.[44] At Johns Hopkins, the greatest advocate of freedom in learning, the number of required hours of instruction in the four-year course increased from

2,662 in 1927–28 to 3,232 in 1935–36.[45] Though material was eliminated from the curriculum, this occurred inefficiently and irregularly.

Medical educators knew they had a good product, but they worked hard to make it better. A healthy spirit of self-criticism was present—one that permeated every study or report of medical education that was published. The first radical curricular reform was introduced by Yale Medical School in 1925. Recognizing that medical students were mature and motivated, the "Yale System," as it came to be known, reduced required course work, increased elective time, eliminated grades, replaced required examinations in each course with comprehensive examinations at the end of the preclinical and clinical periods, and required a dissertation of each student based on original research.[46] Before World War II, no other school introduced so radical a departure. However, the Yale influence was widely felt, and many schools revised their program to provide greater freedom and flexibility. In the effort to achieve an ideal curriculum, truth lay in the search, never in the product in hand.

In seeking to improve teaching, medical schools were limited by the detailed requirements of the state licensing boards. State boards had served a useful function early in the century when many weak schools existed and standards were low. However, after World War I they inhibited flexibility and experimentation, since schools were reluctant to introduce changes in their programs that might make graduates ineligible for a license. Dean David Edsall of Harvard Medical School complained of "the stranglehold that they [State Boards of Examiners] have on the actions of the medical schools, and the way in which, therefore, they gravely hamper the progress of the better schools."[47] In the 1930s medical schools did receive some relief from regulatory bureaucracy. The work of the Commission on Medical Education was especially influential in reducing specific state regulations and providing greater freedom for medical schools to experiment.[48] Yet, the inherent tension between curricular innovation and the need to cover all important subjects was to dominate relations between medical schools and licensing agencies throughout the century.

Probably the most common myth about medical education is that students attained a knowledge of medicine and disease behavior that allowed them to act with certainty in every situation in medical practice. In this inaccurate view, the main purpose of medical education is to replace the uncertainties of the beginner with the certainties of the mature physician. In actuality, physicians in practice regularly encountered dilemmas. Only occasionally did diseases present in the idealized form described in textbooks. In most cases different individuals with the same disease reacted differently, and the physician's task was to try to make sense of each patient complaint. Thus, "chest pain" could result from any one of dozens of causes, not all of which were serious, and not all of which arose from a problem in the heart. Conversely, a patient with a heart problem might have no chest pain at all, or symptoms that mimicked those of a stomach or intestinal illness. After a diagnosis was made, therapeutic decisions also posed challenges, since the desired treatment of one problem could exacerbate another. It was not a trivial matter to decide whether to perform needed surgery on a frail patient at high risk of operative complications. Medical educators understood the nature of medical practice with real human beings. Accordingly, they defined the primary goal of medical education as that of preparing students to deal effectively with the many uncertainties of everyday practice. Sociologist Renée Fox labelled this fundamental aspect of medical education "training for uncertainty."[49]

The best way to train for uncertainty, leading medical educators argued, was to teach how to approach patients in a rigorous scientific way. In their view, the best practitioners were problem-solvers. Hematologist George Minot of Harvard Medical School spoke to students about the vital importance of cultivating an "inquisitive spirit" in which "conclusions must be subjected to adequate test and critical control."[50] Good practitioners and investigators used the same intellectual approaches, he explained. "Every case presents a problem which must be solved."[51]

A second approach to training for uncertainty was to use the clinical clerkships to study a few patients in depth rather than many patients superficially. "Men become educated by steeping themselves thoroughly in a few subjects, not by nibbling at many,"[52] Abraham Flexner wrote in 1925. Scientific method was best taught through the "intensive and thorough study of relatively few patients."[53] The anticipated result was the ability to handle unknowns through the capacity to generalize—the development of "sound methods and habits of study which can be utilized in other and even unfamiliar situations."[54]

Lastly, training for uncertainty was facilitated by keeping one's focus directly on the individual patient, not on idealized stereotypes. The "fundamental fallacy" of medical education and practice, according to the Commission on Medical Education's 1932 report, was that "the human being, who is the unit of medical service, can be regarded as a uniform, standardized organism. The contrary is known to be the case inasmuch as no two individuals are alike, and no two even with the same disorder react in exactly the same way."[55]

Training for uncertainty meant that students would learn to feel comfortable practicing medicine with intellectual freedom. Though they would learn that most patients with a given condition would be approached in a certain way—one that could be described in protocol fashion in a textbook—they would also learn to be alert to the exception, and they would not be afraid to embark on a different course of action when warranted by a patient's particular circumstances. In addition, training for uncertainty, when properly accomplished, resulted in a more "cost-effective" mode of medical practice. Tests would be ordered because they were suggested by a patient's condition, not merely because they were available. The results would be correlated with the patient's condition, and not interpreted literally. Indiscriminate testing made no medical or economic sense.

Though in reality most situations with most patients could be approached in similar ways—no area of medical practice was without its humdrum routine—medicine by protocol was antithetical to informed ideas of what type of practice was best for patients and society. Yet training for uncertainty proved more easily said than done. To achieve this required a mode of medical education difficult for students and faculty alike. Medical education regularly fell short of its aspirations. Faculty often observed that most students were better memorizers than critical thinkers and biological reasoners. Students frequently complained that the curriculum remained bloated with required lectures and courses, with insufficient time for independent thought and elective study. These difficulties never went away. Training physicians for uncertainty became medical education's most elusive ideal.

The Hidden Curriculum

For all the attention paid to it, the formal curriculum represented only part of the educational experience of medical school. The curriculum was concerned with knowledge and facts, reasoning and cognition. Equally important were a physician's attitudes, values, character, and professional identity. These noncognitive objectives of education, though certainly influenced by formal instruction, were also shaped by the grander educational experience that came out of the general culture of medical school. Every individual or group experience that students had molded their attitudes as to what it meant to be a physician. Such learning was latent and implicit, though not at all casual, idiosyncratic, or random. This broader cultural milieu within which the formal curriculum operated has been termed the "hidden curriculum."[56]

What made the hidden curriculum so important in medical education, and other areas of professional education as well, was that students were there by choice, not co-option. Though students certainly had a voice in their education, there was no room in medical school for frank defiance. Students entered medical school because they wanted to acquire what their instructors had to offer. Faculty were always being watched, serving as role models even when they might not have realized they were doing so.

The hidden curriculum operated in several areas. One was the cultivation of a physician's bedside manner. To listen to patients, to be attentive, to inspire confidence, to provide comfort—these qualities of good physicianship required demonstration and reinforcement. So did other important attributes, such as thoroughness, reliability, empathy, and devotion. A good bedside manner was promoted by example, not preaching. No platitudinous lecture on the importance of valuing patients as people could undo the damage if students witnessed their instructors treating patients curtly or abusively, or showing more interest in the laboratory results than in the patients' problems and worries.

Second, the hidden curriculum influenced the gaze with which students viewed patients. It was the primary determinant of whether students learned to view patients as people or as abstract disease entities. Ideally, a good medical education led to the former. However, the fact that so many medical educators of the period worried about this suggested that the worldview of students was becoming much more depersonalized, intellectualized, and medicalized than they wished. The Commission on Medical Education lamented that there was too much interest in laboratory results, not enough in the history, physical examination, and concerns of patients.[57] The dean of the University of Michigan feared that the ideals and values that brought students to medical school in the first place were not consistently being validated by the medical education they received.[58] Of course, numerous contrary examples could be provided. Good data do not exist on the frequency with which the hidden curriculum produced desired results, on how often it backfired, or on how often students emerged relatively unscathed despite institutional obstacles.

Third, the hidden curriculum was instrumental in helping mold professional attitudes, values, and temperament. From the first day of medical school, students experienced a series of critical incidents that resulted in their eventual socialization as physicians: the first anatomical dissection, autopsy, failure in the animal surgery laboratory, exposure to real patients, encounter with nudity, performance of painful or embarrassing procedures, and patient death. Renée Fox constructed a "sociological calendar" of the medical school, which provided "a detailed chronological account of the important attitudinal and cognitive learning that takes place in the classroom and outside of it."[59] The highly patterned events on the calendar, all of which were spinoffs from the formal curriculum, eventually resulted in the development of a professional self-image and of a characteristic temperament combining dispassion with caring that sociologists later called "detached concern."

Lastly, medical schools made implicit value statements by what they left out of the curriculum. The most conspicuous example during this period was preventive medicine, which received only minimal attention at most schools. According to the Commission on Medical Education, a concern for prevention must suffuse the entire medical curriculum. In fact, that hardly happened. Much more typical was the situation at the University of Southern California, where the instructor of preventive medicine lamented "the relative insignificance [to the school] of the course I teach."[60] To students of the hidden curriculum, medical schools were clearly indicating that preventive medicine did not rank high in their value system.

In contrast to the attention given the formal curriculum, the hidden curriculum was infrequently discussed. However, sociological studies in the 1950s clearly demonstrated the enormous influence of the hidden curriculum in shaping the personality, values, and professional identity of physicians, not to mention other professionals as well.[61] Much more needs to be known about the hidden curriculum. Nevertheless, it is clear that to ignore it—whether in seeking to understand medical education historically, or to change medical education for the better today—is to proceed at great risk of failure.

Student Life

If one word could describe the experience of being a medical student, that word would be "consuming."[62] Even the hardest-working, most driven premedical students were hardly prepared for what lay ahead. College undergraduates typically took 15 hours of course credit a semester. The first year of medical school, in contrast, approximated 20 hours of rigorous college credit.[63]

Medical students needed to make attitudinal as well as intellectual adjustments. Advertised as an invigorating educational process, medical education in fact tested physical and mental endurance to the limits and required willingness to submit to a rigidly disciplined regimen. No amount of effort was ever enough. Typically, students began the first year of study eager to "learn it all." They quickly adjusted that view, rationalizing that "you can't do it all." Soon they succumbed to self-preservation, focusing on "what they [the faculty] want us to know." For the duration of medical school, students operated in survival mode.[64]

The experience of medical study required a monastic existence, as students labored from 8 A.M. to late afternoon five and one-half days a week in their preclinical lectures and laboratories, and through sleepless nights "on call" during the clinical years. Unlike college, where a vigorous extracurriculum flourished, extracurricular activities were few—here a yearbook, there a student newsletter. Few students married, and opportunities for a social life barely existed. Students were often told that romance must be postponed. In love, be like an "automobilist," a Cornell professor warned students on opening day in 1935—apply the brakes at the first sign of danger.[65] Such an ascetic existence contrasted markedly with the hedonism of many college students during the Jazz Age and reinforced the public's perception of medicine as a calling.[66]

Medical student life was not always healthy. Few schools had dormitories or recreational facilities, and many students lived in cheap, dingy quarters located near the school, sometimes with undependable sources of heat or running water. Since scholarship aid was scarce, many students from poorer backgrounds had to work for room and board. Faculties worried about the health of many students who repeatedly sold their blood to acquire a few extra dollars to help meet living expenses.[67] Poor housing, diet, and living conditions, combined with exhausting work and occupational exposures, led to major health hazards for medical students. The most notorious was tuberculosis, which claimed a few victims each year at many schools.

From the first day, students knew they were members of the medical school family. They proudly wore their laboratory coats in the preclinical years and white coats in the clinical years, which certified them as professionals. Yet, they were at the very bottom of the medical totem pole. At popular conferences, they were often pushed to the back rows behind faculty and house staff. At ward rounds, they were sometimes shoved to the periphery, too far back to see the patients or hear the conversation among the more senior physicians. Attendance at surgical operations provided the only exercise some students got: holding retractors, often far away from the field of view.

Students often felt vulnerable to forces beyond their control. In the hospital they were frequently exploited as a source of free labor. A nursing shortage or sick house officer could mean more work for an already overburdened clinical clerk. Students occasionally served as experimental subjects in their professors' clinical investigations—sometimes by desire, other times by intimidation or coercion. The quality of their educational experience was not uniform, especially in the clinical rotations, where there was considerable variation in knowledge, teaching skill, and considerateness among faculty members and house officers. Occasionally an instructor or department might terrorize an entire class. The antics of the anatomy department of the Emory University School of Medicine became widely known in the state of Georgia. Department members provided students little help, continually belittled them, and failed an unusually high proportion of the class. One who survived the experience described "how nerve-wracking it was to go through this day after day for eight long months without a bit of help from our so-called 'teachers'. They were more like slave-drivers and seemed to derive a fiendish pleasure from seeing us sweat and squirm under the lash."[68]

The bane of existence for many students was evaluation and grading. Students of this period, especially those promoted to the clinical years, had much less fear of flunking out than their predecessors before World War I. However, students faced a new pressure: the competition for internship. At Harvard, students would get into a "hysterical state of apprehension about the matter."[69] Grades mattered very much in obtaining a good internship, and the pressure to obtain high marks was intense. At some medical schools outbreaks of cheating occurred. After one such instance at Columbia, a faculty member wondered whether "we are graduating a lot of potential crooks instead of the type we ought to graduate."[70] The only relief from the pressure for grades came after internship appointments were announced in the fourth year, at which time many students started to coast.[71]

To students' dismay, testing and grading were hardly exact sciences. Inconsistencies appeared in the grading process everywhere. At Harvard, for instance, the biochemistry department gave higher grades than the anatomy department, and surgery was much more lenient than internal medicine and obstetrics.[72] Students at the school were randomly assigned to different hospitals for their surgical clerkship, yet a marked discrepancy in grades was observed. In one two-year period, 71 percent of the surgical clerks at Boston City Hospital received an A or B, in contrast to 55 percent at the Peter Bent Brigham Hospital and only 39 percent at the Massachusetts General Hospital.[73] To make matters even more arbitrary, medical schools did not all grade alike. Thus, students applying for internships from Cornell, which had a relatively low grading system, often suffered in comparisons with students from schools where higher grades were given.[74]

The period between the world wars witnessed a change in the relationship between students and professors. Until World War I, faculty assumed almost all responsibility for teaching students. After the war, as research, patient care, and residency training grew in importance, faculty attention was diverted, and the closeness between faculty and students began to diminish. Medical schools became less intimate places, and student groups repeatedly issued pleas for more personal contact with faculty.[75] Medical faculties sought ways to retain close involvement with students. In 1937, the Washington University School of Medicine created a Committee on Student Relations so that the faculty "may better know the personal qualities of each student, his fitness for medicine, [and] his interests and inclinations."[76] Such committees did much good, but they also symbolized the problem they were meant to solve. The bureaucratization of intimacy stood as testimony to the enlarging medical school and the relative decline in importance of undergraduate medical education to the institution.

The deflection of faculty attention away from medical students occurred most conspicuously in the clinical departments. There, much of the responsibility for teaching students came to be exercised by house officers. Students saw their attending physicians regularly, but it was the residents and interns whom they saw on a moment-to-moment basis. For students, the quality of a clerkship depended as much on the resident as it did on the faculty attending. A good resident had the power to create a sense of belonging so that the student felt like a true member of the ward team. An insensitive or disdainful resident who provided "scut work" and ridicule instead of teaching and encouragement was a student's nightmare. With difficult residents, students had little choice but to endure, knowing the rotation would end and hoping that in the next they might be more fortunate. If students were lucky, they could learn from these negative examples. If not, they could be scarred for life.

Though medical school was challenging for all, some students encountered special obstacles. In particular, African-American and women students often found that institutional discrimination created barriers between them and the rest of their classmates. Women and black students had a difficult time finding university housing, and when on call they sometimes had to eat in separate dining rooms.[77] Some medical schools did not even have adequate toilet facilities for women.[78] A particularly serious problem was gaining enough clinical experience, especially for African-Americans, who were frequently prohibited from examining nonblack patients. Sometimes a medical faculty would be more liberal than the general society. Thus, at the University of Colorado women students were permitted to work in the male urology clinic—until widespread complaints from patients forced the school to prohibit that practice.[79]

Though student life was stressful, there were many sources of support. Medical schools, despite their burgeoning size, complexity, and formality, cared deeply about their students. This could be seen through the parties, teas, luncheons, and socials that the schools held for students, or through the actions of countless individual instructors who would routinely be accessible or who regularly invited students to their houses for dinner and conversation. Few if any schools were without advising and counselling systems of some sort.

Much of the support system was provided by the students themselves. Sometimes this happened spontaneously or informally—the ritualized obscene pranks in anatomy laboratory, the advice and counsel more advanced students would give to those just beginning, the espirit de corps that evolved among participants in a common struggle. Often the support came through community living, most notably in the fraternities, which played an extremely important role in student life at a time when few schools had enough dormitories. Eating and studying together every night, students saw that others struggled as well. Older students would advise younger, and an alumni network was there to offer assistance finding an internship or establishing a practice. Jews, barred from medical school fraternities as they were from college fraternities, established their own—the most noted being Phi Delta Epsilon. Women students also provided each other support. At some schools they established sororities, such as the Nu Sigma Phi Sorority at the Tufts College Medical School; elsewhere they congregated at informal gathering places, such as the Garrett Room at the Johns Hopkins Hospital.[80] In the effort to cope, no one could let off more steam than medical students. Their capacity to work was matched only by their capacity to release—to the chagrin of proper Victorian faculties that regularly engaged in damage control to mollify outraged neighbors complaining over yet another riotous student party.

As students coped, they asserted themselves in ways that illustrated that student culture represented a dialectic among all participants, not merely a rigorous set of rules imposed by a demanding faculty. Important recent work in social history has demonstrated that vulnerable groups, such as immigrants and workers, had a range of choices about their lives and were hardly passive agents in the tide of history.[81] Similarly, medical students were not abject or powerless. Rather, they exerted a tangible influence over their own environment.

The power of students was apparent even before they started class. Premedical students decided where to apply and, if admitted to more than one school, which school to choose. Medical schools competed vigorously to attract the best students. Cornell worried that its lack of dormitory and scholarships would deter many applicants; Physicians and Surgeons feared that it was losing the best students to Johns Hopkins and Harvard; Harvard established its National Scholarship program for exceptional college undergraduates in 1946 in an attempt "to lure them to Harvard" and stop "the loss of good men who might go elsewhere."[82]

Once students were admitted, their opinion influenced every part of the curriculum. At many schools, students regularly prepared candid critiques of the course of study.[83] Should exposure to a given subject be enhanced or decreased? Was the order of presentation effective? Should the examination period be one week or two, and should tests be multiple choice or essay? What worked and what did not in the pediatrics clerkship? What was lacking in the curriculum or teaching that might be added? As the chairman of anatomy at Cornell pointed out in 1935, "Each class determines to some extent the type of teaching it is to receive."[84]

The ultimate manifestation of student power came in faculty evaluation. As faculty graded students, students graded faculty, and more than a few promotions resulted—and egos were deflated—from student critiques of their professors. Harvard Medical School listened to student criticisms of the great biochemist L. J. Henderson, pushing him out of the medical school in response to student dissatisfaction with his teaching. When the school later tried to get him back, Henderson returned only on the condition that he would never again lecture to medical students.[85] Student opinions were hardly infallible, and students frequently disagreed with each other. Yet, student views, if not always acted upon, were taken seriously.

Perhaps no event was more useful in helping students cope than the class play, productions of black medical humor produced and performed each year before appreciative audiences of fellow students, faculty, and visitors. Legendary in the medical community were the scatological performances put on by the Pithotomy Club of Johns Hopkins, indescribably ribald annual shows that made similar events at other institutions pale in comparison. The annual "Pithotomy"—loosely meaning "to tap a keg"—candidly examined the foibles or pomposity of members of the Hopkins faculty in outlandish plots spiced with bawdy songs and humor. Intended so that we might "see ourselves as others see us," the Pithotomy spared no faculty member from lampooning. The audience was usually indescribably drunk, and attendees would urinate in the alley. Following the show, members of the audience would participate in the "beer slide"—seeing how adeptly they could body surf on a smooth floor well lathered with beer. One distinguished department chairman wore dark glasses the day after the Pithotomy, having sustained a black eye from a wayward mug during the previous night's beer slide.[86]

Throughout the evening—at the Pithotomy and at class plays every-where—students and faculty laughed uproariously with each other. The students vented release from the pressures of medical school while still maintaining their affection for individual professors. In that laughter was acceptance and forgiveness—an acknowledgement that the faculty, for all their foibles, had touched the students and helped shape their futures. In the end students were grateful to those who provided the instruction, guidance, and inspiration to become doctors.

The Limits of Education

The power of medical education to shape the minds and attitudes of physicians could scarcely be disputed. Yet, what was the role of education in influencing behavior? This question perplexed medical educators because they wanted to produce physicians with desirable personal char-acteristics and a social conscience. Could a physician's behavior be molded by the educational experience? Or alternatively, did good physi-cianship ultimately reside in intrinsic characteristics of the individual that could not be modified by any part of the curriculum, formal or hidden?

This debate over educational first principles surfaced with regard to two important issues. The first pertained to the production of caring doc-tors. To some medical educators, empathy, compassion, and social responsibility could be formally taught—either through a premedical training that emphasized the humanities and social sciences,[87] or through courses in medical school in the history of medicine, psychology, sociology, or economics.[88] To others, teaching the art of medicine was the responsibility of the hidden curriculum. Harvard's Richard Cabot, the founder of medical social work, wrote, "This art is to be learned like everything else, by practice and by imitating good role models."[89] Still others doubted whether these qualities could be taught at all. Willard C. Rappleye, dean of the College of Physicians and Surgeons of Columbia University for nearly three decades (1931–1958), believed that character-istics such as compassion, empathy, integrity, resourcefulness, and com-mon sense "are largely individual and apart from those of formal education and training."[90] In this conservative view of the potential of education, if medical schools did anything significant, it was in choosing the right students for admission.

A similar debate emerged over the choices physicians made regarding where to locate. Medical educators were deeply troubled by the growing trend for physicians to practice in cities rather than rural areas. Some thought that medical schools could address the maldistribution issue by admitting more students from rural districts (who might be more likely to return), producing an oversupply of doctors (in the hope that excessive competition would force some to the countryside), or exhorting medical students to serve less populated areas. However, no one could prove that these strategies worked. A careful study sponsored by the General Education Board demonstrated that physicians' choice of a practice site reflected their response to professional, social, and financial incentives, and that in these regards the cities offered many more advantages than rural areas—as they did for so many Americans of the period. The study concluded that interventions such as lowering admission standards, admitting more students, or shortening the medical course would only produce inferior doctors without altering the underlying demographic trends.[91]

These debates in medical education mirrored a broader debate in American education over the capacity of education to influence behavior. The traditional orthodoxy of the American educational system has been the belief that education can shape behavior and mold character.[92] Yet many factors beyond formal education have also been seen to influence behavior. Lawrence A. Cremin pointed out that there have always been limits to formal education as a behavioral force. Behavior, he maintained, is shaped by innumerable "educative" influences—one of which is formal education, but which also include the totality of an individual's upbringing and environment, encompassing such factors as family, friends, neighborhood, religion, and popular culture.[93] The relative roles of educational and educative factors in influencing behavior have never been resolved. This was—and is—education's counterpart to the nature–nurture controversy.

4

The Rise of Graduate Medical Education

IN THE EARLY TWENTIETH CENTURY, most medical schools focused exclusively on upgrading the quality of education leading to the M.D. degree. At a time when the four years of medical school were still thought adequate preparation for the general practice of medicine, undergraduate medical education was the pressing issue of the day. Abraham Flexner's 1910 report did not even mention internship or other hospital training for medical graduates, reflecting the prevailing orthodoxy that the four years of medical school provided sufficient preparation for general practice.

Such a view quickly died out in the years following World War I. Medical knowledge, techniques, and practices were growing and changing too rapidly. Even a superior experience in medical school could no longer prepare a person for private practice. Accordingly, a period of hospital education following graduation—the "internship"—became standard for every physician. In addition, further training was necessary for those who wished to enter specialty practice or pursue academic careers. For these purposes the "residency"—a several-year hospital experience following internship—became the accepted vehicle. By the 1920s, medical educators were observing that the quality of medical practice in the United States was influenced "far more by the mental habits formed by physicians after their graduation than by the knowledge which they acquire as undergraduate students."[1]

In the creation of a system of graduate medical education, the Johns Hopkins Medical School once again played a seminal role. Nevertheless, the university-based, academic model introduced by Johns Hopkins was never to succeed so completely in graduate medical education as it did in undergraduate medical education. Always, the tension between education and service, between university ideals and apprenticeship traditions, wracked even the best intern and residency programs. Moreover, unlike undergraduate medical education, which remained university-based and regulated, graduate medical education became hospital-based and professionally regulated. Many internships and residencies were created in hospitals unaffiliated with medical schools. In graduate medical education, medical schools lost their educational monopoly, even as they were transformed by the enterprise.

The Creation of Internship and Residency

Since the 1870s, American medical schools had been under pressure to increase the length of study to accommodate the ever-growing body of medical knowledge. For over a generation they did so successfully. The 30-year period from 1870 witnessed the expansion of terms from 16 weeks to 32 and the course of study from two years to four. For the typical medical graduate entering general practice, the need for further formal instruction seemed small.

By World War I, however, there was too much to teach even in a four-year course. A rounding-out experience had become necessary for all physicians. Additional study was also required of those who wished to enter a medical specialty or pursue medical research. By the 1920s, the most important issue in medical education had changed from undergraduate medical education to the formal graduate education students received after medical school.[2] (Strictly speaking, medical students were graduate students, but from the point of view of medical education they were undergraduates—hence the terms "undergraduate medical education" to connote the four years of medical school and "graduate medical education" to signify internship and residency.)

What was the best way to complete a physician's education? Some medical educators thought that a fifth year of medical school should be added. During World War I, this concept had many advocates—particularly among many Midwestern medical schools and a few elite Eastern schools.[3] Most medical schools, however, felt that they did not have the physical, financial, or human resources to extend the course. Instead, most medical educators favored a period of graduate training in hospitals, which offered the potential advantage of extensive practical work.

Opportunities for graduate training in hospitals had long existed in America, though such positions were scarce, available only to a tiny handful of graduates. Before World War I hospital appointments went by different names at different institutions: "intern," "extern," "house pupil," "house physician," "resident," "resident physician," and others. All provided a similar experience: a year or two living and working in the hospital, tending to the moment-by-moment affairs of patients and observing the practice habits of eminent physicians of the day.

Before World War I hospital positions had considerable educational deficiencies. They existed as much for the benefit of the hospital as they did for the professional enrichment of house officers. As hospitals became larger and busier, the work of running a hospital increased dramatically. Many of the chores fell to house officers, who received room and board but little or no pay. House officers participated in patient care, but much of their daily routine involved various duties lacking in educational value. Among these were riding in ambulances, maintaining the library, cleaning instruments, ordering equipment, and performing laboratory tests.

During World War I this system of hospital appointments evolved into the internship system. At that time the "internship" became standardized as a hospital-based experience to complete the general education of physicians after their graduation from medical school. Old terminology gave way to new. For instance, at the Massachusetts General Hospital, the term "intern" replaced the earlier, time-honored "house pupil."[4] The Council on Medical Education began examining hospitals to accredit them for "approved" internships with the same vigor with which it had already been evaluating medical schools. In 1919 the Council first published its "Essentials for Approved Internships," and in 1920 it changed its name to the "Council on Medical Education and Hospitals."[5]

The internship reflected both the hospital and the university traditions. As a hospital-based program, it clearly resembled the nineteenth-century system of hospital appointments for medical graduates. However, it also involved the conversion of that system into a formally organized educational program. The many educational features of a properly conducted internship, the Council on Medical Education and Hospitals observed, "definitely stamp this as 'education', not 'on-the-job' training comparable to that of an apprentice garage mechanic."[6] Hospitals that provided an inadequate educational experience stood in violation of the Council's guidelines and could have their internship program removed from the approved list.

Several educational features differentiated the internship (at the high quality programs, at least) from the house positions of the nineteenth century. First, there were conferences, seminars, rounds, lectures, and other types of formal and informal instruction. Second, at hospitals affiliated with medical schools, the presence of medical students offered the opportunity to teach as well as learn. Third, at teaching hospitals, internship provided the opportunity to participate in clinical research. Lastly, the best programs encouraged interns to study patients in detail. At teaching hospitals, interns carried an average load of 9 patients at a time, compared with an average load of 25 patients at community hospitals. The lighter patient load allowed those interns much more time to read about their patients and attend conferences and rounds.[7]

Both medical schools and hospitals encouraged the growth of the internship. Schools regarded the internship as a way to provide students additional training without overtaxing their facilities and resources. Hospitals saw interns as a major solution to their task of providing up-to-date care to growing numbers of patients. Accordingly, the number of internship positions rapidly increased. In 1914, internship positions were available for only one-half of medical school graduates.[8] By 1923, the number of available internships for the first time was large enough to accommodate all graduates of medical school.[9] By the end of World War II, approximately 1,300 hospitals, or roughly one-third of the total number in the country, were approved for internships, and the number of openings far exceeded the number of medical graduates.[10] The most desirable programs were at teaching hospitals, but the spread of internships to community hospitals assured that positions would be available for all.

Internships were offered in three varieties. The most popular was the so-called "rotating" internship, in which interns rotated among all the clinical areas. A certain number of hospitals, particularly those associated with medical schools, offered "straight" internships in medicine or surgery, in which interns spent the entire time in that field. The third type was the "mixed" internship, a cross between the rotating and straight internship, which provided more concentration in medicine and surgery and less time in the various specialties than the rotating internship.[11]

Internship programs varied in length. Most were one year, though many were longer, some as long as three years. Some hospitals offered internships of different lengths. For instance, Mount Sinai Hospital had both a one-year and a two-and-one-half-year internship, the latter being the more rigorous and the more popular among fourth-year medical students applying for positions.[12]

For many years after World War I, medical educators debated whether internship represented the culmination of undergraduate medical education or the first stage of graduate medical education. Some schools required completion of a satisfactory internship before awarding the M.D. degree. However, by 1939 all but 12 schools conferred the M.D. degree at the end of the four-year curriculum, indicating that they considered the internship a phase of graduate medical education.[13] The requirement of the successful completion of an internship for the M.D. degree disappeared after World War II.

The educational ideals of internship were not always realized. Even at teaching hospitals, service functions often overrode educational activities. At Mount Sinai Hospital (New York), interns complained that they were not receiving enough teaching; at Presbyterian Hospital (New York), interns were spending much time doing the work of hospital messengers.[14] Far greater deviation from educational ideals occurred at community hospitals not affiliated with medical schools. At one hospital in Southern California, interns were considered subordinate to nurses and permitted only to take routine histories and administer intravenous medications; didactic rounds, teaching conferences, and other educational activities were nonexistent.[15] In Michigan, many internship programs were thought to "drop below the level of the senior undergraduate year and launch the student into a period of decadence from which he emerges with great difficulty, or not at all."[16] The worst programs were at small community hospitals with fewer than 100 beds. These hospitals provided so little teaching and imposed so much work that they were disparagingly called "the self-teaching types of internship."[17] In view of the wide variation in quality, medical educators generally considered the internship "the most unsatisfactory and uneven portion of the educational scheme of medicine at the present time."[18]

🍎 · 🍎 · 🍎

Though internships varied in quality, on balance they were extremely effective in preparing physicians for general practice. However, additional study was required to enter a specialty. In the 1920s, a standardized system of specialty instruction did not exist. Instead, there were many routes to specialty practice—some educationally sound, others manifestly unsatisfactory. The multiplicity of pathways to specialization was reminiscent of the multiple routes to an undergraduate medical education in the nineteenth century.[19]

Some physicians became specialists by working in an outpatient specialty clinic at a teaching hospital. With time and luck, they could one day receive admitting privileges to the hospital as a specialist in that field. Others worked as assistants to established practitioners who had already become specialists. Postgraduate study abroad represented a third popular route to specialization. Through the early 1930s, approximately 1,000 physicians each year took courses in Europe, particularly in the surgical specialties. Most went to Vienna, where instruction for Americans was provided in English and opportunities to gain practical experience were plentiful.[20] Another common path to specialization was formal course work. Some courses were as short as a week or two; others involved true graduate study and research. Most programs were offered by freestanding graduate medical schools; a few were sponsored by university medical schools. Finally, there was the residency—lengthy periods of hospital training subsequent to the completion of an internship in a limited field of medicine. Many physicians combined two or more of these approaches, such as several years of work in an outpatient specialty clinic of a teaching hospital followed by study in Europe, or a specialty course at a freestanding graduate medical school followed by two or three years as an assistant to a recognized practitioner of that field.[21]

Not surprisingly, with such a potpourri of approaches to specialization, great confusion existed. It was difficult, even for schools and trainees, to keep the various pathways distinct from each other. There was also considerable confusion between "graduate medical education" (formal preparation for a medical specialty) and what later came to be termed "continuing medical education" or "postgraduate medical education" (refresher courses for physicians in practice to review fundamentals or keep up-to-date with new developments in a field). Some refresher courses offered by medical schools or teaching hospitals were more rigorous than many of the programs at freestanding graduate medical schools that purported to train specialists.

The challenge confronting medical education after World War I was the lack of uniformity of specialty training and the low standards of entry to specialty practice. Many so-called "specialists" were self-named and poorly trained. Most had not received broad experience in either the scientific fundamentals or practical aspects of their fields. The most common route to specialty practice was through courses at one of the 30 or so unsupervised graduate medical schools. After a few weeks of study, graduates of such programs would proclaim themselves "specialists." Shortcuts to specialization were especially common in surgery. The consensus among leading university teachers of surgery was that surgical training required a minimum of 1,000 hours of operating time under real conditions with real patients over a six or seven year period.[22] Yet, many graduate medical schools produced "surgeons" through courses of one or two weeks' duration in which various operations were performed on cadavers or dogs.[23]

Graduate medical schools were a diverse lot. A few, such as the University of Minnesota Graduate Medical School, the New York Post-Graduate Medical School, and the University of Pennsylvania Graduate School of Medicine, were respectable academic institutions. During and after World War II, most of these were absorbed by university medical schools. However, the great majority of graduate medical schools were highly commercial, profit-making ventures, as many proprietary medical schools had been before the Flexner report. Among the most notorious of these were the Postgraduate School of Surgical Technique (located in Chicago) and the Chicago Eye, Ear, Nose and Throat College.[24] With so many commercial schools, graduate medical education in the 1920s was in a similar position to undergraduate medical education at the turn of the century.

As medical educators turned their attention to specialization, they sought to eliminate the short commercial courses and make specialty training a true educational experience. However, the best way to do that was widely debated. Some felt that medical schools should develop organized programs of graduate study in the clinical specialties, thereby bringing specialty education into the university. After World War I, some medical schools, including Harvard, Johns Hopkins, New York University, and Columbia, adopted that approach. They established degree-granting programs (most commonly, the Doctor of Medical Science degree), which customarily entailed a minimum of three years of clinical work in a single field, extensive course work in the preclinical sciences, rigorous examinations, original investigative work, and a thesis.[25] Columbia, which apparently had the largest program, enrolled 299 graduate students and awarded 90 Med. Sc. D. degrees from the program's inception in the early 1930s through 1939.[26] These programs provided a genuine graduate education in specialty medicine for mature students.

In the early 1900s, however, another model developed: the residency. This represented a lengthy period of hospital service after internship for physicians who desired to specialize. Like the internship, the residency had its origins in the earlier system of hospital appointments for medical graduates. In the nineteenth century the terms "resident" and "intern" were used more or less interchangeably. However, in the twentieth century, as another example of the German influence on American medicine, the residency was transformed into an intensive educational experience. As one report defined it, the residency, in its "present day concept," had come to mean "a progressive and graduated educational experience designed to enable a physician to make himself proficient in a special field of practice and to give him the educational background for continued development in this field."[27]

The modern residency was introduced to America with the opening of the Johns Hopkins Hospital in 1889.[28] At that time, the faculty used the word "resident" to designate physicians who had completed an internship and were continuing their hospital training to study a specific field of medicine. The hospital initially offered residencies in medicine, surgery, and gynecology. The leaders of the medical staff—William Osler in medicine, William Halsted in surgery—both credited the system of "house assistants" in the German university medical clinics as the inspiration for the residency at Johns Hopkins.[29]

Like its German model, the Hopkins residency was designed to be an academic experience for mature scholars. A resident, in Osler's words, should be "a superior man who wishes to do scientific hospital work."[30] Residents lived in the hospital for a lengthy, indefinite period of time working in a specific field. In addition to their clinical responsibilities, they were expected to conduct original research and remain in close contact with developments in the preclinical sciences. The Hopkins faculty understood that many residents would ultimately enter practice as specialists in a particular field, but they considered the most important objective of residency the training of investigators and teachers. As Halsted explained, "We need a system . . . which will produce not only surgeons but surgeons of the highest type."[31]

During World War I, the Hopkins residency system began to spread to other institutions, much as the Hopkins system of undergraduate medical education had spread to other schools the generation before. Graduates of the Johns Hopkins residency system sometimes facilitated the process. For instance, the neurosurgeon Harvey Cushing, a former surgical chief resident under Halsted, patterned his residency program at the Peter Bent Brigham Hospital after the one at Johns Hopkins. Similarly, George Heuer, another protégé of Halsted, brought the Hopkins model of surgical training to the University of Cincinnati and later to Cornell.

As the residency system spread from Johns Hopkins, it retained its original emphasis on scholarship and inquiry. The residency system assumed many characteristics of a graduate school within the hospital.

At some hospitals, residents were called "graduate students," "fellows," or "graduate fellows."[32] Residents were often encouraged to combine their clinical work with formal study toward a graduate degree, such as an M.S., Sc.D., or Ph.D. Publications by residents were common, and many clinical departments boasted of the number of studies conducted by members of the resident staff.[33] The residency played an analogous role in clinical departments to that played by fellowships in preclinical departments and graduate assistantships in university departments. The common objective was to produce future academic leaders.

With its emphasis on combining clinical study with research, the pre–World War II residency served a dual role. Most conspicuously it provided expert training in a clinical specialty, but it also prepared young physicians for a career in clinical investigation. In this second capacity it helped institutionalize clinical research in the United States, producing the next generation of teachers and investigators in the field. It has long been recognized that one administrative innovation—"full-time" faculty appointments in the clinical departments—contributed to the maturation of clinical science in the United States.[34] Equal recognition should be given to the residency system. Clinical science, the clinical full-time system, and the residency developed hand-in-hand.

Unlike internship, which became available to all medical graduates, residency was reserved for the elite. Usually a strong performance in medical school and internship was required for acceptance into a residency. Some programs imposed the additional requirement of previous research experience in a preclinical science.[35] Acceptance into a residency provided no guarantee of completing the program. Residencies in all fields were structured as so-called "pyramids," the exact shape and slope of the pyramid varying from one program to another. Attrition would occur along the way; only some individuals chosen as "junior assistant residents" would be selected to continue as "senior assistant residents." Ultimately only one would be selected as "resident" (or synonymously, "chief resident")—the crown jewel of graduate medical education in this period. Chief residents would serve indefinite periods as assistants to the department chairman. They would be virtually guaranteed a faculty appointment when a suitable position became available. Kenneth Blackfan, a leading pediatrician of the era, served as John Howland's chief resident for 11 years at Washington University and Johns Hopkins before accepting the professorship of pediatrics at the University of Cincinnati.[36] At the Peter Bent Brigham Hospital, each of the first seven chief residents in internal medicine received academic appointments, compared with only 3 of 20 former assistant residents who were not selected chief resident.[37]

In the 1920s residency programs began to become more widespread. In 1925, the Council on Medical Education and Hospitals of the American Medical Association published its first list of hospitals offering residencies, a list that contained 29 names.[38] In the 1930s, the residency system grew even more conspicuously. Between 1934 and 1939, the number of positions in so-called "long residencies" (that is, three or more years of training) increased from 332 to 1,791.[39] In 1941, there were 30 residency programs in surgery alone patterned after the Johns Hopkins residency.[40]

By the late 1930s the residency had become the favored path to specialization. Most aspiring specialists liked the feeling that residencies provided of being a physician rather than a student, not to mention the fact of not having to pay tuition. Teaching hospitals and medical schools also benefited from the residency system. Hospitals could obtain high-quality medical workers at a low cost, while medical schools could engage in advanced clinical training at a fraction of the expense of operating a separate graduate program in the clinical specialties. During the Depression these were not inconsequential financial advantages to sponsoring institutions.

While the residency was flourishing, fewer and fewer candidates applied for formal graduate study in a clinical specialty. By the outbreak of World War II these programs either had been terminated or had merged with existing residencies. The evolution of graduate medical education at the Columbia-Presbyterian Medical Center illustrated this phenomenon. When the center was built in the 1920s, there was no recognized single pathway of graduate medical education. For several years, the medical school administered both a university-based graduate program and a residency program at Presbyterian Hospital. By the late 1930s, the dean and faculty believed that graduate medical education "can be provided only through internships and residencies."[41] Accordingly, plans were made to end the degree-granting program and merge it with the residency.[42]

In the 1930s, specialty training in the United States began to become standardized and systematized. Much of this work was accomplished by specialty boards, which were comprised of representatives of the Council on Medical Education and Hospitals and the various specialty societies (such as the American College of Surgeons for the American Board of Surgery and the American College of Physicians for the American Board of Internal Medicine). The first specialty board, the American Board of Ophthalmology, was organized in 1917, but in the 1930s specialty boards in many other fields were established (*see Table 3*).[43] The boards were aided by the Advisory Board for Medical Specialties, an umbrella group organized in 1933 whose membership consisted of all the specialty boards.

In the 1930s, by decree of the specialty boards, the "long residency" in an approved hospital became the sole acceptable route to specialization. The exact time required in a residency varied by field, but in no case was less than three years accepted. Each board had its own rules, but in general certification as a specialist required the completion of an approved residency followed by several years of specialty practice, at which time candidates had to pass a difficult examination. Further rationalization of the system would occur later, but by World War II graduate medical edu-

Table 3 · Approved examining boards in medical specialties—1940

Name of Board	Year of Activation
American Board of Ophthalmology	1917
American Board of Otolaryngology	1924
American Board of Obstetrics and Gynecology	1930
American Board of Dermatology	1932
American Board of Pediatrics	1933
American Board of Orthopedic Surgery	1934
American Board of Psychiatry and Neurology	1934
American Board of Radiology	1934
American Board of Urology	1935
American Board of Internal Medicine	1936
American Board of Pathology	1936
American Board of Anesthesiology	1937
American Board of Plastic Surgery	1937
American Board of Surgery	1937

cation in the United States had already taken major steps toward systematization.[44]

As academic and professional leaders sought to upgrade standards of specialty training, their most important goal was eliminating the short courses to specialization. They believed that the public needed to be protected from superficial training and commercialism in graduate medical education, just as a generation before many medical educators felt that the public required similar protection in undergraduate medical education. The reform impulse did not die out in American politics with the official "closing" of the progressive era during World War I; neither did it die in medical education.[45] Like the earlier reform of undergraduate medical education, the reform of graduate medical education assumed many qualities of a moral crusade.

❦ · ❦ · ❦

For medical schools, the rise of graduate medical education was a transforming event. During World War I, the primary educational interest of most schools had been in undergraduate medical education. By World War II, much of their attention had shifted to internship and residency. As new programs were established and existing ones expanded, some schools found themselves responsible for almost as many interns and residents as clinical clerks. By World War II, the educational reputation of a medical school depended as much on its work in graduate as in undergraduate medical education.

Though medical schools provided the intellectual guidance for graduate medical education, they did not control it. Some residencies and most
internships were at hospitals unaffiliated with medical schools. More
important, even at teaching programs, the site of training was not at the
medical school but at the hospital, which provided the patients, conference rooms, laboratory facilities, living quarters, and financial expenses
of maintaining a house staff. As the Massachusetts General Hospital
bluntly noted: "Undergraduate education is directed by the Dean and
Faculty of the Harvard Medical School. The graduate education of the
House Staff of interns and residents is solely a function of the Hospital."[46] Of course, at most teaching hospitals, the service chiefs were
medical school department chairmen. However, in directing their individual residency programs, the chiefs were operating to serve the needs
of their department and the hospital, not those of the medical school as a
whole.

By World War II, control and regulation of graduate medical education
resided with the profession at large through a complex array of regulatory agencies, not with the university or its surrogate organization, the
Association of American Medical Colleges. Medical school faculty, of
course, were exceedingly influential in all these organizations. However,
theirs was not the sole voice, and decisions made by regulatory agencies
were binding on programs that wished to receive accreditation. Even at
the major teaching hospitals, residency programs continually adjusted
details so as to conform with the dictates of the specialty boards. For
instance, at Barnes Hospital, which boasted one of the country's premier
surgical residencies, department chairman Evarts Graham changed the
rotations in pathology and the outpatient department so that "the house
service will meet the demand of the American College of Surgery and the
[American] Board of Surgery."[47] Ironically, Graham himself had spearheaded the effort to create the American Board of Surgery.[48] Medical professors occasionally chafed at the arbitrariness of certain specialty board
policies or at the seeming capriciousness of some of their decisions (especially concerning who passed the oral examinations required at the time
for most specialty diplomas). However, they had no choice but to make
certain that their training programs were in compliance if they wished
their programs to be accredited.

The transfer of control of graduate medical education from universities to the profession occurred by default rather than by design. After
World War I, most members of the profession—including the Council on
Medical Education and the American Hospital Association—thought
internships should be university controlled. For instance, the Intern
Committee of the American Hospital Association believed that the
internship should be required "before granting the degree of M.D. and
that medical schools should accept the responsibilities of the control of
this period."[49] Similarly, many organizations, including some of the specialty societies, thought residency training should be a university respon-

sibility. For instance, a representative of the American College of Physicians stated its position:

> It was felt that both internships and residencies fall within the field of graduate medical training and consequently that they are the direct concern of medical educators and medical faculties and should be managed by educators rather than by professional associations which might be looked upon as exerting an influence analogous to alumni control of universities, and lacking in breadth from an educational point of view. The possibility of acquisition by specialty certifying boards, and similar bodies, of undesirably great influence over postgraduate medical education in the event that the medical schools refuse their responsibility in this direction, was recognized as a definite danger.[50]

Most medical school leaders, however, demurred. They were intent on developing high-quality internship and residency programs at their own teaching hospitals, but, fearing the programs would become unwieldy, they refused to enlarge the size of their programs to include all medical school graduates. In addition, they were reluctant to take responsibility for programs at community hospitals that they could not directly oversee or supervise. A few medical school leaders warned, "If the schools do not take this responsibility [of regulating graduate medical education], then the special certifying boards or other professional bodies will."[51] That is precisely what happened. By default, control of graduate medical education was transferred from the university to the profession at large, in distinction to the university's continued domination of undergraduate medical education. This represented a choice made by medical schools— one that in a later period would return to haunt them.

From Supervision to Responsibility

For all the practical experience gained through clinical clerkships, medical students of necessity remained closely supervised. Yet, it was axiomatic in medicine that an individual was not a mature physician until he had learned to assume full responsibility for the care of patients. It was during internship for general practitioners and residency for specialists that physicians-in-training received the opportunity to develop independence. The assumption of responsibility was the defining educational characteristic of graduate medical education and the feature that transformed students into physicians.

Responsibility for patient management did not automatically accrue to house officers (the generic term for interns and residents). Rather, it was graded in difficulty and earned. Typically, interns and residents began with circumscribed duties that they had assisted with as students. As they proved themselves they received more independence. In a technical field like surgery, responsibility came slowly because of the skill necessary to master operative techniques and develop surgical judgment. In cognitive fields like internal medicine and pediatrics, responsibility for decision-making generally came more quickly. House officers were usually required to demonstrate their competence at making diagnoses before they were given responsibility for important therapeutic decisions.

The assumption of responsibility did not imply lack of oversight. There was regular contact with attending physicians, and advancement in the level of responsibility came gradually. This was especially true in surgery, where residents would wait seemingly interminable periods before being granted operative responsibility. At Johns Hopkins, surgical residents in the 1930s waited years before being permitted to perform their first appendectomy and cholecystectomy. "We had assisted The Resident and the visiting staff so many, many times at operation after operation, that by the time we undertook the procedures on our own, it hardly seemed as if, in fact, we were doing so for the first time."[52] Always there was a person one step more senior working closely with a house officer—a resident with an intern, a senior resident with a junior resident, the chief resident with a senior resident. Backup and support were routinely available, and the greatest moral offense a house officer could commit was not to call for help.

Though house officers were closely watched, they were given far more responsibility than medical students. In clerkships, students were personally supervised, usually by their house officers. In internships and residencies, house officers worked much more independently. It was a "fiction," one surgical chairman declared, to think that all house staff work was done pursuant to the direction of staff and faculty physicians.[53] Help was available to house officers, but they had to ask for it.

Evidence is fragmentary, but the system seemed to work—not only from the standpoint of promoting physician education, but from that of assuring patient safety. A system of tight controls was in place. Charles L. Bosk has pointed out how occupational rituals in house staff education (morning rounds with the attending physicians, departmental teaching rounds, morbidity and mortality conferences, and other similar activities) provided a system of checks and balances, aided supervision of house officers, and helped interns and residents to learn to manage uncertainty.[54] Errors occasionally occurred, but apparently no more frequently than with fully trained physicians. For instance, one teaching hospital found no difference in surgical morbidity and mortality rates between its resident and attending staffs.[55] Though American society at this time was far less litigious than it would later become, through 1944 there were no successful malpractice suits against an intern or resident in the state of New York, and most New York hospitals did not feel the need to carry professional liability insurance for its house staff.[56]

The assumption of responsibility was widely recognized as the most important educational feature of internship and residency. House officers at programs that provided less responsibility were considered not as well trained.[57] For this reason the most prized positions were at voluntary or municipal hospitals with large ward (charity) services, since house officers were given much greater responsibility in managing ward patients than private patients. Many teaching hospitals at this time had separate house staffs for ward and private patients. Invariably, the ward positions were in great demand, while positions on the private services were filled with less able individuals, if they were filled at all.[58]

At teaching hospitals, ambitious interns and residents reveled in the opportunity to assume responsibility for patient care. House officers often competed with each other to perform a procedure or make an important decision. Would the pediatrics intern or resident manage a child's pneumonia? Would a senior surgical resident "give away" the appendectomy to a junior house officer? At Johns Hopkins, senior surgical residents were known to hide cases from the attending physicians so that they might be able to perform the operations themselves.[59] To house officers, the patients were *theirs*, and they eagerly assumed charge of every aspect of their patients' care.

The assumption of responsibility laid bare the fundamental dilemma of graduate medical education. To what degree did a house officer's responsibility to the patient represent a genuine educational opportunity, and to what degree did it provide a source of cheap labor for the hospital? As one experienced medical educator pointed out, if the purpose of internships and residencies were entirely educational, hospitals would not have been so eager to increase the size of their house staffs.[60] Even on the ward services of the major teaching hospitals, house officers were deluged with innumerable duties—performing blood counts and urinalyses, transporting patients to X-ray or physical therapy, drawing blood samples and starting intravenous lines—that hardly required a physician to perform. At community hospitals, where house officer duties were determined mainly "on institutional rather than educational needs,"[61] the balance between education and service was tilted even further toward service. This dual quality of internship and residency—that the experience involved both learning and service; that house officers were both students and hospital employees—represented the fundamental ambiguity of graduate medical education. Achieving the proper balance between education and service would perplex medical educators throughout the twentieth century.

Selecting House Officers

As graduate medical education became important to medical education, it became important to medical students contemplating their futures. A good internship was necessary for all physicians; a good residency, for aspiring specialists or clinical scientists. "Medicine has always been a competitive profession," first-year students at Cornell Medical College were told on opening day in 1935. "Your whole career in medicine is not unlike a race."[62] After World War I, the "race" in medicine included the competition for internship and residency positions.

By the 1930s it was not difficult to find an internship. The number of available positions exceeded the number of medical graduates by 25 percent, and hospitals were continuing to create new internship positions to meet their service needs.[63] However, internships at teaching hospitals were much more difficult to obtain. Competition for these positions was intense, especially at the most prestigious hospitals. For example, in 1942 Mount Sinai Hospital (New York) received applications from 145 candidates for eight intern positions. Most of the eight who were selected were in the top 10 percent of their class, and all were in the top third.[64]

Hospitals debated how to identify the best candidates for internship, just as medical school admissions committees debated how to identify the best applicants to medical school. The emphasis placed on various factors—medical school grades and class standing, letters of recommendation, personal interviews, written or oral examinations administered by the hospital staff to intern candidates—varied from program to program. For instance, Presbyterian Hospital (New York) administered two days of examinations to intern applicants, which were followed by personal interviews, while Barnes Hospital and St. Louis City Hospital made their selections on the basis of the applicants' class standing and general record.[65] Many teaching hospitals reserved most of their positions for graduates of their affiliated medical school. For example, the Hospital of the University of Pennsylvania would hold 11 of its 14 openings for members of the top quarter of the graduating class of the University of Pennsylvania.[66]

To make matters more difficult for students, there was no coordination of appointment dates, and a student's acceptance of an internship offer was considered binding. Many teaching hospitals would pressure students to commit to their program before a competing teaching hospital had made its appointments. This led to a major dilemma for students: to accept a position at a less desirable hospital, or wait to hear from a more desirable hospital, risking the chance of ending up with no appointment at all.[67] Getting the right position was not easy, and anxiety among medical students was intense everywhere.

Compared with internship, residency positions were fewer in number and the method of selection, more informal. William Osler had expressed his preference for choosing residents by personal selection rather than examination. He told the medical board of the Johns Hopkins Hospital: "These young men come in contact with us at all hours and it is absolutely essential that they should be persons with whom we can work pleasantly and congenially. I have suffered so on several occasions, from ungentlemanly residents foisted upon me by the competitive examination plan that I would here enter my warmest protest against it."[68] It was this method that most residency programs followed, especially the leading academic programs. Department chairmen chose young physicians they personally knew, or they relied on the personal recommendations of individuals they trusted. Almost always, those selected for an academic residency had excelled in a competitive internship and had demonstrated promise at research.

Appointment to a residency did not guarantee that an individual would complete the program. Because of the pyramidal organization of most residencies, few rose to the pinnacle. A typical pyramid was illustrated by the obstetrics and gynecology service of the New York Hospital. In the late 1930s the service consisted of eight first-year residents, eight second-year residents, three third-year residents, two fourth-year residents, and two fifth-year residents.[69] The fate of those who were dropped from a residency depended on the prestige of the program and when they were dismissed. Those dropped early from a premier teaching hospital could often find another position; those dropped from a less prestigious program usually became general practitioners. Residents who survived to a higher point on the pyramid, even if not to the apex, might have stayed long enough to qualify for certification as a specialist or even to pursue an academic career. For example, Emil Goetch went to Long Island Medical College and Willis Gatch, to the Indiana University School of Medicine—both as professors and department chairman—without finishing William Halsted's surgical program at Johns Hopkins.[70]

In graduate medical education, like undergraduate medical education, opportunities were limited for African-Americans, women, and ethnic and religious minorities, particularly Jews. Most hospitals excluded blacks from internship and residency positions, even those that allowed African-Americans to work there as medical students. Internship opportunities for African-Americans were mainly provided by "colored hospitals." Very few residency positions for blacks existed, and these were found at only a handful of institutions: Freedmen's Hospital (Howard Medical College), Hubbard Hospital (Meharry Medical College), Harlem Hospital, Provident Hospital (Chicago), Kansas City General Hospital, Number 2, and Homer G. Phillips Hospital (St. Louis City Hospital, Number 2).[71]

Similarly, opportunities for women to receive internships, residencies, and hospital staff appointments were not commensurate with their opportunities as medical students. Many teaching hospitals would not appoint women as interns, no matter how well a woman had performed as a clinical clerk. Residency positions were even harder to obtain. For instance, through World War II, there were no residency positions in surgery open to women in the United States.[72] In 1935, Presbyterian Hospital (New York) passed over for internship a "colored girl" who had performed brilliantly in medical school but appointed an outstanding white man with one arm who had demonstrated he could perform the necessary manual tasks.[73] Race and gender proved greater handicaps in obtaining house positions than physical disability.

Jews also encountered intense anti-Semitism in seeking internships and residencies. The situation at the University of Pittsburgh was typical. There, Jews were accepted as medical students, but when it came to appointing a chief resident in obstetrics, the department chairman wanted an individual who was "a gentile and a protestant."[74] Both private and public hospitals limited the number of Jews on the house staff. By virtue of their wealth, influence, and strong group identity, Jews had an advantage women and blacks did not have: excellent Jewish hospitals. The most important was Mount Sinai (New York), which before World War II became one of the country's leading centers of graduate medical education and clinical investigation, even without a medical school. The hospital, like a magnet, attracted the best and brightest Jewish house officers, specialists, and clinical scientists, many of whom had been denied house staff appointments or admitting privileges at other hospitals.[75] However, the Jewish hospitals could accommodate only a fraction of the qualified Jewish medical students, and many Jewish graduates had to go to less desirable programs.

If internship and residency selection was stressful for students, it was also stressful for hospitals, which had to compete for the best house officers. Community hospitals had the most difficult time at recruitment. With their large patient loads, crushing amount of chores, and scarcity of teaching activities, many of them could not fill their quota of interns. These hospitals often offered financial inducements to prospective interns, but usually to no avail, since students would choose internships on the basis of perceived educational benefits, not on the size of the stipend. "It has generally been found very difficult to fill undesirable internships on a financial basis since interns for the most part are primarily interested in the educational returns,"[76] the American Medical Association noted.

Teaching hospitals had little to fear from community hospitals, but they vigorously competed with each other for the best students. Intense rivalries existed among teaching hospitals in the same city—the Peter Bent Brigham Hospital and the Massachusetts General Hospital in Boston, the New York Hospital and Presbyterian Hospital in New York—as well as among leading teaching hospitals in different cities, such as the rivalry between Johns Hopkins and the Massachusetts General. A network arose in which students were alerted where the best educational opportunities might be found. Graduates of Syracuse, for example, wrote to the school about their internship, advising the dean whether the next year's class should be encouraged to apply to that program or pass it over.[77]

Thus, there were built-in limits as to how far any hospital could deviate from a proper balance between service and education. If service obligations were too great and educational opportunities too meager, students applied to other programs. No hospital could afford to be too complacent about the educational environment or conditions of work it provided its house officers. Students voted with their feet in selecting internships and residencies—demonstrating once again their power to help shape the educational experience.

Stresses and Support

During internship and residency, around-the-clock responsibility meant around-the-clock work. One ethic dominated graduate medical education: house officers should give everything to their patients. A fever spike in a patient at 3 A.M., an intravenous line that had infiltrated, the plating of cultures that arrived at the bacteriological laboratory after the technician had gone home: taking care of such problems was the duty of the responsible house officer. Long hours and fatiguing demands—later so highly publicized by news media—characterized the experience from the beginning.

Much of a house officer's work (at least at the teaching hospitals) was educational. House officers were there to learn (this was the rationale for not paying them a salary[78]), and activities such as conferences, rounds, seminars, lectures, reading, and participation in clinical research formed an important part of their day. However, even at the best programs, the amount of routine work could be overwhelming. At Mount Sinai Hospital (New York), interns spent an "excessive and disproportionate" amount of time on blood counts and examinations of urine.[79] At the Peter Bent Brigham Hospital, surgical house officers were too busy with patient care duties "to find sufficient time for proper recreation, much less for any investigative work or for composition."[80]

Graduate medical education involved total immersion in the institutional culture of the hospital. House officers lived there and spent almost all their time there. They were subject to demeaning rules of personal conduct, a continuation of the nineteenth-century hospital's efforts to dictate the behavior of patients and employees.[81] Teaching hospitals actively discouraged marriage. Although official prohibitions were sometimes rescinded, married house officers were usually expected to live in the hospital with single colleagues. For their labors house officers received token compensation: from nothing to $10 a month for interns, and $10 to $25 a month for residents.

Interns and residents had a more monastic existence than students, who resided outside the hospital and could come and go freely. Interns and residents followed a demanding schedule. Typically they took "call" (that is, admitted new patients) every other night, and they could not leave the hospital when on duty except with special permission. On nights off call, they were expected to return to the hospital residence by 10 P.M. or 12 midnight. Though most hospitals allowed vacations and sick leave, some did not. The University of Colorado, for instance, provided interns no vacation, and time lost from work because of illness had to be made up before interns could receive their certificates.[82]

At most teaching hospitals, complaints about bad food, decrepit living quarters, and inadequate recreational facilities were common. To one surgical chairman, it was "incomprehensible" that mature professionals were required to live in boardinghouse-like cubicles.[83] Conditions were especially trying for women. At Los Angeles County Hospital, the women's quarters were shabby and infected with cockroaches, and two toilets and two baths had to serve 20 to 30 women.[84]

The house staff experience was often influenced by factors determined by chance: the enthusiasm and helpfulness of the medical students, the availability of technical and clerical support, the adequacy of nursing coverage of their assigned floor, or weather conditions (which could influence the number of patients visiting the emergency room on a given admitting night). Especially idiosyncratic were the students. As house officers could enrich or ruin a student's clinical clerkship, students could similarly affect a house officer's experience. Also to be heeded were the nurses, whose practical experience often surpassed that of junior house officers, especially early in the academic year. Though egos of house officers could be bruised if the nurses knew what to do when they did not, only foolhardy interns and residents ignored their help and advice.

Chance also played a role in terms of which attending physicians a house officer worked with. Some faculty were much more supportive than others. Consider the surgical residency at the Peter Bent Brigham Hospital. There, John Homans was a tyrant. "When his mercurial temperament exploded, as it often did in an unpredictable manner, it could give a quick and violent hurt." One former resident remarked, "I first met Dr. Homans when I was filled with youthful romantic illusions. He quickly knocked them out."[85] In contrast, David Cheever, another prominent surgeon at the hospital, was known for his kindness. "In an era of surgical prima donnas he was reserved and imperturbable, even under the most trying circumstances. Always considerate and gracious to his assistants, he never was given to complaint or criticism even when such would have been justified."[86]

Considering their grueling hours and difficult working conditions, it is tempting to liken the plight of house officers to that of labor, which in post–World War I America was successfully organizing to achieve better working conditions from employers. In 1920, the normal work week in America was the six-day, 60-hour week. By 1929, the standard had become a five-and-one-half-day, 48–54-hour week, and many benefits such as paid vacations and shop medical plans had become common as well.[87] However, it would be a mistake to carry the analogy between graduate medical education and the sweatshop too far. House officers viewed themselves as professionals. Though they frequently complained to hospital authorities about their working conditions, they did not organize or unionize, and their protests were almost always polite. Moreover, house officers, unlike many laborers, were there by choice, and they knew that a prestigious, well paying career awaited them.

The visible stresses of house staff training should not obscure the many sources of support that were present. The hospital of this period provided house officers an all-encompassing universe that sustained them physically (literally—with room, meals, and uniforms) and emotionally. The hospital served as a social and intellectual center, where house officers discussed medical and nonmedical matters over dinner or late night snacks. Interns and residents shared every aspect of work and of life, came readily to each others' aid, and formed their own figurative family. At most teaching hospitals the esprit de corps was extraordinary.

Equally important in the support system was the positive impact of having personal relationships with faculty. Faculty were routinely present on the wards, engaging the house staff in clinical research and exemplifying the integration of clinical and scientific excellence. Most faculty took a keen interest in teaching, advising, and mentoring. House officers could not help feeling close to—and supported by—their instructors. The most important faculty member of all was the department head, who typically commanded the unswerving allegiance of his house officers. As one graduate of the Hopkins surgical training program put it, the chairman "was much in contact with the resident staff and I felt his presence on a daily, if not an hourly, basis."[88]

The house staff experience, in summary, contained numerous mechanisms to help house officers cope with the hard work and the assumption of responsibility. The camaraderie among house officers, the metaphorical family that evolved, the closeness and concern of faculty, and the constant availability of help usually allowed the educational and patient-care duties of house officers to be effectively discharged. This is not to suggest that the long hours were justifiable, but the issue of working hours must be seen as part of the larger issue of working conditions. The most pertinent question is the quality of the house staff milieu, the nature of the internal environment, and the adequacy of the educational, technical, and emotional support systems—and not simply the hours of work—if graduate medical education is to be properly understood.

Graduate Medical Education and the Public Interest

In the early twentieth century, specialization became a prominent part of medical practice. Its development was promoted by both scientific and social forces. With the growth of medical knowledge and the increasingly technical nature of certain areas of practice, many physicians were attracted by the satisfaction of mastering a single field. Others were drawn by the shorter hours, fewer house calls, higher income, and greater prestige.[89]

During World War I medical educators began to worry that general practitioners were being eclipsed in the profession by specialists. No one doubted the importance of having well trained ophthalmalogists, obstetricians, urologists, and other specialists available. However, it was not clear that the country needed many specialists since general practitioners could capably manage most medical problems. Precisely how many and what mix of specialists would best serve the public was unknown. Discussion of the topic was extremely subjective and value-laden. Nevertheless, most students of the problem worried that the United States was in danger of becoming overpopulated with specialists.

The controversy over specialization was made more complex because it resurrected the long-standing debate in America between individual liberty and community needs. Traditional individualistic American values favored the absence of any controls on the number or type of specialists produced. The assumption (or hope) was that the sum total of individual choices would somehow be consistent with the larger social need.[90] Yet, after World War I that was not happening. With no system of control, more and more doctors were taking short postgraduate courses and calling themselves specialists.

A major consequence of the establishment of the residency system as the sole route to specialization was that graduate medical education remained in balance with the country's needs for specialists. In 1940, only 24 percent of doctors limited their work to a specialty—a figure that included many older, self-named specialists.[91] Though there was always concern that the number of specialists might become too large, the chief "manpower" issue of American medical practice in the 1920s and 1930s was felt to be the inadequate distribution of doctors to rural areas and small communities, not the overproduction of specialists.[92]

The limitation of specialists reflected in part a response to market forces. Residency programs were controlled by medical school faculties whose main concern was to produce clinical investigators. The number of positions was designed to be small because academic positions were relatively few. Even though it was understood that many residents would enter practice, medical faculties limited the number of positions so that those who desired an academic appointment had a reasonable chance to receive one.

In addition, the limitation of specialists reflected in part the subjugation of individual aspirations to the larger goals of society. Residency was considered a privilege, not a right. All physicians were thought to be entitled to good internship training to round out their general education, but residency and specialization were reserved for the elite or the fortunate. As one report observed, "A man entering his internship has no assurance that he may later be able to obtain a satisfactory residency."[93] In this way, an individual medical graduate's desire to specialize was subordinated to the need of the public for enough general practitioners. Medical educators took it upon themselves to limit the production of specialists.

Though specialization was gaining in popularity among medical graduates, before World War II generalism remained honored at medical schools—a fact that further helped bring about a balanced distribution between general and specialty practice. Prominent specialists and academic leaders, especially in internal medicine, pediatrics, and surgery, defined themselves as generalists first, specialists second, and they would be incensed if anyone were to think differently. The consensus among medical educators was that the study of a specialty should follow a thorough preparation in general medicine. A major report on graduate medical education in 1940 warned of the danger of "premature specialism." A specialist should be "a broadly trained and well-educated physician first and a specialist second."[94]

Medical faculty took this point of view seriously. At the Peter Bent Brigham Hospital, the chief of medicine insisted that the hospital maintain general medical wards rather than establish specialty wards because of the importance of laying "broad foundations for the training of the best type of clinicians."[95] In Cornell's heart clinic, staff cardiologists carefully examined "the whole patient" and boasted of the many noncardiac diseases they diagnosed.[96] Formation of a hematology society in the United States was delayed because "many of the leaders in Hematology, such as [Nobel laureate George] Minot, feel that a separate society would tend to remove workers in the field from General Medicine, and this we consider a bad policy especially for the younger men."[97] Many doctors may have been bitterly disappointed if they did not receive a residency or were dropped too early to qualify as a specialist, but they were not made to feel that general practice was unimportant.

From the standpoint of national goals, therefore, graduate medical education before World War II succeeded in achieving an acceptable balance between general practitioners and specialists. However, in its educational conduct, graduate medical education performed less satisfactorily. Medical educators for decades had stressed the importance of approaching patients in a reasoned, scientific fashion. Tests and procedures were to be done when dictated by a patient's particular circumstances, not merely because they were readily available. The great shortcoming of graduate medical education was that discretion in ordering tests was seldom taught or encouraged. Graduate medical education failed to live up to its own ideals.

Some excessive testing was inevitable and acceptable in teaching hospitals. Patients were often sicker, demanding more sophisticated evaluations and interventions. Clinical studies were being conducted, resulting in a certain amount of testing for research rather than patient management. Moreover, learners had to use tests a number of times to become familiar with their benefits and limitations. As the Council on Medical Education and Hospitals observed, many diagnostic procedures appropriately "are carried out for the education of the physician rather than simply for patient care."[98] Laboratory studies of direct educational or investigative value could hardly be considered contrary to the public interest.

Nevertheless, the level of testing far exceeded that which was necessary for education, research, and the care of sicker patients. This resulted mainly from the way attending physicians taught house officers. The stereotypical attending physician would quickly scold an intern or resident for failing to order a test but rarely explain why certain tests might not be needed. Winford H. Smith, director of the Johns Hopkins Hospital, discussed this problem in detail. He observed that countless X-rays and laboratory tests "are ordered without any particular indication . . . simply because the young house officer is afraid the chief or someone of his superiors will ask for it and will call him down if he hasn't it ready." At the Johns Hopkins Hospital, this was "a source of great extravagance" and the cause of the hospital's operating deficit. The solution lay only in the "careful training of the younger men by the older members of the Staff." "If the younger staff members [house officers] were made to feel that they would be called down by their superiors just as hard for ordering X-rays, electrocardiograms, laboratory examinations, etc., which were not definitely indicated, this would save a lot of time and considerable money."[99]

It would appear that much of the faculties' failure to teach a discriminating approach to testing resulted from the luxury they had of practicing medicine in an environment of abundance. Quantitative data are difficult to find, but qualitative impressions from school and hospital records support this impression. For instance, house officers ordered fewer and more appropriate tests at those unusual times when resources were limited. When X-ray film became scarce at one hospital during World War II, house officers responded by "only requesting radiographic examinations when they are clearly indicated rather than following the [customary] procedure of requesting routine films on all patients."[100] When the supply of film was restored, the number of radiographs returned to the previously high level.

Even during the Depression, house officers usually learned and practiced medicine with unlimited resources. The abundance of training situations created the mistaken sense that resources everywhere were the same. During internship and residency, habits were developed that continued for the duration of a physician's career. Before World War II, the economic consequences of excessive testing were relatively small. Nevertheless, graduate medical education was already fostering extravagant practice styles that in later decades were to have enormous economic consequences for the public that paid the bills.

5

Teaching Hospitals

As the modern hospital matured, teaching of all types occurred at virtually every institution. Even the smallest hospitals were sites of ongoing education through clinical conferences, rounds, staff meetings, and autopsy and chart reviews, not to mention the informal learning that took place whenever doctors sought consultations or discussed cases among themselves. Many small hospitals sponsored internship programs, and some large community hospitals offered residency programs as well. Nevertheless, the term "teaching hospital" was reserved for a select group of institutions—100 to 150 of the roughly 6,800 hospitals in existence—that served as major clinical facilities for medical schools. Though few in number, teaching hospitals were indispensable to medical education as the most important sites of clinical education and research.

Teaching hospitals comprised a heterogeneous lot. Many were private (voluntary); a larger number were publicly owned. Some medical schools, most commonly state schools, owned their teaching hospital; the others had carefully constructed agreements of affiliation. In many cases, a teaching hospital served a single medical school, as in the example of Strong Memorial Hospital and the University of Rochester. In other cases, especially among the municipal institutions, one hospital might participate in the educational programs of a number of medical schools, as Cook County Hospital served several schools in Chicago. Some leading medical educators—including Abraham Flexner—felt that medical schools should have a single hospital. However, as another example that Flexner's influence on medical education was never as strong as some writers have maintained, many schools established affiliations with two or more hospitals to accommodate their growing numbers of house officers and to provide a more diverse educational experience.

After World War I, teaching hospitals championed the same academic ideals as their affiliated medical schools, and the two institutions acted in concert in education, research, and patient care. The relationship between medical schools and teaching hospitals was one of codependency. Medical schools, ever on the alert for clinical facilities, understood that access to the wards of hospitals was essential for teaching and research. Teaching hospitals, in turn, understood that their preeminence in twentieth-century medical practice was a consequence of their participation in medical education.

Though teaching hospitals of the period served as nearly ideal educational laboratories, this did not occur without costs or consequences. It quickly became apparent that teaching hospitals could not be as efficient as nonteaching hospitals, if at the same time they were providing a rich educational environment. In addition, the fact that indigent but not private patients were routinely used in teaching challenged the common belief that medical education resulted in better patient care. Society always needed new doctors, and for this, students and house officers had to learn. Yet society's needs conflicted with those of individual patients, who preferred the most experienced doctors available at the moment. This tension between group and individual welfare was—and is—the fundamental moral dilemma of medical education.

Joining the University

The period between the wars witnessed a confluence of forces in American medical education. As medical schools, with their new responsibilities for patient care and graduate medical education, entered the medical care delivery system, teaching hospitals entered the university. Education and research, once barely tolerated activities, became a central part of the mission of these institutions. For all practical purposes, teaching hospitals became the clinical campuses of medical schools—partners in a collaborative effort to teach, expand knowledge, and elevate the standards of patient care.

After World War I, teaching hospitals embraced education and research as ardently as they had refused to participate in those activities before the war. Teaching hospitals championed better opportunities for student and house staff education. They also provided financial support for clinical research. Thus, Presbyterian Hospital (New York) established a $100,000 fund to help pay for the research expenses of faculty at the College of Physicians and Surgeons; New York Hospital requested that its name be included along with that of Cornell University Medical College on the scientific papers of faculty who held appointments at both institutions; Mount Sinai Hospital (New York) established a journal to publish the research of its medical staff.[1] By deeds, not just words, teaching hospitals showed that they took their new academic role seriously.

For their efforts in teaching and research, teaching hospitals reaped significant benefits. Their medical school affiliations provided them a distinct advantage in the intense competition to attract interns and residents. Association with medical schools allowed hospitals to make their mark in education and research, not just patient care. Benefactors, acknowledging the preeminence of teaching hospitals, usually reserved their largest donations for them. Thus, Presbyterian Hospital attributed its notable success in attracting large gifts to one factor: its affiliation with Columbia University.[2]

Many forces had helped create alliances between teaching hospitals and medical schools during World War I, but after the war none was more important in cementing that relationship than the patient-centered nature of clinical research. To clinical investigators, research was part of practice, and careful observation of patients carried the possibility of learning information that might be of value not only to that patient's care but to the treatment of future patients as well. For hospitals, this meant close attention to their patients by the best doctors. It also meant that hospitals had the opportunity to advance medical knowledge, a purpose many of them now regarded as equally important to the care of the sick. No hospital took that charge more seriously than Massachusetts General, whose leadership in clinical research contributed directly to its eminence in patient care, and vice versa. For instance, in 1936 the hospital described how its accomplishments in the study of hyperparathyroidism, an endocrinological condition, resulted in its becoming the most important center in the world for the clinical treatment of that disease: "The number of patients with hyperparathyroidism admitted is greater than that in any other single clinic in the world for the reason that pioneer work on the diagnosis and treatment of that disease has been done here."[3]

As part of the extended campus of the university, teaching hospitals contributed to the shaping of their affiliated medical schools. For instance, they played a major role in the recruitment and retention of faculty. Clinical faculty of this era were drawn to a school by the promise of wards under their control. A school's competitiveness in this regard depended on the facilities available to it at its affiliated teaching hospital. In addition, teaching hospitals were the sites of innumerable "turf battles" among clinical faculty, such as those between general surgeons and urologists over who would operate on the adrenal gland and between neurosurgeons and orthopedic surgeons over who would be responsible for vertebral discs.

Teaching hospitals faced many issues that the rest of the university, including the medical school, did not. Teaching hospitals had numerous constituencies besides medical professors and students. Each of these groups had its own perspective on the institution and a voice in shaping it. Among these were patients, private physicians, house officers, nurses, administrators, trustees, private insurers (beginning in the 1930s), orderlies, technicians, and workers in such areas as housekeeping, food service, and building maintenance. Teaching hospitals remained firmly anchored in the real world, perpetually facing issues such as nursing shortages, labor unrest, rapid employee turnover, cost overruns, and budgetary shortfalls.

Despite these challenges, the administration of teaching hospitals was relatively simple. Teaching hospitals were large and complex relative to their nineteenth-century antecedents, but they could still operate with small administrative staffs and minimal bureaucratic complexity. For instance, in 1939 the following positions comprised the New York Hospital's entire administrative staff: administrator-in-chief, superintendent, associate superintendent, assistant superintendent, assistant to the superintendent, medical director of New York Hospital–Westchester division, apothecary, assistant to the treasurer, and assistant to the secretary.[4] As late as 1940 the hospital had only a haphazard system of cost-accounting. It knew its total income and deficit but did not have financial information on the component parts of the hospital, such as the income and expenses of the pediatric or surgical floors.[5] Costs were relatively low, with $1,000,000 in the 1920s and $3,000,000 in the 1930s representing an extremely large hospital budget. Many teaching hospitals ran operating deficits, but generous board members often covered the deficit with a single check. Expansion of a teaching hospital depended solely on its ability to raise capital from benefactors or local and state governments. Teaching hospitals did not have to contend with a complex array of regulatory authorities if they wished to acquire equipment or build new facilities.

During this period, many teaching hospitals and medical schools operated as virtually one. Disagreements often occurred, but these were usually readily worked out. The relations between Cornell University Medical College and the New York Hospital represented a model in this regard. The two institutions, located on the same physical site after 1932, were governed by a Joint Administrative Board comprised of representatives of both institutions. Records of both the medical school and hospital reveal continual feuding on even the tiniest of matters, usually pertaining to how expenses of the medical center should be allocated. Yet, on the large issues the medical school and hospital regularly came to each others' aid. In the 1930s, each contributed $175,000 a year to a combined budget to pay for salaries and supplies of the clinical departments.[6] When the hospital incurred a large deficit in 1938, the medical school volunteered to pay some of the hospital's expenses for the next five years, and plans were initiated to undertake a joint fund-raising campaign for the combined institution.[7] Conversely, the hospital helped pay the educational and research costs of the school, and when a crisis in medical student housing occurred in 1942, the hospital offered one of its buildings to alleviate the shortage.[8] Though there was always conflict, the medical school and hospital were drawn together by their common goals, and they believed that "in the last analysis the problem of either institution should be settled for the advantage of both or of the joint institution."[9]

Both medical schools and teaching hospitals were animated by the same purpose of teaching, research, and caring for the sick. As more and more hospitals and schools were constructed in geographic proximity, the two partners were often idealized as a single, unified institution whose laboratories, wards, and clinics were geographically, architecturally, and functionally one. No pair of institutions were more commonly viewed as an integrated whole than the Johns Hopkins Medical School and Hospital. One consultant pointed out that they "were practically one institution, although having different boards" and that "outside Hopkins they [people] did not differentiate between the Hospital . . . and Medical School."[10]

However, the complete union of hospitals and medical schools never occurred. Tensions between the two persisted. Medical schools, arising from university traditions, remained oriented primarily toward education and research, not the provision of patient care. Teaching hospitals, which had arisen from a tradition of charity and patient care, could never forget that their primary role was to provide clinical services. Medical faculties tended to have a cavalier attitude toward costs and expenses that irritated many hospital administrators. Teaching hospitals were under pressure to deliver more and more clinical services, which was distracting to education and research and frustrating to the medical faculties. In the end, medical schools and teaching hospitals retained their separate identities.

Nevertheless, the commitment of teaching hospitals of this period to education and research should not be underestimated. This attitude was exemplified by Presbyterian Hospital (New York), which made clear that clinical services must be kept in balance with academic activities and never pursued for their own sake. The Planning Committee for the hospital declared in 1945 that clinical services "should not be larger than necessary to carry out the fundamental [academic] concepts upon which the Medical Center was put together. *Patient demands in themselves must not dictate our fundamental policy, and no one activity should be dominant.*" The emphasis, according to the committee, should be on the quality of work done and on the promotion of education and research, not on seeing as many patients as possible. "Expansion indicates size and we are not after that in itself. We want *quality* rather than *quantity*. We want proper balance rather than unduly large and unwieldy services. *A thing can become so large that it defeats its own purpose.*"[11]

If there was any doubt that teaching hospitals had adopted academic values, such doubts were laid to rest as the hospitals described how they defined success: not by the volume of patients seen, even less by financial profitability, but by the quality of clinical service and their contributions to education and research. The staff of the hospital of the George Washington University School of Medicine declared that the reputation of a teaching hospital was derived in only one way: "on the basis *of scientific discovery.*" To be great, hospitals must not only teach and practice medicine but "must *make* medicine."[12] The leading teaching hospitals were those most renowned as centers of education and research. Trustees and administrators of teaching hospitals were charged with making their institutions academic leaders, not financial profit-centers. Fiscal responsibility was required for the institutions to do good work, but ultimately teaching hospitals were measured by their academic and professional accomplishments rather than their balance sheets.[13]

The Presence of Time

At first glance, it may have seemed natural for clinical education to be conducted on inpatient wards of hospitals. Medical education must follow the patients, and hospitals had become the center of acute care. Nevertheless, inpatient wards were highly unrepresentative of everyday practice. The typical specialist spent roughly one-third of all professional hours in the hospital. General practitioners spent far less time practicing in hospitals, and some had no hospital appointments at all.[14] That the major site of clinical education became inpatient wards, in distinction to home visits, office practice, the outpatient clinics of hospitals, or other ambulatory settings, represented a deliberate choice.

The emphasis on inpatient teaching arose in part from the educational efficiencies of scale that teaching hospitals provided. A patient with an important physical finding could be examined by many students and house officers, not just a single learner or two working with a solo practitioner. Anyone with a question found expert advice readily at hand. Those available for help consisted of the hospital's entire staff, not just a single preceptor. Laboratories, X-ray facilities, libraries, conferences, and the ongoing opportunity for consultation and discourse were regularly available.

Most important of all, inpatient services offered sufficient time for the objectives of medical education to be met. The ability to solve unknowns and deal thoughtfully with clinical uncertainty could be acquired only if learners had enough time to study patients in depth. They needed to be able to think, read, and talk about their patients and to follow carefully the results of diagnostic studies and therapeutic interventions. Work as an apprentice in a harried practitioner's office did not afford that type of opportunity, nor did rotations in the even more frenetically paced outpatient clinics of most teaching hospitals. Only the inpatient wards provided the right mixture of a rich patient population and abundant time.

Medical educators worked hard to develop the rich educational environment of the teaching wards. For instance, to provide time for learning and study, teaching hospitals hired many more house officers than nonteaching hospitals hired for the same number of patients.[15] In addition, some hospitals restricted the number of admissions so that students, house officers, and faculty would have the time to mingle. The Peter Bent Brigham Hospital was typical in this regard. When the hospital opened shortly before the outbreak of World War I, it decided to limit the number of beds in the institution since the clinical chiefs "considered intimate personal contact in their daily teaching with their junior staff of cardinal importance in perpetuating the high standards envisioned for the institution."[16] Henry Christian, the first chief of medicine, explained that the hospital could not do good educational (or clinical) work if it accepted "more patients than it can satisfactorily handle" and that a large census consisting of routine patients who could find help elsewhere was "the last thing it [the hospital] desires."[17]

The lengthy hospitalizations of the era also contributed to the educa tional richness of inpatient wards. From World War I to World War II the average length of stay fell, but even at midcentury it remained sufficiently long that students and residents could study their patients thoroughly. As late as 1951, the average length of stay for medical ward patients at one teaching hospital was 25.5 days.[18] As a result, learners could observe the full course of their patients' illnesses, acquire a broad education in medical and surgical principles, pursue interesting topics in depth, and develop a sound approach to patient management. For instance, students and house officers learned that maturity and skill in surgery depended on the ability to arrive at an accurate preoperative diagnosis and to determine which patients were likely to benefit from surgery, not on sheer operating technique.

Hospitalized patients were often very sick, and some had life-threatening illnesses, but medical educators considered this an educational advantage even if these patients represented only the extreme end of disease severity. Through exposure to emergencies, students and house officers received firm grounding in the principles of physiology, pathophysiology, and therapeutics. Consider the management of patients with diabetes mellitus. Unstable patients with ketoacidosis (extremely high blood sugar, accompanied by other severe metabolic derangements) were challenging to treat. In this life-threatening complication of diabetes, physicians needed to monitor pulse rate, respiratory rate, blood pressure, and level of consciousness as well as serum electrolytes, sugar, and pH (level of acidity). Intravenous infusions of insulin, fluids, and electrolytes were mandatory. Underlying problems, such as infections and abscesses, needed to be searched for and treated if found. Every step had to be carefully monitored; each decision had to be rapidly made. In contrast, the task of following a stable diabetic's condition in an ambulatory setting, adjusting the diet and insulin dose as necessary, was less stressful and more easily learned. Students or house officers who had mastered the management of ketoacidosis understood diabetes well and found the outpatient treatment of the disease a nonintimidating task. Conversely, those who had never treated ketoacidosis were poorly prepared for medical practice. To medical educators of the era, familiarity with emergencies brought students dividends in terms of knowledge and self-confidence that would last a professional lifetime.[19]

Admission to the hospital was generally unplanned. Hence, chance played a major role in determining what types of conditions a student or house officer would see. In this regard, clinical education might be regarded as adhering to the osmotic concept of education—namely, that through immersion in the life of the wards, students and house officers would eventually see a sufficiently broad range of conditions to be well prepared for the independent practice of medicine. Of note, it was not necessary for learners to admit a patient with a particular condition to experience that condition. Cases of others would regularly be discussed at rounds, conferences, and seminars. Students and house officers could examine those patients themselves or read about the subject in the library. Complaints about inadequate clinical exposure were few.

Though students and house officers were busy, their routine was not as hectic as one might at first surmise. Indeed, by later standards, the pace was sometimes leisurely. At Georgetown University Hospital around 1930, interns could awaken as late as 8:00 A.M. and eat breakfast as late as 9:00 A.M.[20] In the 1920s, two-thirds of teaching hospitals started their scheduled operations at 8:30 or 9:00 A.M., and the other one-third did their surgery in the afternoons.[21] This was a consequence in part of the smaller number of admissions house officers received and the long hospital stays. It also resulted from the absence of intensive care units and high technology medical interventions. Very sick patients either recovered or died, and many patients spent most of their hospitalization in stable condition convalescing after an operation or major illness. Moreover, few house officers were in a rush to leave the hospital by 6 P.M. They lived in the hospital and were already together with their "family." The result was that considerable time was available for discussion, contemplation, and thinking.

Though the inpatient wards of teaching hospitals proved to be an outstanding educational laboratory, they could not facilitate all objectives of medical education. Hospitalized patients were not representative of the ambulatory patients that predominated in office practice. Outpatient care may not have taught the principles of pathophysiology in the same way as the care of medical emergencies, but exposure to ambulatory medicine was necessary and desirable. Harvard's Harvey Cushing was hardly unique in his concern that hospitalized patients hardly resembled "those [with] which the students after graduation are likely to be brought face to face."[22]

Teaching with hospitalized patients carried an additional limitation: it was more difficult to learn to care for the whole patient. In the hospital, the power of patients was diminished, as they were detached from their home, place of work, friends, and family. These unusual circumstances, and the fact that contact with hospital personnel usually ended with discharge, made it difficult for even the most conscientious student or house officer to develop a long-term relationship or acquire an understanding of the whole person. In addition, hospital medicine accentuated medicine's growing reliance on that which could be observed or measured, as opposed to what patients felt or said.[23] Thus, the director of one school's

cardiology service maintained that electrocardiograms, X-rays, and fluo-
roscopy should be obtained on all patients, even if the diagnosis were
already known. "High class clinical records should stress objective findings which are entirely free of personal equation."[24] Though these effects
are difficult to measure, there seems little doubt that the hospital
learner's gaze focused increasingly on the patient as an object, and concerns about the depersonalizing effects of hospital teaching were commonly expressed.[25]

Recognizing the educational limitations of the inpatient wards, medical educators tried a variety of experiments in other clinical settings. The
University of Michigan established a preceptorship program in which
fourth-year students were assigned to community practitioners for a
summer's work.[26] Arkansas and Woman's Medical College of Pennsylvania sponsored programs in which students visited patients in their
homes, particularly to provide obstetrical care.[27] However, the major
alternative to inpatient teaching was the ambulatory clinics of the teaching hospitals. These facilities had a distinguished tradition in medical
education, serving in the nineteenth century as an important site of clinical training. Many twentieth-century medical educators viewed them as
the key to teaching a humane, rounded medicine and to providing exposure to the more common if less serious problems that most physicians
saw in day-to-day practice.

Though the potential of outpatient instruction was widely recognized,
in actuality it was seldom realized. There were too many patients, and
facilities were cramped and overcrowded. Patients experienced long
delays to be seen and brief, frenetic visits when finally called. Clinics
lacked enough clerical and technical help, and there was inadequate
supervision by attending physicians. These and other problems rendered
the outpatient work at most medical schools unsatisfactory for students,
house officers, and patients alike. The Washington University faculty
acknowledged that its clinic work was "thoroughly unsatisfactory,"[28]
and many other medical facilities made similar admissions.

Few medical schools of this era cared if their ambulatory work was
lacking, as long as the inpatient services were strong. The outpatient
department stood low in the hierarchy system of both medical schools
and teaching hospitals. This resulted from many causes, including an
infatuation with the technological nature of scientific medical care, a
rejection of the hospital's traditional welfare function, and a professional
value system that had always accorded much greater prestige to inpatient than outpatient work. Many medical faculties considered the primary purpose of the outpatient departments to be that of serving as a
feeder to the inpatient services to keep the wards filled.

It was not inevitable that educational work in outpatient clinics would
be unsatisfactory. Before World War II, a number of experiments demonstrated that clinic teaching, when properly conducted, could be of great

value. Harvard, Yale, Johns Hopkins, and Cornell, for instance, introduced appointment systems in their ambulatory clinics that reduced waiting for patients and allowed students and house officers more time to spend with each scheduled patient. At the Peter Bent Brigham Hospital, the time allotted for a house officer to see a "new" patient was 30 minutes; for a fourth-year clinical clerk, one to one and one-half hours.[29] The number of patients was limited to those who could be properly handled. The result was greater satisfaction among patients, who lost less time on clinic day and received more thorough evaluations, as well as among students and house officers, who had a rewarding experience in ambulatory medicine.[30]

What allowed these experiments to succeed was that ample time was provided for students and house officers to evaluate their patients and for faculty to supervise the work. As a professor at Cornell observed, for outpatient teaching to be effective, it "should be something more than a casual byproduct of clinic routine."[31] In these experiments, learners benefited from having sufficient time to evaluate patients thoroughly and to discuss cases with instructors. This was in marked contrast to most outpatient clinics, where the hustle and bustle led to poor supervision, little teaching, and the exposure of students to slipshod methods. Time was the irreducible element of good medical education, whatever clinical setting happened to be used.

Of course, good teaching brought about a reduction in the volume of patients that could be satisfactorily handled, both in ambulatory and inpatient settings. Learners needed time to master systematic approaches and faculty needed time to supervise and teach, not just to see their own patients. The director of Cornell's neurology clinic pointed out that six patients in a three-hour session were too many to schedule for even an experienced clinician if teaching were being simultaneously conducted. "During the term when elective students are in the department, it is impossible for the physician, also acting as an instructor, to see a full quota of six patients."[32]

Seeing fewer patients was an acceptable tradeoff to hospital and medical school officials of the era, who routinely defined success in terms of the quality rather than the quantity of work done. As Christian put it in 1928: "The more time given to each patient, the less the total number of patients that we can handle per day or per year. Still, it is more important to do good work than to handle many patients."[33] Medical education, by its very nature, did not allow teaching hospitals to be efficient in terms of seeing the most patients in the shortest time. Educational quality could be maintained only in an environment that allowed sufficient time for teaching and learning. Medical school and teaching hospital officials rejoiced in the choice they made to do the work well—at least on the inpatient services. If they had to accept certain production inefficiencies to maintain educational quality, that was a concession they gladly made.

The Ward Service

As time was essential for clinical learning, so was exposure to a wide variety of patients. This teaching hospitals of the era also provided in great abundance. However, not all patients were used in teaching. Rather, it was the poor patients treated on the indigent wards—variously called the "ward services" or "pavilion services"—who provided most of the "clinical material" for teaching and research. In keeping with a long-standing tradition in Western medicine, these patients received free medical care in exchange for their participation in the educational activities of the institution.

After World War I, teaching hospitals provided care to many individuals who were not poor, both a large number of private (paying out-of-pocket) and a small number of semiprivate (insured) patients. However, these patients were used sparingly in education. Students could take their histories and perform physical examinations, but little more. The Council on Medical Education and Hospitals observed, "They [paying patients] may be shown as a rare jewel, a flower, or a curiosity; but medical students will never be allowed to follow through a disease and learn its course on such patients."[34] Similarly, house officers were not given any real responsibility for their care. Residents were not permitted to perform surgery on private patients or make important therapeutic decisions, and occasionally, not even to do complete physical examinations or write notes in charts.[35] Private patients were regarded as "belonging" to their private physicians, and it was made clear to students and house officers that they should not intrude.

For medical education to occur, the ward service was necessary. Here students were permitted to be active learners and house officers allowed to assume meaningful responsibilities. Here also were conducted most of the clinical studies that allowed some teaching hospitals to become nationally or internationally known. The professional reputation of a teaching hospital arose almost exclusively from its teaching service. This was why one clinical chief of Massachusetts General Hospital declared, "The MGH's soul lies in its teaching wards."[36]

It is likely that the care of ward patients benefited from their being used in teaching programs. They were conscientiously treated by energetic house officers and students, under the supervision of the best medical minds in the country. Discussions of their cases at rounds and conferences regularly resulted in new ideas that were helpful in management. Many ward patients profited from the emotional support of students, house officers, and nurses, who acted zealously as their advocates and often defended them against seemingly impersonal hospital forces.

Nevertheless, the fact remained that private patients, who had a choice, did not allow themselves to be used in the main educational activities of teaching hospitals. No amount of supervision, oversight, and backup—and all these checks and balances were present—could obscure the basic dilemma that what was needed for education fundamentally conflicted with what was needed for the immediate care of patients. It was in the patient's interest to have the most experienced surgeon perform the operation; it was in society's interest to allow a learner to operate. To a nation that has perpetually struggled with the dichotomy between individual rights and community needs, it should be no surprise that medical education was faced with the same issue.

6

Academic Medical Centers and the Public

THOUGH MEDICAL SCHOOLS AND TEACHING HOSPITALS were separate entities, they operated extremely closely, and their individual successes depended very much on their collaboration. In the late 1920s, the
term "medical center" came into use to describe arrangements in which a
medical school and teaching hospital occupied adjoining physical sites.
The term was first used in conjunction with the opening of the Columbia-
Presbyterian Medical Center in 1928 and the New York Hospital–Cornell
Medical Center in 1932. After World War II these complexes came to be
called "academic medical centers."[1]

Though no two were exactly alike, the centers typically consisted of a
medical school, a university-owned or controlled hospital, and affiliated
specialty hospitals or institutes. For instance, the Columbia-Presbyterian
Medical Center was initially comprised of the College of Physicians and
Surgeons of Columbia University, Presbyterian Hospital, the Sloan Hospital for Women, the Vanderbilt Clinic (an outpatient facility), the Neurological Institute, and Babies Hospital.[2] Conceptually, the most important
principle was that the various components of a center would not merely
operate side by side but would collaborate in teaching, research, and
patient care. One medical school dean in the late 1920s attempted "to so
intermix the budgets of the medical school and hospital that the university would never be able to separate them."[3] The public often found it
difficult to distinguish between the medical school and teaching hospital,
so closely were the two associated. For many purposes the new term
"academic medical center" became a more useful reference than "medical
school" or "teaching hospital" alone.

The constituency of academic medical centers, like that of the university, went beyond those individuals who taught and studied there. Like
the university, the academic medical center had a place in the larger soci-

ety, and there were always broader aspects to its work than teaching and research. Medical faculties felt a responsibility to physicians in practice, not merely to students and house officers. Through consultations and various programs of continuing medical education, academic medical centers assisted doctors not associated with the centers, thereby helping to elevate the standards of practice in the community. In addition, medical faculties provided large amounts of charity care, mindful that this had been a venerable tradition of teaching hospitals. Finally, academic medical centers were at the center of efforts to improve the quality of medical care and the health of the people, thus rendering service to the nation at large. In short, academic medical centers, like their parent universities, accepted the duty of utility—that is, of providing service to the society that supported them and allowed them to pursue their scientific interests.[4] Though there were always conspicuous strains of discord in the external relations of the academic medical centers, just as there were in their internal operations, few members of society in this period were dissatisfied with what medical education was contributing to the larger good.

Town and Gown

After World War I, medical faculties became increasingly concerned about the professional growth of physicians in practice. It was estimated in 1937 that without systematic study, an average practitioner would be professionally deficient in 5 years and hopelessly out of date in 10 to 15 years.[5] The ethos of medical education stressed the importance of self-learning. However, no medical educator was so naive as to believe that harried practitioners, particularly in rural or solo practice, could keep up-to-date without help.

Discussion of the educational needs of practitioners arose slowly because the problems of undergraduate and then graduate medical education were so pressing. Before 1920, the emphasis was on remedying the deficiencies of doctors who had received inadequate training. The primary vehicles for this were the various proprietary "polyclinical" medical schools ("undergraduate repair shops,"[6] Abraham Flexner had called them). After 1920, continuing medical education was frequently confused with graduate medical education. However, with the rise of internship and residency, the separate identity of continuing medical education became clear. By the 1930s, its mission of helping well-trained physicians keep up-to-date was widely understood.[7]

Continuing medical education was never as high a priority to medical faculties as the education of students and house officers, in part because many state and county medical societies also sponsored programs. Nevertheless, in the 1920s most schools began to take this responsibility seriously. Many schools offered formal courses. Some of these were short; others, long. Some were conducted in clinics and wards; others, in auditoriums and lecture rooms. In 1940–41 a typical school, New York University, offered 19 courses and had 159 registrants.[8]

Much continuing medical education was informal. Conferences and lectures at medical centers were open to the medical public, and schools took pride in the attendance of large numbers of private practitioners not affiliated with the center. At Mount Sinai Hospital (New York), standing room only crowds were attracted to the major weekly teaching events. The staff proudly noted how "In this manner the Hospital has steadily expanded its influence on the practice of medicine outside its walls."[9]

Recognizing that it was often difficult for busy practitioners to come to a medical center, some schools took their courses to the practitioners, offering continuing medical education instruction at community hospitals in cities, towns, and rural areas. The University of Michigan, Albany Medical College, and Tufts College Medical School were leaders in this regional approach to continuing medical education.[10] Their behavior in this respect was reminiscent of the "Wisconsin idea" of university service, one element of which was the extension movement, whereby university classes were held throughout the state.[11]

Medical faculties were also concerned with assisting practitioners with difficult cases. Sometimes this could be handled through a telephone call or letter. More commonly it meant seeing challenging patients in consultation and, if necessary, admitting them to the hospital for evaluation or treatment. Afterwards, patients would be returned to the referring physician with a report of the findings, assessment, and recommendations. In providing consultations, medical professors were using their expertise to benefit the community in a fashion similar to many other university professors, particularly in areas like law, engineering, business, and agriculture.

Referrals represented a small but important part of the clinical work of academic medical centers. The Columbia-Presbyterian Medical Center, now the "diagnostic center of the community," experienced a "flood of inquiries of diagnostic assistance of all degrees," ranging from a "professional specialty opinion" to a "full diagnostic work-up."[12] At the University of Michigan, the large number of referrals was highly conspicuous at the school's hospital. The dean observed: "The practice of medicine at University Hospital is not the routine variety encountered in the average private physician's office. Nearly every one [sic] who comes to us [by referral] is a difficult and obscure medical or surgical problem that taxes the skill and strength of our clinical staff."[13] Professors were kept mentally sharp by tackling the most difficult cases; community practitioners were served by the assistance they received with patients they could not adequately manage on their own.

The relationship that developed between community practitioners (or "town") and full-time faculty (or "gown") proved to be mutually beneficial. Private practitioners understood that their high status in society derived from the education they had received at the academic medical centers and from the fact that medical faculties stood behind them once they had entered practice. Conversely, medical faculties needed private practitioners to translate their work into demonstrable achievement so that the public would continue to be willing to support medical education and research. The goodwill of private practitioners often proved helpful to medical faculties in recruiting students to a school, attracting house officers to a teaching hospital, or securing funds from a municipality or state legislature. No part of the "town" was more important to a faculty than its own alumni, whose political and financial support could be indispensable. In recognition of this, many medical schools began creating alumni offices to help foster the continued loyalty of their graduates.

Nevertheless, relations between town and gown were not always smooth, primarily because private practitioners often worried that academic medical centers would steal their patients. In 1925 the chief of medicine at the Peter Bent Brigham Hospital acknowledged, "Unfortunately, at times, misunderstandings do arise and a physician feels that he has been badly treated because his patient does not return to him."[14] Such worries were accentuated during the difficult economic years of the Depression. Controversies in which the school of medicine was charged with unfairly competing with the local medical profession erupted in many places, including Cincinnati, where the medical society deeply resented perceived intrusions by the University of Cincinnati, and Chicago, where private practitioners similarly resented the University of Chicago for seeing large numbers of paying patients in its clinics.[15]

However, before World War II academic medical centers never posed a serious economic threat to private practitioners. The number of teaching hospitals was small, as was the size of the full-time faculties. Most important, few medical faculties wished to compete for paying patients. They were already very busy overseeing the care of large populations of charity patients. Except for referrals, emergencies, and patients in need of specialized services or of particular teaching interest, most medical faculties did not seek out private patients. As the University of Pennsylvania faculty put it, it was their intention not to be "a competitor of private physicians."[16]

Records of medical schools and teaching hospitals reveal instances where this policy was violated. However, those episodes represented the exceptions. Faculty who treated private practitioners poorly—by arrogance, condescension, tardiness in sending reports, or failing to return patients—were vulnerable to discipline. At the University of Colorado, one staff member received a three-month suspension from the Department of Urology for "soliciting a patient from the Outpatient Department for his own private practice" and was placed on probation after his return.[17] Temple University School of Medicine scrutinized its outpatient work to avoid "dispensary abuse," that is, providing free care to patients who could afford to see a private physician.[18] Henry A. Christian stated the issue the most succinctly of all. The Peter Bent Brigham Hospital, he wrote repeatedly, had too many patients to do its work well, and if it could return some of its patients to local practitioners, it could do much better work.[19] It was simply not part of either the educational or charitable mission of academic medical centers to see many private patients.

Thus, the relationship between town and gown was generally harmonious. Tensions were always present, and feuding would periodically erupt, but the overall tenor remained cordial. The key to a cohesive profession lay in continuing medical education, the provision of medical consultations, and the avoidance of competition for patients. In this fashion town and gown cooperated, rather than competed, in making medical care available to the American people.

This cooperation allowed significant efficiency in the delivery of medical care, even without formal coordination or planning. As Daniel M. Fox has discussed, sophisticated technologies and services were available at most academic medical centers, but only rarely at other hospitals. Academic medical centers served as referral sources for a city, region, or state; few community hospitals attempted to compete with them in providing these specialized services. From the academic medical centers, new medical information was disseminated throughout the region, and the centers exerted an influence that helped upgrade the standards of practice in the community.[20] Academic medical centers represented only a small part of the country's medical care delivery system, but they represented the engine that allowed the rest of the system to operate.

The Care of the Poor

As teaching hospitals collaborated with medical schools after World War I, their traditional charitable mission remained at the foreground. Of course, paying patients were treated as well. Full-time faculty needed beds for referral patients; voluntary faculty needed accommodations for their own private patients. However, most teaching hospitals continued to provide vast amounts of free care. In this way, academic medical centers served not only the medical public—that is, the practitioners of a region as seen in the previous section—but the general public as well.

The amount of charity care varied from one academic medical center to another. University teaching hospitals in less populated regions, such as the University of Vermont and the University of Kansas, tended to have smaller charity services than hospitals in densely populated urban areas. The greatest amount of charity care was provided at the large municipal hospitals that had established affiliations with medical schools, such as Bellevue Hospital, Los Angeles County Hospital, and Cook County Hospital, where nearly 100 percent of patients were charity cases. Urban voluntary (private) teaching hospitals, such as Barnes Hospital, Presbyterian Hospital, and the Peter Bent Brigham Hospital, usually reserved 60 to 80 percent of their beds for free care. Through the 1940s, for instance, the ward service at the Peter Bent Brigham Hospital comprised 80 percent of the hospital's inpatient census.[21] It would be an embarrassment to a voluntary hospital if its ward service dropped below 50 percent of the beds. When that happened briefly at Barnes Hospital, some of the staff felt that the hospital was doing only "a trifling amount of work" and did not deserve any further philanthropic support until it had restored the ward service back to its usual size.[22]

From the standpoint of the country's medical care system, the amount of charity care provided at academic medical centers was enormous. In Baltimore, for instance, the Johns Hopkins Hospital carried nearly 50 percent of the city's outpatient indigent load and provided more free care than the city's entire municipal hospital system.[23] The monetary value of this care was equally impressive. Precise figures are difficult to come by, but the value of the charity included both the hospital care and the foregoing of professional fees by the full-time and voluntary faculties. One study at midcentury estimated that the magnitude of free professional services at teaching hospitals, exclusive of hospital costs, exceeded $100,000,000 a year. The authors described academic medical centers as one of the greatest categories of philanthropic institutions in the country.[24]

Providing so much charity care was not easy. Teaching hospitals would usually be reimbursed by local governments for treating indigents of their jurisdiction, but invariably the governments would pay less than the actual cost of the care. In 1940, for instance, Presbyterian Hospital incurred a loss of $350,000 for care it gave to indigents of New York City.[25] Deficits would have to be made up from endowment income and gifts. Nevertheless, academic medical centers felt obligated to provide as much free care as possible. As the Hospital of Woman's Medical College of Pennsylvania put it, "We have always exceeded [the] State allowance for free work *because* we are a teaching hospital [italics mine]."[26] Academic medical centers were service-maximizers, not profit-maximizers, and deficits incurred from providing charitable care were considered a sign of doing good work.

Eligibility for treatment as a ward patient varied from hospital to hospital, each of which had its own specific rules. However, the principles were the same everywhere. As much as possible, teaching hospitals tried to restrict free care to residents of their geographic region. Patients were questioned about their income and financial resources. Only individuals below a certain income level were accepted as patients. Most teaching hospitals had a rating scale that further categorized patients according to the degree of financial need, the type and severity of illness, and the ability to withstand the financial hardship of losing time from work.[27] Many patients received free care; others were asked to contribute something, though less than the actual cost. For instance, at Presbyterian Hospital (New York), the average ward patient in 1942 paid $3.12 daily for $8.81 worth of care.[28] Teaching hospitals were keen to prevent abuse of the system by patients who could afford to see a private physician or pay for a hospital room. However, hospital administrators also knew that some patients were too proud to reveal their financial plight, and they would try to identify such individuals and not let them pay.[29]

Ward patients received good medical care. Yet, throughout this period academic medical centers adhered to a professional definition of "quality," not a consumer definition. They evaluated care by its technical merits, not by the amenities or creature comforts. The Medical Board of the New York Hospital found it "unfortunate that too much emphasis is placed on food served in the hospital." Why should patients be concerned with food, the board wondered, "when the medical and surgical treatment is the very best?"[30]

All patients endured certain indignities and discomforts: bedpans, food trays, noxious medicines and treatments, repeated examinations, needle sticks, instrumentation, bed baths, alcohol rubs, and dressing changes. Most of these were relatively unimportant to patients who entered sick and came out well. However, ward patients experienced far greater indignities than private patients. In the outpatient department, ward patients seldom received appointments and typically had long waits in noisy, overcrowded corridors. If admitted to the hospital, they were sent to large wards with 20 or more beds. There the patients were subjected to a lack of privacy, commotion, the house diet, unpleasant odors, and strict limitations on visits. Sometimes they were treated rudely by hospital personnel. The experience of the ward could be especially unpleasant at municipal hospitals, which were chronically underfunded, understaffed, overcrowded, and poorly maintained.[31] Private patients, in contrast, were given individual rooms (sometimes lavishly appointed), better food, soundproofing, extra toilets, sitz baths, showers, more liberal visiting privileges, and sometimes a sitting room for relaxation or greeting guests. As still another example of the class system of American society manifesting itself in the inner workings of the hospital, it was considered inappropriate to mix charity and private patients on the same inpatient floor or outpatient corridor.

Frank racism was not uncommon at teaching hospitals, particularly those in southern or border regions. Many teaching hospitals had segregated wards for African-American patients, including those who could afford to pay for a private room. Some hospitals conducted student teaching only on the black wards. At the Johns Hopkins Hospital, even "the highest type Negro" was frequently addressed by first name, while the Hospital of Woman's Medical College of Pennsylvania preferred having empty beds to putting white and black patients together in the same room.[32] Once again, teaching institutions reflected the discriminatory practices of society.

The provision of charity care caused many educational leaders to ponder the medical school's role in the university. Of the three primary missions of the university—education, research, and utility—it has always been utility that has engendered the greatest debate. This has been especially true for the medical school, which is the only branch of the university to practice what it teaches under university auspices. The medical school, like the rest of the university, must serve the broader society—but without becoming so inextricably involved that it loses its commitment to academic values or its capacity to serve as a moral critic.

No one gave more thought to this issue than Abraham Flexner, considered by Clark Kerr to be one of the greatest critics of the American university, not just the American medical school.[33] In a classic treatise on higher education in 1930, Flexner discussed the dilemma of utility. He acknowledged that "universities exist, partly at least, in order that they may influence the direction in which thinking and living move." However, he warned that "participation is wholesome only when subordinated to educational function."[34] Flexner concluded that medical professors had the duty to see patients, but only insofar as this work contributed to their teaching and research. Medical professors who would see patients for the sake of seeing patients—that is, participate in the ordinary practice of medicine—would no longer be discharging their responsibility to the university.[35]

In this context, the provision of charity care posed a perplexing problem for academic medical centers. The university ideal was that they should see enough patients to promote education and research, but not so many that academic pursuits would be overshadowed. However, this balance was always more easily talked about than achieved. The demands on academic medical centers for charity care were great, and growing numbers of private patients were also seeking treatment at university centers.

Nevertheless, most academic medical centers succeeded in keeping their university functions at the foreground. Several factors allowed this to happen. One was economic. At this time medical schools were not financially dependent on revenues from medical practice to pay for school expenses. A second pertained to values—the staunch commitment of both medical faculties and teaching hospitals to academic ideals. This typically resulted in the professional brakes being applied whenever the balance shifted too far in the direction of clinical service. Lastly, the vision of service remained focused on individuals and not on whole populations of patients. In the early 1940s, Mayor Fiorello H. LaGuardia of New York City asked Cornell University Medical College to provide care for a large portion of the city's population that would be receiving medical coverage under a proposed new insurance plan. The college refused.

"The function of the medical college is one of medical education," the dean explained, and not that of assuming responsibility for "an extensive program of the administration of medical care."[36] Through these various ways, academic medical centers managed to discharge their charitable role without often losing the balance among education, research, and patient care.

Medical Education and the Nation's Health

As World War II loomed, Americans were spared at least one anxiety they had had before the outbreak of World War I: the quality of the country's doctors. American medical schools had become the best in the world, and American physicians, the best prepared. A strong system of graduate medical education and specialty certification had also been created, assuring that all specialists would be thoroughly trained in their particular field.

Medical science was continuing to make great strides. The ability of medicine to "conquer" disease was symbolized by the successful treatment of President Franklin D. Roosevelt's son in 1936 with a new sulfa drug for a life-threatening streptococcal infection. Twelve years before, the son of another president, Calvin Coolidge, had died of "blood poisoning" resulting from a tennis blister.[37] By the advent of World War II, medicine and public health had achieved impressive success in their historically most important task: the understanding and control of infectious diseases.

American physicians were effectively bringing the new medical knowledge to the care of patients. Confidence in medicine had never been higher, and by the 1940s the once tarnished image of physicians in America had turned decidedly heroic.[38] Doctors were widely perceived as working on behalf of the public interest. Though the trend toward specialization had started, most physicians were still general practitioners. The house call had not vanished, accounting for four of every ten encounters between doctors and patients in 1930.[39] Physicians were perceived as advisers and counselors who knew their patients and families well. Few people resented medical incomes. Though greed was hardly absent, a spirit of charity pervaded the profession, as manifested by the enormous amount of free care doctors provided. No one knew exactly how much charity work they performed, but the monetary value was immense, and it was estimated that at least 50 percent of hospitalized patients paid no professional fees.[40] Though some specialists had very high earnings, most doctors were not getting rich. The median net income of physicians in private practice in the early 1930s was $3,800, or three times the income of the average wage earner.[41]

Medical care continued to be perceived as essential to the fiscal health of the country. Numerous studies pointed out the economic impact of disease—its role as a major cause of poverty and its deleterious effects on the nation's productivity. Medical care, at roughly $2.5 billion a year in the early 1930s, or slightly more than 3 percent of the gross national product, was not inexpensive. However, it was considered a smart investment that could result in handsome returns. "Medical care is essential," one study concluded in 1932. "While it requires substantial expenditures, its absence or inadequacy involves still greater costs."[42]

At the heart of the nation's medical care system were the academic medical centers. It was there that medical knowledge was discovered, technologies were developed, and new or improved medical practices introduced. It was also at the academic medical centers that all physicians received their undergraduate medical education and many their graduate training. Through consultations, conferences, lectures, and formal course work, medical centers also provided practicing physicians help with difficult cases and assistance in keeping current. As one medical dean wrote, it was the work of academic medical centers that "ultimately determines the standards of medical care."[43]

It was considered a truism that medical care would be only as good as the individuals practicing it—that is, that the quality of medical education determined the quality of medical practice. However, as another manifestation of the technocratic ideal in American culture, medical practice came to be considered the key to protecting the nation's health. Among doctors and the public alike, health was generally equated with the medical care available, not with any social or economic determinants. Many reformers of the era worried about the high rates of disease that occurred in some parts of the country or among certain parts of the population, but from this they inferred the need for more doctors and medical care, not improved nutrition, better housing, more efficient sanitation, a less toxic environment, safer and healthier working conditions, or better opportunities for education and employment.

Typical in this regard was the *Final Report of the Commission on Medical Education* (1932)—a major survey of undergraduate medical education organized by the Association of American Medical Colleges, but, reflecting its Depression roots, a document concerned as much with creating a healthier people and better medical care system as with medical education per se. In the view of the Commission, "The greatest health problem of the country is that of making modern medical services available to the entire population."[44] This meant maintaining the proper balance between specialists and general practitioners and redressing the geographic maldistribution of doctors that was already depriving many rural areas of physicians. To the Commission, America needed more medicine, not less, and any additional financial burden would be worth the cost. "The essential feature of a well conceived program [of medical care] is the quality of the service rendered. The organization and the methods of financial support should be formulated to improve and maintain that quality, not merely to provide a service at low cost."[45]

Being considered indispensable to the health and economic productivity of the nation represented heady expectations of medical education. Were these expectations realistic? Was there more to the nation's health than good medical care provided by well-trained doctors? Did good medical care guarantee the economic competitiveness of the country? These assumptions, though challenged in a later era, at the time were questioned by few. For the moment, individuals concerned about the health of the American people, or critical of the system of delivering medical services, wanted more medicine, not less—that is, more of the doctors, discoveries, and oversight of practice provided by the nation's academic medical centers.

7

World War II and Medical Education

MEDICAL SCHOOLS HAD LONG BEEN RESPONSIBLE for the quality of care rendered civilians, but during World War II they took direct responsibility for the military's medical care as well. The proportion of faculty that enlisted in the armed services was much higher than that of the general profession.[1] At the country's 52 general hospital units and 20 evacuation hospital units, the medical personnel, which numbered about 2,500, came almost entirely from academic medical centers.[2] At home, schools were extremely short-staffed, but they nonetheless increased the production of doctors to meet both military and civilian needs. In addition, they conducted an extraordinary amount of war-related medical research that enabled a dramatic reduction in death and suffering among troops in combat.

Medical school faculties were hardly the only doctors who assisted the war effort. Ultimately, approximately 46,000 physicians (roughly 30 percent of those in active practice) served at home or abroad in the Army Medical Corps.[3] In addition, nurses, dentists, veterinarians, technicians, and other health care professionals also served in large numbers. However, academic physicians provided the leadership. Medical schools emerged from the war with even more influence and prestige than before, and the sacrifices and contributions of their faculties reinforced the public's view that medical education was serving society's needs.

World War II resulted in no major lasting changes for medical education. Rather, its legacy was to affirm the quality of American medical schools, validate the importance of medical research, and whet the nation's appetite for more doctors and medical care. After the war, as before, the country continued to conflate the health of the people with the amount of medical care available, ignoring the behavioral, environmental, and social roots of illness. To meet the new challenges arising from the growing prevalence of chronic diseases, the answer seemed the same as always: turning to basic medical research to find the solutions. The public emerged from the war wanting more medical care, not less—or, stated another way, more of the knowledge, doctors, and services provided by the academic medical centers. For the next generation, it would seem as if medical education and research could get from a grateful public whatever it wished.

Mobilization for War

Even before the bombing of Pearl Harbor, many medical schools began to prepare for the possibility of war. For instance, in October 1939 the Harvard faculty began discussing strategies for education, research, and patient care in the event that war would call away many of the staff.[4] In October 1940, the faculty established three military base hospitals, in accordance with the surgeon general's request.[5] By March 1941, 12 members of the school's teaching staff were on active duty, and another 110 held military reserve commissions.[6] A number of other medical schools also organized military hospital units prior to the country's entry into the war.

Mobilization in medical education began in earnest following Pearl Harbor. Immediately the Association of American Medical Colleges recommended that the four-year undergraduate medical course be covered in three years.[7] Almost all schools complied. Other steps quickly followed as medical faculties strove to meet their dual task of producing more doctors and providing medical care in the theaters of war abroad.

The mobilization of Johns Hopkins was typical. By early 1942, the Hopkins faculty had assumed responsibility for two military hospital units overseas. In April 1942, 38 faculty members went into active duty; a year later, 92 faculty members were in uniform. The school's research program was severely curtailed, and much of the remaining research was geared toward projects having a direct bearing on the war. The school began offering a course on venereal disease control to medical officers of the army and navy, and many faculty members accepted important government advisory posts. Entrance requirements to the school were eased. Only two years of college were expected, and the requirement of a foreign language was suspended. The school eliminated summer vacations and electives for students and adopted an accelerated program of instruction. Internship at the hospital was also reduced in length, and residency positions were decreased in number and duration. The hospital operated on short supply. Not only were there fewer attending physicians and house officers, but there were fewer nurses and paramedical personnel as well. Supplies were rationed. Only with great difficulty could the hospital obtain meat, coffee, pharmaceuticals, and certain medical and surgical devices.[8]

The country's medical mobilization was an especially complex task because civilian medical needs also had to be met. The wartime medical work involved members of the profession at large, not just the faculties of teaching centers and new medical graduates. Private practitioners served the war effort in diverse ways: taking on public health duties, examining new recruits for the selective service, and caring for the civilian population at home. However, leadership of military medicine devolved to the teaching centers, which assumed responsibility for each of the wartime hospitals and medical camps (for instance, the 1st General Hospital Unit, manned by personnel from Bellevue Hospital, and the 20th, by doctors from the University of Pennsylvania).[9] Many practitioners from the community, particularly those under the age of 45, also served in uniform, but they usually had positions subordinate to the teachers and specialists from the academic medical centers. And of course, only the academic medical centers possessed the means to produce the new doctors that were needed at home and abroad.

For medical school faculties, mobilization for war posed a difficult dilemma. They did not object to the extra work—either the demanding service in the military hospitals, or the challenge of running a medical school and teaching hospital with a skeleton staff. However, they were deeply troubled by the lower educational standards of the accelerated programs. Munitions manufacturers would not intentionally ship defective explosives, and defense contractors would not ship substandard planes and tanks. Medical schools felt they had a similar obligation not to send out poorly trained doctors. The dean of the University of Michigan expressed the widespread concern: "We view with anxiety the effect of the accelerated program upon medical education. The rapid schedules adopted by most schools will make an immediate contribution to the war effort, but their effects upon the quality of medical education are inviting decadent trends."[10]

However, the urgency of war proved too great. Under continual pressure from military and government authorities, medical schools capitulated to the demand to increase the production of physicians. For the duration of the war they energetically, if uneasily, pursued the accelerated program.[11] Everywhere, entrance requirements were relaxed, and the 9-9-9-9 accelerated curriculum became standard. Of medical students admitted during the war, 55 percent were under contract to the army and 25 percent to the navy, leaving 20 percent for civilian service, largely women and men designated "4-F."[12] The result was the graduation of approximately 25,000 doctors during the war (an increase of 5,000 over peacetime), approximately 80 percent of whom directly entered the military after internship or residency.[13]

The war exacted a great toll on all who participated in medical education. Faculty who served abroad exchanged their privileged life at home for two or three years of uncomfortable and sometimes dangerous assignments in one or another of the military hospitals. Medical schools had the prerogative to declare certain faculty members as "essential," thereby allowing them to receive deferments, but many "essential men" voluntarily enlisted. At some medical schools, up to 60 percent of the clinical faculty served in the military.[14] From Harvard alone, a school with a large voluntary and full-time faculty, over 300 doctors ultimately participated in active war service.[15] Nationwide, by 1 July 1943, 5,637 faculty members were in active military service, and that number grew even larger as the war progressed.[16]

Faculty members remaining at home faced the imposing task of carrying on with vastly depleted personnel. With the accelerated curriculum, the amount of undergraduate teaching was 25 percent greater. The logistical problems of shortening the curriculum, rearranging classroom schedules, and finding facilities for lectures, laboratory instruction, and clinical work proved to be a minor administrative nightmare.[17] As many patients needed to be cared for as before, yet the number of clinical faculty had been greatly reduced, and there were fewer interns and residents to help. Many faculty members also had important wartime committee or consulting assignments. To accommodate these responsibilities, medical research was severely curtailed, except for war-related investigations. Life was "an awful ratrace [sic],"[18] a faculty member at a typical school recalled.

Medical students were taxed to the limits of physical endurance. With the reduction of admissions requirements, students were younger, less mature, and not as thoroughly prepared. They received no concessions because of the brevity of the course of study. As one dean put it, "While we have accelerated our program, the content of our curriculum has not been shortened."[19] Though some material was eliminated, other subjects of military importance were added: tropical medicine, first aid and traumatic surgery, the handling of gas casualties, industrial hygiene, and more emphasis on public health and venereal disease. To cover the material, teaching was often conducted beyond regular hours. For instance, junior students at Cornell received their 20 lectures in radiology from 5:00 to 6:30 P.M.[20] Because there were too few instructors for the size of the classes, lectures often substituted for laboratory and clinical work, and faculty had less opportunity to provide individualized instruction or engage in Socratic dialogues. Students had little time to contemplate, engage in research, or pursue topics of interest in detail. The result, one writer noted, was "greater superficiality in learning, less tenacity of retention of what was learned, and a minimum of that contemplation and discussion from which spring habits of independent thought."[21]

The frenzied pace of the accelerated curriculum took a great toll on many students. In a typical program, students received only one two-week break in the course of a year, usually sometime in June. Among the consequences were a greater number of scholastic casualties and an increase in the amount and severity of student illness.[22] Financial pressures on less affluent students increased since it was now much more difficult to work while in school. The army and navy paid the tuition of students who agreed to enter the service upon graduation, but that could be a mixed blessing since the students had to submit to military drills and routines, as if they did not already have enough to do learning medicine.[23] Moreover, students labored under great anxiety about their futures. No one could tell them how adequate their internship would be, whether they would get a residency, what their military assignment would be, how long they would remain in the service, whether they would be able to resume hospital training after returning from duty, or whether they would be crowded out after the war by new, better-trained generations of students.[24]

The war also exacted a great toll on graduate medical education. Internship was reduced to nine months—a change that no one was happy with, or even tried to defend educationally, but which was considered "a regrettable wartime necessity."[25] After a series of preliminary reductions, residency positions in 1943 were decreased to 50 percent of the prewar level, and the length of a typical residency was cut in half.[26] The academic, not the service, components of graduate medical education represented the parts most quickly reduced. For instance, the extensive experience residents in obstetrics and gynecology received in pathology was eliminated.[27] Research fellowships were discontinued, and for several years most scientific training programs in both preclinical and clinical departments had few if any graduate students or fellows. The country emerged from the war with a shortage of young medical teachers and investigators, similar to the shortage of instructors that developed in other scientific fields.[28]

The exigencies of war caused a number of other adjustments. Greater opportunities occurred for women to enter medical school as well as to receive advanced graduate training. Harvard Medical School finally became coeducational, and Massachusetts General Hospital noted that "throughout the hospital women are appearing in the intern and resident ranks in steadily increasing numbers."[29] Students and house officers were given new duties and responsibilities caring for private patients. Wartime shortages fostered the development of the "subinternship"—an advanced clinical elective in which senior medical students substituted for interns on vacation or illness leave. As previously noted, new courses and subject matter were added to the undergraduate curriculum, particularly on topics of wartime significance.

At the war's conclusion, the return of medical education to normal posed logistic challenges of its own, though the administrative headaches of deceleration seemed relatively minor now that the war had been won. Resuming the four-year curriculum and accommodating both new graduates and returning veterans in internships and residencies required extremely careful planning. On the other hand, the return of faculty and restoration of residency programs facilitated teaching and patient care and allowed the resumption of medical research.[30]

World War II produced no major changes in medical education. Rather, the war allowed a demonstration of the effectiveness of the system as well as of the patriotism and public-spiritedness of the faculty, students, and house officers who worked in it. After the war, the subinternship and the increased use of private patients in clinical teaching persisted; the addition to the curriculum of subjects directly pertinent to military medicine did not. The gains of women in achieving access to medicine proved fleeting, as they did in the workforce as a whole. More lasting advance of the cause of women would have to await the civil rights and feminist movements.

In contrast to industry, the increased wartime production of doctors by medical schools was modest. In almost every industry, extraordinary gains in efficiency and productivity were realized. Between Pearl Harbor and D-Day, the time needed to produce a ship decreased from six months to 12 days, while synthetic rubber production increased 100-fold.[31] By these standards, the 25 percent increase in the number of physicians produced was modest. This observation has led one author, in an otherwise discriminating article, to deem the accelerated curriculum and wartime work of medical schools a "failure."[32]

Such criticism is to misunderstand the nature of medical education and to draw erroneous analogies with industry. Certain similarities between medical schools and industrial corporations can legitimately be drawn, but industrial analogies work only to a point. The great increases in industrial productivity that occurred during the war resulted from automation and new technologies.[33] Medical education, on the other hand, remained labor-intensive and time-demanding. It continued to require personalized instruction, frequent discussions between learners and teachers, and time for students to develop problem-solving skills and the capacity to deal with uncertainty. From this perspective, the increased output of doctors was impressive.

Medical training did come under severe criticism during World War II. Complaints arose not from the military but from the medical faculties themselves, which throughout the war remained dissatisfied with many aspects of the accelerated program. They felt that in the haste to produce more doctors, educational standards were being compromised. Since the quality of medical practice depended on the quality of medical education, they were not convinced that they were doing the country an unequivocal favor. They were also aware that no other nation was accelerating the training of its doctors during the war.

Such sentiments were widespread among medical educators, pervading the discussions of the Executive Council of the Association of American Medical Colleges, the Council on Medical Education and Hospitals, the faculty meetings of numerous schools, and the published writings of prominent medical educators. No one had an "objective" or quantitative measure of the deleterious effects of accelerated medical education, but the uniform impression of dedicated teachers who actually taught was that educational quality was suffering. They were concerned about many things, including hurried teaching, the overuse of lectures, the falling use of the library, and the elimination of elective and research opportunities. Most of all, they were troubled by the loss of time, which made it much more difficult for students to reflect, assimilate material, and develop reasoning skills, problem-solving capacity, and independence. Willard C. Rappleye, chairman of the Executive Council of the Association of American Medical Colleges, concluded from a study of U.S. medical schools in 1943 that "the danger signal of a breakdown in scholastic standards is flying."[34]

In this context the greatest legacy of World War II for American medical education was in creating a resolve never again to risk compromising standards. Producing doctors was not the same as manufacturing bombs, rubber, ships, or airplanes. If the country were to need a larger number of doctors in the future, other ways must be found than taking so much time out of the education of a physician. This view prevailed when the Korean War broke out. A joint committee of the Association of American Medical Colleges and the American Medical Association recommended against adopting another accelerated program: "The price of acceleration has proved to be lowered quality of graduates, exhaustion of faculties, and serious curtailment of research. . . . The rapid production of half-trained men will make statistical charts look better but will not improve the health of the nation."[35] The committee felt that a vigorous effort should be made to increase the number of doctors—but not at the expense of quality. For much of the rest of the century, medical schools' commitment to educational quality would remain.

The War Against Disease

Historically, the soldier's greatest foe has been disease. Until the twentieth century, the mortality caused by illness vastly exceeded the number of deaths resulting directly from combat. With deprivation, exposure, overcrowding, malnutrition, and poor sanitation, military camps were routinely ravaged by epidemic diseases. Many were lethal; others (infectious diarrhea, for instance), debilitating. Moreover, battle injury carried a grave prognosis. Countless wounded soldiers did not survive their injuries because of tetanus or sepsis. Innumerable others found themselves permanently maimed because of the inability of doctors to perform even the most basic reparative surgery. By World War I conditions had improved significantly, but the influenza pandemic of 1918–19, which decimated fighting troops in Europe and claimed tens of millions of lives worldwide, served as a terrible reminder of the power of disease.[36]

As World War II began, science was considered the key to the country's defense. The government had turned to science during past wars, but never on the scale that it did now. The most pressing military needs at first seemed to be of a technological nature. In response, the National Defense Research Committee, comprised of eminent civilian scientists, was created. This committee was ultimately responsible for such developments as radar, proximity fuses, amphibious vehicles, and the atomic bomb. However, it quickly became apparent that medical science was equally vital to the war effort. Accordingly, President Roosevelt ordered the formation of a committee with similar responsibilities in medicine: the Committee on Medical Research, chaired by Alfred Newton Richards, an eminent pharmacologist at the University of Pennsylvania. The National Defense Research Committee and the Committee on Medical Research together formed the Office of Scientific Research and Development, which coordinated all defense-related scientific work.

As the physical sciences were vital to national security, so were the medical sciences. The example of physiology was typical. Because American soldiers were fighting in arctic, desert, and tropical climates, the effects of heat, cold, humidity, excessive dryness, altitude, and pressure had to be understood, and the proper food and clothing for a worldwide military force had to be determined. Soldiers in the Pacific needed uniforms light enough to keep cool yet strong enough to protect against insects, torrential downpours, and the threat of chemical warfare. The use of sophisticated aircraft required an understanding of human reflexes and fatigue and the effects of high altitudes. Through contracts with universities, medical schools, teaching hospitals, and research institutes, the Committee on Medical Research recruited physiologists to help with hundreds of such problems, and workers at almost every medical school participated.[37]

Not just physiology but virtually every medical field contributed to wartime research. The results of this vast effort, which resulted in thousands of papers and reports, almost defy imagination.[38] In the words of Richards:

> Among the many problems with which we were concerned were: protection against influenza, pneumonia, dysenteries, and gas gangrene; prophylaxis and treatment of streptococcus infections and of venereal disease; discovery and use of a substitute for quinine (taken from us by the Japanese) in the treatment of malaria, the number one menace of the tropics; acceleration of convalescence; prevention and control of bacterial infections of wounds and burns; avoidance and treatment of shock; methods of restoring blood volume after hemorrhage and preservation of whole blood for transport from this country to combat theaters; nerve regeneration and nerve repair following nerve injury; protection of aviators against lack of oxygen, cold, and 'blackout'; means for better adaptation of men to extremes of heat, cold, and humidity; protection against poison gases; insecticides and repellents with which to avoid malaria, typhus, and the other insect-borne tropical diseases.[39]

Much of the work had civilian as well as military value. Lasting contributions included vaccines against influenza, typhus, and cholera, new drug treatments of malaria, the development of the insecticide DDT, and the separation of human blood plasma into therapeutically useful constituents (albumin, globulins, and clotting factors) for the treatment of shock and control of bleeding. Probably the most important contribution of the program was the development of methods of mass-producing penicillin. At the time of the war's outbreak, the antibiotic was used only experimentally. In less than three years, through a massive collaboration involving biologists, chemists, physicians, government scientists, and the pharmaceutical industry, the scale of production increased from one-liter bottles to 15,000-gallon tanks.

The war against disease paid off spectacularly in terms of saving lives, alleviating suffering, and helping the wounded recover. During World War II, the army death rate from disease was 0.6 per thousand, compared with 14.1 per thousand during World War I. More impressive, only 3 percent of wounded soldiers died, and new surgical techniques and rehabilitative procedures allowed much speedier recoveries and much less permanent dysfunction.[40] Equally remarkable, the work of the Committee on Medical Research had been conducted at a total cost of approximately $24,000,000, or the price of financing the war for three and one-half hours.[41]

The war on disease was not without its problems. The pressure was understandably intense to develop solutions to immediate military problems. Fundamental, curiosity-driven medical investigation was severely curtailed. In addition, with the atrophy of training programs, the nation's supply of young medical scientists was depleted, resulting in serious postwar shortages. These lessons were not lost upon influential scientists charged with the development of the country's postwar science policy. As Richards put it, one consequence of the war was the universal recognition of the value of pure research as a national asset. "Most, if not all, of the useful results which have come out of medical scientific war efforts are in no real sense discoveries; they are rather the developments of discoveries made long before the war in laboratories where knowledge is pursued for its own sake with little regard for utility."[42] Accordingly, scientific leaders developed a postwar science policy that emphasized fundamental research and the training of young investigators through well-supported fellowship programs.[43]

Nevertheless, medical science during World War II brilliantly succeeded at what it was asked to do. The success of the war on disease stands as an important corrective to the widespread misperception that American medical science was immature prior to the postwar expansion of the National Institutes of Health. Rather, American medical research had already become the best in the world. The accomplishments of the war on disease would not have occurred had American medical research not already been sufficiently mature, any more than the atomic bomb would have been developed without a strong endogenous base in physics and engineering. In response to a huge infusion of federal funds, the size of America's medical research establishment was to grow enormously after the war. However, the intellectual and institutional infrastructure to make good use of those funds was already in place.

The Apotheosis of Medical Optimism

Despite inevitable continuities, the United States after World War II was a distinctly new society. The war had dramatically altered American culture, values, and aspirations. In foreign affairs, the country occupied a new position of international leadership. Domestically, the war contributed to the acceptance of a much larger, more active federal government. America ended the war a more urban, technological, and industrial nation, and the seeds of radical social change had been planted.[44]

Medicine, too, faced a new world. After the war there was considerable discussion of new methods of financing and delivering medical care. Group practice was appearing, voluntary private medical insurance plans were spreading, experiments in comprehensive medical care to individuals and communities were underway, and a national campaign for compulsory medical insurance had started. The demand for medical care was increasing, and medical care was more and more perceived as a basic right of all citizens.

The scientific challenges confronting medicine were also changing. Life expectancy in the United States had increased from 47 years in 1900 to 65 years in 1945, but people were dying of different diseases. Cardiovascular diseases, including stroke and vascular causes of renal failure, had supplanted infectious diseases as the number one killer. Other leading causes of death included cancer and degenerative conditions associated with aging. More Americans died each year from any of the most prevalent chronic diseases than died in battle during World War II. Many other chronic maladies, such as peptic ulcer, arthritis, mental illness, asthma, and hay fever, accounted for considerable suffering and disability, even if they made little impact on mortality statistics.[45]

The public was not alarmed. The experience of the war against disease during World War II suggested that these problems, too, could be solved by medical research. In his famous report to President Roosevelt, *Science, The Endless Frontier*, Vannevar Bush, Roosevelt's science adviser and director of the Office of Scientific Research and Development, outlined the approach that the country would soon adopt. Progress in combating disease, he wrote, depends upon "an expanding body of new scientific knowledge." What was needed to address chronic illnesses was a broad-based program of fundamental research since "progress in the war against disease [the report was full of military metaphors] results from discoveries in remote and unexpected fields of medicine and the underlying sciences." Bush recommended that the government begin the large-scale support of basic medical research.[46]

The Bush report found a receptive audience among federal officials, the scientific community, and the lay public. Medical research had proven itself during the recent conflagration. Why now should it not conquer chronic diseases, given enough money and support? As in the creative period of American medical education, imaginations began to soar, and popular expectations of what medical research might accomplish often took on a utopian quality. This attitude was illustrated by the World Health Organization's expansive definition of health in 1946 as "a state of complete physical, mental, and social well-being, and not merely the absence of disease or infirmity."[47]

For academic medical centers, such medical optimism represented a double-edged sword. It was beneficial in winning federal dollars for medical research, but it created the danger of disillusionment and backlash if the high expectations were not met. Medical scientists knew that progress in the control of many chronic diseases would be slow in coming since so much fundamental knowledge needed to be accumulated. As one authority wrote regarding cancer, "A $2,000,000,000 Manhattan Project on cancer—where the basic leads are not yet clear—would probably only waste large sums of money if it did not do more positive damage."[48] In addition, as important as good treatment was to those already sick, there remained nagging concerns that more was necessary to achieve a healthier population than merely making available the therapies flowing from scientific research. What was needed in guiding policy was humility and statesmanship—humility, to recognize the many broad social and behavioral determinants of health; statesmanship, to foster legitimate hope and seek appropriate support without misrepresenting the possibility of an immediate practical return. How well such leadership would be provided remained to be seen.

PART II

Medical Education in the Era of the Multiversity

The Growth of
Research and Service
in a Period of Abundance

8

The Ascendancy
of Research

IF ONE WISH DOMINATED many medical faculties from the
beginning of the modern era, it was the desire to do research. American medical schools, like their parent universities, were created and
molded by aspiring scholars with strong disciplinary identities. To educate most effectively, to determine the standards of patient care, and to
improve the level of practice for future patients, it was necessary for
medical schools to be staffed by creative faculties actively engaged in
scholarly inquiry, or so it was firmly believed. The small size of American
medical research before World War II resulted from the relative scarcity
of funds and not from any lack of faculty interest in research.

The ties formed between the federal government and academic medical centers during World War II irrevocably altered the scale of medical
research in the United States. Over the next two decades, staggering
growth in the research enterprise occurred, the result of a massive infusion of federal dollars. Although some schools received much more
money than others, ultimately all were transformed. To many observers,
the 1950s and 1960s were "the day of the 'researcher'," as research grew
to overshadow teaching and clinical practice at many academic medical
centers.[1]

The ascendancy of American medical research occurred as part of the
more generalized expansion of science and higher education in the
United States produced after the war by federal spending. Government
aid to medical research was paralleled by its aid to scientific research
through the National Science Foundation, established in 1950.[2] Federal
support transformed American universities, as it did American medical
schools—particularly the few dozen academically prominent universities
that had earned the designation of "research universities."[3] In 1960,
higher education received $1.5 billion in federal support, a 100-fold
increase from 1940, most of which went toward research.[4] The hypertro-

phy of research, the enormous growth in university size, the development of many constituencies within the university, and the university's increased involvement in the life of society led Clark Kerr, then the president of the University of California, to popularize the term "multiversity" to describe the research university in 1963.[5] What was new was not the existence of federal aid to higher education but the scale of that aid, the creation of a federal grant university sharply focused on research, and the transformation of the university into a prime instrument of national purpose.

In the pursuit of medical research during this period, one characteristic remained unchanged from the first half of the century: the commitment of workers to the public good. Medical scientists were hardly without ego, ambition, or entrepreneurial skill, but their value system remained the same as before. The objective was professional recognition, not personal financial profit (or glory, not gold, as Franklin Mall had originally put it). Medical faculty reveled in their new opportunities to pursue their curiosity in an unfettered fashion and to earn a good salary in the process. However, they also made clear their position that academic medical centers should remain socially committed institutions devoted to furthering the public good.

The Age of Federal Beneficence

In the 1940s, a great transformation in the scale of American medical research began. This growth started during World War II, as schools began receiving government contracts and grants from the Office of Scientific Research and Development. After the war, primarily as a result of continuing federal appropriations, the amount of research continued to increase. Cornell, for instance, spent $1,153,000 on research in 1950, compared with $170,000 in 1939; the University of Southern California, $595,333 in 1949–50, compared with $31,787 in 1939–40.[6] Nationwide, from 1940–41 to 1950–51, spending on research increased 900 percent at state schools and over 700 percent at private schools. For comparison, other expenditures during that time rose only 200 percent at state schools and 100 percent at private schools.[7]

Nevertheless, the public still demanded more medical research. The war against disease during World War II had yielded impressive results, raising expectations as to what a federally sponsored war against chronic diseases might accomplish during peacetime. Public support for medical research was fostered by many aspects of the cultural climate of the 1940s and 1950s: the industrial expansion and general economic prosperity, the country's outward tranquility and optimism, the acceptance of a larger role for the federal government, and the new consensus that viewed the university in general and scientific research in particular as central to the national purpose.[8] A strong lay lobby, led by Mary Lasker, the wife of advertising mogul Albert Lasker, and Florence Mahoney, whose husband owned an interest in the Cox newspaper chain, helped make medical research an important issue in Congress.

One result was the development of the National Institutes of Health (NIH). Administratively, the NIH can be traced back to a tiny public health laboratory established in 1887 on Staten Island, New York, and moved in 1891 to Washington, D.C. The responsibilities of the laboratory were gradually broadened, and in 1930 its name was changed to the National Institute of Health. That year its congressional appropriation was $43,000. In 1937 the National Cancer Institute (NCI) was organized as an independent unit; legislation in 1944 resulted in the NCI being joined to the NIH. In 1948, additional legislation empowered the surgeon general to establish separate institutes to address major disease problems. The first of these new institutes, the National Heart Institute and the National Institute for Dental Research, were created in 1948, and the singular "institute" was changed to the plural "institutes" in the name of the NIH. Each institute was instructed to conduct research within its field on the NIH campus in Bethesda, Maryland ("intramural" research), and to support research at medical schools, universities, teaching hospitals, and other sites through a program of grants and contracts ("extramural" research).[9]

Initially, many academic leaders opposed the idea that the government should continue supporting biomedical research. Their chief concerns were that federal sponsorship would distort scientific priorities and that investigators would shape projects to conform with what they believed were the aims of granting agencies. However, as the empowering capacity of federal dollars became apparent, and as intellectual freedom appeared to be preserved, most academic leaders changed their view. According to one former dean, the voices of dissent soon became "so faint that their message was completely lost in the noise of the applause from the majority (myself included), who rejected any argument against more and larger grants for research and training."[10]

Enabled by federal support, the 1950s and 1960s became a golden era of American medical research. Congress could not give the NIH enough money, and executive branch requests for allocations were routinely exceeded. This made possible an unprecedented expansion of the scale of research. The most prominent schools became even larger and stronger, and extensive research programs arose at virtually every school. To a well-known dean in 1960, "Most of our schools have changed from schools of medicine to research institutes."[11] As one sign of the nationalization of research, journals from individual institutions declined in importance relative to national specialty journals. By 1961, the most important institutional journal of all—the *Bulletin of the Johns Hopkins Hospital*—was encountering serious difficulties because it was receiving fewer and fewer submissions from members of the Hopkins faculty.[12]

The growth in research funding during the first 20 years of the NIH proved staggering. In 1947, the nation expended $87 million on medical research, of which $27 million came from the federal government and $8.3 million from the NIH. In 1966, the nation spent $2.05 billion on medical research, independent of construction and training, of which $1.4 billion came from the federal government and $800 million from the NIH. Correcting for inflation, that represented a 15-fold increase in the total dollar amount invested in medical research during that period.[13] Though no school ever admitted to having enough money, by the 1960s they all enjoyed a much healthier financial status than ever before, and some were considered rich. By 1972, medical schools accounted for 10 percent of the total expenditures of higher education and employed about 10 percent of all personnel, even though they enrolled only about 0.5 percent of students.[14]

The support of medical research following World War II was not confined to the federal government. State legislatures generously supported their medical schools, foundations and private donors continued to make sizeable gifts, and corporations increased their ties with medical schools. Yet, federal sources came to exceed all others combined. In 1968, the U.S. government accounted for 58 percent of the income of medical schools.[15] Foundations saw their role change from that of the principal patrons of medical research to advocates of special causes (for instance, the American Cancer Society and the National Foundation for Infantile Paralysis) or sponsors of innovative experiments in education, research, or the delivery of care that, if successful, could be emulated by others. In this latter category, the Commonwealth Fund played an especially important role in the 1950s and 1960s, as in its support of the development of a highly influential, organ-based medical curriculum at Western Reserve University.[16]

A large amount of federal money went into the infrastructure of research. For instance, at midcentury buildings and equipment were aging, and space was severely constrained. It was said at the time that "if people were not working in closets, and if apparatus were not placed in the corridors, the laboratories were not being properly utilized." Under the Health Research Facilities Construction Act of 1956, the federal government provided matching funds for equipment and facilities—an offer that few schools failed to take advantage of.[17] Similarly, the NIH appropriated sizeable funds to support training programs in medical research. A host of new or expanded opportunities arose, such as M.D.–Ph.D. training programs for scientifically oriented medical students and a variety of fellowships for Ph.D. and postdoctoral study. By the early 1960s, some schools, such as Yale and the University of California, San Francisco, had more graduate students working toward Ph.D. degrees than undergraduate medical students.[18]

Medical schools and faculty benefited in diverse ways from federal research grants. For instance, in the 1950s NIH regulations began permitting faculty to use their grants for salary support, not just the expenses of research. This policy provided significant financial relief to medical schools, allowed faculty salaries to rise, and fostered further expansion. Similarly, the NIH continually liberalized payments to medical schools and universities for the indirect costs of research (items such as utilities, mortgage payments, and the upkeep of the buildings and laboratories). From 8 percent in the early 1950s, overhead was increased to 15 percent in the mid-1950s and 20 percent in the early 1960s. Thus, if an investigator in the early 1960s were to obtain a $50,000 grant, his sponsoring institution received an additional $10,000. Federal grants also paid for personnel such as secretaries, glassware washers, animal care assistants, and laboratory technicians. This relieved investigators from most of the mundane tasks of research.

The postwar growth of research proceeded relatively undisturbed by many important events of the period. McCarthyism, for instance, exacted a major toll on many university campuses.[19] However, scarcely any evidence of the inquisition can be found in medical school records, perhaps because of the absence of political radicalism on medical campuses and the public's satisfaction with what medical research was contributing to the common good.[20] Similarly, the Korean War exerted little effect on medical schools. Faculties were attuned to the possibility of another extended conflict, and they had publicly declared their resolve not to allow teaching or research to be shortchanged. Fortunately, however, they did not have to be put to the test.

Though many cultural forces influenced the growth of research, individuals also mattered. At the national level, no scientist was more important than James A. Shannon, who, as director from 1955 to 1968, led the NIH through its years of greatest expansion. At the institutional level, individuals also made a difference. Thus, the postwar transformation of Baylor University College of Medicine into a major research center can be attributed in large measure to the work of the surgeon Michael De Bakey, and that of Southwestern, to the nephrologist Donald W. Seldin. Similarly, the rapid rise to elite status of the University of Washington School of Medicine, which was not even established until after the war, owed much to the leadership of the endocrinologist Robert Williams. At the disciplinary level, individuals once again made a difference. In internal medicine, for instance, no person was more important that Eugene Stead, the long-standing chairman of the department of medicine at Duke, who transformed a good department into an outstanding one and whose residency program became famous for the large number of trainees who subsequently became prominent department chairmen.

The explosion of research funding produced profound changes at each of the nation's medical schools. Physical plants, faculty sizes, graduate training programs, and operating budgets grew enormously, and most of the growth pertained to research. By the 1950s, many schools were spending more money on research than on all other activities combined.[21] "The teaching staff would be small if it were not for the research projects supported by outside organizations,"[22] a medical school dean observed. By 1954, 65 of 80 medical schools employed full-time faculty; a decade later, that practice had become universal.[23] From 1951 to 1966, the number of salaried faculty at U.S. medical schools increased from about 3,500 to more than 17,000.[24] Every school enjoyed dramatic growth, but none as much as Harvard Medical School, which became the wealthiest of all. Federal support, a school official observed, has "enriched Harvard beyond anything that private sources had ever accomplished."[25] The income of Harvard Medical School from government sources rose from a little over $1,000,000 (26 percent of the school's total budget) in the early 1950s to nearly $26,000,000 two decades later (64 percent of the total budget).[26]

Of course, even in the federal era American medical schools remained a diverse group. In 1963, medical schools spent on average $5 million for research, but the range was $1.2 million to $16.1 million. The ten highest "haves," as they were called, averaged $11.3 million; the ten worst-off "have-nots," $1.7 million.[27] Schools remained conscious of their special missions and distinctive local traditions. For instance, Woman's Medical College and Howard continued to emphasize the education of women and African-Americans, respectively. The Catholic medical schools met regularly to discuss their mutual problems, particularly the challenge of remaining competitive in a more liberal social environment that provided greater opportunities for Catholics.[28] Outstanding state schools, such as Michigan, Minnesota, Wisconsin, and Colorado, wrestled with how to serve as national institutions through research while at the same time fulfilling their obligation to produce practitioners for the state.

Nevertheless, the distinct consequence of federal spending was greater homogenization of medical schools. By the 1960s even the least well-funded schools had developed thriving scientific programs. At Jefferson, still considered a clinical school, research activities had increased five-fold from 1946 to 1960, and plans were underway to expand the research program still further.[29] At Woman's Medical College, the number of full-time faculty by 1967 had grown to 75. This was about one-half to two-thirds the complement of the average medical school at the time, but it was still a matter of pride to that persistently underfunded school.[30] At Temple, research grants increased from virtually nothing in the late 1940s to $1,300,000 in 1958–59 and to $5,370,894 in 1968–69.[31] By the 1968-69 fiscal year, Arkansas was spending over $2,500,000 on scientific research and training—more than ten times its entire budget at the end of World War II.[32] Few schools could rival the scientific capacity of Harvard or Johns Hopkins, but even the lower tier schools were just as committed to promoting research.

In these expansionary times, competition among medical schools was fierce, especially to acquire and retain leading faculty members. Though scientific training programs had grown everywhere, job opportunities had mushroomed even more, creating a bull market for academic medicine. In 1960 there were 851 unfilled full-time positions in the country's medical schools, an increase of 196 from the year before.[33] In the race for faculty members, schools engaged in what one dean called "jungle warfare."[34] No school was immune from raids on its faculty. Competitors would woo a medical professor with offers of higher pay, more space, new equipment, a larger number of research fellows or graduate students, more internal funding, and fewer institutional responsibilities that might interfere with research.

All aspiring medical faculty benefited from the bull market, but none as much as Jewish medical scientists, whose opportunities in academic medicine now flourished with the quiet end of institutional anti-Semitism. Federal agencies allocated research grants on merit, not religion, and many of the most impressive proposals came from Jewish investigators. To most schools, hungry for talented faculty who could bring in large grants with lucrative overhead payments, religion ceased to matter. Ironically, the increased opportunity for Jewish investigators worked to the disadvantage of Mount Sinai Hospital, long a haven for Jewish medical scholars. As opportunities for Jews increased at medical schools, fewer and fewer sought positions at Mount Sinai. In the 1950s the hospital found its stature within medicine waning, even as the Jewish influence within the profession was rising.[35]

In the intense competition for money, faculty, and resources, no school fared better than Harvard. The school's position as the country's most prestigious medical school resulted mainly from its success at research and its productivity in training investigators who subsequently joined the faculty at other institutions. In the 1950s a handful of schools were net exporters of faculty (seven schools produced more than 50 percent of the nation's full-time teachers), but none was more successful in this regard than Harvard. Fifteen percent of the nation's full-time medical teachers had received all or some of their training at Harvard or its affiliated hospitals.[36] A cachet developed around the school—one that many Harvard doctors worked to enhance by speaking regularly of "Harvard medicine." Though the school eminently deserved its high reputation, the Harvard ego was not small and the faculty could be smug. Thus, when the school offered a talented assistant professor of anatomy a promotion to associate professor, a faculty supporter wrote, "The fact that he has recently been considered for the chairmanship of the departments of anatomy at Southwestern, Vanderbilt, and Colorado, clearly indicates that he has the scientific stature to merit consideration for . . . [an associate professorship] at Harvard."[37]

The ascendancy of research placed the medical school in an ambivalent relationship with the rest of the university. In some ways it brought the two closer. The university spirit, everyone recognized, represented a state of mind in which scholarship stood as a high institutional priority. From this perspective, the increase of research at medical schools and the strong disciplinary identities of faculty members reinforced the position of medicine as a university field. In 1949, the Washington University medical faculty felt so much a part of the university that they voted to donate a portion of their income to the university to help offset a budgetary shortfall faced by the liberal arts campus.[38]

On the other hand, the growth of research also increased the independence of many medical schools from their parent universities, in large part because of their growing ability to support themselves. Sometimes medical schools acted with impunity, making decisions without consulting the university or even in defiance of the university's wishes.[39] There was far less interaction between unversities and medical schools than many had hoped, even where the two shared the same location. Tensions often flared, especially over the higher salaries that medical school faculties typically received. It was extremely irritating to many university faculty to be paid less than comparably trained medical faculty doing the same type of work, as, for example, in biochemistry.[40]

As medical schools grew, there was usually little planning. Most research grants went to individual faculty members pursuing their particular interests, not to medical schools for institutional purposes. The typical result was that new research programs were simply added on to old in piecemeal fashion, and little thought was given to terminating programs that might have outlived their usefulness. Moreover, it was hardly unknown for an investigator or a school to make an application simply because money in Washington was available. One of the few who worried about these issues was Milton S. Eisenhower, the president of the Johns Hopkins University and brother of President Dwight D. Eisenhower. "Is there an optimal limit or rate to this rapid expansion?" he asked in 1960. He feared that "the system of project grants, rapidly increasing year by year, essentially without total perspective and purpose, is pulling us unconsciously in an undesirable direction."[41] Another contemporary critic from the Massachusetts General Hospital also expressed his dismay at the recalcitrance of medical schools to plan for optimum size or to develop a coherent research strategy: "No matter how much space can be built it will be filled. I guess the question is with what."[42] Such concerns went largely unheeded, however, as most medical schools were content to go wherever the money could be found.

Though some may have worried about the unbridled growth, all admired the achievements of medical research. Among the important events were the birth of molecular biology, the description of sickle cell anemia as the first identified molecular disease, the expansion of knowledge in immunology, and the development of the technique of radioimmunoassay (the use of radioactive materials to detect and measure very small amounts of protein particles—an analytical technique of great importance in medical and biological research). Much of immediate therapeutic value was also discovered. An array of new antibiotics was developed, as were cortisone, the polio vaccine, and effective new drugs for the treatment of high blood pressure, heart disease, and certain types of cancer. The era witnessed remarkable events in surgery: cardiac catheterization, open heart surgery, and the beginning of organ transplantation. High technology entered medicine with the creation of the extracorporeal pump (the heart-lung machine), renal dialysis (the artificial kidney), and mechanical ventilators.

Throughout this period, the traditional conviction of experimental medicine that fundamental study yields practical results seemed vindicated. This was illustrated by the development of the polio vaccine. The names Jonas Salk and Albert Sabin were lionized for their vaccines, but their work was made possible by the tissue culture technique developed by John F. Enders, Frederick Robbins, and Thomas H. Weller. This technique, the product of much basic research, allowed poliovirus for the first time to be cultivated. Only then could a vaccine against it be developed. It was Enders, Robbins, and Weller—and not Salk or Sabin—who received the Nobel Prize.[43]

Despite these accomplishments, chronic and degenerative illnesses were proving strong adversaries. By 1960, the average life expectancy in the United States had risen to over 70 years. However, of the 23 years gained since 1900, only 4½ had been added to the lives of persons over 45.[44] This placed medical scientists in a difficult position politically. They understood the power of experimental methods, and they recognized that effective treatments would not be developed except by rigorous laboratory research. Yet they also knew that the problems of cancer, heart disease, stroke, arthritis, and neurological diseases—not to mention aging itself—were not amenable to quick or easy cures. When it came time to appeal to the public, cautious optimism lost out. Most public representatives of medical science became expansive in their portrayal of what research might accomplish, if only given more money. Thus, the Association of American Medical Colleges, testifying before Congress in 1969, declared, "It is interesting to speculate about the medical advances which might have occurred in the past decade if a sum equal to that invested in space exploration had been spent on health research."[45]

A few leading investigators warned against encouraging unrealistic expectations. Alfred N. Richards, who had headed the successful war against disease during World War II, warned in 1957 that money alone would not guarantee results. "You can't get a baby in one month by making nine women pregnant."[46] René Dubos, an outstanding biologist and medical scientist at the Rockefeller Institute for Medical Research, argued against "the illusion that perfect health and happiness are within man's possibilities." Human beings, he wrote, like all living things, are in equilibrium with their environment. Eliminate one disease, and another will take its place. If a human should be so fortunate as to enjoy a healthy life, death will still ultimately occur. "Complete and lasting freedom from disease is but a dream remembered from imaginings of a Garden of Eden."[47] However, in the prosperous and optimistic era before the Vietnam War, Richards and Dubos represented the exception. Few dared—or cared—to be cautious.

To most medical school officials in the 1960s, the expansion of federal support had been a godsend. Federal dollars had allowed the growth of medical research and the development of medical schools beyond anyone's wildest expectations. Moreover, scientists themselves had generally been responsible for allocating the funds, which alleviated much of the earlier concern that politics would direct research. Of course, support from any external source always carried the risk of interference. However, after two decades, the federal record in this regard compared favorably with money from alumni, philanthropists, foundations, industry, and state legislatures. Most educators concluded that on balance federal support had accomplished much good. As a consultant to one school wrote, "If a faculty member opposes this practice on the basis of academic idealism, it shows that he has not been faced with the facts of economic realism concerning the financing of the college."[48]

Nevertheless, after a generation of federal support, medical schools—and multiversities—found themselves more vulnerable than before. Federal funds, like any external support, did not assure continuing growth and development since grants end and support can be withdrawn. As medical schools began to pay less and less of their own way, almost imperceptibly they began to lose control of their own destiny. They had always been dependent on external help, but never before had they been in a situation where as much as two-thirds of their operating budget came from a single outside source. As the ratio of "soft" to "hard" dollars grew each year, few medical schools worried. They were becoming wealthier, and to some it seemed that federal support would continue to grow forever. Yet, what medical schools gained in resources, they lost in autonomy, for they became dependent on one patron.

Changing Intellectual Directions

If medical research grew in size after World War II, it also shifted in intellectual direction. As the atom was smashed in the 1940s, so was the cell. After the war, medical research became much more reductionistic than before—that is, the emphasis turned to the subcellular and molecular level, and life processes were increasingly understood in physical and chemical terms. Medical research merged with general and theoretical biology—hence the growing use of the new term "biomedical." These trends had been underway since before the war, but in the 1950s and 1960s they achieved much fuller expression.

Underlying the transformation of biomedical research was the molecular revolution that was transforming the whole of biology. At the core of this revolution was the growing recognition that all biological events can be explained by fundamental chemical and physical laws governing the spatial arrangements and interactions of atoms and molecules. The most important examples related to genetics and protein synthesis. A universal genetic code was uncovered in which all genetic information was stored in predictable form in deoxyribonucleic acid (DNA). The DNA molecule, which represented a series of genes, transmitted its information to ribonucleic acid (RNA), which in turn guided the production of specific proteins. Such work was made possible by powerful new investigative tools like electron microscopy, X-ray crystallography, and radioimmunoassays. A growing unity of biology evolved that made observations in even the smallest living organisms, like viruses, applicable to humans.

At the medical school, these changes were most apparent in the scientific departments. The focus in anatomy shifted from gross anatomy and microscopic histology to the morphology and function of subcellular elements detected by the electron microscope. Biochemistry turned from nutrition and intermediate metabolism to enzyme systems and biochemical and molecular genetics. Physiology moved from mammalian organ function to fundamental cellular processes like nerve conduction and membrane permeability. Bacteriology evolved into microbiology, the study of all microbial organisms, with a particular focus on microbial physiology and genetics. The emphasis in pharmacology shifted from the effects of drugs on intact animals to the effects of chemical agents at the cellular and membrane level.[49] Before the war, these departments were collectively known as the "preclinical" departments, but by the 1950s they were generally called the "basic science" departments, reflecting their divorce from clinical medicine and their new focus on matters of interest to theoretical biology.[50] As another manifestation of the growing unity of biology, the intellectual borders among these disciplines began to break down, and cross-disciplinary fields, such as immunology, cell biology, and molecular genetics, began to flourish.

Fueled by NIH funds, the basic science departments began to look more and more like university science departments. Many expanded their graduate programs, and some took on the appearance of independent research institutes. By 1963, for instance, the Department of Microbiology at Cornell had about 30 graduate students—more than were enrolled at the whole medical school 10 or 15 years before.[51] Basic science faculties, which had employed growing numbers of Ph.D.s before the war, now came to be dominated by Ph.D.s. The National Board of Medical Examiners, which conducted the examination that most students took for medical licensure, began using mainly Ph.D.s to write questions in the basic sciences.[52]

A similar scientific maturation occurred in the clinical departments. By the 1950s, the observational approach to clinical investigation had passed its era of peak usefulness, as there were only so many clinical entities to be uncovered and described. Instead, the analytical or physiological approach became dominant. As discussed earlier, this approach had started before World War II, but after the war it came to define the field. Clinical investigators increasingly employed laboratory methods to delineate the biochemical mechanisms of disease (or "pathophysiology") and develop rational therapies. Gynecologists, who once published articles primarily concerning operative techniques, now studied cytology, endocrinology, and metabolism. Obstetrical research expanded to encompass reproductive biology, including contraception and infertility. Surgeons studied the physiological changes induced by anesthesia, which resulted in much greater attention being paid to pre- and postoperative care. Clinical investigators from internal medicine, pediatrics, and surgery studied the immune system, including mechanisms of inciting and suppressing an immunological or inflammatory response. The *Journal of Clinical Investigation*, the most important journal of clinical research, began to look more and more like a journal of applied biochemistry.

Clinical investigators after the war were much more thoroughly trained in bench research than workers in the field before the war. Instead of a relatively brief time in a laboratory to pick up whatever scientific skills they needed, an experience often combined with residency, they now spent several years studying one or more of the basic sciences. Some took Ph.D. degrees along with their medical training, others worked for several years in a basic science laboratory at the NIH, still others spent several years in a research laboratory of a clinical department, and some did all three. Conventional medical study simply did not teach how to design experiments in the same rigorous fashion.

As knowledge increased and techniques proliferated, clinical science became more specialized, and the number of subspecialty divisions in clinical departments grew rapidly. This was especially true of internal medicine, where a major department in the 1960s might have ten or more subspecialty divisions or units. However, subspecialists in the different fields had much in common, as manifested by the fact that the most important meetings in clinical research were not the subspecialty society meetings but the Atlantic City meetings, which continued to bring together clinical scientists of all interests.[53]

Though clinical scientists of the 1950s and 1960s were highly sophisticated scientifically, they shared important characteristics with clinical scientists of the observational era: the focus on questions of immediate bearing to patient care and the capacity to excel as clinicians and teachers. Clinical investigators now required research laboratories of their own (their work was too complex to allow them to use hospital diagnostic laboratories, as before), but, of great symbolic importance, their laboratories were usually located within the hospital and not in a separate facility. The leading clinical scientists—in internal medicine, George Thorn, W. Barry Wood, A. McGehee Harvey, Carl Moore, Cecil Watson, Fuller Allbright, Max Wintrobe, Paul Beeson, Eugene Stead, Robert Williams, and William Daughaday, among many others—were notable for their ability to combine scientific and clinical excellence. Daughaday, for instance, rose to prominence for fundamental work in endocrinology and later was elected to the National Academy of Sciences. Yet he always maintained an active clinical practice, appeared repeatedly on lists of the nation's best doctors, and excelled at clinical teaching. To students and house officers, the eminent clinical scientists were still the master clinicians and clinical teachers. Many worried that the new demands of clinical research might lead to an atrophy of clinical acumen, but as yet that had not widely happened.

The success of biomedical research was not without problems for medical education. As both basic and clinical research matured, it was no longer reasonable to assume that research scientists could be produced as a by-product of the education of physicians. James Shannon remarked in 1957, "Unlike the university-trained Ph.D. candidate, these individuals [M.D.s] have little or no training in research methodology, procedure, and theory, and so they are handicapped in proceeding effectively to advanced research."[54] Biomedical research acquired an independent quality, no longer requiring the presence and stimulation of medical students. For many faculty, the joy and excitement that was once associated with teaching medical students began to migrate upward along the training path to graduate students, fellows, and postdoctoral students who could more fully appreciate the nuances of their projects.

In addition, the perpetual challenge to correlate basic science with clinical teaching became more difficult than ever. In every clinical field, tensions arose between research on one hand and clinical care and teaching on the other. These strains were evident every time a chief resident selected a topic for grand rounds. Should the topic be clinical or scientific? Should a case be presented, or was the topic so scientific that it would be better to proceed directly to the talk? These strains were also apparent every time a new department chairman was to be appointed. Should the new chief be primarily a scientist or a clinician—a rat doctor or an eminent clinical master? The biochemist-clinician controversy raged invariably whenever a major clinical appointment was to be made.[55]

Despite these problems, for the time being most rejoiced in the theoretical and practical results of biomedical research. Medical educators retained their traditional conviction that research, patient care, and teaching go hand-in-hand and cannot be separated without loss. If basic scientists were increasingly removed from the problems of clinical medicine, clinical scientists could forge that bridge, since they fluently spoke the language of both science and patient care. The most distinguished faculty in all departments still taught medical students, even if sometimes grudgingly. For the moment, the intellectual harmony among research, education, and patient care remained intact. However, the balance was delicate, and the forces drawing them apart were growing stronger.

The Decline of Academic Gentility

With the easy availability of federal funds, the many successes of biomedical research, and the adulation of the public, the two decades following World War II represented a "golden age" for medical schools. Yet, during this period the quality of academic life gradually changed. American medical schools evolved from modestly sized educational institutions into large, multifaceted organizations. The earlier sense of family, intimacy, and institutional loyalty declined, and their administration became challenging and often frustrating.

For faculty, the postwar period was one of unbridled opportunity, as departments and schools began to recruit at an unprecedented level. Most departments retained their pyramidal structure—that is, the higher the academic rank, the fewer the positions. However, to accommodate the rapidly enlarging pool of talented faculty, departments for the first time increased the number of appointments at the senior level. For instance, the Department of Medicine of Washington University in 1955 had 10 full-time full professors in addition to the chairman and 20 full-time associate professors.[56] In this bull market, income levels rose (see Tables 4, 5, and 6),[57] as did faculty perquisites such as better retirement plans, insurance benefits, and college tuition assistance for their children. In the mid-1960s, Columbia was paying $3,155 in fringe benefits on a $20,000 salary.[58] Such developments for the first time allowed a widespread sense of financial security to pervade academic medicine.

Faculty opportunities varied from school to school and field to field. Typically, appointment and promotion were easier in a less competitive field, such as anesthesiology, or at a less prestigious school. Many schools allowed clinical faculty up to ten years to be promoted to associate professor, compared with the strict "up or out" rule of seven years at universities (though medical schools frequently found themselves at odds with the American Association of University Professors on this issue).[59] Promotions invariably came more easily to those being wooed by other institutions. Thus, the rapid advancement of the surgeon W. Gerald Austen at Harvard Medical School to associate professor in the winter of 1964–65 (and to full professor a year and a half later) resulted not only from his outstanding qualifications but also from the fact that Harvard did not want to lose him. Johns Hopkins had offered him a full professorship, and he was a leading candidate for at least two departmental chairmanships.[60]

Though opportunities for faculty were growing, such opportunities did not come without cost. With support increasingly provided from "soft" (that is, neither guaranteed nor permanent) money, medical scientists found themselves on a treadmill to support themselves. Faculty members were under intense pressure to obtain grants, and often they had to find funds from multiple sources. Consider the support of an assistant professor of pediatrics at Harvard Medical School who was undergoing review for promotion to associate professor:

> With respect to the financing of Dr. P's immediate future, there are several pathways. For next year, he has the Fellowship from the Cerebral Palsy Foundation and we have proposed to supplement this from the training

Table 4 Comparison of average maximum salaries paid to full-time faculty members of the rank of instructor or above in 34 four-year medical schools for fiscal years 1940–41 and 1949–50

	Medical basic science faculty, 34 schools				Clinical faculty, 32 schools			
	Number of schools	*1940–41*	*1949–50*	*Percent increase*	*Number of schools*	*1940–41*	*1949–50*	*Percent increase*
Professor								
Tax-supported schools	13	$6,042	$10,035		13	$7,520	$11,785	
Privately supported schools	21	8,528	11,067		19	11,125	15,632	
Average	34	7,578	10,702	41	32	9,580	14,069	47
Associate Professor								
Tax-supported schools	13	4,268	6,747		13	5,333	8,627	
Privately supported schools	21	4,756	7,217		19	7,020	9,010	
Average	34	4,579	7,037	54	32	6,378	8,862	39
Assistant Professor								
Tax-supported schools	13	3,565	6,007		13	3,914	6,811	
Privately supported schools	21	3,631	5,953		19	4,574	7,801	
Average	34	3,606	5,974	66	32	4,274	7,372	72
Instructor								
Tax-supported schools	13	2,408	4,014		13	2,735	4,810	
Privately supported schools	21	2,597	4,210		19	3,008	5,925	
Average	34	2,526	4,133	64	32	2,918	5,527	89

Note: The figures given for average salaries of full-time faculty members of the teaching staffs of the medical schools represent very roughly that amount which is paid by the medical school itself. In many institutions the so-called "full-time" faculty member is allowed to supplement his income by consultations, either private or in government or industry. In other institutions full-time faculty members receive a part of their stipend from hospitals or from university teaching appointments outside the medical school. In the past this has been especially true of the clinical years, with some institutions relying entirely on volunteer or part-time instruction in these years.

Of these 34 schools one had no full-time clinical faculty members and one had only one instructor. These schools are therefore not included in figures for clinical faculty.

Table 5 Faculty salaries at a medical school: University of Maryland, 1954

	Base Salary	Total Salary
Basic Science Departments		
Professor and Head	$12,000	No Limit Set
Professor	9,500	$12,000
Associate Professor	8,000	9,500
Assistant Professor	6,500	8,000
Instructor	5,000	6,500
Junior Instructor	3,500	4,700
Assistant	3,000	4,000
Clinical Departments—Absolute Full-time		
Professor and Head	$15,000	$18,000
Professor	12,750	14,250
Associate Professor	10,500	12,750
Assistant Professor	8,250	10,500
Associate	6,000	8,250
Instructor	5,000	7,000
Assistant	3,500	5,500

Clinical Departments—Geographic Full-time with Compensation

	Base Salary	Earning Limit	Net Total
Professor and Head	$12,000	$9,000	$21,000
Professor	9,400	7,125	16,525
Associate Professor	8,500	6,375	14,875
Assistant Professor	7,000	5,250	12,250
Associate	5,500	4,125	9,625
Instructor	4,666	3,500	8,166
Assistant	3,666	2,750	6,416

Table 6 Faculty salaries, 1965 (medians)

	Strict				Geographic			
	Dept. Chairman	Professor	Associate Professor	Assistant Professor	Dept. Chairman	Professor	Associate Professor	Assistant Professor
Basic Science	21,500	17,500	14,500	11,500				
Pathology	27,000	23,000	20,000	16,000	24,186	19,500	17,250	14,000
Medicine	30,250	23,928	19,000	15,500	27,000	19,500	16,400	13,500
Surgery	32,000	28,000	22,000	17,500	25,872	20,000	17,000	14,000
Obs.-Gynecology	30,000	25,000	20,000	16,000	24,986	20,453	16,695	14,172
Pediatrics	28,000	23,000	18,090	15,000	26,000	21,000	17,500	14,014
Psychiatry	30,000	23,500	20,000	15,575	24,209	20,000	17,250	14,900
Anesthesiology	30,000	27,000	22,000	20,251	23,852	22,502	16,000	15,000
Radiology	31,000	28,500	23,000	19,000	26,982	21,468	18,768	15,500
Public Health–Preventive Medicine	23,500	20,000	16,875	14,000	24,000	21,500	16,200	13,625
Other Clinical	24,500	21,250	18,218	15,000	20,578	18,325	15,000	12,950

grant that is held by Max Finland and myself. . . . A salary for an Assistant Program Director to be affiliated with each of us was included in the training grant program, with a sum of money insufficient for full-time support, but sufficient to act as a supplement to other sources of support. After the forthcoming year is under way, we would hope to submit P for a Research Career Development Award from the United States Public Health Service. At the same time, we are in the process of submitting a proposal for a rather extensive program having to do with the role of perinatal factors in development. . . . P would be listed [as a participant in the study]. . . . He is preparing an application for grant support to cover his growing interest in the physiology of endotoxin.

To this, the department promised to contribute another $1,000 per year of its own funds.[61]

To add to faculty concerns, the grant application process became increasingly complex and time-consuming, as did the requirements for reporting from successful applicants. The dean of Cornell complained, "The annual requirement of intensive foraging for funds, preparation of reports, and supporting data exhausts a great deal of the energy of investigators which could be spent with more profit in other activities."[62] Biomedical research had become a demanding taskmaster. Whereas before the war medical scientists had been bench workers surrounded by a few colleagues in modest quarters, they were now increasingly forced to become entrepreneurs.

Academic life for faculty became more and more frenetic. Not only did they face the continual problems of seeking funds and reporting on the use of those funds, but the competition became keener. In an era of expansion, there was always someone new coming along, challenging one's work or ideas. Moreover, faculty had to endure the constant uncertainty that a new grant might not be found. For now, most schools minimized this possibility and came to regard NIH funds as almost as "hard" as income from endowments and tuition. It was tempting to view NIH funds as a way to increase the size, salary level, and research support of the faculty without drawing on institutional funds.[63] Yet, as a few administrators recognized, there was never any guarantee that additional funds would be forthcoming. George P. Berry, the dean of Harvard Medical School, observed in 1961 that investigators working on grants "simply do not have the security and peace of mind they would have on University funds."[64]

With the ascendancy of research, institutional loyalty diminished. The executive committee of the New York University College of Medicine observed, "The fact that many more members of the faculty are dependent upon outside granting agencies, not only for the support of their research projects, but also for their salary, undoubtedly weakens the ties to the school."[65] Research grants could be used for salary support only for the portion of a faculty member's time spent in research. This gave many faculty members the leverage to demand and receive "protected" time—that is, time for research that was protected from teaching, clinical duties, and administrative service to the school. Most research grants were portable, allowing faculty members to move readily from one school to another if a better opportunity could be found. Moreover, the growth of research resulted in numerous extrainstitutional duties: serving on the editorial boards of journals and governing councils of specialty societies, reviewing grant requests for the NIH or private agencies, consulting for government or industry, and lecturing at professional meetings, symposia, conferences, medical schools, teaching hospitals, and other gatherings around the world. "Cosmopolitan professors" (faculty who spent considerable time away from home) had existed before World War II, but the growth of the research enterprise, the increased availability of travel funds from research grants, and the growing popularity of airplane travel greatly increased their numbers. Francis D. Moore, Mosely Professor of Surgery at Harvard, observed:

> The present-day professor readily becomes a member of the jet set. He loves to go and take airplanes. We have members of this Faculty who do not spend a single week entirely at home in the course of an entire academic year. They will accept any and all invitations at other universities. . . . But it is very difficult to get them to attend a student session here.[66]

In the age of the multiversity, traditional "turf battles" among and within departments became more intense. Departments and divisions vied mightily to receive the most space, money, and opportunities. In the basic sciences, anatomy departments continued their relative decline in influence, biochemistry departments saw their stature continue to increase, and new fields like human genetics and molecular biology provided important political and intellectual capital to the department that managed to expropriate those subjects for themselves—here biochemistry, there physiology or microbiology. In the clinical fields, the forces toward subspecialization continued to grow. This was most pronounced in internal medicine but was also conspicuous in pediatrics and surgery. The strength of the various clinical departments varied from school to school, depending mainly on the intellectual and personal qualities of the department chairs, but in general internal medicine and surgery remained the dominant departments.

At most medical schools, the rapid growth in faculty size, the frenetic chase for grants, and the increasing competitiveness of biomedical research led to a loss of the close association with colleagues that had characterized faculty life before World War II. As early as 1947 the executive committee of the University of Pennsylvania School of Medicine observed that "the members of the faculty did not now know each other"[67]—a situation that only intensified with time. Medical school events that once drew large crowds were now often poorly attended. Faculty newsletters were established to disseminate information that at an earlier time everyone knew as a matter of course. Many faculty knew few people outside their department, basic science and clinical faculty were frequently at odds (in no small measure owing to the extraordinary growth in size and power of the clinical departments), junior faculty frequently felt that their views and concerns were irrelevant to those who governed the institution, and even full professors often felt they had little say in school affairs (unless they were department heads). The esprit de corps and sense of common purpose began to decline—slowly in the 1950s, more rapidly in the 1960s. Of course, there were always exceptions. Robert Loeb, an eminent internist and longtime chairman of the department at Columbia, managed to retain the loyalty of a group of able senior faculty who chose to stay with him rather than to accept lucrative offers to chair other departments at far higher salaries.[68] Nevertheless, such examples were increasingly rare. Fewer faculty retained a strong feeling for the institution as a whole, and individual interests gradually became stronger than group interests.

Among those who suffered the most from the decline of community at medical schools were the voluntary (part-time) clinical faculty members. With the ascendancy of research and the growth of clinical specialization, part-timers at many schools found themselves being replaced by full-timers for the major clinical positions. At the Massachusetts General Hospital, for instance, the part-time faculty felt more and more removed from the institution as "research men with little interest in part-time staff activities" were being appointed chiefs of the various clinical units.[69] Voluntary faculty continued to teach, but increasingly they were given the less prestigious assignments (teaching physical diagnosis to second-year medical students, for instance), and their influence and stature at most schools decreased. Once an integral part of the metaphorical medical school family, voluntary faculty now often felt that the schools had become insensitive to their needs and unappreciative of their efforts.

Medical school deans also found their positions becoming more demanding with the ascendancy of research. Before World War II, the deanship had not been easy, but at many medical schools it was still a part-time job. The transformation of medical schools into big businesses posed major new organizational and administrative challenges, and the responsibility for meeting those challenges fell mainly to the dean. The deanship universally became a full-time position, and many new positions under the dean were created: assistant or associate deans for admissions, curriculum, student affairs, research, community relations, continuing medical education, and hospital relations. As operating budgets grew larger, issues of fiscal management became paramount, and the business manager often became the most important member of the dean's staff. Whereas before the war professional skill and leadership ability had been considered the most important attributes of a good dean, by the early 1950s the most important quality was considered administrative ability.[70]

Despite the additional administrative support, these responsibilities took a toll on the morale of deans, many of whom still thought they could combine deaning with research, teaching, practice, or even chairing a department. The frustrations of the position became enormous, and the turnover of deans increased dramatically. "As if he were an isotope, the dean is often referred to in terms of his half-life,"[71] one successful dean, Robert J. Glaser, then of Stanford, observed in a classic address in 1969. From 1949 to 1959, there were 11 new deans at U.S. medical schools. However, from 1959 to 1969, there were 67 new deans (exclusive of the appointments of deans of new medical schools), and at the time of Glaser's address 9 deanships were unfilled. From 1962 to 1969, the average tenure of medical school deans fell from seven to four years.[72] One typical ex-dean spoke of "the damage to my nervous and vascular systems" that the deanship had inflicted on him.[73]

One reason that the deanship had become so trying was that the office had lost much of its earlier authority. Before World War II, most medical school funds came from internal sources that were controlled by the dean, and the major decisions about educational policy, faculty hiring, the allocation of space, and the development of new programs were usually his to make. With the development of a grants economy, most new funds went directly to the primary investigator or department, bypassing the dean. Departments became increasingly financially self-sufficient, and it was not uncommon for department chairmen to make decisions about appointments, promotions, research programs, and major expenditures without consulting the dean. Always, of course, the specific dynamics of a school reflected local traditions and the personalities of those in power—here a forceful dean, there a strong executive faculty. Nevertheless, the general thrust was centrifugal, as power and authority increasingly resided with the department chairmen.

With the ascendancy of research, the role of department chairmen also changed. Although they enjoyed more autonomy and power than before the war, their administrative duties increased enormously. As a result, it was increasingly difficult for chairmen to continue their own active scientific careers, particularly in the clinical departments, where the administrative load was usually the highest. Accordingly, the chairman's role changed from doer to facilitator. Chairmen made their mark by the leadership they provided, the intellectual and professional standards they maintained, the individuals they appointed to the staff, and the decisions they made about educational and investigative directions for the department. The most effective chairmen were shrewd judges of people, choosing the best individuals available to serve as division chiefs and full professors, and making the wisest decisions regarding appointments and promotions. The position required maturity and generosity of spirit, for the rewards came not from their own original work but from helping others succeed.

Though much in medical schools had changed with the ascendancy of research, one thing had not: the conviction of most faculty that they were university professors. This was illustrated in discussions concerning salary. Few subjects generated as much emotion as that of compensation, and real or perceived inequities of pay were a continual source of friction. Faculty could be lured to other institutions by money. However, no one entered academic medicine expecting a high income. Medical professors were paid well on a university scale, but an academic career continued to pay significantly less than private practice. The executive committee of one medical school observed: "If the individual physician was interested in high monetary income, he should accept private practice. If on the other hand he prefers an academic appointment, he should choose that. There should be no obligation on the part of the Medical School to see that he has both."[74] Salary levels were often the lowest at the most prestigious schools. Thus, Nathan B. Talbot was appointed Professor of Pediatrics at Harvard Medical School and Chief of the Children's Service at the Massachusetts General Hospital in 1962 at a salary of $22,000; Paul Beeson's salary in 1965 as Chairman of the Department of Medicine at Yale, the highest in the department, was $28,000.[75]

Rather, the most important factor in attracting and retaining faculty members at an institution was the provision of space and facilities. As the University of Southern California observed, "Unless the research facilities are provided the faculty cannot be recruited."[76] Similarly, Hahnemann, a school that lost more than it won in the recruiting wars, explained, "In today's market, you cannot get first-rate faculty without first-rate [laboratory] accommodations."[77] Bargaining with faculty was much more on the basis of the square feet of laboratory space, the provision of graduate students and fellows, and the amount of "protected" time for research than on the dollar amount of the salary.

If the expectation of faculty that they would not get rich as medical professors was one continuity with pre–World War II medical education, medical schools' disdain for commercialism was another. World War II had demonstrated the importance of being able to bring scientific discoveries to rapid commercial development, and as a result relations between medical schools and industry grew much closer. Nevertheless, medical schools continued to refuse to engage in profit-seeking behavior. This was once again illustrated by their attitudes toward patents. It was still the universal policy that investigators should not benefit financially from patents resulting from their work. By now, some schools accepted patent rights for discoveries or inventions of their faculty, using the royalties to support further research at the school. However, many schools considered even this small step to be inappropriate. One critic was Harvard, the most important research school of all, which believed that no individual or institution should profit from medical research, even if those monies were used to support additional research. The dean explained:

> It [our patent policy] is based on our belief that discoveries and inventions in the fields of medicine and health should, by their very nature, be used to promote the public welfare. Thus it seems improper to us that individuals or institutions should profit from discoveries or inventions. At Harvard, therefore, no efforts are made to obtain patents except in those instances when it is deemed necessary to do so in order to prevent others from obtaining a patent for private gain.[78]

In short, after World War II medical schools continued to see themselves as public trusts serving the public interest. Of course, medical schools were hardly without self-interest. Like universities, they represented a curious mixture of selfish and selfless concerns, of institutional aggrandizement coupled with a commitment to service and the public good. However, on balance, the service motif continued to dominate.

9

The Expansion of Clinical Service

A S THE UNITED STATES GREW MORE COMPLEX after World War II, so did its universities. The research university idealized by Abraham Flexner in 1930, it now seemed, exemplified the innocence of American higher education before the war.[1] In the words of Clark Kerr, Flexner's university was a "one-industry town"—that industry being research and scholarship. The postwar multiversity, in contrast—Kerr's "city of intellect"—was a pluralistic intellectual metropolis. Advanced teaching and research were at its core, but superimposed were a host of new constituencies and duties as an anxious, expectant public increasingly turned to its universities for guidance, leadership, and practical aid in coping with the problems of a complex society.[2]

No branch of the multiversity better illustrated the new practical demands imposed on it than the medical school. Throughout the twentieth century medical schools, through their teaching hospitals, had been involved in delivering medical care to large segments of the population, particularly the urban poor. After World War II, they continued their traditional charitable work. In addition, they began serving the middle class, who had become empowered to seek private medical and hospital care through the rise of private insurance.

The expansion of clinical service in the two decades following World War II created strains within academic medical centers, largely because of the distractions that patient care inevitably placed on teaching and research. Nevertheless, few academic medical centers lost sight—at least for long—of their unique role as educators of future physicians and producers of new medical knowledge and technologies. They worked hard to preserve the learning environment of the teaching hospital, even as that environment came under pressure from changing social, economic, and demographic circumstances. After the war, the strength of American medicine continued to reside in its academic medical centers—the collaborations of medical schools and teaching hospitals that generated knowledge, produced doctors, served as the ultimate arbiters in complicated clinical cases, and defined the standards of excellence in patient care.

Academic Medical Centers and the Rising Demand for Medical Care

In postwar America, the public's demand for medical care grew rapidly. In part this resulted from the fact that modern medicine and surgery worked. The skepticism of earlier generations of Americans toward scientific medicine became barely discernible. The growing demand for medical care also reflected the country's affluence. As commentators in the 1950s and the 1960s pointed out, only abundant societies enjoyed the prosperity and stability to allow a national search for personal security—medical or otherwise.[3]

In the changing social climate, medical care increasingly came to be regarded as a basic right. This attitude gave rise to a variety of experiments in financing and delivering medical care: sickness insurance, comprehensive care programs, neighborhood health centers, group practice, health maintenance organizations (called prepaid group medical practices at the time), and even a serious flirtation with compulsory national health insurance. (Of course, some of these experiments had started before the war.) The innovation that most shaped the practice of medicine was private medical insurance, which was obtainable from the Blue Cross organizations and other insurance companies. Private hospitalization insurance originated in the 1930s but became widespread in the late 1940s and 1950s, mainly because of the insistence of organized labor and the tax benefits that employers began to receive for offering such insurance to employees. For the middle class, private insurance, whether through group or individual policies, became the major method of paying for hospital care.[4]

As patients became empowered with private insurance, hospitals became much busier places. To meet the rising demand, hospitals had to be renovated and expanded, and new hospitals were needed as well. In 1946, Congress passed the Hospital Survey and Construction Act (popularly known as the Hill-Burton Act after its sponsors, Senators Lister Hill and Harold H. Burton). By 1971, the federal government had disbursed $3.7 billion in Hill-Burton funds for hospital construction and had generated $9.1 billion more in state and local matching funds.[5] The Hill-Burton legislation, like the National Institutes of Health (NIH), reflected the government's desire to make medical knowledge and scientific medical care more accessible to the American people.[6]

Of the country's 5,684 acute-care general hospitals, none was more affected by the public's rising demand for care than the 227 "major" teaching hospitals, which were defined as university-controlled hospitals that were used extensively for medical student teaching.[7] In the postwar era, the public not only expected these hospitals to set the standards of medical care as before but also to be responsible for large population areas. The philosophy underlying postwar federal health policy was that each region of the country should be served by one or more major teaching hospitals, which would provide consultations to smaller hospitals in the region and specialized hospital care to any patient in the region who needed it.[8]

The growing demand on teaching hospitals for clinical services was hardly an accident, for they were universally regarded as the hospitals that delivered the best patient care. Teaching hospitals possessed the latest diagnostic and therapeutic technologies, including many that were unavailable even at very large community hospitals. In addition, they consistently attracted the finest physicians (nowhere was it more difficult for physicians to receive admitting privileges than at a teaching hospital), as well as the best interns and residents. The spirit of education and research that permeated them kept the professional staff at the forefront of knowledge and prevented patient care from deteriorating into perfunctory routine. For those reasons professional and popular lists of the nation's "best" hospitals were consistently comprised exclusively of teaching institutions.

Precisely how far teaching hospitals stood above the rest was open to conjecture. A number of studies purported to show that teaching institutions provided the best care, but these studies were not well controlled or free of bias.[9] Nevertheless, few argued with the general conclusion. John H. Knowles, the outspoken director of the Massachusetts General Hospital, portrayed teaching hospitals as unrivaled islands of medical excellence. He once offended many doctors, including some former members of the Massachusetts General Hospital house staff, by publicly stating that there were only a few hospitals in the country where he would allow himself to be treated if he were sick.[10] Most medical educators, though less disdainful of community medicine than Knowles, felt equally strongly that teaching hospitals provided the best patient care.[11] So did the federal government, which through the Veterans Administration (VA) gave its imprimatur to the idea that education and research enhance patient care. After World War II, the VA constructed dozens of new hospitals, many of which were given affiliations with medical schools. To the VA, the purpose of these affiliations was simple: to allow veterans to receive "the highest quality of medical care."[12]

With their high reputations, teaching hospitals easily attracted many new patients. For instance, the New York Hospital admitted 28,459 patients and provided 293,227 patient-days of care in 1966, compared with 13,467 admissions and 189,571 patient-days of care in 1934.[13] Most teaching hospitals operated at nearly full occupancy. This situation was an administrator's delight if enough beds were occupied by paying patients, but it was extremely frustrating for voluntary and full-time physicians trying to schedule their private patients for elective admissions. At Presbyterian Hospital (New York), staff doctors in 1967 encountered four- to eight-week delays in getting their elective patients into the hospital.[14] Teaching hospitals also assumed numerous responsibilities that many community hospitals would shun. For instance, in the early 1950s the University of Arkansas Hospital admitted large numbers of patients with acute poliomyelitis since the other Little Rock hospitals refused to accept those patients. The University of Arkansas Hospital also provided most of the care for African-Americans in the Little Rock area, since few private hospitals in the city would admit black patients, even those who could afford to pay.[15]

At many teaching hospitals the pace of activity reached frenetic levels. For instance, the volume of patients seen in the emergency rooms grew tremendously, as did the task of quickly differentiating the acutely ill patients from the majority with nonemergent problems.[16] Emergency rooms were made even more chaotic by the frequent unavailability of beds for patients requiring hospitalization. At the New York Hospital, a "holding unit" in the emergency room was established to keep patients temporarily until a bed became available; at the Johns Hopkins Hospital, chief residents were given the authority to admit ward patients to private rooms and private patients to ward beds, if necessary.[17] The deluge of patients posed major problems for the medical records departments, many of which began running out of space and were forced to start placing patient records on microfilm.[18] Laboratory facilities were also stressed to the hilt. At one typical teaching hospital, the number of blood tests performed in 1968 was ten times greater than in the 1930s.[19]

In the postwar era, teaching hospitals continued to serve large numbers of indigent patients. However, except for the VA and municipal hospitals, the proportion of charity patients gradually fell. Instead, semiprivate patients (patients with hospital insurance who would share a room with another patient) became their primary constituency. The example of Presbyterian Hospital (New York) was typical. In 1939, 10 percent of its patients had Blue Cross coverage; in 1949, over 30 percent; and in 1960, over 50 percent.[20] Teaching hospitals, like other hospitals, became fully integrated into the country's new system of hospital insurance plans.

With larger numbers of private patients coming to teaching hospitals, full-time faculty began to engage in more clinical practice. As one measure, the professional income they generated from patient care rose dramatically. At Washington University, the full-time faculty earned $195,400 in professional fees in 1946–47, compared with an average of $12,000 per year in the 1930s; at Johns Hopkins, $279,438 in 1952–53, compared with $32,500 in 1929–30.[21] In the 1950s and 1960s, the level of faculty practice grew still larger, upsetting the voluntary faculty at some schools.[22]

As teaching hospitals entered the market for paying patients, they benefited from their reputation for upholding the highest standards of patient care, which in turn resulted primarily from the quality of their medical staffs. To assure that they could retain their competitive advantage, teaching hospitals, like medical schools, began to pay less attention to religion, gender, and ethnicity in their staff appointments—a policy reinforced by the popular revulsion against racism that followed the disclosure of Nazi atrocities during World War II. Of all the groups that had suffered from quotas, Jews benefited the most, as hospital after hospital that had once closed its doors to Jewish house officers and physicians became much more accommodating. For instance, the Boston Lying-in Hospital, whose earlier refusal to grant hospital privileges to Jewish doctors forced the nearby Beth Israel Hospital to develop an obstetrical service of its own, at last began to appoint Jews to its staff.[23]

Though larger and busier, teaching hospitals faced many familiar problems. They continued to be beset by troublesome management issues such as nursing shortages, labor unrest, potential employee unionization, the disruptions and inconveniences caused to patients by teaching, and the decrepit, overcrowded conditions in the outpatient departments. The emergency rooms and clinics of many teaching institutions served as a barometer of changing social conditions: the increase of unwed motherhood, or the changing ethnographic composition of the neighborhood. The wards and clinics still served as battlegrounds of academic medicine, as departments vied for the same ward or laboratory space, or as several medical schools in a city competed for privileges and opportunities at a municipal hospital that was shared among them.

As before the war, most teaching hospitals continued to be perceived as impersonal places. A self-study conducted at one teaching hospital in 1960 found that its patients considered it to be technically excellent but personally cold—a finding that undoubtedly could have been made at almost any teaching institution of the era.[24] Teaching hospitals were not unconcerned with the courtesies and amenities afforded their patients. However, throughout the 1950s and 1960s they remained focused on the quality of medical care rather than on the comfort and convenience of patients. In a preconsumer, pre–Civil Rights era, they felt that the best way to attract patients was through professional excellence. As a staff member at Massachusetts General pointed out, the key to a full census was in "attracting men of ability and stature to the practicing staff. . . . If we have enough outstanding men drawing patients to the hospital, our beds will be continually filled."[25]

As teaching hospitals grew, new problems in their administration also arose. Like medical schools, they became big businesses. In 1964, for instance, Massachusetts General Hospital had an operating income of $23,163,000, compared with $2,084,000 in 1940.[26] As medical technology became more costly, the challenge of managing a teaching hospital grew accordingly, for the common attitude was that if a device or a machine was good, the hospital must have it regardless of cost. "The first principle and the principal goal is to improve service in the care of the sick and the prevention of disease," Knowles wrote. "Any saving of money is a secondary gain."[27] In the era of private insurance, hospital finances depended increasingly on third-party reimbursement. The percentage of annual income derived from endowment and gifts fell sharply—at one teaching hospital, from 21 percent in 1950 to 2.8 percent in 1975.[28] In a poor financial year, losses could reach millions of dollars. Gone were the days when a wealthy benefactor could easily write a check to cover a hospital's operating deficit.

Teaching hospitals became not only bigger but more complex. A delicate operation, such as resection of a coarcted (narrowed) segment of the aorta, required, in addition to a skilled surgeon, elaborate preoperative testing, a well-trained anesthesiologist and operating team, and skilled personnel to tend to the innumerable details of postoperative care. Malpractice insurance, once carried by neither physicians nor hospitals, became de rigueur. Technological aids to communications were introduced, such as Centrex telephone systems, radiopagers, and computer billing systems. Teaching hospitals had to deal with a host of payers and regulatory agencies. To manage such complex technical, financial, legal, and regulatory matters, the administration of teaching hospitals became a profession in itself, as evidenced by the establishment of the Organization of University Health Administrators in 1957.[29]

Of all the problems teaching hospitals faced, the most severe was that of continuing to provide free care to indigent patients. By the 1960s, the proportion of ward patients had fallen substantially, as many former ward patients had acquired medical insurance of their own. However, as costs mounted, free care represented an even greater financial burden on hospitals than before. In 1964, for instance, Massachusetts General Hospital provided nearly $4.3 million of charity care—a ten-fold increase in dollars from 1940.[30] Reimbursement for indigent care from local or state agencies continued to be far less than the actual costs of care, causing many hospitals to hemorrhage financially. New York Hospital, for instance, lost $2,460,000 in 1960 for care provided on its ward pavilions.[31] Through the 1960s, many teaching hospitals still took pride in never having turned away a needy patient, but they could do so only by what was termed "the Robin Hood" method of care—charging insured and self-paying patients a premium to help underwrite the costs of caring for the poor.[32]

By the mid-1960s, academic medical centers had become extremely active in the delivery of care to paying patients. However, a cloud was on the horizon, for as disease was being controlled, the medical care delivery system was becoming increasingly diseased. Some worried about access to care; others worried about the fragmentation of services resulting from growing specialization; still others worried about an overemphasis upon the treatment of disease rather than the maintenance of health. But most worried about the growing cost of medical care, which was rising faster than any other part of the cost-of-living index. In 1964, Senator Abraham

Ribicoff called the high cost of hospital care the most important health problem facing the nation. "If contemporary medical marvels are priced out of the range of the average American, our brilliant conquest of so many illnesses will prove to be a hollow victory."[33]

To some in academic medicine, the emergence of problems in the medical care delivery system represented another opportunity for university medical centers to serve the public. The Kennedy–Johnson years represented a time of high expectations of the university to solve the social and economic problems of the country. To many, it represented the height of folly for academic medical centers, which boasted of their responsibility for ensuring the health of the nation, not to turn their attention to the study of the methods by which medical services were distributed to the public. As the dean of Harvard Medical School wrote, "Without in any way minimizing the continuing promise of the medical sciences, let me venture to predict that it is in the area of the redefinition of the social responsibilities of medicine that the greatest change and progress will be made in the next few decades."[34] How well that prediction would be fulfilled remained to be seen.

The Persistence of Academic Values

Since the early twentieth century, a symbiotic relationship had existed between medical schools and teaching hospitals. Medical schools could be no stronger than their affiliated hospitals, which provided the clinical workshops for students, house officers, and faculty. Conversely, the clinical preeminence of teaching hospitals was the result of their participation in medical education. By education was meant not merely the literal instruction of students, house officers, and fellows, but something far more: the attraction of the leading medical minds to the attending staff and of the best medical graduates to the house staff; the spirit of critical rigor that made teaching hospitals superior places for the diagnosis and treatment of difficult medical problems; and the continuous monitoring of patients and challenging of assumptions that resulted not only in outstanding care of individuals but also the frequent discovery of something new that could benefit patients in the future.

Through education and research, teaching hospitals had a special creative function in contemporary medicine. In business terms, their mission was to serve as the research and development arm of the medical industry—continuously testing and reshaping medical practice, and displaying a standard of care and style of critical analysis that learners would strive to emulate. The creative essence of teaching hospitals was described in an address by Walter Bauer, the chief of the medical service at the Massachusetts General Hospital, who spoke of their "razor-edged scientific analysis, probing, observing, recording, doubting, alert to every aberration from the patient's demeanor to the enzymes in his serum." To Bauer, teaching hospitals had "grave and inescapable" responsibilities, for "what we do and think in our teaching hospitals will influence the thought and practice of our colleagues everywhere, and, in turn, the health and happiness of our generation."[35]

After the war, as before, teaching hospitals represented a diverse group—all the more so in the 1950s and 1960s because of the addition of many Veterans Administration hospitals to their ranks. Some teaching hospitals were public, others were private; some were university-owned, most were independently chartered. While the relation of some teaching hospitals with their affiliated medical school or schools was decidedly close, others experienced considerable strains in those relationships. Nevertheless, as a group, teaching hospitals in the 1950s and 1960s continued to be remarkably supportive of education and research. This was true of both public hospitals, such as Los Angeles County, which in the 1950s energetically aided the educational and research activities of the University of Southern California, and private hospitals, such as Mount Sinai, which set aside $2 million of endowment funds in 1956 to support education and research.[36] Teaching hospitals understood that they could not occupy the pinnacle of American medicine without a strong academic program and a close relationship with a medical school. Dean A. Clark, the general director of the Massachusetts General Hospital from 1949 to 1961, spoke to this point in 1955: "Quite recently I was asked by the Chairman of the Board of Trustees of a prominent teaching hospital in another city, 'What single factor do you think has been most important in making the Massachusetts General Hospital the dynamic, vitally active, enthusiastic institution that it is today?' Fortunately, the answer is easy and I could give it at once: 'The Harvard Medical School.'"[37]

Teaching hospitals of the 1950s and 1960s exhibited a relentless commitment to quality—both in the professional care rendered their patients and in their academic mission. Success was defined not in terms of the size of the institution, the number of patients seen, or the condition of the financial ledgers but by the professional standards and scientific work. This attitude permeated the fierce rivalry between Peter Bent Brigham Hospital and Massachusetts General Hospital, two outstanding teaching hospitals affiliated with Harvard Medical School. In a heated meeting between representatives of the two in 1968, John H. Knowles, who had succeeded Clark as general director of the Massachusetts General Hospital, spoke disparagingly of the smaller size and budget of the Brigham. Outraged leaders of Peter Bent Brigham claimed that the opposite conclusion should be drawn: that Massachusetts General had grown too big, and that its larger size reflected too much clinical work that distracted the hospital from its university mission. To leaders of the Brigham, that hospital's smaller size was its chief asset in remaining truer to high clinical and academic standards.[38]

Though Knowles later apologized for his remarks, he had no reason to apologize for Massachusetts General as a teaching hospital. No other American hospital of the era made more notable contributions to education and research. Prior to World War II, the hospital's research budget, like that of other leading teaching hospitals, was small, amounting to scarcely $50,000 in 1935.[39] With the growth in federal research funding after World War II, Massachusetts General prospered as much as any single institution. The 1950s represented an especially propitious decade for the hospital. By 1960, 15.1 percent of the hospital's total available space was devoted to research activities, as was 23.2 percent of its total budget, or well over $5 million—an amount more than that spent on research by many medical schools.[40] Because of its geographic distance from Harvard Medical School, the hospital established a number of "basic science" research units of its own, which produced fundamental research of very high quality—including the work of Nobel laureate biochemist Fritz A. Lipmann.[41] The Massachusetts General Hospital, Dean George P. Berry of Harvard noted, regarded itself *"not* as a 'University Hospital' but a medical university in its own right."[42]

Though medical schools and teaching hospitals had many common concerns, the interests of the two were not identical. As before World War II, strains existed in the relationships of even the closest medical schools and teaching hospitals. Thus, authorities of Harvard Medical School spoke of "the Massachusetts General Problem," while trustees of Massachusetts General referred to a temporary "treaty" they had negotiated with the medical school.[43] Many of these tensions reflected traditional administrative disputes, such as how income and expenses should be allocated or what the proper reporting structure should be. However, the main source of conflict continued to arise from the fact that the two had separate origins and missions. Medical schools, with their university roots, were primarily future-directed. Their chief task was to educate doctors and develop sounder methods of practice for tomorrow. Teaching hospitals, in contrast, arose from a service tradition that defined their main responsibility as caring for patients in the immediate present. Teaching and research, in the last analysis, belonged to the medical school; the care of patients, to the hospital. As Berry put it, "The primary objective of a hospital is to care for sick people, that of a medical school to produce good doctors."[44] Even Massachusetts General Hospital, the most conspicuous example of an academic hospital, acknowledged that teaching and research were subsidiary to the hospital's primary duty: "the care of the patient."[45]

In this context, the expansion of clinical service at academic medical centers in the 1950s and 1960s—and in particular, the full-time faculty's more prominent role in private practice—created a major dilemma. Achieving the proper balance at medical schools among education, research, and patient care had always been a difficult task requiring Solomon-like wisdom. That challenge became even more difficult now because of the growing possibility that practice interests would overshadow academic interests. A prominent faculty member at Johns Hopkins worried that "the employment of the full-time staff as money makers" contained "the germ of self-destruction" of academic life—that is, the loss "of the leisure for thought, study and investigation for which full-time was created."[46] Dean Berry of Harvard Medical School wrote, "When the earnings of the professor are used to support the show, whether it be the university or the hospital or even a department, the results are destructive to the academic scene—teaching and research suffer."[47] A report on medical education in 1953 pointed out that some schools were already assuming unduly large service responsibilities, at the cost of research and teaching. "If students and professor are not to be unduly hurried in their studies, then the number of patients must be limited. . . . These ideal teaching conditions are almost impossible to meet when the hospital must assume the responsibility for the care of too large a number of patients."[48] A special committee of the Association of American Medical Colleges appreciated the financial gain that could accrue to a medical faculty through institutional group practice, but it worried that the widespread adoption of these programs "may portend retrogression toward a proprietary type of school."[49]

As academic medical centers expanded their service role, battles frequently erupted between medical schools, which usually sought to restrain the amount of private practice, and teaching hospitals, which typically tried to meet the demand for increased service. Thus, at Michigan the faculty complained bitterly that the administration of the hospital "was more interested in filling the hospital than in meeting teaching requirements."[50] In general, medical faculties lost most of these disputes. Administrators of teaching hospitals could point not only to the immediate public service the academic medical center would be providing by expanding faculty practice but also to the increased revenues the hospital and medical school would be receiving.

Nevertheless, the commitment of medical schools and teaching hospitals to academic values remained strong. For instance, as the University of Pennsylvania made plans to increase the volume of its faculty practice in 1947, it declared that "the Staff must not lose sight of the fact that this is a teaching institution and a harbor of research, and for those reasons it cannot become overloaded with a diffuse clinical practice."[51] Similarly, as Johns Hopkins organized its faculty group practice more formally in the 1950s, the school emphasized that the amount of private practice by the full-time staff "would always be kept within limits determined by the educational programs of the institutions."[52] The challenge of preserving the proper balance between service and educational activities was discussed in great detail at the Columbia-Presbyterian Medical Center, which wanted to play "its full part" in the national trend toward expanded community service without losing sight of its university mission. The solution, it felt, was to keep private practice subordinate to education and research. "We shall play a much more useful and important part in the medical education of the present and the future if we adhere to our original concepts and fit the various phases of this community service into our picture than if we allow these things to dominate our policy."[53]

As a result, academic medical centers in the 1950s and 1960s remained true to university principles, even as their private practice increased. They usually succeeded in applying the brakes whenever they stood in danger of engaging in too much patient care. Thus, despite a growing faculty practice, Washington University continued to make staff appointments based on research ability and not on clinical earning power.[54] At Johns Hopkins, the director of the Private Patient Clinic complained in 1959 of "insufficient professional participation" by full-time faculty in the school's group practice.[55] Presbyterian Hospital declined a request from the city of New York to accept more ambulance cases to its already overcrowded emergency room because it feared that a deterioration of teaching standards would occur.[56] At medical centers everywhere, full-time faculty—to the great chagrin of hospital administrators—demonstrated their indifference to financial matters by their frequent failure to bill for professional services rendered.[57]

As another indication that medical schools retained a strong academic focus, they repeatedly refused requests from community hospitals to establish formal affiliations. This was not easy for schools to do, for they needed more hospital facilities to accommodate the growing numbers of full-time faculty, residents, and postdoctoral fellows. However, throughout the post–World War II era they granted affiliations only to highly select hospitals. The policy of New York University was typical. There, affiliations with community or specialty hospitals were approved only if they could be shown to be "of value to the Medical School for teaching or research purposes."[58] Most applications, to New York University and medical schools around the country, were rejected.

If there were any doubts that most academic medical centers were able to preserve scholarly values, those doubts were laid to rest by the generally favorable relationships they continued to enjoy with private practitioners of the community and region. "Town-gown" relationships represented an excellent barometer of the amount of group practice by medical school faculties, for private practitioners were exquisitely sensitive to any organized competition from the medical schools, real or perceived, for private patients. Most private practitioners, despite occasional misgivings, remained friendly toward academic medical centers. The situation at the University of Pittsburgh was typical. There, an inspection in 1957 found that "despite the initiation of full-time clinical faculty positions which can be a source of irritation to physicians in private practice . . . relations are good between the medical school and the medical profession locally and in the state."[59] Though town-gown feuds periodically erupted, the feuds were usually short-lived, and on balance academic medical centers were thought to be supporting private practitioners and not competing with them.

This situation resulted from the strength of academic medical centers' ongoing commitment to teaching and research. The dean of the Cornell University Medical College pointed out in 1956 that 75 percent of the hospital medical care in the United States was given in hospitals of less than 100 beds. "I can assure you that no sane or responsible medical school administration would want to be responsible for the staffing or other problems of more beds than are absolutely necessary for the clinical instruction of students."[60] The general director of the Massachusetts General Hospital pointed out in 1958: "The main reason why this competition from teaching hospitals, though legitimate, is no real threat to the medical profession is that it is, *per se*, very limited competition. The teaching hospitals' only competitive desire is to have available enough patients of all varieties for the necessities of medical education, internship, and residency training."[61] After the war, as during the first half of the century, medical faculties helped elevate and maintain the standards of medical practice in the community without becoming unduly competitive for private patients.

The Preservation of the Learning Environment

Progressive medical education had always imposed great demands upon learners, who were expected to take considerable responsibility for their own education. Yet, students and house officers were not expected to proceed without help. Medical educators had the obligation to provide a learning environment that would stimulate, nurture, and support them in their educational journey. In the clinical arena, this meant making available a diverse array of patients, a cohort of skilled teachers, and sufficient time to study patients in detail and pursue problems in depth. Before World War II, teaching hospitals offered such an educational laboratory.

After the war, the rich learning environment of the teaching hospital was placed in jeopardy. The most immediate threat arose from the conversion of large numbers of charity beds to semiprivate beds. As noted earlier, the ward services had been indispensable to good teaching because students and house officers were given much more responsibility with indigent than private patients. However, hospital costs were soaring, and charity care represented a growing financial burden. With the spread of private insurance, voluntary hospitals everywhere began converting ward beds to semiprivate beds. For instance, administrators at the Johns Hopkins Hospital decreased the amount of free care given in the outpatient clinics because of large operating losses, despite knowing that a reduction in the size of the clinic population would be harmful to the educational program of the school.[62] At the Peter Bent Brigham Hospital, ward patients occupied only 50 percent of the beds in 1953, compared with 80 percent just a short time before.[63]

To faculty everywhere, the encroachment upon the ward service represented a serious obstacle to their ability to educate students and house officers, however delighted some hospital administrators might have been to have more paying patients. George W. Thorn, physician-in-chief of the Peter Bent Brigham Hospital, felt that the "most serious problem facing the privately endowed university hospitals is the dwindling ward population."[64] The chairman of surgery at Cornell warned, "Teaching medical centers which emphasize primarily private patient care in an attempt to be self-supporting soon lose their academic atmosphere, and their capacity for teaching and research."[65] Faculty at the University of Pennsylvania acknowledged the importance, both financially and socially, of treating more private and semiprivate patients. However, they maintained that to do so at the expense of the ward service was contrary to the purpose for which their hospital was founded. "You cannot maintain the highest type of teaching without adequate ward facilities in a University Hospital."[66]

No one argued that students and house officers had little to learn from private patients. Certain conditions were more common in middle and upper class patients, and the inclusion of this group in medical education made for a broader educational experience. The use of private patients also allowed students and house officers greater exposure to rare or unusual diseases, which were a frequent cause of referral to the specialty services of teaching hospitals. Some also thought that experience with paying patients would help students learn to take better medical histories. In a statement reflecting many typical presuppositions of the pre–Civil Rights era, the dean of one medical school declared that both clinic and private patients were needed. "The lower social and economic classes are far less communicative but far more available to physical examinations. The reverse is true for the upper social and economic groups."[67]

Nevertheless, the use of private patients continued to have many limitations in medical teaching. As before World War II, private patients, whether self-paying or insured, were under much less duress to have students and house officers involved with their cases. At Georgetown, to the outrage of interns and residents, it was common practice for private physicians to write orders in patient charts without any discussion with the house officers, thereby depriving them of the opportunity for a genuine learning experience with those patients.[68] At Woman's Medical College of Pennsylvania, some physicians were unwilling to allow their private and semiprivate patients to be examined by students.[69] At the New York Hospital, house officers were periodically reminded "not to intrude into the area of the private physicians," and students and house officers were frequently not permitted to perform genital and rectal examinations on private patients.[70]

The use of private patients was less consequential for undergraduate medical education since students were closely supervised and not permitted to act on their own. To students, it usually made little difference if they had private or ward patients. However, the use of private patients was much more problematic for interns and residents. The cardinal tenet of graduate medical education, as discussed earlier, was the assumption of responsibility. This objective could not be satisfactorily met when a patient's private physician assumed direction of the case. At Johns Hopkins, where the modern American residency arose, the Medical Board warned that the growing dearth of ward patients was "an exceedingly serious problem, and if unsolved will spell the doom of The Johns Hopkins residencies."[71] The general director of the Massachusetts General Hospital predicted that the use of private patients would cause residency to "deteriorate into a kind of second-rate apprenticeship."[72] Reports from many medical schools similarly warned that the displacement of ward patients was injurious to graduate medical education.[73] Residencies in all specialties were affected, but the problem was greatest in the surgical fields, where legitimate fears arose that with private patients house officers might not receive enough operative experience to qualify for board certification.

Alarmed by these developments, many medical schools took measures to guarantee that their trainees would continue to receive sufficient exposure to ward patients. Some, like Jefferson, began using endowment income to pay for indigent care.[74] This approach did not provide a permanent solution because of the growing costs of hospitalization, though it did illustrate the resolve of medical faculties to protect their teaching service as much as possible. A common and more successful approach was to redefine the criteria for being a ward patient. In the 1950s, most teaching hospitals negotiated arrangements with Blue Cross and other insurers by which certain semiprivate patients could be used in teaching. Typically, these were patients without a private physician of their own on either the full-time or voluntary staff.[75] In 1954, such patients accounted for 34 percent of the patient-days on the ward services of one typical teaching hospital.[76] Another common approach was for medical schools to expand their teaching activities at municipal and veterans hospitals, where patients were used freely in house staff education. Indeed, despite their skewed gender and age grouping, veterans hospitals often became as desirable places for teaching and research as the main university hospitals. And lastly, many teaching hospitals, especially by the 1960s, began to confer more responsibility on house officers in caring for private patients—for instance, by allowing only interns and residents to write orders in the charts. Through these various devices, most university residency programs retained the ability to provide their house officers sufficient responsibility in patient care.

The opportunity to assume responsibility was only one feature of the learning environment of teaching hospitals. Had this quality been sufficient, municipal hospitals without close university affiliations would not have encountered so much difficulty attracting house officers. Rather, good teachers were also necessary to provide instruction and supervision and to demonstrate high standards of critical thought and professional comportment. However, many faculty were already spending much more time in research, owing to the postwar boom in federal research funding. Now, with the expansion of clinical service, faculty were being asked to see more private patients as well. With only 24 hours in a day, faculty often found themselves cramped for time, and it was easy for teaching or resident supervision to be shortchanged.

Here, too, medical schools were able to preserve the quality of the clinical learning environment. Though full-time clinical professors found themselves torn in many directions, the number of clinical faculty had grown several-fold, so that no scarcity of capable instructors existed. In addition, as before the war, most medical schools had a cohort of able and conscientious voluntary faculty who contributed greatly to the teaching efforts of the institution. The dedication of this group was often inspiring. For instance, one member of the voluntary faculty at the Massachusetts General Hospital devoted over 25 hours a month to hospital meetings (most of which pertained to educational matters), not to mention the considerable time he spent directly in teaching.[77] At no teaching hospital were excellent instructors and role models in short supply.

The most important feature that made the traditional ward service such a rich educational laboratory was the presence of time—time to observe longitudinally the natural history of disease, to make a diagnosis and monitor the response to treatment, to read, think, inquire, and pursue topics in depth, to develop reasoning and problem-solving skills, and to get to know patients and their families (including circumstances at home, work, or school that might allow more empathetic or effective treatment). In the two decades that followed World War II, the time available to spend with individual patients decreased, as changes in medical practice led to shorter hospital stays. The use of penicillin and other new antibiotics markedly decreased the number of hospital days for patients with infectious diseases, and the new custom of early ambulation had a similar consequence for patients with many other medical and surgical conditions.[78] The average length of stay varied from hospital to hospital, from the private service (where it was typically shorter) to the ward service (where it was customarily longer), from one clinical service to another, and even from one year to another on the same service of the same hospital. Nevertheless, the universal trend was toward shorter hospital stays. At the University of Michigan Hospital, for instance, the average length of stay decreased from nearly 18 days in 1946 to less than 12 days in 1963.[79] *Figure* 2 graphically illustrates the national trend toward shorter stays.[80]

In addition, as medical technology became more sophisticated, life on the wards became more hectic. Many new surgical procedures were much more complex than older operations. For example, kidney transplantation, usually listed as one operation, in fact required two operating teams, two operating rooms, and a total of about 14 hours.[81] Powerful new drugs, such as corticosteroids and various cancer chemotherapies,

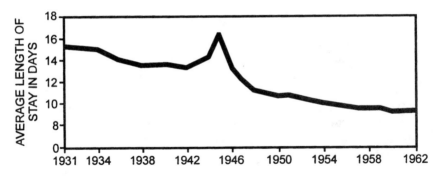

Figure 2   *Length of stay at general and specific hospitals, 1931–1962*

carried an increased risk of toxic reactions and side effects. The development of technologies like mechanical ventilators (artificial lungs), extracorporeal circulatory pumps (heart-lung machines), hemodialyzers (artificial kidneys), and cardiac pacemakers imposed more work on the medical staff and required the cooperation and assistance of highly trained supporting personnel. The development of complex electronic equipment, particularly machinery for monitoring the electrical impulses of the heart, led to the creation in the 1960s of intensive care units. With sicker patients, more things to do, and a greater turnover of patients, house officers and students were busier than ever, and time for study and reflection became scarcer.

Nevertheless, there was still sufficient time to allow the educational qualities of the inpatient wards to be preserved. The 11- or 12-day hospitalization of 1965 was long enough to afford learners ample opportunity to study most patients and their diseases. Though sicker patients required more work, teaching hospitals responded by providing the resident staff more assistance: blood drawers, intravenous (IV) starting teams, laboratory technicians, and other supporting personnel to help with many of the routine tasks.

Most important, neither Blue Cross nor any other insurer imposed significant limitations on what doctors could do with their patients or on how long patients could remain in the hospital. Partly as a result of discussions with representatives of academic medical centers, patients could be admitted for diagnostic workups, not just treatment of a known condition, and patients could remain in the hospital as long as medical circumstances dictated. Only in the mid-1960s did Blue Cross begin to question excessive hospital stays (defined at the time as exceeding 21 days in duration), and even in those cases full payment to the hospital was usually forthcoming if there was a satisfactory explanation for the days in the hospital beyond three weeks. Considerable inefficiencies continued in the management of many patients—for instance, the common practice of admitting a patient on a Friday or Saturday for an operation the following Monday. Though third-party payers frequently bristled at such practices, they did not punish by withholding payment, with the consequence that students and house officers still had enough time to learn.

Despite the above accommodations, the learning environment of teaching hospitals was not perfect. The primary deficiency lay in the inpatient wards, which, though rich in "clinical material," were becoming even less representative of the spectrum of serious illness than before. Many chronic diseases—high blood pressure, for example—were usually treated satisfactorily in an ambulatory setting; only especially severe or complicated cases warranted hospitalization. Advice about health promotion (adopting healthy dietary and living habits) could be better performed in an office than in a hospital, as could important screening procedures like blood pressure checks, sugar and cholesterol determinations, and heart, prostate, breast, and rectal examinations. Ambulatory settings were also the preferred location for the diagnosis and treatment of most common but minor conditions. In the view of some medical educators, more and better ambulatory education was needed to complement the opportunities provided on the inpatient wards.

Nevertheless, most medical educators of the era continued to regard the inpatient ward service as the best site for students and house officers to study medicine. In their view, outpatient teaching continued to be haphazard—too few cases of serious or "interesting" illness amid the mass of minor complaints. Moreover, as discussed earlier, the skills best taught in the hospital were considered the ones most fundamental to medical practice, even if the majority of care was delivered in an office. It was on the wards where learners had the most time to study problems in detail and the best opportunities to learn pathophysiological mechanisms, the natural history of disease, and the principles of physical diagnosis, differential diagnosis, and therapy. This point was addressed by David P. Barr, chairman of the department of medicine at Cornell, who wrote, "While it has been shown that a general Out-Patient Department in a large metropolitan hospital can offer valuable instruction, it has not as yet been demonstrated either to students, house officers, or attending physicians that this is superior or even equivalent to the teaching which can be given in relation to the wards of a hospital." He acknowledged the importance of the sociological teaching that could be done in the outpatient clinics, but "it is by no means apparent as yet how much of such teaching can be introduced without limiting or mutilating the teaching of anatomical and chemical pathology and the traditional therapeutics."[82] What made Barr's comments so telling was that he was the director of Cornell's Clinic for Comprehensive Care and Teaching, the most important experiment in ambulatory medical teaching of the 1950s and 1960s.

By 1965, American teaching hospitals were much different places from what they had been a generation before. There were more patients to be seen, the turnover of patients was greater, the patients tended to be sicker, and powerful new medicines and technologies had greatly extended the capacity of hospital medicine to diagnose and treat illness.

The prosperity of the country and the spread of private hospital insurance had resulted in a contraction of the ward service. The country had changed, and so had teaching hospitals and medical practice. But one thing had not: the commitment of medical educators to providing learners the best possible educational opportunities. Medical education had to alter many of its long-standing ideas, traditions, and approaches. However, it did so in a way that enabled the quality of the clinical learning environment to be preserved.

10

The Maturation of Graduate Medical Education

THE EXPLOSION OF KNOWLEDGE in all academic disciplines after World War II shattered traditional approaches toward scholarship. Throughout the university, the fragmentation of disciplines and academic specialization occurred. Scholars from different departments—and even from within the same department—found that they had less in common to talk about. The gulf between the scientific disciplines and the humanities grew particularly large, as C. P. Snow described in his classic 1959 essay "The Two Cultures and the Scientific Revolution."[1]

In medicine, a similar fragmentation of knowledge and practice occurred. The movement toward specialization had been underway for many decades, but as biomedical research progressed, the growth of specialization and subspecialization rapidly accelerated. Areas such as internal medicine, surgery, and pediatrics—long recognized as fundamental medical specialties—increasingly became regarded as general disciplines that were preparatory toward careers in a specific subspecialty. In internal medicine, for example, physicians increasingly concentrated in one of the growing number of recognized subspecialties, such as cardiology, gastroenterology, or endocrinology. Within a subspecialty, a physician might choose to concentrate still further. For instance, within endocrinology, a doctor might subspecialize in diabetes or thyroid diseases. Of course, medicine did not become as fragmented as many other academic disciplines. All medical practice was based on the same scientific infrastructure, and specialists needed to cooperate with each other to provide the best care. A complex heart operation required the coordinated efforts of the patient's pediatrician or internist, cardiologist, radiologist, cardiac surgeon, and anesthesiologist. Yet, by the 1950s medicine had evolved from a single broad area of practice into a federation of diverse disciplines.[2]

Though general practice did not disappear after World War II, its attractiveness as a career to physicians in training markedly decreased. Following internship, more and more medical graduates sought residencies to pursue a specialty, and after residency, many sought postdoctoral training in a clinical subspecialty as well. Teaching hospitals quickly met the increased demand for specialty training. Residency positions, previously reserved for only a small portion of each graduating class, became available to all who desired one, and postdoctoral fellowships became easily obtainable as well. Graduate medical education, once only a secondary interest of medical faculties, became one of their primary concerns. At many medical centers, the number of interns, residents, subspecialty residents, and clinical fellows grew to exceed the number of medical students. As the multiversity began to swell with graduate student training programs (from 1946 to 1970, the number of graduate students in American universities increased from 120,000 to 900,000[3]), the postwar academic medical center became home to a vastly expanded program of graduate medical education.

By the mid-1960s, graduate medical education had accomplished most of its major objectives, but new forces had also been set in motion. With its maturation, the harmony that had previously existed between individual choices and the nation's perceived "manpower" needs came to an end. No one doubted that changing medical practice required more specialists, but by the 1960s many began to believe that medical education had overshot the mark, producing too many specialists and too few primary care physicians. Moreover, as academic medical centers produced more specialists and subspecialists, they began to lose their traditional monopoly on specialized services. Upon completing their residency or fellowship, most trainees chose to enter practice rather than pursue academic careers. By the mid-1960s, academic medical centers had produced so many specialists and subspecialists that for the first time private practitioners in the community could begin to compete with them in providing specialized care.

The Democratization of Residency

Before World War II, only a minority of doctors became specialists. However, the war irreversibly altered physicians' attitudes toward specialization. The first *Directory of Medical Specialists* was issued in 1940, clearly differentiating those who had been certified in a specialty from those who had not. In the military, physicians with specialty certification, or those who had been taken from an advanced stage of a residency, received higher rank, more pay, greater professional responsibility, and preferred assignments. Professional assignments had little to do with seniority, age, or experience. General practitioners who had been practicing for years received lower commissions, less pay, and less important duties than much younger doctors recruited directly from a residency. Suddenly and dramatically, the prestige of specialists was upgraded and that of general practitioners, downgraded, by no less an authority than the federal government.[4]

The result was an unprecedented demand for specialty residency positions among doctors who had served in the war. This caught most medical educators by surprise. They had thought that the greatest educational need of returning medical veterans would be for continuing medical education courses to become more familiar with scientific developments of the past several years. However, two-thirds of physicians in the military indicated their strong desire to receive residency training to become certified specialists when the war was over—including many older doctors who had already been in general practice.[5] A surprised Council on Medical Education and Hospitals admitted in 1945 that the demand of thousands of veterans for specialty residency positions had greatly exceeded its estimates.[6] As the war ended, teaching hospitals everywhere expanded their residency staffs. University Hospitals of Cleveland increased the size of its house staff by 25 percent to around 120 house officers, while the Johns Hopkins Hospital, which before the war had 66 resident positions, increased the number to 96.[7]

The demand for residency positions proved not to be a transitory phenomenon. In the late 1940s and 1950s the majority of medical students sought "straight" internships followed by residency positions in a medical specialty. As early as 1947, an official of one medical school noted the conspicuous trend among students at the school "to decry preparation for general practice."[8] By 1959, another major medical school observed that the proportion of its graduating class seeking specialty residencies had reached 80 percent.[9]

The reasons for this switch were not hard to find. The rapid expansion of medical knowledge and growing procedural complexity of medical practice made specialization in many fields an intellectual necessity.[10] In addition, in postwar America, the disparity in income and social prestige between specialists and general practitioners continued to grow. Lastly, generalist role models began to disappear from the teaching wards. Before the war, the typical attending physician on the ward service was a generalist within his specialty: a surgeon who would perform a cholecystectomy one day and set a compound fracture the next; an internist who would manage all patients with only occasional requests for consultation. After the war, more and more attending physicians were NIH-trained subspecialists (cardiologists and rheumatologists in internal medicine, for example) who were much more inclined to obtain consultations for problems outside their area of special interest. Students saw fewer examples of physicians comfortable managing a broad range of illnesses on their own.[11]

The increasing desire of medical students to specialize was met by a growing demand of teaching hospitals for specialty residents. As noted earlier, the democratization of medical care through private insurance, together with the growing technical capacity of hospital-based medicine, led to greatly expanded demands on teaching hospitals for clinical care. Before the war teaching hospitals could operate efficiently with relatively small numbers of residents, but now they needed many more house officers to tend to the vast amount of moment-to-moment work. As a result, the number of residency positions offered by U.S. hospitals increased from 5,796 in 1940 to 46,258 in 1970.[12]

The growth in the number of house officers was also promoted by medical schools. The presence of a mature, responsible resident staff to tend to patient care allowed faculty much more time for research, private practice, consulting, and other activities. As residents began to care for more private patients, most hospitals permitted their admission and progress notes to serve as the legal record, thus freeing full-time and voluntary faculty from the time-consuming task of writing notes of their own. Residents were continually present, not only for routine chores but also to make important decisions and perform most procedures. Only for unusual problems would attending physicians need to be called for their patients outside of formal attending rounds. Residents were also assigned more formal teaching duties with medical students and greater responsibilities in outpatient departments. In recognition of this, many medical schools began granting residents the faculty title of "assistant" and listing them in the medical school catalogues.[13] Small wonder that clinical departments, in the face of their own expanding educational, research, and service functions, perpetually put pressure on hospital administrators to increase the number of house officers, or that departments competed vigorously with each other for priority in receiving any new house staff positions that a hospital might allocate.

The growth of residency training at the Columbia-Presbyterian Medical Center illustrated the attractiveness of residents to clinical departments. From 1941 to 1959, the number of residents increased from 125 to 247, while the combined ward, semiprivate, and private bed capacity increased only from 1,259 to 1,498. A committee of the medical board identified two factors that had led to the remarkable growth of the residency staff. One was the increased work load of the clinical services, which reflected sicker patients, a more rapid turnover of patients, and a rising number of technically sophisticated procedures. The second was the greater involvement of residents in medical student teaching.[14] House officers had become the key to keeping academic medical centers running, just as graduate students had become essential for the smooth operation of the multiversity.

For academic medical centers, the growth of graduate medical education was a transforming event. Through World War II, residency staffs had intentionally been small, with most positions reserved for individuals considering academic careers. After the war, the number of house officers at most academic medical centers grew to exceed the number of medical students present in the hospital at any one time. The New York Hospital–Cornell Medical Center was typical. By 1955, there were 178 interns and residents on the staff of the hospital, which was more than the number of third- and fourth-year students enrolled in the medical school. In addition, the medical center was assuming a much larger role in graduate scientific study and in the education of allied health professionals. In 1955, the medical center had 400 nursing students, 149 students in programs such as occupational and physical therapy, and a large number of clinical fellows and graduate students working toward M.A. or Ph.D. degrees.[15]

Though some new residency programs were created, most of the growth occurred from the expansion of existing programs. Residency training became democratized. The strict pyramid that had existed before the war gave way to a parallel system in which junior residents progressed up the ladder to become senior residents, thereby meeting board requirements for specialty certification. When the first list of approved internships was published in 1927, there were three times as many interns as residents in the country. By the 1960s, there were three times as many residents as interns.[16] The only specialty that maintained a pyramidal structure was general surgery. In other fields, acceptance into a residency usually assured the opportunity to finish. As a result, specialty training and certification became standard for the rank and file of the profession, not merely for a few selected physicians seeking to become academic leaders.

The maturation of graduate medical education posed new challenges for academic medical centers. For individual faculty members, ward teaching became more difficult, now that a "team" regularly included individuals ranging in experience from third-year students to house officers in a fourth, fifth, or sixth year of residency. Where and how to place the emphasis in teaching became a challenging pedagogical task. Students often resented discussions beyond their level of comprehension; mature house officers easily became bored with teaching aimed at beginners.[17] For medical schools, the growing number of house officers and specialty fellows, together with the larger number of full-time clinical faculty, created the need for more space and "patient material." As noted earlier, many schools expanded their clinical network beyond their original teaching hospital to establish affiliations with veterans hospitals, municipal hospitals, specialty hospitals, and selected community hospitals, where medical faculty were given laboratories and offices and students and house officers assigned clinical duties.

Although the growth of graduate medical education occurred most conspicuously at academic medical centers, the centers did not have a monopoly on internship and residency training, any more than they did before the war. Many community hospitals unaffiliated with academic medical centers continued to offer freestanding internships (internships unattached to any residency program). Some of the larger community hospitals sponsored residencies. In 1959, nearly 20 percent of the hospitals in the United States had either interns, residents, or both.[18]

However, in the fierce competition among hospitals to attract house officers, teaching hospitals still held a distinct advantage, owing to their rich educational environment and the greater clinical autonomy they typically provided house officers. Teaching hospitals nearly invariably filled their positions. Conversely, hospitals without a medical school affiliation often struggled to fill their allocated positions, and some could not fill even half their quota.[19]

As the demand for house officers increased, a shortage developed, especially for interns. In 1958, there were 12,325 approved internship positions but only 6,861 graduates of American medical schools.[20] Accordingly, many hospitals lacking an affiliation with a medical school began to recruit foreign medical graduates to their house staffs. From 1950 to 1959, the number of foreign medical graduates serving as interns or residents in the United States increased from 2,072 to 9,457.[21] Even with this influx, the demand for house officers could not be fully met. By the late 1960s, 20 percent of approved internship and residency positions were still unfilled, even though by that time 32 percent of interns and residents in the U.S. were graduates of foreign medical schools.[22]

In the competitive world of graduate medical education, competition existed not only among hospitals to attract house officers, but also among specialties to attract the brightest residents. Fields that were perceived as the most intellectually exciting had the greatest advantage. For instance, the relative popularity of ophthalmology and unpopularity of otolaryngology had little to do with factors such as income, lifestyle, or social status and much more to do with the greater technological capacity of ophthalmology as a discipline. As one surgical chairman commented, "It is difficult to get good house staff in otolaryngology as the field is not sufficiently challenging."[23] Among the fields encountering the greatest difficulty in attracting top ranking students were radiology, anesthesiology, and surgical subspecialties like urology and orthopedics. The specialty that attracted the highest proportion of good students was internal medicine, which in the 1960s was selected by up to 80 percent of students elected to Alpha Omega Alpha (the medical honorary society) at some schools.[24]

Control of internship and residency, as before the war, was fragmented among a large and confusing array of agencies: the Association of American Medical Colleges, American Medical Association, specialty boards, and residency review committees, among others. Medical schools and universities exerted considerable influence on graduate medical education, but they did not assume institutional responsibility for it, so that graduate medical education remained hospital-based rather than university-based. In the 1960s two widely publicized reports—the Millis report, sponsored by the American Medical Association, and the Coggeshall report, sponsored by the Association of American Medical Colleges— urged universities to assume greater corporate responsibility for the entire continuum of medical education.[25] However, these exhortations largely went unheeded. Even at academic medical centers, residency programs were considered departmental, not institutional, matters. Responsibility lay in the hands of the service chiefs, who were influenced primarily by the needs of their own program and the requirements of the specialty boards and residency review committees. There was little consideration of the broader institutional needs of the medical center or of the desirability of better coordinating graduate medical education with the other phases of medical education.

The democratization of residency transformed the contour of medical education in America. The multiplication of residency positions, together with the rising quality of clinical clerkships for medical students, squeezed the internship from above and below. Two-year internships disappeared, and teaching hospitals gradually abandoned the rotating internship. This led to the decision in 1970 to eliminate the freestanding internship. Effective 1 July 1975, internship became the first year of an integrated residency program; it ceased to exist as an independent, often culminating, educational experience.[26] The democratization of residency also reduced the importance to medical schools of continuing medical education. It was difficult to find a school that did not offer continuing medical education programs, but faculty members typically considered the activity unprestigious, and many refused to participate. At the University of Michigan, always one of the most dedicated schools in this arena, it was feared that unless faculty attitudes quickly changed the school "will have no faculty on which to call to perform the services required."[27] Increasingly, the leadership of continuing medical education came to be provided by specialty societies, state and local medical organizations, and pharmaceutical companies.

The ready availability of internship and residency positions after the war cast into sharp relief the fundamental ambiguity of graduate medical education: Was it education or service? As innumerable observers pointed out, it was impossible to separate the educational from the service components of graduate medical education, for the fundamental pedagogical principle of internship and residency called for house officers to develop independence by receiving responsibility and providing service. Yet, the economic exploitation of house officers was widespread. This occurred particularly often at hospitals unaffiliated with medical schools, but in more muted form the same phenomenon occurred at teaching hospitals as well. Even at Massachusetts General Hospital, house officers often found themselves "weighted with the routine tasks of clinical care that have little or no educational value."[28] Medical educators were usually quick to label internship and residency as important educational experiences, but their actions often betrayed them, and the fundamental ambiguity of graduate medical education remained unresolved.

The democratization of residency represented the success of the free enterprise system and the triumph of the individual's right in a democracy to choose his or her own career. Individual hospitals and residency programs sought house officers on the basis of their particular service and educational needs, while students sought the specialty that interested them the most. Program directors, hospitals, and students all made decisions on the basis of their own desires and requirements, not on the basis of the national need for any particular specialty. As long as the national interest was felt to be served, medical school graduates could continue to expect free choice in specialty training, and residency programs could anticipate having the opportunity to recruit as many house officers as they wished.

In the 1950s and 1960s, however, the sum of individual choices resulted in a precipitous shift toward specialization and a decline in general practice and comprehensive primary care. According to one study, in 1931, 84 percent of physicians in practice classified themselves as general practitioners; in 1960, 45 percent; and in 1965, 37 percent, half of whom were over 65 years of age. In 1967, only 15 percent of students were planning to enter general practice.[29] The harmony that had once linked individual decisions by students and residency programs to the national objective of producing a proper balance of physicians had ended. What was beneficial for individual physicians and residency programs was not so clearly beneficial for the nation as a whole.

Knowledgeable observers spoke with humility about the "needs" for different types of doctors. Such determinations were extremely value-laden and often based on miscalculations or erroneous assumptions. However, few felt comfortable with the specialty mix that was now occurring. A major challenge to graduate medical education became that of reconciling the desires of individual physicians and programs with national goals. How to do that posed a perplexing problem, especially in a democracy, which traditionally favored the individual in the ongoing tension between personal liberty and community needs. However, many began to believe that the pendulum had swung too far and that medical education must try to find a way to establish a specialty mix that better served the nation as a whole. As one editorial suggested in the specific context of surgical subspecialty training, "If these points cannot be determined by surgeons, they most likely will be decided by the government."[30] Physicians a generation later, long accustomed to a high degree of autonomy, would be stunned by the accuracy of that prediction— though ultimately it would be the market rather than government that wielded the greatest power.

The Rise of Subspecialty Training

Before World War II, the residency represented the culmination of medical education. After World War II, however, residency training became insufficient to achieve its traditional goals. Clinically, it no longer brought house officers to the cutting edge of specialty care. With the proliferation of medical knowledge, broad competence over fields like internal medicine, surgery, and pediatrics was no longer attainable. Even the most gifted clinicians had to subspecialize if mastery of a particular area was their objective. For instance, ophthalmologists began subspecializing in problems of the retina or cornea; surgeons, in fields like plastic surgery and orthopedic surgery; and obstetricians and gynecologists, in infertility or high-risk pregnancy.

After the war, residency also lost much of its value as preparation for an academic career. The pace was much busier, leaving less time than before for reflection and clinical research. In addition, the growing sophistication of clinical research required much more extensive laboratory training than a residency could provide. Lastly, as a consequence of the democratization of residency, proportionately fewer residents entered training with an academic bent. Residency was now for the rank and file, not just for those aspiring to leadership in the profession. As with the democratization of higher education that occurred at this time (from 1946 to 1970, college enrollments in the United States increased from two million to eight million[31]), the democratization of residency provided educational opportunity to many who previously would have been denied it. On the other hand, as the bachelor's degree lost its ability to signify a liberally educated individual,[32] specialty certification became more reliable as a sign of vocational rather than academic preparedness.

The emergence of formal subspecialty training following World War II provided a vehicle both for the mastery of a clinical subspecialty and the cultivation of research skills for those contemplating investigative careers. Subspecialty training after the war came to represent much of what residency training had represented before: an additional educational experience for mature physicians to become expert in a defined area of clinical medicine and to acquire the research skills necessary for an academic career. The route to acquiring subspecialty training depended on the field. In the surgical subspecialties, the subspecialty residency became the standard mode of entry. After two or three years of preliminary preparation in a general surgery program (one year of surgical internship followed by one or two years of surgical residency), graduate physicians would spend another three to five years in a surgical subspecialty residency like neurosurgery or urology, which provided both clinical training and research opportunities.[33] In other fields, the clinical fellowship became the conventional way to obtain subspecialty training. For instance, following a residency in internal medicine, graduates would spend another two or three years as subspecialty "fellows" in fields such as rheumatology, cardiology, hematology, or endocrinology. Here, they would acquire advanced clinical training and be provided protected time for research.

As the final stage of formal medical education, fellowship training was the most atomized and variable. It was the most atomized in the sense that fellows selected a program on the basis of one division of a department (or even one investigator), in contrast to residents, who came to an entire department of a medical school, or students, who came to all the departments of a school. Fellowship also became the most variable aspect of formal medical education because it provided the greatest flexibility to accommodate an individual's particular interests and needs. Many aspiring clinical investigators complemented their clinical fellowships with additional research work at a medical school, the National Institutes of Health (NIH), or both. The role of clinical fellows varied from school to school, department to department, division to division, and mentor to mentor—depending on the interests of the fellow and research adviser and on the source of funding.

Though it was understood that subspecialty training would provide advanced clinical experience—gastroenterology fellows would become skilled at performing endoscopies and liver biopsies; pulmonary fellows, bronchoscopies and ventilator management—the primary objective of the fellowship was to prepare future clinical investigators. Hence, most fellowship programs had strong academic emphases. As one reflection of this, the majority of fellowship programs were supported by training grants from the NIH, in contrast to residency programs, which were supported almost entirely from clinical revenues.[34] Fellows often received their paychecks from the medical school or university, while residents were customarily paid by the hospital. It was now subspecialty training, not residency, that was intended to prepare future academic leaders for the profession.

The two decades that followed World War II were as conspicuous for the proliferation of subspecialty fellowship programs as for the democratization of residency. At many teaching hospitals, the number of clinical fellows grew to exceed the number of interns and residents. At the Massachusetts General Hospital, for instance, there were 246 subspecialty fellows in 1964–65, compared with 180 members of the resident staff.[35] The presence of so many subspecialty fellows enhanced the excitement and scholarly atmosphere of academic medical centers. Their presence also created considerable confusion, particularly on the clinical side, where questions of jurisdiction and responsibility frequently arose. In theory, interns and residents were the primary care physicians, subspecialty fellows, the consultants. In practice, however, subspecialty fellows often tried to usurp control of patient management for themselves. Among the turf battles in the inner life of teaching hospitals were those between residents and subspecialty fellows for the control of cases.

For many fellows, subspecialty training was an invigorating experience. Every moment of internship and residency had been consumed with clinical learning or patient care; now they had leisure time for scholarly contemplation and original research. However, subspecialty fellowships were not just for aspiring scholars. In the 1950s and 1960s, subspecialty training, like residency, was democratized. Fellowship positions became readily available to virtually all who sought them—if not in one's desired field, then in another; if not at a preferred institution, then at a second or third choice. As with residency, most trainees sought fellowships because they wanted advanced clinical training, not preparation for an academic career. If a year or two of research was the initiation price for subspecialty credentials, it was a price they gladly paid.

By the early 1970s, many leaders of academic medicine were concerned that so few subspecialty trainees were pursuing academic careers. In the early 1970s, the NIH instituted a payback provision for the stipends it paid subspecialty fellows. For each year of NIH fellowship support, fellows were obligated to "repay" with a year contributed to medical education.[36] However, these provisions were weakly enforced and did little to alter the prevailing pattern. In the mid-1970s, even in internal medicine departments, only 6 percent of fellows were serious about an academic career.[37] Though many fine clinical investigators and teachers emerged from fellowship programs, the overwhelming majority of clinical subspecialists ultimately entered private practice.

In many respects, the production of so many specialists and subspecialists represented a public service. In 1932, the Commission on Medical Education had declared that the most important challenge to medical education was "that of making the benefits of modern medical knowledge available to the entire population."[38] Through the democratization of graduate medical education, that was more or less accomplished. Yet, at the same time the stage was set for an enormous irony: academic medical centers were training their clinical competition. University-trained subspecialists, skilled with the latest technology and gadgetry, could—and did—successfully demand that their community hospitals acquire the necessary equipment and supporting personnel so they could practice in the suburbs what they had learned at the university. Even so venerable an institution as Massachusetts General Hospital noticed that "the small suburban and out-of-town hospitals are putting up increasingly stiff competition."[39] In the 1960s, such competition was small, so strong was the position of academic medical centers, so young were the subspecialty training programs, and so cordial were the relations of academic medical centers with community physicians. Nevertheless, the seeds of a new equilibrium had been planted.

The Changing Life of the House Officer

In many respects, the lives of house officers after the war were similar to what they had been before. Many of the traditional stresses continued unabated: the hard work, long hours, sleepless nights, sense of vulnerability to unpredictable forces like nursing shortages, and total commitment to every aspect of their patients' care. Many of the traditional sources of support were also present: the camaraderie among the house officers, availability of immediate help, and exhilaration of being aware that one's medical competence was growing perceptibly on an almost daily basis. Complaints about the ordeals of internship and residency were common, but most physicians had positive memories of this phase of their training and with hindsight viewed the experience nostalgically.[40]

No two house officers ever had precisely identical experiences. Even within the same residency, the experience differed. House officers would admit different patients, they would be assigned different students and attending physicians, and they would work on different floors and units, some with an abundance of helpful nurses and ward clerks, others with staff shortages or paramedical personnel that liked to see house officers squirm. From the house officer's perspective, one night on call could be easy; the next could be horrendous, a sleepless nightmare with a flood of new admissions or innumerable cross-coverage dilemmas. There were notable differences between the programs of community and teaching hospitals, as well as among the programs of teaching hospitals, each of which had its unique traditions and personality. The particularity of each house officer's individual experience remained an important feature of graduate medical education.

Nevertheless, after the war some conspicuous changes began to occur in the lives of house officers. At all programs, the family-like quality of graduate medical education started to disappear. In part this resulted from the growing size of house staff programs. By the late 1940s, the number of house officers had become too large to allow them all to continue to reside in the hospital. With great reluctance, hospitals began to provide living allowances to house staff in place of the long-provided room and board. At first chief residents, then married house officers, and ultimately, any house officer who wished was permitted to live outside the hospital.[41] The total immersion in hospital life—the intimacy of knowing everyone, the habit of eating together, the late night discussions—diminished. As academic medical centers developed affiliations with other hospitals, house officers would be spread among two or more hospitals—further diluting the traditional sense of association of the house staff experience. Relations with faculty also tended to grow more distant, another consequence of the larger size of the programs.

Other factors also contributed to the decline of community. The 1950s and 1960s witnessed a liberalization of lifestyle and a heightened concern with leisure and personal indulgence. Men no longer regularly wore hats when going downtown, or women, gloves, and American society became increasingly consumer-oriented, consumption-driven, and swayed by the power of advertising and the mass media.[42] These trends manifested themselves in graduate medical education. Marriage and children, once verboten among house officers, became common as interns and residents no longer felt an obligation to delay personal gratification for professional education. To the postwar generation, the paternalistic rules and behavior guidelines that had once governed house officers could no longer be justified. House officers, of course, remained productivity-driven, not hedonistically oriented. However, they had come to feel that they were entitled to lives of their own. As that happened, the centrality of the hospital to their lives diminished.

A second major difference in the experience of house officers, particularly at teaching hospitals, was the increased assignment of private patients. To medical educators and house officers, as noted earlier, this was a disturbing educational trend because of the diminished responsibility house officers received with private patients. As the number of private and semiprivate patients grew, and as the proportion of ward patients fell, tensions often mounted, particularly at hospitals that before the war had had the largest and proudest ward services. At Massachusetts General Hospital, for instance, house officers regarded the encroachment upon the ward service by private patients as an invasion of their sacrosanct territory. House officers were often cool toward the voluntary faculty, whom they resented for usurping the teaching beds. Many private physicians, in turn, disliked uppity attitudes among the house staff, who would sometimes make major decisions on private physicians' patients without consulting them, or even "steal" their patients for the ward service (for instance, by admitting a private patient in the emergency room to the ward service and notifying the private physician only after the patient had been discharged).[43]

Though the rising number of private patients was educationally disturbing, interns and residents also reaped certain gains: for the first time, they received salaries. This resulted from the policy of private insurers to reimburse hospitals for the costs of house staff coverage.[44] Accordingly, house officers at last began to earn living wages. At Massachusetts General Hospital, for instance, salaries in 1963 ranged from $3,000 for an intern to $6,000 for a fifth-year resident. In 1950, interns there had received only room and board, and fifth-year residents, a stipend of $1,200 plus room and board.[45] What house officers lost educationally from private patients, they gained financially.

After the passage of Medicare and Medicaid (1965), which generously reimbursed hospitals for the costs of graduate medical education, house staff compensation increased even more dramatically. Between 1965 and 1969, the median house staff salary for each level of training (intern, first-year resident, etc.) doubled, and no end was in sight. In 1970 the median salary for an intern was $7,040 and for a fifth-year resident, $10,070.[46] Medical educators were pleased that house officers were receiving living wages, but some began to wonder whether the rapid escalation of salaries would ever stop. At the University of California, Los Angeles, the dean expressed the "gnawing fear" that house staff salaries will "continuously climb and *never* reach an endpoint." He was glad that "the old and somewhat unjust tradition of starvation wages for house staff members was breaking down," but he worried that house staff salaries might exceed those of junior faculty.[47]

Though the presence of private patients allowed house staff salaries to rise, competition among hospitals for house officers and the demands of house officers for higher stipends also played a role. Salary became a weapon in the efforts of teaching hospitals to recruit the best house officers, particularly when they were competing against hospitals in the same city or geographical region. Thus, teaching programs in cities like New York, Philadelphia, Chicago, Boston, and Los Angeles continually had their eye on each others' pay scales. Jefferson Medical College, for instance, repeatedly raised its house staff pay scale in response to competition from the other Philadelphia teaching programs.[48] Students and house officers reveled in this competition. In voices that were more muted than those of the protest era of the late 1960s, they made their desire for higher incomes known, and leaders of even the most prestigious programs had to listen.

For house officers, the appearance of stipends could not have occurred at a better time. It was financially onerous to delay earning an income when the length of graduate medical education was shorter. Now, with so many years of residency and fellowship training, the opportunity costs of graduate medical education would have been even greater without salaries. Stipends thus facilitated the democratization of graduate medical education since many house officers and fellows would have been unable to pursue their education without them. Even with salaries, indebtedness was often a problem, particularly since many house officers were marrying and starting families. In 1968, it was estimated that the average indebtedness among residents at one major Eastern teaching hospital at the end of three years of residency was $5,300.[49] Many house officers, especially residents and fellows, took to moonlighting, despite official prohibitions against that practice at virtually every program. Examining insurance applicants was an especially popular form of moonlighting, since it interfered the least with a house officer's schedule.[50]

A third important difference in the lives of house officers was the more hectic pace. With research typically moved to the fellowship phase of training, there was less of a sense of scholarly adventure. On the other hand, there was more to do for the moment. Sicker patients, together with the availability of new technologies and procedures, resulted in much more work in the daily care of patients. House officers had greater responsibility for teaching medical students and staffing the outpatient clinics. These activities were in addition to the traditional chores ("scut work") of internship and residency: drawing blood samples, starting intravenous lines, transporting patients and laboratory specimens to and fro, obtaining supplies, hanging blood for transfusions, and placing laboratory results in the chart. There was so much to do that at many programs, the attendance of house officers at conferences fell.[51] Handwriting was frequently so illegible that at least one teaching hospital instituted a course in penmanship.[52] The appearance of radiopagers in the early 1960s served as a constant reminder to house officers that they could never get away, at least while on duty. Small wonder, then, that innumerable instances can be found of house officers acting out: insensitivity to nurses and patients, rude and abusive behavior toward other hospital personnel, intentionally disconnecting the telephones in their call rooms while on duty, taking parking spaces that were not theirs or hospital food meant for patients, and perpetual delinquency in dictating their discharge summaries. At the New York Hospital, one frustrated resident ripped the handle off a door, another broke a lock, and many regularly left their hospital-owned apartments "in a deplorable condition."[53] Such examples, though not representative of house officers and difficult for a historian to quantify, nonetheless indicate the conditions of extreme stress that all house officers were working under. This view is reinforced by one small published study of sleep deprivation among medical interns, which observed that not only impaired efficiency of performance but also negative mood swings and transient psychopathology could result.[54]

The busy pace of house staff life once again cast into sharp relief the fundamental ambiguity of graduate medical education: Was it service or education? There was no way that voluntary and full-time faculty could have cared for more than a fraction of their private patients were it not for the work of interns and residents. Without house staff, no teaching hospital could have operated, short of spending a prodigious amount on professional replacements. The hectic pace also created a major pedagogical challenge: devising a way to allow house officers responsibility for patient care yet at the same time providing sufficient supervision so that avoidable mistakes would not be made. At most programs, the degree of supervision was often less than ideal, especially in the emergency room and outpatient clinics, where house officers spent considerable time working independently.[55]

Though many aspects of graduate medical education had changed, one thing had not: the failure of medical educators to live up to their ideals about teaching a thoughtful approach to the management of patients. David P. Barr, the chairman of the department of medicine at Cornell, reiterated these principles in 1954 when he wrote that in the proper evaluation of patients "discrimination is necessary at every turn"—not only in the application "but also in the well-considered omission" of diagnostic and therapeutic procedures.[56] Yet at every turn, house officers could be found engaging in a profligate practice style without ever being educated or taken to task for that behavior. At Johns Hopkins, for instance, one committee in 1959 found that "there is no mechanism on any service at the present time to evaluate the appropriateness of admission or of the duration of stay, or of the necessity for the various examinations and tests which are performed."[57] Indeed, faculty pressure usually operated in the opposite direction—encouraging rather than discouraging unnecessary tests and examinations. John H. Knowles, the general director of Massachusetts General Hospital, pointed out in 1964, "Medical faculties have not taught by rewarding restraint and thoughtfulness in the use of tests but usually have condemned the house officer when he has missed one determination."[58]

Medical faculties after the war were no more lax in their failure to train house officers properly for medical uncertainty than they had always been, but the consequences were much greater now. Scientific research had produced a much larger and more expensive menu of tests and procedures. House officers, accustomed to an environment of abundance in which virtually anything they considered was available and paid for, could easily succumb to the fallacy that good medical care involved doing everything imaginable. In the 1950s and 1960s, medical costs were already rapidly spiraling upward, but few physicians, house officers—or medical teachers—seemed to realize that careful actions on their part could help mitigate the problem.

11

The Forgotten Medical Student

AMERICAN MEDICAL SCHOOLS OF THE 1960s were larger, more complex institutions than they had been a generation before. Indeed, they bore no more resemblance to pre–World War II medical schools than the multiversity did to the smaller and simpler American university of the 1930s. However, despite growing responsibilities, what made a medical school a medical *school*—in distinction from a research institute or group medical practice—was the presence of medical students. The period after World War II was significant for undergraduate medical education, as the curriculum continued to evolve, new experiments in medical education were undertaken, and many changes occurred in the lives and experiences of medical students.

Despite the attention undergraduate medical education received, by the 1960s a striking phenomenon had occurred: the teaching of medical students had evolved from the central mission of prewar medical schools to no more than a byproduct of what academic medical centers were now doing. Amid the pressures of research, graduate medical education, and the provision of increased patient care, the education of medical students had become merely a passing concern. In ignoring undergraduate students, medical schools were not alone. The problems of the multiversity Clark Kerr discussed—its preoccupation with research, consulting, government service, and graduate training, to the neglect of undergraduate education—afflicted medical schools as well.[1] As medical schools accommodated a diverse array of important activities, medical students became their forgotten members.

The Evolving Curriculum

If there was one constant in the medical curriculum, that constant was a broad mandate to change. The curriculum was intended not only to incorporate the most important new knowledge and ideas (and to discard the unimportant or incorrect) but also to accommodate the larger changes affecting medical practice: the new disease patterns seen in an older and more affluent population, the new methods and technologies of diagnosis and treatment, and an appreciation of the broad cultural changes affecting the organization, financing, and delivery of medical services.

The process of curricular revision, so apparent before World War II, continued unabated after the war. In addition to the yearly rearrangement of details, faculties periodically reexamined the entire curriculum, instituting major overhauls in the subject matter, organization, and presentation of the material. Harvard Medical School, for instance, introduced major curricular revisions in 1957, 1965, and 1968, the primary thrust of which was to attempt to achieve better integration of the scientific and clinical subjects.[2] Always, departments competed vigorously for more time in the curriculum—in part out of excitement for their fields, in part because departments with heavier teaching loads had greater claim on the dean for money and resources, and in part because exposure to students offered the opportunity to attract new recruits to the discipline (the "apostolic mission" of teaching[3]). For every victor in the curricular wars, there was a loser. Witness the frustration of Cornell's department of pharmacology in having its teaching hours reduced in 1949.[4] Medical education was a national enterprise, and major innovations or experiments at one school often had repercussions elsewhere. Thus, in introducing multidisciplinary laboratories to its basic science teaching in 1962, the University of Southern California "naturally leaned heavily on the experience of Western Reserve, Harvard, Albert Einstein, Florida, and many other medical schools in our planning."[5]

In the details no two curricula were precisely alike. Even at the same school, students had different experiences, depending on the particular laboratory instructors, section leaders, house officers, and attending physicians to whom they were assigned. In addition, the educational atmosphere differed from one school to another. The elite schools saw themselves as the producers of scholars and specialists. Other institutions, particularly many of the state schools, regarded their mission as producing doctors who would enter practice, preferably in the state.

Nevertheless, the similarities in the course of instruction greatly outweighed the differences. The evolution of the curriculum tended to proceed in tandem from one school to another, in the end producing a standard product. This was manifested (and influenced) by the rise in importance of the National Board of Medical Examiners (NBME), which after World War II became the dominant organization in medical licensing. Previously, to receive a medical license, a graduate needed to complete an internship and pass the examination of a state medical board. Most states had reciprocity agreements with each other, though no state had an agreement with all other states. The NBME, in a much more professional examination procedure, administered its tests in three parts:

Part I, on the basic sciences at the end of the second year of medical school; Part II, on the clinical subjects at the end of the fourth year of medical school; and Part III, at the end of the internship. Eligibility for a medical license depended on passing all three parts. Students in all states took the same set of examinations, and all but a few states came to accept the results of the NBME for a license.[6]

The more important differences among medical schools related not to what was taught but to intangible factors such as the enthusiasm and teaching ability of the faculty, the motivation and talent of the students and house officers, the opportunities for creative work, and the traditions and ambitions that permeated the institution as a whole. Hematology taught by someone like Maxwell Wintrobe of the University of Utah or Carl Moore of Washington University, both builders of the field, might well be at a higher level of intellectual excitement than that taught by an ordinary board certified hematologist. These intangibles were difficult if not impossible to measure, but their importance was widely appreciated. The faculty of Harvard Medical School pointed this out while preparing for its curricular revision of 1957. "Teachers are more important than courses. Students should meet the best instructors—and be exposed to them for significant periods of time."[7] Medical faculties understood that the organization of the curriculum was only the beginning of what was meant by "medical education."

As the formal curriculum evolved, the most notable development was the establishment of the course in pathophysiology (the molecular, bio-chemical, and physiological mechanisms of disease). Robert H. Ebert, a former dean of Harvard Medical School, considered this course, usually taught during the second year, to be "the only important curricular change" of the period.[8] Instruction in pathophysiology provided students a greater appreciation of the scientific underpinning of medical practice as well as the fact that clinical investigation could contribute to an understanding of fundamental biological issues. Of note was that the course was taught mainly by clinical scientists, not basic scientists, thus providing students role models of how clinical and scientific expertise could be achieved by one individual.

The greatest deficiency of the medical curriculum, as judged from the persistent complaints of students, educators, and official commissions, was its narrow, technical focus. The curriculum provided the scientific foundation of medical practice, but it gave scant attention to issues such as preventive medicine, occupational medicine, the doctor-patient relationship, and the changing social and economic environment in which physicians practiced their art. One instructor of occupational medicine complained bitterly of how she had "been talking almost to my self" about the importance of the subject.[9] A major goal of medical education was for each physician "to become an educated and well-balanced man or woman in the University sense."[10] Few observers felt that medical education achieved that objective.

Though the subject matter continued to evolve, the pedagogical issues confronted by medical educators remained remarkably similar to those encountered all century long. Curriculum committees at every school wrestled endlessly with a variety of important challenges: achieving a better coordination between premedical and medical study, defining the core basis of medical knowledge that all physicians needed to know regardless of future specialty choice, eliminating redundancy in the course work, integrating the scientific and clinical teaching more effectively, lessening the crushing weight of detail, providing more elective time, encouraging compassion and empathy, and extending students' gaze past the individual patient to include the family as well as community health needs. Medical educators also continued to confront the perennial problem of how to emphasize reasoning and analysis rather than rote memorization, or what sociologist Renée Fox, as previously noted, termed "training for uncertainty."[11]

An especially thorny problem was how to evaluate students fairly and objectively. It was through addressing this concern that the NBME assumed leadership in the field of evaluation. In 1950 the NBME introduced standardized multiple-choice "objective" tests, which it developed in consultation with the Educational Testing Service (the agency that administered the college entrance examination and medical college admissions test). The NBME was quick to point out the difficulties of constructing a proper objective test. "It is not enough to jot down a large number of multiple-choice questions and call it an examination." Rather, developing a test "is an expert and laborious task" in which rigorous statistical methods must be used "to choose and pretest the items and subject them to critical analysis."[12] Medical schools everywhere began developing objective tests of their own or retaining the NBME to construct tests for them. Some schools simply used NBME examinations in place of their own. These practices, not surprisingly, led to another set of troubling questions. What precisely did objective tests measure: memory, or understanding and the ability to reason? How should schools regard students whose scores on the NBME examination were at sharp variance with their grades? Should a degree be granted to a poor student who passed the National Board examination, or denied a good student who failed the examination? On these troubling questions there was no consensus—especially since no correlation had been shown between performance on the NBME examinations and future performance as a physician.[13]

The above pedagogical problems had long concerned medical educators, but after World War II they assumed greater urgency. The information explosion was accelerating, producing even more new knowledge to be added to an already overcrowded curriculum. The enlarging scientific foundation of medicine, the sharp line in the curriculum between preclinical and clinical study, and increasing specialization helped obscure the ultimate goal of medical education: producing up-to-date doctors capable of providing compassionate care. The conditions of medical practice were also rapidly changing—not only from the spread of group practice and private medical insurance but also from more fundamental forces: the steep rise in population since the turn of the century; the sharp increase in the number and proportion of children and older individuals, each with special medical needs; the urbanization of America and movement of many city dwellers to the suburbs; the growing conviction that medical care was a right; and the increased ability of an affluent society to pay for that care. These and other changes, both internal and external to medicine, led to a number of important curricular experiments that went far beyond the scope of ordinary curricular revision.[14]

One set of ventures attempted to achieve better integration of university and medical education. By the 1950s medical education had become rigid and lengthy, particularly if graduate medical education was taken into consideration. The average physician was in his or her early 30s before entering practice. Many feared that the long period of study was preventing able individuals from entering medicine. This concern led Johns Hopkins, Northwestern, and Boston University to introduce programs that more closely coordinated medical with premedical study, thereby shortening the length of study leading to the M.D. degree. In 1959, Johns Hopkins began a program in which selected students were admitted to medical school after completing the sophomore year of college ("Year I" at the Johns Hopkins School of Medicine). Year I consisted of intense scientific study, after which students entered the conventional first year of medical school ("Year II"). The Hopkins program thus shortened college and medical study from eight years to seven. In 1961, Northwestern and Boston University began admitting students from high school into special programs that allowed them to complete their premedical and medical work in six years. This was accomplished by carefully designed instruction in the fundamental sciences, which allowed the premedical requirements to be met in two years instead of four. Anecdotally, graduates of these programs seemed to perform as well in medical school as students who had taken the standard four years of college, though many faculty felt that good performance in medical school did not represent an adequate justification for shortening the liberal arts phase of a physician's education.[15]

Another approach was initiated in 1959 by Stanford, which extended medical school from four years to five. Here the objective was not that of coordinating premedical with medical study but achieving a fuller realization of medical education as a university endeavor. More elective time was provided in each year, while the third year was designated for research or elective study anywhere in the university in accordance with the student's interests. Before Stanford's experiment, medical educators all century long had unquestioningly accepted the view that the curriculum should fit into an immutable four-year period of study. The Stanford faculty was the first in this century to suggest that the size of the box should depend on its contents.[16]

A second set of experiments attempted to help students better understand the patient as a whole. This issue, always a concern to medical educators, became more pressing in the postwar era because of increasing specialization and the shortening length of hospital stay, which made it more difficult to get to know patients and their families. Accordingly, four schools—Cornell University Medical College, the University of Colorado School of Medicine, Temple University School of Medicine, and the University of North Carolina School of Medicine—introduced experimental programs in what was termed "comprehensive medicine." The programs differed in emphasis and detail, but all employed a common approach. Fourth-year students participated in a general medical clinic that admitted both pediatric and adult patients, and continuity of care was provided so that students followed patients for several months. The programs emphasized preventive medicine, concern for the patient (as opposed to the disease), attention to the emotional and environmental factors of illness, and instruction in fields like psychiatry, psychology, sociology, and social medicine. However, no lasting impact of these programs on student attitudes could be shown. By the late 1960s they had been discontinued, owing to the withdrawal of financial support, the lack of student interest, the skepticism of many faculty that the programs made a difference, and, in the case of Colorado, political difficulties between the medical school and the city of Denver.[17]

The most important experiment of the era was the reorganization of the teaching program at Western Reserve University School of Medicine (which became Case Western Reserve University in 1967, following the merger between Western Reserve University and the Case Institute of Technology).[18] This experiment came most squarely to grips with the fundamental pedagogic challenges in medical education: the information overload, the inadequate cultivation of analytical as opposed to retentive skills, and the lack of integration between the basic sciences and the clinical clerkships. The new program emphasized principles and fundamental concepts, reasoning and understanding, and the development of problem-solving skills. The standard curricular structure of the time, two years of basic sciences followed by two years of clinical clerkships, was abandoned for a curriculum divided into three parts. The first phase, one year in duration, studied normal structure, function, and development. The second phase, lasting one and one-half years, turned to the aberrations of structure, function, and development that occur in disease. The third phase, also lasting one and one-half years, consisted of the clinical clerkships. The greatest departure occurred during the first two phases. There, teaching was conducted on an interdepartmental, interdisciplinary basis that came to be called "organ based teaching." Instruction on the circulatory system, for example, was provided by anatomists, physiologists, cardiologists, and hematologists. New multidisciplinary laboratories were introduced for this part of the curriculum. Instead of being assigned to a department's student laboratory when that subject was taught, students were given laboratory facilities of their own that were used for all the laboratory courses. In addition, the program introduced other important changes, such as the abolition of grades and class rankings, the implementation of a preceptorship system that lasted the entire four years of medical school, early contact with patients, and much greater amounts of elective time, especially after the completion of the first year of study.

Western Reserve introduced its new curriculum in 1952. The idea of innovating in medical education had been the brainchild of Joseph T. Wearn, an internist who had become dean of the medical school in 1945. Wearn assumed leadership of the institution at a time that proved propitious for embarking on a major educational experiment. During his first five years as dean, the school lost 10 of 13 department chairmen through death or retirement, and Wearn replaced them with individuals sympathetic to his commitment to educational reform. Wearn also involved the larger faculty of the medical school at all stages of the planning. A newly created General Faculty of approximately 200 members devoted considerable time and thought to developing the new program. The enthusiasm of the faculty at large was later thought to have been a critical factor in the success of the experiment. Indeed, this was considered to have been the most radical change that occurred. The actual amount of curricular change was small, if measured in terms of time given to the various subjects, but a major attitudinal shift had made the needs of learners a matter of central importance to the faculty.[19]

Though Western Reserve introduced modifications over the years, the educational philosophy and teaching methods of the experiment remained intact. The new program received national and international attention, and the school attracted some of the brightest and most highly motivated students in the country. The school influenced medical education nationally, both through emulation and the recruitment of faculty or graduates of the school to other institutions. No school adopted the Western Reserve program in toto, but the philosophy of interdisciplinary teaching and the tool of multidisciplinary laboratories influenced many existing schools and played an even more important role in shaping the new medical schools created in the 1960s.

None of the above programs would have occurred without financial assistance from private foundations. The most important was the Commonwealth Fund, which underwrote the experiments at integrating university and medical education, teaching comprehensive care, and reforming the curriculum at Western Reserve.[20] However, other foundations also took a major interest in medical education, and they supported many programs in medical education for which federal funds could not be obtained. As a former medical dean wrote, "It is difficult to identify any significant development in medical education in which a foundation grant did not play an important role."[21]

The curricular experiments of the era demonstrated several major points. One was the importance of the enthusiasm of the faculty. The Harvard faculty noted this in reflecting on its 1957 reforms. "These men [those who reorganized the curriculum] enjoyed the experience, and their enthusiasm has been passed along to the students. Therefore, perhaps the value of curricular change was to stimulate the interests and broaden the views of those doing the teaching rather than any absolute gain in the amount or nature of the material presented."[22] When the faculty was supportive, as at Western Reserve, the experiment seemed to work. When the faculty was more skeptical and less involved, as with Cornell's comprehensive care program, the experiment was more easily abandoned.

In addition, the curricular experiments of the era made clear that a faculty could engage extensively in educational matters and still excel at research. This was demonstrated at Western Reserve, long a distinguished research school, which saw its productivity and reputation in research increase still further following the introduction of its integrated curriculum. In the 1950s very few instructors left the school because of dissatisfaction with the program, and over a dozen faculty members were recruited by other schools to be department chairmen or deans.[23]

Lastly, the curricular experiments made apparent the need to devise strategies to evaluate curricula and teaching methods. This became especially obvious after the initiation of the Western Reserve experiment, which was introduced without a meaningful evaluation component. Accordingly, in the 1950s medical educators began making attempts to apply the tools of educational psychology to the development and testing of curricula and teaching methods. By 1970 roughly half of the medical schools had established units or divisions of research in medical education. The work of George E. Miller and colleagues at the University of Buffalo (later called the State University of New York at Buffalo) and the University of Illinois College of Medicine was especially important to the development of this field.[24]

Though the curricular experiments of the postwar period were notable, by the mid-1960s it was clear that not much had changed in medical education. The 1950s, one writer observed, were a decade of "relative calm in medical education."[25] Everywhere, the same educational ideals—the importance of active learning, of understanding rather than memorizing, and of developing problem-solving skills—were continually professed, yet everywhere complaints could be found that these ideals were not being realized. In 1962 a noted educator remarked, "Medical education has remained remarkably conservative over the years . . . I am aware of no medical school which has fully exploited the great untapped potential of 'self-education by a medical student' as a major theme of its education policy."[26] Students were also dissatisfied. In 1967 more than 80 students at Tufts signed a petition criticizing the curriculum of the first two years for containing too many lectures, providing too much detail, and emphasizing rote memorization. "In short, the educa-

tional process through which we are put tends to foster intellectual stulti-
fication and emasculation and not emotional growth and maturation."[27]
Such sentiments among medical students were widespread.

Thus, American medical education in the 1960s occupied a curious
position. The medical schools were unquestionably doing an excellent job
of teaching. They were producing outstanding doctors, and no United
States citizen who could gain admission to an American school would
even think of going to a foreign country for medical study (excluding
elective work at certain established British or Continental schools). Yet, a
lingering feeling persisted that American medical education could and
should be doing even better. To medical educators, the problems and criticisms of the curriculum sounded remarkably similar to those heard all
century long.

The Changing Medical Student

Like graduate medical education, undergraduate medical education was
built on a base that was firmly in place by World War II. Hence, it should
be no surprise that the experience of being a medical student retained
much in common with that of the first half of the twentieth century,
even as the subject matter and organization of the material evolved.
Hard work still dominated the lives of students. To cover the necessary
ground, one medical faculty observed, the medical student "must fit 25
hours into a 24 hour day."[28] In the clinical clerkships, the line between
education and service continued to be blurred, as exhausted house officers frequently forced medical students to perform many of the innumerable chores of patient care. A student report from the University of
Michigan stated candidly, "When the junior year is mentioned, a discussion of scut work is immediately forthcoming."[29] If there was any relief
in the ordeal, it was during electives, especially those of the fourth year.
Indeed, faculty records suggest that fourth-year students on electives frequently regarded them as vacations.[30]

Medical school continued to represent not only hard work but considerable stress, much of it revolving around grading. Many medical students who had been at the top of their high school and college classes
now found that they were competing against classmates equally intelli-
gent and disciplined. The fear of flunking out was low, especially after
students reached the third year.[31] However, medical students tended to
be high-achieving, goal-oriented individuals who knew that there were
additional educational steps still ahead. The competition to do well in the
course work was keen, and this was accentuated by the fine detail with
which most medical schools ranked their students. Cornell, for instance,
ranked its students from number one to number 84, while the University
of Michigan calculated grade point averages to the fourth decimal point
in determining class standing.[32] Small wonder, then, that the majority of
Cornell students would skip seminars in histology and embryology (in

the faculty's view, the best and most important part of the teaching) to study for upcoming examinations, or that a Michigan student bitterly protested to the chairman of the bacteriology department that he was entitled to one more point on a recent test, which would have raised his score from 94 to 95.[33]

What made grading so distressing to many students was its apparent arbitrariness. Medical faculties generally tried hard to be fair and constructive, but, as one medical school dean observed, "Grading students is not an exact science."[34] Inconsistency and unevenness of standards persisted in this period, as it had in the interwar period. Different grading scales also continued to be found from one school to another, giving students at schools with more lenient grading standards a competitive advantage in applying for internship. To help alleviate these problems, some schools continued to adopt pass-fail grading systems—only to discover that many of the best students disliked them because academic accomplishments were less apparent on transcripts.[35]

The degree of stress in medical school, or how stress might have differed from earlier eras, was difficult to measure. Certainly, the work was demanding and the pressures intense. The vastness of medical knowledge, the student's imperfect mastery of what was currently known, the limitations of medical knowledge, and the huge responsibility involved with providing care to another person created uncertainties that plagued all students. These stresses were compounded by the pressures of evaluation and the hunt for a good internship. In 1966, 30 percent of Harvard Medical School's first-year class sought psychiatric help from the student health service.[36]

Educators debated whether the emotional demands of medical education had increased or whether the fiber and backbone of students had weakened in a less individualistic, less self-reliant age. To David Seegal, professor of medicine at Columbia University and co-editor of the *Journal of Chronic Diseases*, the solution for anxious medical students was "a self-kick in the seat of the pants." What was needed were "such homely qualities as rigorous self-examination, self-discipline, and self-reliance" so that the student might make an effort "to work out his own minor emotional problems." John H. Knowles, the general director of the Massachusetts General Hospital, agreed. He told Seegal: "Your general statement . . . is a firm plea for a continuation of the so-called Protestant Ethic, individualism, self-reliance, etc. It, of course, is in direct opposition to the present trend which has been aptly stated as the Freudian subversion of the American character which says that all of us are utterly dependent on and need help from everyone around us." Others, of course, disagreed. Three psychiatrists wrote, "Instead of being a sign of weakness, it is most often a sign of strength that the student who really needs help can admit this need and comes to the psychiatrist for help."[37] Suffice it to say, the debate continued unresolved.

As always, students were not without voices or influence. They made decisions regarding where to apply for medical school and internship and provided feedback to the faculty about every aspect of the curriculum. Reflecting the outer calm of the 1950s and early 1960s, student voices tended to be polite and nonconfrontational, but they could still be caustic and direct. Cases in point are irreverent student publications such as the University of Southern California's *Borborygmi* (literally meaning the rumbling noises caused by the propulsion of gas through the intestines), which found no subject or individual too sacred to lampoon.[38] Medical schools frequently implemented changes on the basis of student opinion, even though they remained aware that opinion within a class could vary considerably and that students' perceptions often changed with time.[39]

Although much of student life was unchanged after the war, there were conspicuous differences. Postwar changes in American culture and medical education affected the lives of medical students in a similar fashion as those of house officers. Students continued to work exceedingly hard, but no longer was the medical center their total universe. The earlier sense of being part of a cohesive family disappeared. More and more students lived away from the medical school, the fraternity system declined, and in the clinical years students rotated through several hospitals. On the wards, students' experience was increasingly shaped by contact with interns and residents rather than faculty. Students had outside interests and lives of their own, most conspicuously, dating and marriage. By the 1960s, over 50 percent of the students in many graduating classes were married.[40]

The experience of searching for an internship also changed. Before the war, each program had its own decision date, which pressured students into making binding decisions before they knew all their options. This problem was resolved by the institution in 1951–52 of a new system for selecting interns: the National Intern Matching Plan (or "Match"), which was established as a joint program of the Association of American Medical Colleges, the American Medical Association, and the hospital associations. Under this system students ranked the hospitals to which they had applied, while the hospitals ranked the applicants to their programs. On a certain date the lists were matched, and students and hospitals were informed of the results, which were binding. The new system proved popular, and it quickly became entrenched.[41]

In terms of their academic backgrounds, medical students were similar to students from before the war. Premedical requirements changed little; hard-working admissions committees continued to struggle with the difficult task of selecting the most promising applicants.[42] However, the student body in the postwar period became much more heterogeneous, especially with respect to the religious backgrounds of students. Quotas against Jews and Catholics disappeared, just as appointments to medical school faculties and many house staff programs became less restrictive. Major increases in the number of women and African-Americans admitted did not occur at this time, but prejudice where it existed was usually manifested by the failure to take positive steps to recruit women or blacks rather than overt discrimination in the admissions process.[43]

If medical school became more democratic with the ending of quotas, it became more exclusionary in terms of social class. Medical education was increasingly expensive, and scholarship funds were limited, especially in comparison with the amounts available for college and graduate study. The average cost of a four-year medical education (tuition and expenses) for members of the class of 1959 was $11,440. The mean annual income of parents of medical students that year was $9,734, compared with $5,557 for white urban families nationwide.[44] Forty percent of medical students enrolled in 1959 came from families with annual incomes of greater than $10,000, or the top 8 percent.[45] Part-time work was available, but there were limits to how much students could work without jeopardizing their studies. Half of the medical students who graduated in 1959 were in debt, with the greatest debt loads being found among students from lower income families.[46] More than ever, medicine was becoming a profession accessible mainly to the well-to-do.

Medical schools were troubled by this situation, but with scholarship and loan money in short supply, there was little they could do. It was estimated that full tuition paid for less than one-third of the actual costs of instruction.[47] Accordingly, even strong schools often took into account students' financial status in making their admissions decisions.[48] Some schools admitted students regardless of their ability to pay, but without financial aid many of these students either went to less expensive schools or decided not to pursue medicine at all.[49]

As before the war, medical schools competed vigorously with each other for students. The school in the strongest position was Harvard. In 1958–59, over 8 percent of the national applicant pool, or 1,274 of 15,170 total applicants, applied to Harvard. On various measurements, such as college grades and scores on the Medical College Admissions Test, Harvard medical students rated the highest in the nation.[50] Even rival Johns Hopkins conceded Harvard's superiority in attracting the best students.[51] To Johns Hopkins's chagrin, Harvard was consistently selected by the vast majority of students accepted to both schools.[52] The easiest school in the country to get into (for state residents) was the University of Arkansas, which one year received only 225 applications for a class of 105—a ratio of 2.2 applications per position, the lowest in the country.[53] Students at the school had a "distressingly high failure rate," and the school lobbied the state legislature to permit at least 10 percent of enrollees to be out-of-state students if qualified Arkansas residents were not available.[54]

However, it also became clear in the postwar period that medicine was in competition with other fields, including science, education, law, government, and business, for the best college graduates. After World War II, with so many veterans applying, medical schools were inundated with applicants. In 1949–50, there were 24,434 applicants to U.S. medical schools, or more than 3.4 applicants for each available position. In the early 1950s the number of applicants to medical school remained high, though at lower levels. In 1957, however, interest in medicine among college students sharply plummeted after the Soviet Union launched *Sputnik*. Large numbers of college undergraduates started seeking careers in the physical sciences, mathematics, and engineering rather than medicine as part of the country's concentrated effort to win the space race. The nadir was reached in 1961–62, when only 14,381 individuals applied for admission to medical schools in the United States, or fewer than 1.7 applicants for each available position nationwide.[55] This trend reversed itself only in 1962, when the growing number of college graduates and the excitement generated by so many important scientific breakthroughs led to renewed interest in medicine as a career.

The decline and subsequent resurgence of medicine's popularity as a career suggested that cultural factors influenced the decision to apply to medical school and the characteristics of those who did apply. This view received confirmation from a study published in 1978 by Daniel H. Funkenstein, a psychiatrist at Harvard Medical School, who found that the values, aspirations, and personal characteristics of medical students varied over time in ways that reflected changes in American society and culture. Funkenstein identified five distinct student eras: the specialty era (1940–1958), the scientific era (1959–1968), the student activism era (1969–1970), the doldrums era (1971–1974), and the primary care and increasing governmental control era (1975–). Of particular note was his observation that factors outside of medical school, such as prevailing cultural attitudes and economic incentives, were the major determinants of the career choices of medical students. These factors were found to have influenced career choices much more significantly than anything that happened during medical school.[56]

Observations of changing values and aspirations among medical students threw into sharp relief a question of basic importance to medical education: Who are the students? A fundamental blindness (some would call it a conceit) of medical educators throughout the twentieth century was their faith that medical education, through manipulations of the curriculum and the environment of learning, could influence the behavior, values, and choices of physicians. Funkenstein's studies forced a reconsideration of that view. Agnes G. Rezler, for instance, found little evidence to support "the optimistic assumption of medical educators that people's attitudes can be changed fundamentally." If proper attitudes and values are to be developed among physicians, she wrote, then faculties must select students "who possess certain [desirable] attitudes prior to entrance . . . instead of trying to develop such attitudes in students after they enter medical school."[57]

This blindness to the power of cultural forces was not confined to medical educators. Teachers and administrators throughout the educational system had traditionally expressed their faith in the ability of the schools to mold behavior and character, "Americanize" immigrants, and create a homogeneous "melting pot" out of an ethnically, religiously, and racially diverse society.[58] It would be a mistake to accept the extreme view—that teachers and ideas, mentors and role models, and values and traditions imparted through the educational process do not matter. Abundant evidence can be mustered to attest to the power of formal teaching and the capacity of the "hidden curriculum" to influence the values and attitudes of medical students.[59] Nevertheless, to ignore the character of students and the influence of culture would be to create exaggerated expectations of the power of medical education.

Producing More Doctors

Medical schools had always had a dual obligation to the country. First and most conspicuously, they had the responsibility to provide a superior education to those seeking to become doctors. In addition, they had the responsibility to train enough doctors to meet the medical needs of the public. The quantity as well as the quality of doctors mattered if schools were to be of greatest service to the community and nation.

Since World War I, the issue of the number of doctors had received little attention. During the Flexnerian period, conventional wisdom held that the country suffered from a surplus of poorly trained doctors. Educators and policy-makers of the period commonly used the slogan "fewer but better doctors" to characterize their views. In the aftermath of the Flexner report, many substandard medical schools closed, and the output of doctors dropped to dangerously low levels. However, by 1930 the number of doctors produced each year had returned to pre-Flexnerian levels, as had the ratio of doctors to the general population. After 1930, the number of graduates each year gradually rose, keeping pace with the overall population increase of the country (*see Figure 3*).[60] Throughout this period, there was much concern about the geographical maldistribution of doctors but little worry about the overall supply. Accordingly, most of the growth in physician numbers, both before and after World War II, resulted from the establishment of new medical schools in areas of the country that had undergone substantial population growth but were without medical schools of their own. Examples of these schools included Duke University, the University of Florida, the University of Miami, the University of Kentucky, and the University of Washington.

In the late 1940s, however, the public began to demand a still larger supply of physicians. Such pressure came from a variety of sources. Swelling college enrollments resulted in a greater demand among college undergraduates for places in medical school. It became something of an embarrassment to medical educators to have so few positions relative to the number of qualified applicants. Pressure to increase the supply of physicians also came from many rural and medically underserved communities, which could hardly be persuaded the country had enough doctors when they were without access to physicians. Most important, the increased demand for physicians reflected the growing health consciousness of the American people. As medical care came to be regarded as a basic right, the demand for more doctors and medical services grew accordingly.

Medical educators found themselves in a quandary. They generally sympathized with the objective of producing more doctors but knew that standards could not be lowered without doing the country an extreme disservice. There were only three ways to increase the output of doctors: accelerate the curriculum, expand class sizes at existing schools, or establish new medical schools. The experience of World War II—which had demonstrated the educational unsoundness of an accelerated curriculum—was very fresh with them. To most educators, shortening the standard length of training at a time of logarithmic increases in knowledge was simply unacceptable.[61]

A better approach in their view was to expand class size or establish new schools. However, these were viable options only if the financial means could be made available. As educators, they understood the enormous effort and expense necessary to assure excellence in medical education. Each school knew precisely how many students it could accommodate without compromising standards, based on the capacity of its classrooms and laboratories, the number of cadavers it could obtain for anatomy and dogs for physiology, the size of its faculty, and the clinical facilities it controlled. They believed that more students could be taught only if new facilities were acquired and additional faculty hired.

To acquire the necessary funds, medical school leaders began to look to the federal government. This was not a uniformly popular idea at first, in large part because the expanded role of the federal government was so new, and many worried that federal aid to medical education might result in centralized control or loss of the flexibility to innovate. A survey of medical school deans in 1950 found that an appreciable minority (22 percent) actually opposed direct federal aid to medical education for these reasons.[62] However, a decade later such concerns had largely disappeared. The federal government had supported biomedical research without interfering with academic freedom, and the schools had grown accustomed to dealing with the federal government as a patron. By the late 1950s most leaders of academic medicine favored federal aid to medical education, even though the American Medical Association did not endorse the idea until a decade later.

Though concern about an inadequate supply of doctors had been growing since the end of World War II, the issue achieved center stage upon the publication of a report by the Surgeon General's Consultant Group on Medical Education in 1959. This report came to be known as the "Bane report" after Frank Bane, the chairman of the consultant group and a former executive director of the Council of State Governments. The

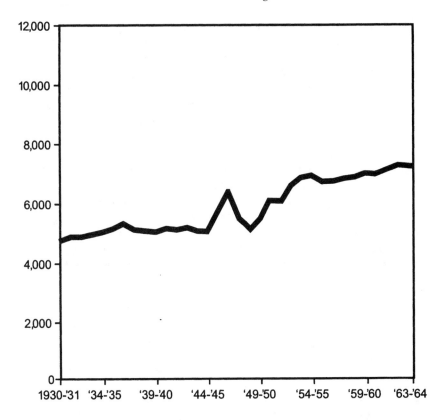

Figure 3　*Graduates of American medical schools, 1930–1964*

Bane report shocked the public by projecting a nationwide shortfall of nearly 40,000 physicians by 1975. According to the report, for the nation's health to be protected, medical and osteopathic schools needed to increase the number of graduates from the current 7,400 a year to 11,000 by 1975. The report offered a blueprint for expanding existing schools and creating new ones to avert the impending doctor shortage.[63]

The Bane report quickly became the most influential and effectual report on medical education since Abraham Flexner's report a half century before. It proved instrumental in shaping public opinion and mobilizing Congress to act. The immediate legislative consequence was the Health Professions Educational Assistance Act of 1963. This bill provided existing schools federal matching funds for the construction of new educational facilities, provided that they increase the size of their entering class by 5 percent or five students, whichever was greater. (Many schools increased their class sizes by much more.) New schools were awarded two federal dollars for every dollar raised on their own. The legislation also made federal loan money available to medical students. This bill was followed by revised legislation in 1965 (and still more generous legislation in 1968 and 1971) that provided schools so-called "capitation payments" (a specified sum per student) as incentives to increase enrollments. For instance, in 1967–69, schools that agreed to undertake a one-time increase of their enrollment by the greater of five students or 2.5 percent were eligible to receive a base grant of $25,000 plus $500 for each student enrolled.[64] Capitation payments were attractive to schools because they could be used for operating expenses, not just construction costs.

Federal legislation had a great impact on both the number of schools and the number of students. In the 1960s, 15 new medical schools were opened, and by the end of the decade plans were underway for a dozen more. By 1980, 126 medical schools were in operation, compared with 86 in 1960. The majority of these schools were state-supported institutions since even with federal subsidies, few private universities had the financial resources to construct and operate a new medical school. Many of the new schools became known as "community-based medical schools" because they had smaller faculties and used community hospitals for clinical teaching. Compared with traditional medical schools, commu-

Table 7   Growth in medical schools, entering class sizes, and M.D. graduates, academic years 1960–61 to 1980–81

Year	Number of Schools	Entering Class Size	Number of M.D. Graduates
1960–61	86	8,298	6,994
1961–62	87	8,483	7,168
1962–63	87	8,642	7,264
1963–64	87	8,772	7,336
1964–65	88	8,856	7,409
1965–66	88	8,759	7,574
1966–67	89	8,964	7,743
1967–68	94	9,479	7,973
1968–69	99	9,863	8,059
1969–70	101	10,401	8,367
1970–71	103	11,348	8,974
1971–72	108	12,361	9,551
1972–73	112	13,726	10,391
1973–74	114	14,185	11,613
1974–75	114	14,963	12,714
1975–76	114	15,351	13,561
1976–77	116	15,667	13,607
1977–78	122	16,134	14,393
1978–79	125	16,620	14,966
1979–80	126	17,014	15,135
1980–81	126	17,320	15,985

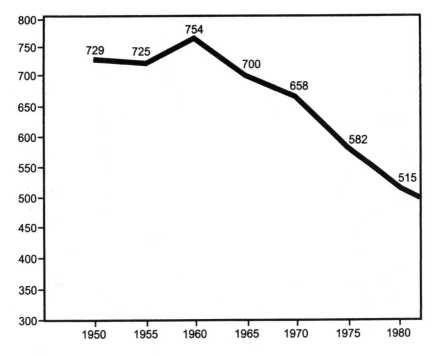

Figure 4 *Number of people per physician in the United States, 1950–1980*

nity-based schools tended to be more open to curricular experimentation, more sensitive to issues of community health, and more likely to profess an interest in producing primary care practitioners. The new medical schools and larger enrollments at existing schools produced a sharp increase in the number of physicians. By 1970, 11,348 students were enrolled in the first-year classes of medical schools, compared with 8,298 a decade before. By 1980, after all the new schools had become operational, the number of entering students had increased to 17,320, while the ratio between the general population of the country and the number of doctors had fallen substantially (*see Table 7* and *Figure 4*).[65]

The movement to produce more doctors reflected an interplay between medical schools and society. Established medical schools would not have expanded their class sizes had they not been subjected to strong pressure from the federal government and enticed by the promise of financial assistance. On the other hand, medical schools campaigned effectively to make certain that educational quality would be maintained while increasing enrollments. A case in point was their refusal to abbreviate the curriculum to produce more doctors. Similarly, new schools were approved only if adequate resources could be guaranteed, and the schools had to demonstrate that they were developing within the environment of a strong university or liberal arts college. As medical educators acquiesced to society's demand for more doctors, they were able to preserve high standards in undergraduate medical education.

The need to preserve quality in medical education at a time of rapid expansion thrust the agency that accredited medical schools, the Liaison Committee on Medical Education (LCME), into a position of new power and importance. The LCME had been established in 1942 as a cooperative effort of the Association of American Medical Colleges and the Council on Medical Education and Hospitals of the American Medical Association. Prior to 1968, the LCME had no more than a casual relationship with the federal government, but in 1968 the United States Office of Education formally recognized it as the official organization for the accreditation of medical schools and began appointing public representatives to the committee. As medical schools increased their enrollments, the LCME made certain that the schools did not move too quickly—that is, that the schools maintained an appropriate balance between the size of the enrollment in each class and the total resources of the institution. The LCME also established the financial, physical, and educational criteria for new medical schools and assumed responsibility for reviewing and choosing among the many proposals that were made to develop new schools.[66]

Since the 1940s, the federal government had been the dominant patron of biomedical research. With the passage of the Medicare and Medicaid legislation in 1965, the federal government assumed a similar role in the financing of medical care. Now, with the steps taken to avert a doctor shortage, the federal government was directly influencing undergraduate medical education. It became clear to medical educators that the center of power and financial support had moved from a local-state axis to a federal axis. Accordingly, in 1968 the Association of American Medical Colleges, which had been headquartered in Evansville, Illinois, moved its national office to Washington, D.C., where it could have ready access to Congress, federal agencies, and other organizations involved with higher education. The Association also reorganized its staff so that it could assume a more active lobbying role on issues of medical care and health care policy.[67]

The movement to produce more doctors was part of a broader cultural change in which medical care came to be viewed as a basic right. Social Security had been established. Now, many felt that medical security needed to be established as well, and an abundant supply of well-trained doctors was deemed necessary to achieve that objective. Underlying the movement was the traditional assumption of American health care policy: that the health of the nation was determined primarily by the quality and quantity of doctors. As the Association of American Medical Colleges put it, "The future health of the people will depend in considerable measure upon the continuing supply of competent physicians."[68]

In the 1960s, as in earlier decades, no one doubted that medical care would be only as good as the individuals practicing it—that is, that good medical care depended on having good doctors. On the other hand, some began to wonder whether there might be more to achieving a healthy nation than simply having capable doctors tend to the sick and injured. The dean of the University of Michigan School of Medicine observed that no clear relationship had been established between the number of doctors and the state of health of the population. He pointed to the lessons of World War II, when the national experience "showed continued improvement in the public health statistics even though the number of physicians available to the civilian population was sharply reduced."[69] Some even began to wonder if there might be a downside to producing more doctors. Economist Eli Ginzberg spoke of the difficulty of determining the "proper" proportion of physicians to the general population. He worried that the demand (as opposed to the need) for medical care might be limitless and that producing more doctors might increase the costs of medical care without appreciably improving the health of the people.[70] But once again, such cautions went unheeded and traditional assumptions, unchallenged. At the level of national policy, the tradition of equating the health of the nation with the number and quality of doctors continued unabated.

The Devaluation of Teaching

As events discussed in this chapter have shown, the period after World War II can hardly be called inactive in undergraduate medical education. Nevertheless, as medical schools grew in size and complexity, the instruction of medical students became a small part of their work. By the 1950s, the instruction of students was already often dwarfed by the training of house officers, clinical fellows, and graduate students.[71] In addition, medical schools had greatly expanded their responsibilities in research and patient care. Academic medical centers had evolved into big businesses with complicated organizational structures and ever-growing financial needs. As early as 1953, one major report on medical education maintained that many schools were building "large empires" at the cost of educating medical students. "Philosophers have pointed out that when size transcends quality that is the beginning of decadence."[72]

Of the many activities of medical schools in the postwar period, by far the most dominant was biomedical research. At the Cornell University Medical College, for instance, expenditures on student teaching rose from $449,170 in 1933 to $1,081,130 in 1956, or 140 percent. During the same period, expenditures on research rose from $88,510 to $2,837,054, or 3,100 percent.[73] By 1960, 56 percent of faculty time at the school was devoted to research, while only 14 percent was spent on undergraduate medical education.[74] Figures such as these can be misleading because they can give the false impression that research is separate and exclusive from other efforts of the faculty. Even so, the ascendancy of research and deemphasis of undergraduate teaching was unmistakable.

The rise of research was not intrinsically harmful to undergraduate medical education. Indeed, throughout the century educators had commonly maintained that research invigorated teaching by enabling a scholarly atmosphere for the study of medicine. Students were exposed to the reasoning skills of the finest medical minds, and they became aware of the tentative nature of even the seemingly most secure pieces of medical knowledge. The presence of research kept medical educators from going overboard teaching practical details instead of fundamental principles and reminded educators that students needed time to think, digest, and wonder.

Nevertheless, at many postwar medical schools, as throughout the multiversity, teaching experienced a decline in the value structure of the institution, while research enjoyed a concomitant rise in importance. It became increasingly clear that issues of undergraduate medical education mattered less and less to many instructors and administrators. The construction and supervision of the curriculum, once the primary responsibility of the dean and department chairmen, was delegated to an assistant or associate dean for curriculum and representatives from the different departments. Though many exceptions existed, faculty often voiced little interest in students or enthusiasm for teaching—especially the typical medical students planning careers in practice rather than research. At New York University, members of the executive committee had to urge the faculty to treat students "as individuals rather than en masse."[75] At the University of California, Los Angeles, administrators were embarrassed when an aerial photograph of the audience at commencement showed only 24 faculty members sitting in a faculty section of 200 chairs.[76] It was not the declining percentage of the budget or the growth of other important duties of academic medical centers that led to the forgotten medical student. Rather, it was the fact that student affairs occupied a position of diminishing importance in the institutional value system.

Any doubt that teaching was subordinate to research could be laid to rest by examining the reward system of medical schools. Everywhere, promotion and academic advancement resulted mainly from research. The "publish or perish" phenomenon was as strong at medical schools as it was elsewhere in the multiversity.[77] Promotion documents of medical schools typically listed teaching as an important criterion for advancement. However, as a department chairman at the University of California, Los Angeles, declared, the recognition of teaching skills on paper merely represented "lip-service."[78] Indeed, as John H. Knowles pointed out, at some schools being known as a good teacher could even be "an obstacle to advancement."[79] In the feverish race to publish as many papers as possible, much insignificant research found its way into print, and the trend toward the devaluation of the published article, the standard unit of academic currency, continued unabated from before the war. An eminent Harvard surgeon decried the increasingly common practice of engaging in "the repetitive publication of the same data in minor journals or the 'rewarming' of the same facts and figures in a variety of different publications."[80]

The high value placed on research permeated lower tier and special mission schools, not just the research elite. In 1958, the faculty of Woman's Medical College of Pennsylvania voted to convert a large number of ward beds to semiprivate beds to help raise $2,500,000 for a new research wing. The faculty knew that the loss of the ward beds would hurt its educational program, but they felt that establishing a research presence was a higher priority.[81] At these schools promotions typically came more easily than at the elite institutions, but here, as elsewhere, the most important criteria were publishing papers and winning grants.

Research was also the primary determinant of a school's standing among other schools. The most prestigious schools were those most successful at advancing biomedical knowledge and producing new faculty members. Perceived teaching quality was the least important factor in determining an institution's reputation.[82] Schools took great pride in having high numbers of graduates become professors and deans. They carefully noted the percentage of their graduating classes that took internships at good teaching hospitals or that subsequently pursued research careers. As the Department of Medical Microbiology at the University of Southern California School of Medicine said in the evaluation of one outstanding student: "Should be recruited for academic medicine. This is our highest praise."[83] Faculty raids were often a source of pride to the raided school. Thus, Hahnemann Medical College, frequently overlooked in discussions of American medical schools, took consolation when its professor of surgery was lured away by the offer of a chair at Yale. "The better this institution becomes, the more will we be called on to supply good men to good places, and seen in its proper light, this is not a cause for anguish but of pride."[84]

Herein lay the primary obstacle many schools experienced in trying to institute genuine curricular reform: time spent teaching was incompatible with institutional values that gave priority to research. It was difficult to entice faculty members to give much attention to students when they were seldom rewarded by the institution for doing so. At medical schools, as throughout the multiversity, academic reputations of faculty were national or international and presumed to depend on universal criteria. In contrast, teaching reputations were primarily local. Hence, the frequent neglect of undergraduate students—whether at the medical school or at the liberal arts campus of the multiversity.[85]

Though absorption with research could easily lead to the neglect of undergraduates anywhere in the multiversity, the problem was particularly severe at medical schools. External support was readily available for research, but funds that could be used for education were in scarce supply, even taking into account the federal programs of the 1960s to expand the production of physicians.[86] To help pay for education, many schools freely admitted to having "'bootlegged' funds from research and patient care."[87] Tuition fees, which accounted for more than 70 percent of the income of medical schools in 1910, provided only 28 percent of income in 1948 and 7 percent in 1968, despite substantial increases.[88] Research grants, now the dominant source of income, had a distorting effect on many schools, for well-funded instructors who generated their own support often refused any institutional responsibilities. For practical purposes, many instructors became voluntary faculty: if they so desired, they could refuse to teach.[89]

Though the ready availability of research funding diminished the importance of teaching at many medical schools, in the last analysis the emphasis on research was consistent with faculty values and aspirations that had been apparent since the time that academic medicine emerged as a full-time career in the United States. From the beginning, many faculty members valued the local recognition they received for excellence in teaching, but they valued even more the national and international honors they could garner for research. This value system posed the chief obstacle to true curricular reform. Teaching, when done well, was time-consuming and labor-intensive, requiring close personal contact with students. Good teaching required a generalist and synthetic orientation that in an era of increasing specialization took greater and greater effort to provide. The learning environment, in short, had to be carefully constructed with the individual needs of students kept foremost. This was contrary to the development of American medical schools, which as institutions evolved in such a way as to meet the needs of the faculty first.

These remarks are not to deny that good—indeed, inspired—teaching regularly occurred, or that the ranks of every faculty contained dedicated, gifted teachers. Rather, these observations are to suggest that good teaching in the modern medical school, as in the proprietary school so harshly criticized by Abraham Flexner, was frequently by accident rather than by design. The institutional obstacles to redressing that situation were formidable. Had A. Lawrence Lowell, who in the 1920s had been unable to persuade Harvard Medical School to divert some of its rapidly growing resources from research to education, been alive, he would undoubtedly have been dismayed but not surprised.

PART III

Breaking the Social Contract

The Erosion of University Values, the Decline of Public-Spiritedness, and the Beginning of the Second Revolution in Medical Education

12

Medicare, Medicaid, and Medical Education

IF THERE WAS ONE SINGULAR CHARACTERISTIC of the American medical school during the generation that followed World War II, that characteristic would be its intensely academic nature. The period between 1945 and 1965 represented the scientific era at its peak—not merely in work accomplished, for many stunning scientific discoveries were made before and after—but in how a commitment to biomedical research dominated the institutional mission and in how the public strongly supported that mission through munificent appropriations and popular approbation. If teaching sometimes was forgotten amid the drive to expand knowledge, that was an affliction medical professors shared with professors in all branches of the multiversity.

With the passage in 1965 of Medicare and Medicaid, a new era began—one in which the clinical activities of medical schools began to hypertrophy, swelling out of proportion to their other duties. This effect was not expected at the time Medicare and Medicaid legislation was enacted, nor did it happen immediately. Nevertheless, in the years that followed, clinical service rapidly grew to become their most conspicuous activity and most important source of income. In the process, their link to the university weakened, their commitment to academic values decreased, their tradition of charity eroded, and they became enmeshed more firmly than ever in the health care delivery system. If research had once been the master, that role at most medical schools was increasingly assumed by patient care—to the increasing subordination of both research and teaching.

The Escalation of Faculty Practice

Since World War II, with the spread of private medical insurance, medical schools had greatly expanded their activities in patient care. Nevertheless, faculty practice before 1965 was modest in scale relative to the academic functions of medical schools. In 1965–66, of total medical school revenues of $882 million, medical service provided $49 million.[1] Faculty practice had become an important activity, but medical schools were hardly dependent on it financially.

In the mid-1960s, however, the finances of medical schools began to appear more tenuous, primarily because federal grants for biomedical research became more difficult to obtain. The astounding expansion of the National Institutes of Health (NIH) could not have continued indefinitely, but the acceleration of the Vietnam War caused the growth rate of NIH appropriations to diminish abruptly. Of note, the cutbacks in NIH appropriations were in the rate of growth, not in the absolute level of dollars (though rescissions in funds for construction and training did occur). Nevertheless, a mood of despair pervaded academic medicine, as medical leaders complained of "unconscionable" cutbacks in federal support for biomedical research.[2]

Fortunately for the finances of medical schools, the federal government in 1965 enacted the landmark Medicare and Medicaid legislation. Medicare provided substantial federal health benefits to individuals over the age of 65 and to disabled persons of any age, while Medicaid, a shared federal-state program, provided health benefits to poor persons who passed a means test. This legislation placed beneficiaries on a similar fee-for-service basis as other private patients. Academic medical centers began receiving payment for virtually every service they had formerly provided free or below cost to many indigent patients. Doctors and hospitals everywhere benefited in a similar fashion, but none as much as the medical faculties and teaching hospitals, which had been providing the lion's portion of charity care. The result was the creation of a major new source of revenue for academic medical centers.

The roots of Medicare and Medicaid lay in the growing technical capability of medicine, the accelerating demand for medical care, the federal government's increasing involvement in domestic affairs, the rising level of prosperity in society, and the evolving belief that medical care is a right. By 1965, approximately 75 percent of the population was covered by private medical insurance, which had become an important fringe benefit of labor contracts. However, large pockets of the population did not have access to private medical care—especially the elderly and persons living in poverty, precisely the groups most in need of medical services. The publication in 1962 of Michael Harrington's best-selling book, *The Other America*, drew widespread attention to the urgency of poverty in the United States and the growing discrepancy between the "haves" and "have-nots." In the optimistic, expansive mood of the Kennedy–Johnson era, one result was Medicare and Medicaid. These programs were important parts of the "Great Society"—the outpouring of social legislation in the 1960s that included major initiatives for public welfare, civil rights, mass transit, public housing, federal aid to education, and urban renewal.[3]

The benefits of Medicare and Medicaid were immediate and widespread. Millions of Americans were brought into the private health care system, resulting in greater utilization of medical services than ever before. From 1965 to 1980, the number of admissions to nonfederal short-term general hospitals rose by 50 percent, an increase that was particularly marked among individuals over 65. In 1965, 16 percent of patients discharged from short-term general hospitals were 65 or older; by 1985, that figure had grown to 30 percent.[4] Medical institutions also profited from the new programs—especially Medicare, which did not depend on the willingness or ability of a state to fund its component of the program. Medicare proved a bonanza to doctors and hospitals because of its liberal payment schedule and willingness to reimburse hospitals for capital costs. Medicare had a multiplier effect, for once the federal government became a payer of medical services, private insurers usually followed Medicare's decisions about allowable expenses and rates of reimbursement. Though Medicare and Medicaid were enacted at the same time, it was Medicare that had the greatest impact on academic medical centers.[5]

After the passage of Medicare, medical faculties rapidly increased their clinical work. The most conspicuous activity occurred at first with Medicare patients. However, it quickly became clear that a private patient was a private patient, regardless of which particular insurer was paying the bill, and faculties soon began to see many more traditional private patients. The volume of private practice among faculty rose dramatically—in teaching wards and clinics, private hospital wings, and separate faculty offices designated for private ambulatory care. Many patients seen by clinical faculty were utilized in teaching, but a growing portion of faculty practice was independent of student or house staff education.

The administrative vehicles for faculty practice were the so-called "faculty practice plans," organized group practices consisting of the full-time and voluntary clinical faculty of the medical school. Faculty practice plans first appeared in the 1950s in response to the growth of private medical insurance, and in the 1960s the number of schools operating such plans increased. After the passage of Medicare, such plans became universal. In a typical plan, full-time faculty would sign an authorization card, which allowed the administrator of the plan to bill in their names for services rendered to private patients, including Medicare and Medicaid patients. Plan administrators could also bill for the professional fees of full-time and voluntary faculty for the supervision they provided house officers on the teaching services. Monies received were deposited in a general account, to be used in ways specified by the particular faculty practice plan.

No two faculty practice plans were identical, since each was organized to fit the needs of the particular institution. In some cases, the plans were schoolwide; in others, they were organized at the departmental level. All were governed by complex legal agreements that specified a wide variety of differing details such as administrative and reporting procedures, fee determination, billing and collection practices, compensation schedules, and income distribution. Generally, however, membership in the school or department's practice plan was required of full-time faculty, and most plans covered all clinical income, no matter what the nature of the service or where provided.[6]

In the years following the introduction of Medicare and Medicaid, the growth of faculty practice was nothing short of extraordinary. The experience at Johns Hopkins was typical. In 1970–71, the clinical income of the full-time staff amounted to $1,901,000; by 1974–75, that figure had reached $6,130,000; and by 1983–84, $60,000,000.[7] Nationwide, the income generated from faculty practice showed a similar rate of increase. By 1980–81, practice income had become the largest source of revenue for medical schools (*see Table 8*).[8]

For full-time faculty, the escalation of faculty practice represented a bonanza, since a major use of clinical income was to improve faculty compensation. At public medical schools, professional fees in the 1970s provided 30 to 40 percent of the salary of the average faculty member; at private schools, the percentage was even higher.[9] Faculty salaries, traditionally modest relative to the earnings of private practice, began to rise dramatically. Benefits were most marked in the clinical departments, but salaries rose throughout the medical school as clinical earnings were also channeled into the support of basic science faculty. By 1975, salaries in clinical departments had risen to levels approaching those of practicing physicians (*see Table 9*).[10] To compete successfully for faculty, medical schools now had to offer competitive reimbursement, not research opportunities alone. Even the most prestigious schools were not immune from

Table 8   Revenues, U.S. medical schools (dollars in millions)

Year	Medical Service	Federal Research	Total, All Sources
1960–61	28	133	436
1965–66	49	350	882
1970–71	209	438	1,713
1975–76	609	823	3,389
1980–81	1,729	1,487	6,481
1985–86	3,773	2,229	11,096
1990–91	9,406	4,039	20,991

Table 9 Median faculty salaries, strict full-time appointment, 1975–76

Department	Instructor	Assistant Professor	Associate Professor	Professor	Chairman
Basic Science	15,000	19,000	24,000	31,000	40,000
Anesthesiology	35,000	42,000	48,000	52,000	64,000
Dermatology	17,000	26,000	30,000	45,000	50,000
Family Practice	21,000	35,000	39,000	41,000	49,000
General Surgery	20,000	36,000	45,000	53,000	65,000
Medicine	20,000	30,000	38,000	45,000	58,000
Neurology	18,000	30,000	36,000	45,000	51,000
Neurosurgery	18,000	32,000	48,000	52,000	66,000
Obs–Gynecology	18,000	32,000	43,000	47,000	59,000
Ophthalmology	18,000	35,000	37,000	50,000	64,000
Orthopedic Surgery	20,000	40,000	48,000	56,000	59,000
Otolaryngology	17,000	35,000	30,000	34,000	64,000
Pathology	18,000	28,000	36,000	43,000	55,000
Pediatrics	18,000	28,000	34,000	41,000	54,000
Plastic Surgery	15,000	37,000	45,000	65,000	
Preventive Medicine	17,000	22,000	27,000	35,000	43,000
Psychiatry	17,000	25,000	34,000	42,000	55,000
Radiology	23,000	37,000	46,000	55,000	66,000
Thoracic & Cardiovascular Surgery	22,000	39,000	50,000	64,000	
Urology	18,000	38,000	45,000	59,000	55,000

the pressures to raise faculty salaries. Leaders at Johns Hopkins acknowledged that without a remunerative professional practice plan the school would be at a "serious handicap" in faculty recruitment.[11]

Another important use of clinical revenue was to cross-subsidize academic activities. Specifics of how this was done varied, but virtually everywhere the principle was the same: to use surplus practice income for the scientific and professional development of the institution. Thus, research did not suffer as NIH funding leveled off, for at every institution practice income enabled the recruitment of faculty, establishment of training programs, construction of buildings, and purchase of equipment and supplies. Clinical practice, in essence, became the medical schools' core business, one which was used to subsidize their central academic mission.

Teaching hospitals also entered a new age of prosperity. They could bill Medicare and Medicaid for hospital charges, and they received payment for both the direct expenses of graduate medical education (house staff salaries) and the indirect expenses of maintaining a house staff program, such as adjustments for a sicker mix of patients, compensation of teachers, and recovery of the costs of maintaining call rooms and teaching facilities (the so-called "education passthrough").[12] By the 1970s, the typical teaching hospital had become a gargantuan complex with revenues running into many tens of millions of dollars.

Not surprisingly, innumerable problems arose regarding the disposition of clinical income. Decisions had to be made about how much of the money to use for faculty salaries and how much to use for research directly. Decisions also had to be made regarding the proportion of clinical fees that would be retained by the individual, division, or department that earned the money and the percentage that would be made available to others in the institution. The common result was disagreements and feuding that pitted one part of the medical school against another. High clinical earners like surgeons and radiologists were especially likely to seek to retain the professional fees they generated. Clinical faculty based at municipal or veterans hospitals, where government regulations typically imposed income restrictions, were often envious of the higher compensation received by colleagues who happened to be located at other hospitals. Many basic scientists, despite seeing their salaries rise, were angry at the growing discrepancy between their salaries and those of the clinical faculty. A department chairman at the University of Michigan echoed the prevailing view when he said that the use of clinical income was "the most important and potentially destructive current issue within the Medical Center."[13]

For medical schools the escalation of faculty practice was transforming. To handle the large sums of money generated by faculty practice, schools needed to adopt better administrative methods, with the result that the organizational evolution of medical schools into efficient, large-scale businesses was accelerated. Typical in this regard was the University of Colorado, which in 1978, using older, haphazard methods, found itself with a low collection rate and an average delay between billing and collection of 240 days. Accordingly, the school introduced a computer billing system and revised other administrative procedures to improve efficiency.[14] Nationwide, the administration of faculty practice plans became an exacting occupation with managerial responsibility assigned to trained business executives who reported to the department chairman, dean, or chief administrator of the academic medical center.[15]

In addition, the arrival of Medicare and Medicaid hastened the erosion of the charitable mission of academic medical centers. The need for charity care hardly ended, of course, since millions of individuals under the age of 65 were too well off to qualify for Medicaid yet unable to afford medical insurance or pay for private care. Medical faculties and teaching hospitals continued to set the standard for American medicine in eleemosynary behavior. Nevertheless, with clinical revenues so high, the losses most academic medical centers incurred from charity work became much smaller as a percentage of income. Historically, academic medical centers had provided great amounts of free care. Now, they were transformed into vendors of services.

With the advent of Medicare, medical faculties found they had much wider responsibilities than before. Medicare carried many implications for academic medical centers in terms of expanded community service and the provision of nonhospital services such as home care, hospice care, and nursing home care. Many teaching hospitals developed their own nursing home facilities, many medical schools established departments of community medicine, and medical faculties began to engage in a variety of experiments with neighborhood health centers, mental health clinics, and substance abuse programs. With chronic diseases continuing to rise in prevalence, medical faculties also began speaking of prevention as well as cure and of health promotion as well as treatment. This broader agenda was also influenced by the intense social activism of the era. Though these activities ultimately remained marginal to the activities of most academic medical centers, their importance was symbolically recognized by the increasing frequency with which academic medical centers were called academic health centers. In name, if not always in action, academic health centers acknowledged their enlarging responsibilities.[16]

As the volume of faculty practice escalated, the financial worries of the late 1960s were soon forgotten. The huge growth of clinical income made medical schools less dependent on the vagaries of research funding. On the other hand, medical faculties were now vendors of services, and like all vendors of services, they were vulnerable to the whims of purchasers and payers. As one noted surgeon wrote, "The power to pay for services is the power to regulate those services."[17] Initially, medical schools were not troubled by that notion, so generous were the reimbursements from Medicare and private insurers. In a fee-for-service environment, medical schools grew rich beyond their wildest expectations. However, as clinical income became their dominant source of revenue, their fate became allied to that of the health care delivery system. Their continued prosperity now depended on how favorably the health care delivery system would continue to smile upon them.

Toward a One-Class System of Care

The United States, like most Western nations, had traditionally had a two-class system of health care. Private health care, for those who could pay for it, was patient-oriented, personalized, and based on continuity of the doctor-patient relationship. It offered patients minimal waiting time to see their physicians and convenient, comfortable, personalized service in both ambulatory and hospital settings. In contrast, the "clinic" mode of care, for those who received charity medical services, was depersonalized, somewhat inefficient, and sometimes degrading—even if the same technical quality of care was rendered. Typically this care was provided by the interns, residents, and fellows of a teaching hospital under the supervision of a member of the medical faculty, who was not the patient's personal physician. Continuity of care was often broken by the regular rotation of house staff and faculty.

Since World War II, however, as part of a growing civil rights movement, American attitudes toward the poor had been undergoing fundamental changes. Increasingly, the American public recognized the dignity of the individual regardless of race, creed, or financial capacity. Such an attitudinal change contributed to the emerging view that health care was a right, not a philanthropic favor. As a result of this cultural shift, it became increasingly difficult to justify the physical or mental inconvenience of patients on the grounds that they were being treated in a clinic. Accordingly, in the 1950s some medical schools and teaching hospitals began to question the appropriateness of the two-class system. For instance, in 1960 the Columbia-Presbyterian Medical Center rehabilitated its Vanderbilt Clinic and revised scheduling and admitting policies to make the facility more user-friendly to the poor patients it served.[18]

In this context, Medicare and Medicaid provided more than a mechanism for financing health care. They also embodied the culmination of a social revolution. The legislation was the product of the same White House administration that had sponsored the Civil Rights Act of 1964 and the Voting Rights Act of 1965. Architects of the legislation believed that there needed to be one system of care for all patients. In their view, separate systems inevitably tended toward inequality and did not deserve public funds. The goal of Medicare and Medicaid was to bring the elderly and the poor into the same health care system that served the more affluent.[19]

The passage of Medicare and Medicaid prompted academic health centers to move toward a system that treated all patients with courtesy and dignity. Outpatient departments were renovated and updated, as were inpatient facilities. Appointment systems were introduced in ambulatory clinics, and the vast inpatient wards began to disappear in response to Medicare requirements that patients be assigned to semiprivate rooms having two, three, or four beds. Terms such as "ward service," "clinic service," and "teaching service" were abandoned for various euphemisms—here, the "university clinical service"; there, the "semiprivate service." These linguistic changes were symbolically important, much as the substitution of "black" for "Negro" and "health care" for "medical care."

From the standpoint of education, what was most important was that Medicare patients were required to be treated as private patients. This meant that an identifiable, senior physician had to assume responsibility for management of the case. Typically the responsible physician was expected to be the attending physician, who was now asked to be more than just a supervisor of house staff. The precise definition of a "private physician" for billing purposes was continually debated, and Medicare regularly sent out clarifications of the conditions that had to be met for teaching physicians to be eligible for reimbursement. Nevertheless, the underlying principle was always the same: payment for the professional services of salaried full-time clinicians under Part B of Medicare would be made only when a private patient relationship existed.

Medical educators found themselves on the horns of a dilemma. They rejoiced that Medicare would pay medical schools professional fees for the work of the faculty in a teaching setting. However, they worried that the conversion of Medicare (and Medicaid) patients to private patient status might destroy the ward services of teaching hospitals, thereby critically damaging the teaching programs. Educators understood that learners could develop independence only when they had the opportunity to assume real responsibility for patient care. In the past this could not be done with private patients. Many educators feared that with Medicare, medical faculties might thrive but medical education might wither.[20]

Threats to the ward service from changing patterns of medical practice were not new. As noted earlier, the number of ward patients had fallen in the 1940s and 1950s in response to the spread of private medical insurance. However, for a while it appeared that the erosion of the ward service under Medicare would be carried much further. For instance, soon after the implementation of Medicare, 90 percent of patients on the ward services of the Johns Hopkins Hospital were private patients covered by some form of insurance or public payment program.[21] Before the enactment of Medicare, a physician at the Massachusetts General Hospital had predicted that governmental medical care programs for the aged might "wipe out the medical ward teaching service with a stroke of the pen."[22] Now many educators feared that view might prove to be correct.

Ultimately, an accommodation was reached satisfying Medicare and Medicaid authorities that beneficiaries were receiving private medical care and yet leaving the graduate training system essentially intact. This was accomplished by allowing house officers to be delegated major responsibilities for patient management as the representatives of the attending physician, who was now the private physician of legal record. Attending physicians, as before, would round regularly with their house staff. It was expected that the resident would immediately contact the attending physician if help were needed. Attending physicians would document their participation in the patients' charts, typically by writing a brief admitting note within 48 or 72 hours of admission or, alternatively, by countersigning the resident's admitting note. At some institutions, attending physicians would countersign residents' progress notes as well. Medicare and Medicaid would pay the professional fees of faculty, provided that such documentation was in the chart.

Medical educators were pleased with this system because undergraduate teaching and house staff training were left undisturbed. In particular, with patients on Medicare and Medicaid who did not have a private physician, house officers were allowed to retain the supervised independence that they had traditionally received with ward patients. House officers were the first to see new patients on admission, and they were the ones contacted about any changes or problems. The decision of what constituted an "emergency" requiring the immediate notification of the attending physician was left to their discretion. In essence, the major change that resulted was that attending physicians now documented their involvement in the hospital charts. Ward patients, called by new names and housed in more comfortable quarters, were still treated primarily by the house staff. Accordingly, the quality of the learning environment on the teaching services remained high.

If medical education escaped relatively unscathed, that was because a truly one-class system of care was never fully achieved. Major steps had been taken in that direction, but full egalitarianism in medical care did not occur, any more than it did elsewhere in American society. Not all private patients were treated the same—as evidenced by the ease with which patients with their own private physician but not patients on the teaching service could receive prompt radiological examinations or priority scheduling in the operating room. Similarly, after discharge, patients on the teaching service continued to encounter difficulties in receiving long-term follow-up and good continuity of care, even if they were on Medicare or Medicaid.

The movement toward a one-class system of care once again highlighted the intrinsic ethical dilemma of medical education. It was in the interest of society for house officers to assume major responsibility for patient care so that the country could have well-trained doctors in the future; it was in the interest of the individual to be treated by someone experienced. Throughout history, the answer had been easy: use poor patients for teaching in exchange for free care. However, that was the social contract of poverty, not of an affluent society aspiring toward egalitarianism.

The question of how to teach medicine effectively with private patients perplexed medical educators, and a variety of approaches was entertained. Some pointed to the high professional quality of care on teaching services, arguing that private patients would consider it a "privilege" and "opportunity" to be used in teaching, if only they were properly informed. Others argued that private patients had an ethical duty to allow themselves to be used in teaching since they were benefiting from the earlier training their own physicians had received—much as ethicists might argue that no one should be entitled to enjoy a potluck dinner without having brought a dish of his own. Still others contended that private patients might be persuaded to be used in teaching if greater precautions were provided—for instance, by lengthening the time of training and thus conferring responsibility to house officers more slowly.[23] Nevertheless, this debate remained theoretical, for Medicare and Medicaid did not eliminate the opportunities for house officers to assume high levels of responsibility with certain groups of patients. If medical educators and society escaped having to determine how to provide house officers responsibility in a one-class system of health care, that was because the country's rhetoric of human dignity and social equality continued to outstrip the reality.

The Inversion of University Ideals

If one theme more than any other characterized American medical education for the first two-thirds of the twentieth century, it was the effort of faculty and administrators to make the medical school a true branch of the university. The medical school's claim to a place in the university arose from its commitment to advanced education and research. The instruction of medical students (and later, house officers, clinical fellows, and graduate students) could not effectively proceed without the same attention to curriculum, learning opportunities, and intellectual freedom as education in any other university discipline. Similarly, creativity and productivity in every branch of biomedical research required that investigators devote their full time to university work. Well-trained clinicians, masters of the here and now, could provide practical instruction and participate in some descriptive clinical studies, but the future of medical knowledge and practice rested in the hands of those with fertile minds and scientific preparedness who had the opportunity to approach their subject as university scholars.

Another important mission of medical schools was the provision of patient care. Without an active clinical practice, medical schools could neither teach nor engage in clinical research. Accordingly, the search for clinical facilities had been another dominant theme in the history of American medical education. An active clinical practice allowed medical faculties to substantiate their claim as the standard-bearers of medical care and to serve their community by accepting difficult cases in referral.

Moreover, the large volume of free care that medical faculties provided validated the role of medical schools and teaching hospitals as important philanthropic institutions.

If unchecked, of course, patient care could easily interfere with the creative work of faculty members. The practice of medicine makes demands on physicians' time and energy that are difficult to control. Once the responsibility of patient care is assumed, the freedom to pursue research and teaching is often compromised, for the needs of patients become paramount. Some medical practice is necessary for clinical skills to remain sharp, but too much practice jeopardizes teaching and research and endangers the overall academic reputation of an institution. Precisely how much medical practice could be combined with academic pursuits varied from specialty to specialty. Clinical work was more readily combined with scholarship in the surgical fields, where the operating room was essential to teaching and the advancement of surgical knowledge. In internal medicine and pediatrics, where so much research had become laboratory-based, much smaller amounts of clinical work intruded on academic productivity.

One of the most difficult tasks confronting American medical schools throughout the twentieth century was discharging their patient care responsibilities without losing sight of their academic mission. As seen already, there was never a time when clinical practice did not intrude on teaching and research. Before World War II, the bustling charity clinics of teaching hospitals severely tested the ability of medical faculties to provide care without losing a scholarly orientation. After World War II, as the number of insured patients seeking treatment at academic medical centers increased, the demands on medical faculties to provide clinical services grew even stronger.

Nevertheless, before 1965, most medical schools managed to remain focused on their university duties. This was possible in part because at many schools the full-time clinical faculty received considerable help from the voluntary staff, who provided much of the clinical teaching and charity care. More important, medical faculties were not dependent on clinical income to meet the operating expenses of the school. As a result, they were not under economic duress to see every paying patient seeking their services. Rather, they could confine their clinical activities to charity work and to private patients of interest to them in relation to teaching and research.

The passage of Medicare and Medicaid dramatically altered the equilibrium at medical schools between academic and service functions. With Medicare, many charity patients formerly used in teaching became financially attractive to private practitioners and community hospitals. Unless medical schools competed for Medicare patients—and other private patients as well—they stood in danger of losing their "clinical material," with irreparable damage to their academic programs. As one medical school observed, "The Medicare legislation of this year puts the medical schools in direct competition for teaching material with the practitioners of medicine."[24] In this sense the escalation of faculty practice was congressionally mandated, for schools were left with little choice but to join the race for patients.

However, it did not take medical schools long to adjust to the new rules of the health care delivery system. Immediately upon implementation of Medicare, medical schools began receiving generous reimbursement for clinical services once rendered for free, and the schools could see little reason not to accept the money—particularly in light of the ending of the NIH's "golden era." As medical faculties earned more and more clinical income, they discovered that they liked it, and for the first time they vigorously began to seek paying patients. Quickly, the volume of patient care they provided increased, and academic health centers became even busier than before.

As faculties scurried to provide private medical care, they found it increasingly difficult to keep their academic mission in focus. As always, significant local variation could be observed. At some schools, clinical practice became more dominating; at others, it remained less obtrusive. However, virtually everywhere escalating clinical practice had an erosive effect on university values. At the University of Michigan, the dean noted that "in some of our clinical departments there is now absolutely no opportunity for faculty members to think or to have time for scholarly effort."[25] At Georgetown, overinvolvement of the faculty in clinical practice was having "an adverse impact on the quality of teaching and the extent of scholarly effort."[26] At Howard, the faculty feared "subtle or direct pressure may be exerted to increase practice income," to the detriment of teaching and research.[27]

The transforming effects of the escalation of clinical practice could be seen clearly at Johns Hopkins, the pioneer of university medicine in the United States. When Milton Eisenhower assumed the presidency of the university in 1956, the budget of the medical school was $4,100,000, and the school's program was well balanced among the objectives of teaching, research, and clinical service. When he left the presidency in 1967, the budget had grown to $22,000,000, reflecting mainly the growth in federal research support. However, in Eisenhower's opinion, the growth had been well managed and the balance reasonably maintained. When he resumed the presidency in 1971, the budget had grown to $42,000,000, primarily from the infusion of clinical practice dollars. In Eisenhower's judgment, the school's program had lost its balance, and clinical practice had started to undermine academic pursuits.[28]

The growth that occurred at medical schools after the passage of Medicare and Medicaid was enormous. However, as one manifestation of the inversion of university ideals, most of the growth occurred in clinical rather than academic activities. To generate more money, additional full-time clinical faculty were necessary. By 1980, the number of full-time faculty at American medical schools had increased to 50,536, from roughly

17,000 in 1965, with most of the increase occurring in the clinical departments.[29] Unlike faculty growth during the era of the multiversity, the increase had less to do with the development of research programs than with the specialty practice of medicine and the oversight of graduate training programs in the various clinical disciplines. Scarcely a school could be found where the faculty was not growing much larger than needed to sustain the school's academic work or where concerns were not raised that the faculty as a whole was spending too much time in patient care rather than teaching and research.

As another manifestation of the inversion of university ideals, the preponderance of income from faculty practice plans was used to raise faculty salaries, particularly those of members of clinical departments. For instance, a study in 1974 of seven sample schools found that the majority of practice income (nearly 80 percent at two of the sample schools) was used for faculty salaries and fringe benefits, leaving a much more modest percentage for investment in construction, equipment, program development, teaching, and the direct support of research.[30] Before Medicare, medical faculty were content to live on professors' salaries in exchange for the opportunity to teach and to conduct research. Now, clinical faculty were major income-generators for the institution, and increasingly they felt that they deserved salaries at or near those of private practitioners in their respective fields.

The strengthening ties of medical schools to the health care delivery system disrupted many traditional relationships. For instance, the escalation of faculty practice was disturbing to many voluntary faculty members and did much to chill their relations with the medical school. Traditionally, as noted earlier, the unsalaried volunteer faculty at many medical schools had provided an enormous amount of clinical instruction. However, by the 1970s the full-time clinical faculty, which had grown enormously in size, had displaced the private faculty from many important teaching duties. Moreover, as faculty sizes grew in the face of limited hospital beds, full-time faculty usually received priority in admitting their patients, thereby diminishing the role of volunteer faculty in the clinical operations of medical schools. The goodwill that had long existed at most schools between volunteer and full-time faculty began to erode.

Similarly, the increasing involvement of medical schools in the health care delivery system was disruptive of traditional relationships between the scientific and clinical branches of medical schools and between the medical school and the rest of the university. Here, Johns Hopkins is again illustrative. As faculty practice grew, the escalating salaries for clinicians were viewed as having "a very destructive effect on the relationship between the clinical and basic science departments," and disturbed members of the basic science departments felt that they were becoming "'second-class citizens' financially."[31] Yet, even the basic science faculty were highly paid relative to other university faculty, leading university officials to worry that the growing salary differential between the liberal arts campus and the medical school would disrupt the salary structure of the entire university.[32] With the escalation of faculty practice, academic health centers grew into self-supporting, far-flung empires whose budgets often exceeded the budget of the rest of the university combined and whose unprecedented autonomy frequently led to resentment among other university departments.

As faculty practice escalated, medical schools openly—some would have said brazenly—began competing for patients with community doctors and hospitals, something they once vowed they would never do. The case of the University of Arkansas was typical. In the 1950s the medical school, lacking adequate hospital facilities, embarked on an arduous campaign to persuade the state legislature to appropriate funds for a new medical center. The effort was successful largely because of the support of the medical practitioners of the state.[33] In enlisting the support of the local profession, the school promised that "the competitive practice of medicine by the full-time faculty" and "the care of private patients in the Medical Center" would be specifically precluded.[34] Yet, such protestations were quickly forgotten a decade later, when a new dean, pushed by the passage of Medicare, declared that private practice by the full-time faculty in the university hospital was now "absolutely necessary."[35] Earlier promises to the contrary, the University of Arkansas began competing with the local profession.

In assessing the impact of the escalation of faculty practice on the institutional balance of medical schools, it would be inaccurate to suggest that they lost sight of their academic mission. Though most clinical income was used to support salaries, large sums were left to underwrite scholarship. Moreover, an academic value system was clearly retained, as evidenced by policies regarding promotions and rewards. High clinical earners, because of market conditions, were usually paid the most, but productive investigators received the lion's share of promotions, honors, and peer recognition. In addition, it is not unreasonable to speculate that the higher salaries now available to all medical faculty were instrumental in attracting to academic careers many excellent workers who in previous generations might have been deterred from research by paltry academic salaries—again, to the ultimate benefit of biomedical research as a whole.

Nevertheless, as medical schools became squarely entrenched in the health care delivery system, their ties with the university correspondingly weakened. As Robert Ebert wrote, "By the end of the sixties the centrifugal force generated by medical center size, fiscal autonomy, and substantial salary differentials began to exceed the centripetal force of academically oriented physicians wanting to maintain close ties to the university."[36] Clinical faculty at many schools spent more and more time in patient care, often routine, rather than in teaching and research. The key element in the transformation from an academic to a clinical orientation had not been the increased volume of patients treated per se but the economic dependence on clinical income to meet the operating expenses of the schools. This Abraham Flexner could have predicted. In 1930 he had written that there was no safety for academic medicine if a faculty were dependent upon its earning power. "If the scientific budget of a clinical department is once dependent upon the earnings of the clinical staff, that staff will in all probability have to earn the requisite amount— by doing what it is interested in, if it can, by doing other things, should that become necessary."[37] In the era of the multiversity, research had been the master, and if the faculty sometimes became distracted from teaching, it was to pursue their research. After the passage of Medicare and Medicaid, the master increasingly became patient care, to the subordination of both teaching and research and to the inversion of the university ideals upon which the modern medical school had been founded.

13

Medical Education in an Era of Protest and Civil Rights

IF MEDICAL EDUCATORS OPERATED under any single illusion after World War II, it was the illusion of autonomy. The remarkable growth in wealth, size, power, and influence experienced by academic health centers created the deceptive view that academic health centers controlled their own destiny. In the 1960s and 1970s, however, America was rocked by social unrest, as the antiwar and civil rights movements tore at the fabric of American society. The passions, moral fervor, and discord swept through the medical schools, undermining their confidence. Student rebellions, house staff unionization, and the clamor of women and minorities, especially African-Americans, to receive a place in medicine challenged the traditionally staid and self-confident medical faculties. It became clear that medical schools, as all institutions in society, were vulnerable to external social conditions that they could not control. Though medical schools emerged from the protest era little changed, the myth of autonomy had been exposed as false.

These disparate events each revealed fundamental features of American medical education. Student activism, and faculty reaction to it, demonstrated the fundamentally conservative nature of medical schools and their student bodies. House staff unions once again placed in sharp relief the fundamental ambiguities of graduate medical education: the tension between education and service, and the debate over whether house officers were students or employees. And the struggles of women and minorities reaffirmed the importance not of entry alone but of the internal organizational environment if true equality of opportunity in medicine—or any field—were ever to be achieved. In the last analysis, the protest era was more significant for what it revealed about American medical education than for any specific reforms or changes that resulted.

Student Activism

Throughout the history of American medical education, students had influenced the educational environment. Nevertheless, with the exception of the class play, where rules of propriety were temporarily suspended, medical students traditionally spoke in polite, deferential voices. Medical school attracted few radicals, and success in school required a high degree of conformity and absorption with the work. Medical schools were not dissimilar from the rest of the university, where a high degree of decorum remained, and where rebellion was defined by fraternity pranks, not by student takeovers of university buildings.

In the 1960s, fueled by the civil rights movement and the strong sentiment against the Vietnam War, a new era of student discord erupted on university campuses. Student radicalism seized national attention in the fall of 1964 with the Free Speech Movement at the Berkeley campus of the University of California. After that, confrontations between students and university administrations became common. As one measure, from 1964 to 1967, the number of campus chapters of Students for a Democratic Society (SDS), a radical organization at the forefront of the student protest movement, grew from 29 to 247. By the spring of 1968, a mood of intense foreboding pervaded American society and college campuses, as the Vietnam War dragged on and as the assassination of Martin Luther King Jr., precipitated a new round of urban rioting. Campus protests became angrier, more frequent, and, for the first time, violent. In the spring of 1968, student radicals captured several buildings at Columbia University; in April 1969, armed black militant students seized the student union building at Cornell; in April 1970, students at Yale University went on strike in support of an indicted leader of the revolutionary Black Panther party; and in May 1970, National Guard troops shot and killed four students at Kent State University during an antiwar riot in which university protesters had burned the campus ROTC building. In 1968 and 1969, violent protest occurred on about 150 campuses, including many of the nation's most prestigious universities.[1]

Even at the height of the protests, only a small minority of students was actively radical. However, large numbers of liberal sympathizers could easily be mobilized to sign petitions, participate in rallies, and engage in demonstrations, especially in the wake of a catalyzing political event. Reinforcing political activism among students was the emergence of a widespread youth counterculture that defied authority and social convention by distinctive speech, appearance, and music and by its celebration of sensual experience, immediate gratification, and personal liberation, particularly through psychedelic drugs and sex. The counterculture was a social rather than a purely political phenomenon, but one that clearly fostered political activism.

While the protests on university campuses were raging, a parallel student movement emerged at medical schools. The climax occurred between 1968 and 1970—in part because of the turbulence of those years and in part because of the entry into medical school of many students who had participated in campus protest movements as college under-graduates. At times medical students could be raucous and confronta-tional, as when students disrupted the American Medical Association House of Delegates in June 1968 and the Council of Deans in February 1969, but in general their protests tended to be orderly. Even so, as uni-versities were shaken during the protest era, so were medical schools.[2]

Student protest at medical schools, like that at university campuses, was not a single movement and hence could not be easily defined or characterized. What Diane Ravitch has said of the university protest movement could be said equally well of the medical school movement: "It could be likened to a series of concentric circles, whose numbers expanded or contracted in response to the political climate and specific issues on a given campus."[3] Student organization was encouraged by the general social turbulence of the 1960s, but of all the factors, according to Fitzhugh Mullan, a former student activist who has written thoughtfully on the subject, the Vietnam War was paramount.[4]

Activism among medical students usually expressed itself in one of three independent but mutually supportive ways. The first was political protest. Students rallied and campaigned in behalf of a host of issues— the environment, feminism, homosexual rights, nuclear disarmament, and poverty—but mostly in protest of racism and the Vietnam War. At Columbia, students staged a rally to raise bail money for incarcerated members of the Black Panther party; at Tufts, members of the first- and second-year classes persuaded the school to suspend classes for five days to allow students to participate in political campaigns; at Boston Univer-sity, students held a teach-in against the Vietnam War.[5]

The second category of student activism involved efforts to make the medical school more responsive to the health needs of the community, particularly the poor. Activism in this area shared several common char-acteristics: the students' desire to "do something" immediately, their recognition of the failures of existing institutions, their efforts to make the medical center more socially responsive, and their impatience with the requirement that they become adequately acquainted with the basic sci-ences before being allowed to participate in the study and care of patients. At the Mount Sinai School of Medicine, first- and second-year students supported a strike of Local 1199, the hospital union, against the hospital.[6] At Columbia, many members of the first- and second-year classes demanded that the school establish programs for the treatment and rehabilitation of drug addicts and increase the hiring of minority groups at the medical center.[7] At Michigan, students organized a confer-ence on the health problems of the poor.[8] At Harvard, 278 students peti-tioned the school to establish a commission to seek ways to improve the quality, availability, and utilization of health services in the neighboring black community.[9]

In many cases, concern for community health needs led students into direct involvement in the health affairs of the impoverished and disadvantaged. At the forefront of such efforts was a new national coalition of health science students known as the Student Health Organizations (SHO), which provided an important link between student organizing at the local and national levels. The SHOs grew out of political activities of students at the University of Southern California, some of whom had spent the summer of 1965 working with the Medical Committee for Human Rights in Mississippi. With the cosponsorship of the medical school, student leaders at the University of Southern California obtained a demonstration grant from the Office of Economic Opportunity to provide fellowships during the summer of 1966 for 90 medical, dental, nursing, and social work students from 40 institutions in 11 states. The goals of the summer project were to provide health services to the community, educate students in issues pertaining to the health care of the poor, and stimulate the community to work for social change. Enthusiasm among students for the project resulted in the creation of SHO chapters at a number of medical schools. At its peak in 1968, loosely confederated SHOs had been organized at approximately 70 schools, and a national assembly in February of that year attracted over 600 health science students from 40 states. That summer student health projects were conducted in eight cities, and over 500 health science students participated.[10]

The third area of student activism encompassed efforts to promote educational reform. Student clamor arose on virtually every issue affecting their lives: admissions, the curriculum, teaching, grading, faculty recruitment and promotions, tuition, room rents, the condition of the residence halls, the adequacy of recreational facilities, the quality of food in the cafeteria and snack bar, and the prices in the vending machines. Their gaze was not just on student affairs but on all aspects of institutional policy. At Boston University, for instance, students organized a Student Committee on Medical School Affairs to investigate allegations of institutional racism and sexism.[11]

Students had always exerted some influence on medical school affairs. What was new was their stridency, impatience, and frequent confrontations with the faculty—here a statement of grievances, there a disruption of classes with tardiness or noise. Like other university students, medical students (including many who might not have been particularly political) often wore the uniform of protest: long hair, mustaches or beards, and disheveled clothing that did not include a tie. Student appearance served only to shock further conservative, traditional faculty. "Their slovenly appearance with dirty, long hair touching wounds, with offensive body odors, dirty hands and nails, and nondescript and inappropriate clothing belies their professional medical goals,"[12] one distressed instructor wrote. Many faculty were also shocked by the brazen language with which students sometimes voiced their complaints. Thus, *The Weekly Flatus*, a student newspaper at the University of Southern Califor-

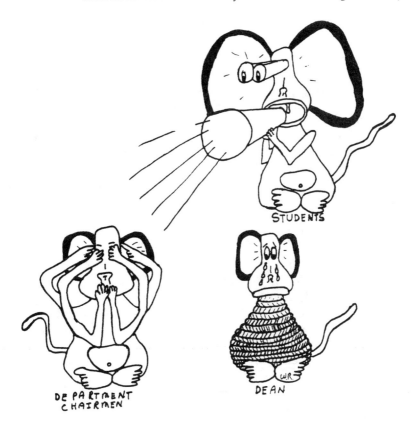

STUDENTS

DEPARTMENT
CHAIRMEN

DEAN

Figure 5

nia School of Medicine, put faculty on notice: "We feel if we are given shitty lectures, the rest of the school ought to be aware of it too."[13]

Also new to the protest era was student insistence on becoming part of the formal decision-making structure of medical schools. Students of the era often demanded—and frequently received—the opportunity to serve as voting members of faculty committees. One study in 1969 found that students at 51 of 83 medical schools participated in institutional affairs in a determinative rather than a consultative way—that is, through direct involvement in institutional governance.[14] As an instructor at the University of North Carolina School of Medicine put it, "Medical students seem to essentially be telling us how to run the medical school, which may not be so bad, but is certainly new."[15] Faculty and administrators were sometimes satirized as cowering under to student demands (*see Figure 5*).[16]

In their protests, students were not without sympathizers at medical schools. The political causes that magnetized students—particularly the Vietnam War—aroused many house officers and faculty as well. In addition, students often found themselves with considerable faculty support on matters of educational policy. Improving medical education was a shared goal, and faculty frequently found the suggestions of students to be insightful and constructive. At the University of Maryland, the curriculum committee was so impressed with the ideas of the first-year class that the committee voted unanimously to add students to its membership.[17]

On the other hand, shared goals could not prevent the development of a generation gap between students and faculty. Many faculty were disturbed by the outspokenness of students and their defiance of authority. In contrast to previous generations of students, who adapted themselves to the system, students of the protest era were determined to change the system and became impatient with any delay. Hence the degree of conflict and mistrust between students and faculty reached unprecedented levels.

Even at the height of the protest era, medical students were never as unruly or disruptive as students on many college and university campuses. Generation gap aside, medical students identified with the medical profession, unlike many university-based radicals, who openly disavowed the establishment. Student activists at medical schools wanted to change medical schools, not do away with them. They criticized the schools for their insularity and aloofness from society, for their preoccupation with research and disinterest in community health. This differentiated them from university radicals, who attacked the university for being too much a part of society, for serving as a willing accomplice of the military-industrial establishment. Medical schools, in short, had many student activists but few revolutionaries.

After 1970, the most intense student rebellions abated, and by the time the war was over, medical schools had once again become quiet places. SHO chapters faded away, students concentrated on their studies, relationships with the faculty normalized, and faculties and administrators breathed collective sighs of relief that they had weathered the storm. For instance, at Harvard Medical School, which had been the scene of considerable student activism in the 1960s, students by 1974 were exhibiting little overt antagonism toward the "system." If Harvard students had any principal interest outside of study, according to the dean, it was now in their personal and family life and in the quality of their lifestyle, not in politics or social activism[18]—thus giving some support to the widely observed emergence of a "Me generation" following the Vietnam War.

Though by the early 1970s the protest era had ended, it was not without lasting consequences. Student voices—at least some of them—remained more vocal, challenging, and questioning of authority than before. At most schools students retained the rights they had won to serve on faculty committees, particularly those pertaining to admissions, education, curriculum, and student affairs. Students at many schools showed a heightened sense of voluntarism, as manifested by participation in a wide variety of service projects: feeding the hungry, aiding the homeless, providing science instruction at inner-city high schools, tutoring disadvantaged children. At the national level, the Student American Medical Association (SAMA) was revitalized as a relevant forum for social and educational concerns. In the mid-1970s, as a demonstration of its independence from the more conservative American Medical Association (AMA), SAMA changed its name to the American Medical Student Association (AMSA) and appropriated some of the liberal ideology of the defunct SHO. In addition, the Organization of Student Representatives (OSR) was established in 1971 as a permanent part of the governing structure of the Association of American Medical Colleges.

Nevertheless, after the protest era was over, student interest in social issues and the problems of the health care delivery system, in general, waned considerably. By the mid-1970s, two investigators found medical students to be more politically conservative than their predecessors and attributed the "liberal shift" of the protest era to a period effect.[19] Such conservatism, on the whole, has persisted. When this author visited the Mount Sinai School of Medicine in preparation for this book, graffiti in the student locker room poked fun at Local 1199. "How many 1199 workers does it take to screw in a lightbulb? 1199. None to do it and 1199 to watch and say ooo-ahhh! Plus one more to ask for a raise." This was a far cry from the support students at the school had provided the union when it went on strike at the hospital 16 years before. Faculty also became absorbed once again with their academic and clinical duties. Concerns about serving the health care needs of the community or addressing the problems of the health care delivery system, important issues to some faculty during the Vietnam War, were now as forgotten by most faculty as they were by most students. Of course, in a war-weary nation, the impulse for social activism was everywhere muted. Yet, from the perspective of using the intellectual and political power of the academic health center to address the broad health care needs of society, medical schools had become not just quiet but virtually apathetic. The fundamental conservatism of the medical school—and medical profession— seemed undeniable.

House Staff Militancy

If the voices of students had always been discernible in medical education, so had those of house officers. After World War II, house officers became bolder, as they spoke out frequently on matters relating to patient care, the conditions of work, and salaries. At Boston City Hospital, 270 interns and residents (over 90 percent of the house officers at the hospital) signed a petition of protest to the mayor of Boston decrying the deteriorating conditions of patient care encountered there.[20] At George Washington, house officers protested the cramped call rooms, inadequate number of blood drawers and ward clerks, and other work conditions at the university hospital.[21] At the University of California, Los Angeles, house officers engaged in "lengthy and acrid debate" with hospital administrators on the subject of their salaries.[22] No teaching hospital could afford to ignore house staff complaints. Hospitals that were slow to raise salaries or hire more support personnel risked becoming less competitive in the next round of house staff recruitment.

In the protest era, however, the voices of house officers for the first time became shrill, their rhetoric radical, and their methods confrontational. Much house officer unrest, like that of medical students, was precipitated by external political events, particularly the Vietnam War. In the late 1960s house officers everywhere could be found signing antiwar petitions, joining marches, and participating in teach-ins and demonstrations. In addition, much house staff protest was aimed directly at the medical school or teaching hospital. To socially conscious house officers of the era, concerns for patient care, patient dignity, and the academic health center's role in the community assumed a new urgency.[23]

House staff militancy took a different form from that of medical students. Student activism peaked in the late 1960s. House staff militancy, in contrast, became most strident in the 1970s, after campus unrest had largely subsided. Student activism focused on a variety of social issues. House officers concentrated mainly on training concerns, particularly levels of pay and hours of work. Indeed, the distinctive characteristic of house staff militancy was the establishment of house staff associations for collective bargaining on salary, working conditions, job security, and hours—precisely the bread and butter issues of most trade unions.

House officers had good reason to speak out on matters of pay and conditions of work. Their position had always been an ambiguous one—part student, part employee. Academic health centers had long used the educational component of graduate medical education to justify trifling salaries and the use of house officers as cheap labor. To a large teaching hospital in the 1960s or early 1970s, the use of house officers for routine chores could easily save hundreds of thousands of dollars a year from not having to hire more support personnel. In the 1960s, house staff salaries did rise and ancillary staffing was improved, but only because assertive house officers and students made known their intention to seek programs with more competitive salaries, benefits, and working conditions and not because of any intrinsic generosity of teaching hospitals. Even so, as house officers were fond of pointing out, on an hourly basis they remained poorly paid.[24] In addition, many house officers distrusted hospital administrators, whom they often found condescending, unappreciative of their efforts, and insensitive to their welfare.

Issues of pay and working hours assumed a much greater importance to house officers in the late 1960s. Reflecting broader cultural changes, marriage, family, and "personal time" had become accepted rights of house officers. Matters of compensation and hours accordingly became more important. One survey in 1968 found that few married house officers could live in any degree of comfort without borrowing money or having their spouses work.[25] Moreover, residency and fellowship training delayed by several years the ability of trainees to begin earning a full professional living.

In the 1960s, house staff demands for higher salaries were typically made informally. During that time, however, initial steps at unionization occurred. Pioneering the movement was the Committee of Interns and Residents (CIR), formed in New York City in 1958. The CIR laid much of the groundwork for organizing house staff into unionlike groups and for encouraging a much more militant approach in their dealings with hospital administrations. By 1972, the CIR represented nearly 1,200 interns and residents in New York at 18 municipal hospitals; it also negotiated the contracts for house staff at seven voluntary (private) nonprofit hospitals. CIR had a full-time staff, collected dues, published a newsletter, and exercised substantial influence in local and state government.[26]

In the still tempestuous early 1970s, with many former campus activists now house officers, the unionization movement spread. Across the country interns and residents organized into local house staff associations that claimed the right to speak on behalf of all house officers at the institution. By 1972, house staff associations had been organized at 70 percent of all hospitals with graduate training programs and at 81 percent of hospitals run by local and state governments.[27] House staff associations varied considerably in their militancy. For instance, at Freedman's Hospital (the former name of Howard University Hospital) house officers engaged in a work slowdown in January 1973 because of unhappiness with salaries and fringe benefits. However, the house staff ended the slowdown after the hospital explained its financial plight to them.[28] At many other institutions the house staff would not have been so accommodating. In general, house staff associations tended to be more organized and militant at hospitals without close affiliations with a medical school, which suggested to some that the unionization movement was more pronounced in situations where house officers felt they were not receiving much faculty attention or good teaching.[29]

House staff associations had diverse objectives. They addressed a broad mixture of issues encompassing both training and social concerns—higher pay and more time off on one hand, better patient care and a more socially responsive academic health center on the other. The diffuse array of house staff interests was apparent in March 1971, when more than 200 interns and residents from all parts of the country took part in a three-day conference in St. Louis to provide a national forum for house staff concerns and to attempt to lay the groundwork for a national union. The conference took a stand on a host of issues. It opposed any discrimination based on race or sex and the war in Southeast Asia, and it supported universal health insurance, community control of health services, new programs to treat substance abuse, and written labor agreements between hospitals and house staff that would call for higher pay, better fringe benefits, more vacation time, and a limit to the number of hours on duty. Each of the topics engendered considerable discussion, and on no issue was there full agreement within the group.[30]

Though many house staff associations professed an interest in health care and social issues, the employee issues of salary and working hours quickly became paramount, and the larger concerns were soon relegated to a minor position in discussions. This development was observed in a survey of house staff associations in 1971, which found that the associations placed an "overriding stress" on pay. At one association after another, house staff groups were found putting most of their effort into their own salary and benefits package—often espousing a broad set of goals in their public statements and a narrower one the bargaining table. The survey concluded that "the drive toward house staff unity is prompted not by a sense of social commitment nor by a desire to right health-delivery wrongs, but rather by a—dare we say it?—selfish drive for 'what's coming to us' in the form of higher pay, parking privileges, and free lunches."[31] This pattern was typified by events at Los Angeles County Hospital, where the house staff association in 1970 organized a heal-in to protest what it considered overcrowding and inadequate treatment at the hospital. The heal-in ended after a few weeks, when most members of the association voted to accept a 35 percent increase in pay. The president of the house staff association, a dedicated social activist, complained bitterly of the ready abandonment of the larger cause. "Most house officers at the hospital 'are very nouveau riche and so they seduce themselves out of worrying about hospital conditions.'"[32]

Underlying the house staff union movement was the fundamental question of graduate medical education: Were house officers students or employees? Academic health centers repeatedly argued the former; house staff associations, the latter. Medical educators and hospital administrators liked to call house staff pay an "educational stipend"; house officers chose to call it a "salary." Typically, house officers were labeled as "students" or "employees" depending on the vested interests of the party doing the labeling, who would conveniently forget that house officers were in fact both.

House staff militancy assumed a new level of intensity in the summer of 1974, following amendments to the National Labor Relations Act that allowed employees of institutions in the health care field to organize for purposes of collective bargaining. Local house staff associations became more insistent in their demands for higher pay and fewer hours, while the Physicians' National Housestaff Association (PNHA), whose membership came primarily from city, county, and state hospitals, accelerated its efforts to establish a national house staff union. The local house staff associations had been very successful at promoting their members' financial interests. By 1976, the average house staff salary in the United States ranged from $12,329 for an intern to $15,557 for a resident in the fifth postgraduate year.[33] However, they felt there were many more gains to be made in the area of reducing the hours of work. On this issue, the most militant union of all, the CIR, went on strike in March 1975 against 21 voluntary and city-run hospitals in New York City, the first strike of its kind in the country. At least 1,000 of the union's 3,000 members failed to report for work during the strike, which ultimately was resolved when the hospitals conceded to the union's terms.[34]

During the CIR strike, it was apparent that an enormous generation gap in medicine had developed. The union went on strike over work schedules said to run up to 100 hours a week with stretches of up to 50 hours at a time. The CIR demanded a limit of 80 hours a week to allow time for rest and family life. Hospital officials decried this demand as demonstrating a lack of professionalism and a move toward a "shift mentality." "When I was a boy," one medical director complained after the strike had ended, "we worked two out of three nights, and now they're working only one out of three."[35] The hospitals contended that although interns and residents were often on duty for long hours, they usually found the time for proper sleep. The hospitals also contended that hard work was part of the practice of medicine and that the residency experience set the tone for what would follow. To this, house officers retorted that senior hospital officials had lost touch with the realities of modern hospital practice. The greater number of admissions, the presence of sicker patients, and the use of so many sophisticated procedures had made life on call much more challenging and fatiguing than in the past. One young physician stated succinctly: "Hospitals are complex places. There's a lot more to do now."[36] House officers also were quick to point out that few Americans would interpret a distaste for 50-hour shifts as a sign of lack of dedication to medicine.

Many educators feared that house staff unions would bring about the end of a system of training, not to mention the end of medicine as a calling. In this, their fears were unfounded. There existed ample room to make call schedules more humane, not to mention safer for patients, without sacrificing the traditional educational opportunity provided by internship and residency to immerse oneself in clinical work. None of the house staff associations proposed lazy schedules that would have made medicine appear an easy or attractive career to those not deeply committed. An every third night call schedule—the result of the CIR strike—could be positive for learning, allowing more time to read, think, relax, and refresh.

Yet, there was considerable hypocrisy in house staff demands for fewer hours. Many house officers used their free time not for reading, rest, or family life, as they claimed, but for moonlighting—that is, the outside practice of medicine, typically by working in an emergency room or intensive care unit at another hospital. Since the 1950s, house officers had regularly engaged in moonlighting, but in the 1970s the prevalence and scale of moonlighting dramatically increased—even though salaries had been substantially raised, and even though the average debt load of house officers was still relatively small. To many first-hand observers, house officers often seemed more interested in moonlighting than in learning medicine, teaching students, or caring for patients.

Examples of rampant moonlighting were widespread. Medical students at the Mount Sinai School of Medicine complained to the dean that all the house officers wanted to do "was get out at 4 or 5 P.M. so they could moonlight."[37] At the University of Michigan, faculty found repeated instances of slipshod performance in patient care by house officers who were tired from the previous night's moonlighting. "We cannot have quality tertiary care programs when our house officers neglect reading, and neglect research, to moonlight at local emergency rooms."[38] In the CIR strike, the union won the right to moonlight for most of the house staff it represented, even as it struck for shorter work weeks on the grounds of exhaustion and sleep deprivation.[39] Nationwide, 78 percent of residents in the third year of postgraduate study engaged in moonlighting, according to one survey in 1977.[40] Another study estimated that the average extracurricular work week of the moonlighter was 58 hours.[41] Residents in specialties like otolaryngology and orthopedics were often permitted to take evening or weekend call from home since most problems could be handled by telephone. It was not uncommon for residents in those fields to carry their beepers with them to another hospital so they could moonlight while officially on duty. Such levels of moonlighting provided incomes that allowed many house officers to enjoy a luxurious lifestyle, not merely pay off loans or support a young family.

If medicine as a calling was threatened, it was not from house staff unions per se but from the underlying culture of affluence, consumption, and self-indulgence that helped give rise to high house staff salary expectations. The 1970s, as many writers have pointed out, was a time that glorified self-fulfillment and immediate gratification—the "Me-Decade," to use Tom Wolfe's phrase. Yippie leader Jerry Rubin became a Wall Street broker; student radical Rennie Davis began selling insurance.[42] House officers were no more immune to these cultural influences than anyone else. Indeed, sociological studies have indicated that house officers of the mid-1970s, like medical students, were less idealistic and more conservative politically than their predecessors.[43] In this context it is not surprising that house staff associations emphasized wages and working hours or that moonlighting became so widespread. One contemporary observer described what he saw happening: "Well paid house officers have cars, apartments, wives, money for entertainment, ski trips, etc. In our affluent society, the distractions thus afforded and the search for 'fulfillment' have tended to displace the dedication, the determination, [and] the quest for learning and skill."[44] The history of house staff organizing is in need of further study, but when that happens, writers will undoubtedly detect a pronounced influence of the cultural values of the decade.

Ultimately, house staff militancy abated. In 1976, the National Labor

Relations Board decided that interns, residents, and clinical fellows were students rather than employees with regard to their petitions to be recognized as bargaining units, and therefore that they were ineligible to engage in union organization under the jurisdiction of the National Labor Relations Act. After various appeals, the decision was upheld in 1980, when the United States Supreme Court refused to review the matter. Most house staff associations dissolved or became inactive, faculty-house staff relationships normalized, and academic health centers were spared further threat of strikes or collective bargaining.

Officials at academic health centers breathed a collective sigh of relief. They had legally won their point: that education, not service, was the raison d'être for graduate medical education, and that house officers should be considered primarily students. Senior faculty and hospital administrators, who remembered an earlier era when house officers and faculty were part of a closely knit professional family, could scarcely comprehend what had led to a confrontational "we versus they" attitude and were delighted to see the return of collegial relationships. House officers, too, were generally content with what had transpired. They had lost their legal effort to be declared employees, but they had achieved their primary objectives: higher salaries and less onerous call schedules. By 1980, with the turmoil of the protest era over, house officers were glad to be in an educational environment, not in an adversarial labor-management relationship with hospital and medical school officials.

Nevertheless, the fundamental ambiguity that had allowed the unionization movement to proceed—the question of whether graduate medical education was education or service—was not resolved by the National Labor Relations Board. House officers since the 1970s have enjoyed better pay and shorter hours. However, at every training program, the tension between educational and service needs has continued. The legal edict that house officers are students did not end—and may have encouraged—their frequent abuse as cheap labor, while the many subsequent efforts to shorten hours created new worries that something of educational importance was being lost, namely the benefits resulting from assuming total responsibility for one's patients. In fact graduate medical education is both education and service, for service is indispensable to learning. The challenge of creating the proper balance, however, has remained as elusive to achieve as always.

Minorities

Following World War II, as noted earlier, medicine became a more open profession. However, not all groups shared in the growing accessibility of medicine as a career. In particular, African-Americans and other racial minorities continued to encounter severe problems. Indeed, not until 1966 were all medical schools desegregated. In the 1950s and 1960s, between 2 and 3 percent of entering U.S. medical students were black, at a time when 10 percent of the total population was black. Statistics prior to 1971 for Mexican-Americans, mainland Puerto Ricans, and Native Americans (the other groups designated by the Association of American Medical Colleges [AAMC] in 1970 as "underrepresented minorities") do not exist, but their numbers were far fewer. At this time racial discrimination in medicine was hardly confined to medical schools. Thus, it was difficult for minority physicians to obtain residency positions or hospital staff appointments, and many professional organizations would not admit or elect black members. Even the federal government was a party to racial discrimination. In 1947, 24 of the 127 Veterans Administration hospitals had separate wards for black patients, and full desegregation of these facilities did not occur until 1955.[45]

In the 1960s, the civil rights movement rapidly gained momentum. Popular protest against racial discrimination was intensified by the assassination of Martin Luther King Jr., in 1968. In response to these events, the AAMC established its Office of Minority Affairs in 1969 and convened its first task force on minorities in medicine the following year. The task force articulated the goal that minorities should be represented in medicine in proportion to their numbers in the overall population. The objective was to increase minority medical student enrollment from 2.8 percent of the student body in 1970–71 to 12 percent by 1975–76.[46]

In the late 1960s, new programs of affirmative action swept through medical schools, as they did in other branches of higher education. This reflected both a sincere conversion of medical faculties to the cause and their desire not to be subject to public criticism. Schools located in African-American or Hispanic communities showed particular sensitivity to increasing minority enrollment, motivated at least in part by concern for achieving better community relationships in an era of urban riots. Many schools came under intense pressure to increase minority enrollments from their own students. In Philadelphia, the Student Health Organization demanded that each of the city's medical schools increase the enrollment of black students to one-third of the class.[47] Some saw in affirmative action a way to improve the health conditions of minority and impoverished citizens, since a number of studies showed that black physicians primarily treated minority patients.[48] In this regard, however, James L. Curtis, a prominent African-American psychiatrist and a leader of the effort to increase minority enrollments, warned that this was a poor reason to increase the number of black physicians. In his view, the real goal was a color-blind health care delivery system in which black doctors would regularly treat patients of all races.[49]

Admissions represented only one part of most affirmative action programs. Typically, schools also provided a variety of supportive services for minority students: a dean of minority affairs, student support groups, tutoring and counseling services, and remedial and enrichment programs. Many schools began outreach programs into the community—for instance, creating summer programs for promising minority high school and college students—in the hope of arousing an interest in health care careers among these students (and in the hope that some of them might later seek admission to the school). Financial aid represented a singularly important part of successful affirmative action programs. With assistance from a number of private foundations, most notably the Josiah Macy, Jr. Foundation, the Commonwealth Fund, the Alfred Sloan Foundation, and the Robert Wood Johnson Foundation, the amount of scholarship money available to minority students increased substantially. By 1974, the National Medical Foundation, the major source of private scholarships for minority students, made $2,280,000 in awards, compared with $195,000 in 1968.[50]

Competition among medical schools to attract minority students was intense. Schools tried all sorts of recruitment devices: advertising, visits to college campuses (particularly black colleges), and follow-up letters and telephone calls to applicants—or even to those who had requested applications and had not yet sent them in. The fundamental problem was that the pool of qualified minority candidates was small. Because of their prestige and larger pool of scholarship funds, the wealthy, research-intensive schools enjoyed the most success in attracting applicants. Weaker schools often complained of this. Thus Hahnemann Medical College spoke bitterly of what it called the "black brain drain"—"affluent ivy league medical schools attracting many applicants of high calibre and thus reducing the pool for the predominantly negro [*sic*] schools and schools such as Hahnemann which lack the financial resources to offer ample scholarships and loan funds."[51]

In the competition to recruit minority students, most medical schools relaxed their admission standards. In a typical year (1978), African-American applicants nationwide had science grade point averages of 2.60, compared with 3.31 for whites, and scores on the Medical College Admissions Test (MCAT) that were one and one-half standard deviations lower.[52] To admit minority students, medical schools had to dig much deeper into the applicant pool. In some cases, minority students were admitted despite known academic handicaps, such as inferior preparation in the premedical science courses or severe reading deficiencies. At Howard, for instance, some students were admitted with "pitifully low" reading abilities—200 words per minute, compared with the average graduate student's ability to read light material at 350 to 450 words per minute.[53]

On the other hand, no school relaxed its graduation requirements. Even as affirmative action spread, schools remained bound by their fiduciary duty to society to graduate only competent physicians. Accordingly, schools accepted the fact that some students would require extra help and additional time. Most schools liberalized their policies regarding the repetition of individual courses or entire years of study in the event of failure. A few schools established special programs that allowed promising minority students with weak credentials to complete the first year of study in two years.[54]

The need to maintain high standards for the M.D. degree placed medical schools in an awkward position. How far should they go in providing remedial work to those of disadvantaged backgrounds for the sake of rectifying social injustices? Most schools went much further than a few years before. Everywhere, faculties could be found devoting extra hours of effort to remediation for students. Few schools, however, were confident that they knew exactly how much extra help and how many extra chances to give. Typical dilemmas occurred at Michigan, where the faculty wrestled with such problems as what to do with an emotionally disturbed black student who had barely passed the first two years of medical school after four years of study, or another minority student who had failed Part I of the National Board examination three times.[55] Though graduation standards were rarely compromised, many schools showed a propensity to give repeated chances that would have astounded earlier generations of medical educators.

Though many minority students required extra help, the results seem to have justified the effort. Overall, they performed less well in the basic science courses than white students. Their rate of academic failure during that part of the curriculum was 10 to 15 percent, or several times that of the rest of the class. However, their performance in the clinical years was generally indistinguishable from that of nonminority students.[56] Moreover, many minority students did very well throughout the four-year course without receiving special help, despite low MCAT scores and mediocre college grades that for white students would have predicted academic disaster. At the University of Maryland, for instance, 70 percent of minority students with low "objective" test data had no noteworthy difficulty in medical school.[57] Such observations reminded medical educators of the lack of predictive power of their measuring instruments and of the possible cultural biases of standardized tests.

Though affirmative action enjoyed many early successes, it was not without troubling consequences. In the effort to help minority students, disadvantaged white students seemed to be overlooked. Medical schools, like many other institutions of higher education, found themselves at the center of a political morass, the focus of attack from both proponents and opponents of affirmative action. For instance, the New York University School of Medicine was simultaneously sued by a group of black students alleging discrimination in its admissions process and a white student alleging "reverse discrimination."[58] Many longtime supporters of civil rights, including some black leaders, were disturbed by the new direction affirmative action brought to the civil rights movement. Affirmative action, Diane Ravitch has written, "symbolized the shift in government policy from color-blindness to color-consciousness, from individual rights to group rights, and from a government policy forbidding specific acts of discrimination to a government policy relying on statistical disparities among groups as presumptive evidence of discrimination."[59]

Most ironic of all, the position of minority medical schools diminished, even as the opportunities for minority students in medicine increased. In 1969, Howard and Meharry enrolled 75 percent of all African-American medical students; in 1979, only 20 percent.[60] These schools found it more difficult to recruit good students now that all medical schools were competing for minority enrollees. Howard, the stronger of the two schools, found that its ability to attract the best prepared and brightest black students "has been eroded by affirmative action programs at public schools with lower tuitions and at private medical schools with large scholarships and loan endowments."[61] Even worse was the predicament of black teaching hospitals, once the most important site for the training of African-American interns and residents. Many of these hospitals were forced to close, the victims of inadequate financing and the preference of African-American physicians to train and practice at university teaching hospitals when given the opportunity.

The first phase of minority recruitment lasted until 1974. In the late 1960s and early 1970s, a substantial increase in the number of minority medical students occurred (*see Figure 6*).[62] By 1974, underrepresented minority groups represented approximately 10 percent of all entering students, up from 3 percent in 1968. The proportion of African-Americans in the entering class had increased from 2.7 to 7.5 percent, while the number of Mexican-Americans had risen 11-fold, and the numbers of Native Americans and mainland Puerto Ricans more than 20-fold. These results, though short of the AAMC's goals, represented nothing less than a demographic revolution.[63]

After 1974, however, minority enrollments underwent a period of stagnation. The number of students admitted remained about the same, but the minority population in the U.S. continued to grow. Accordingly, the representation of minority students as a proportion of the minority population fell (*see Figure 6*). This relative decline in minority enrollments occurred despite sincere efforts of most medical schools to recruit qualified applicants and despite the opening of a third black medical school, Morehouse School of Medicine, in 1981.[64]

Several factors accounted for the relative decline in minority enrollments in the latter 1970s and the 1980s. Funds for scholarships fell, while tuition began to rise steeply. Students of all backgrounds were affected by those changes, but none more than minority students, who generally had fewer financial resources. In addition, affirmative action suffered a major defeat in the case of *Bakke v. the University of California* (1978). The U.S. Supreme Court held that the use of specific quotas based solely on race was not permissible, and for this reason ordered that Allen Bakke should be admitted to the University of California, Davis, School of Medicine, a school that had twice rejected the 34-year-old white engineer. Ironically, the court ruled only against quotas, not against the use of race as a factor in the admissions process, thereby legitimizing the essential principle of most affirmative action programs. Nevertheless, the decision had what

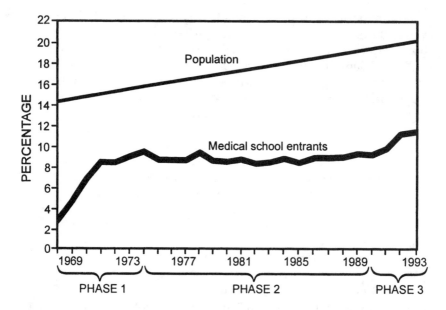

Figure 6 *Members of underrepresented minority groups as a percentage of the U.S. population and of students entering U.S. medical schools, 1968 through 1993. Underrepresented minority groups are defined here as blacks, Mexican-Americans, mainland Puerto Ricans, and American Indians*

AAMC officers called "a chilling effect" on minority recruitment to medical schools.[65]

Most important, the relative decline in minority enrollments resulted from the fact that the number of qualified minority applicants was not expanding rapidly enough. The problem of minorities in medicine was deep-rooted, arising from educational, cultural, and economic deprivation that dated to the earliest years of childhood. In the 1980s the public became increasingly aware of the inadequacies of the country's school system, which in the words of one influential report made the United States "a nation at risk" because of its failure to prepare students for the increasingly technical world in which they would live.[66] Minority students, particularly those from economically disadvantaged backgrounds, typically attended some of the worst public schools.[67] For medical schools this meant an insufficient number of academically well-prepared minority applicants. The pioneering educators Abraham Flexner and Henry Pritchett, who had repeatedly pointed out the dependence of medical schools on the lower tiers of the educational system, would not have been surprised.

Concern about the deficient educational pipeline led the AAMC to launch a new initiative in 1990, "Project 3000 by 2000," whose goal was to achieve an enrollment of 3,000 minority students in U.S. medical schools by the year 2000. The strategy involved establishing partnerships between medical schools and elementary schools, high schools, and colleges to expand the number of well-prepared minority group applicants. What was new in the initiative was the concerted effort to persuade medical schools to attack the problem directly—not merely by summer enrichment programs for minority college students planning to enter medicine, but by direct involvement with local school districts and colleges to improve the quality of science education at high schools and colleges and even at elementary and junior high schools. Some conspicuous early successes occurred, as manifested by successful community partnerships established by the University of California, San Francisco, Baylor College of Medicine, the University of Kentucky, and the University of Tennessee, among others. In the early 1990s, the percentage of minority student entrants again began to rise (*see Figure 6*), leading the AAMC to hope that a third phase of minority enrollment was beginning.[68]

From their inception in the late 1960s, affirmative action admission programs had an understandable focus: increasing the entry and retention of underrepresented minority students in medical school. From the standpoint of education, such a focus was incomplete, for it did not take into account the experiences of minority students once admitted. From this perspective, there was much work to be done at virtually every medical school—and problems in this area could not so readily be ascribed to a deficient educational system or the lack of scholarship support. Many medical schools, including those with high proportions of minority students, did poorly at creating a welcoming, supportive atmosphere.

The problems facing minority students were severe. Some students had to overcome academic handicaps; all had to overcome the psychological handicap of being part of a small, visible group amid a large body of white students and faculty, many of whom believed that the minority students were there only because of the color of their skin. Minority students, with relatively few living role models or heroes from the history of medicine, commonly felt like tokens, and they spoke frequently of their feelings of isolation and alienation from the rest of the school. Even worse, institutional racism was common. Skeptical white students and faculty frequently expected minority students to fail, white patients occasionally refused to be examined by black students, and minority students would sometimes walk through corridors observing walls scrawled with racial epithets.[69] Students of the "hidden curriculum" could readily understand the profound effects of such a climate in undermining self-esteem and academic performance.

In addition, the ultimate goal of affirmative action was to increase the entry of underrepresented minorities into medicine, not medical school. Here, too, there remained much work to be done—and this work was at the level of the medical school and the profession, not the educational system at large. African-Americans and other underrepresented minorities aspired to be not only practitioners but also teachers, researchers, and managers of the health care system. Yet, long after the launching of affirmative action, the representation of minority physicians in these positions remained low. For instance, in 1994 only 2.4 percent of faculty members at U.S. medical schools were black.[70] Equality of opportunity in medicine, in short, ultimately required not only a sound educational pipeline but a profession and society that welcomed all qualified individuals and recognized that it was in the national interest to make good use of all the country's human capital.

Women

Women, like racial minorities, also encountered major difficulties pursuing medicine as a career. In the 1960s, between 6 and 7 percent of doctors in the United States were women, a figure that had been stable for decades. This compared favorably with the percentage of women in other professions—for example, 2 percent in law and less than 1 percent in engineering. However, it was far less than the percentage of women doctors in European countries—for instance, 30 percent in Germany, 20 percent in the Netherlands, 25 percent in Great Britain, and 75 percent in the Soviet Union.[71]

Overt discrimination in admissions occurred less commonly with women than racial minorities. After World War II, every medical school but Jefferson admitted women, and in the fall of 1961 Jefferson became coeducational. Women who applied were accepted into medical school at the same rates as men, and their performances in medical school were comparable.[72] Though women, including single women, were found to work fewer hours than men, studies found that over 90 percent of women physicians engaged in full-time medical work, including 82 percent of married women.[73] Studies also showed that most patients of both sexes were receptive to being treated by women doctors.[74]

However, women in general were not encouraged to enter medicine. Indeed, from the earliest days of childhood, women were discouraged from considering careers in any demanding field. The stereotypical "feminine" role was reinforced by childhood readers, the curricula of elementary and high schools, guidance counselors, the popular media, and a culture that rewarded girls for politeness and submission and boys for winning and achievement. In college, intellectually capable women often received little encouragement to enter medicine or science from their teachers and advisers. Moreover, it was known that once in medical school women encountered other obstacles, particularly the growing length of time required by residency and fellowship, which made it difficult to combine medical training with starting families. Accordingly, the number of women applicants remained low.[75]

In the late 1960s, the number of women medical students began to soar. Primarily this was the result of the revival of the feminist movement, which created opportunities for women in medicine, just as the civil rights movement did for racial minorities. The women's movement in its diverse guises stimulated the ambitions of women, raising their sights and encouraging them to enter nontraditional fields. As traditional sex stereotypes began to change, women's causes received legal protection by the enactment in 1972 of Title IX of the Higher Education Amendments, which banned sex discrimination in educational programs receiving federal funds. In 1969–70, 929 women entered medical school, or 9.9 percent of new entrants. A decade later, first-year women students had increased to 4,575, or 27.8 percent of matriculants. By 1993–94, 6,851 women started medical school, or 42.0 percent of the first-year class.[76]

The increase in the number of women was accomplished with much less trauma than accompanied the affirmative action programs for racial minorities. The educational pipeline for women applicants—most of whom were white—was just as good as for the men who were applying. Unlike the case of racial minorities, whose numbers plateaued in the mid-1970s, the number of women matriculants continued to grow. As one sign of how rapidly women entered the medical mainstream, Woman's Medical College of Pennsylvania found that there was no longer a large demand for a separate women's medical school. In 1969–70 the school began admitting men and changed its name to Medical College of Pennsylvania.

To discriminating eyes, however, the decline of visible barriers to medical school unmasked another set of problems: the subtle but severe informal barriers that women faced in achieving full gender parity in medicine. As with racial minorities, the challenge of educating women physicians involved not merely admissions but also creating an environment that provided them equal opportunity in all branches of practice, research, and teaching. As in the case of minorities, the obstacles were formidable—reflecting in part the perpetuation of sex stereotypes and gender bias, and in part the reluctance of a male-dominated profession to make structural allowances in medical education to accommodate the special needs of women bearing and raising children.

At the student level, sexism in medical school was clearly apparent.[77] Admission committees would frequently ask women, but not men, detailed questions about their plans for marriage and children. Counseling and advising services were poor, few schools provided time off for pregnancy, day care services for women with children were scarce, and gynecological services at student health clinics were often substandard. Women students were subject to insensitive, condescending remarks by faculty, and patients often mistook them for nurses. Sexual harassment was widely known.[78] Problems of on-call lodging and other accommodations for women were frequently severe. For instance, in surgical clerkships, male students used the same locker room as the surgeons while female students typically used the nurses' locker room. This practice excluded women from the informal but important locker room discussions between the surgeon and male students. (However, no one knew quite what to do about that situation.) Problems of clinical teaching also regularly arose. For example, women often received little practical experience in the male genitorectal examination.

Many problems experienced by women at medical school, though real and substantial, were difficult to measure or quantify. Janet Bickel, who has written widely about women in medicine, has popularized the concept, arising from recent feminist scholarship, of "microinequities" to describe these inapparent but real slights. Examples include sexual humor disparaging to women, focusing on a woman's appearance while downplaying her professional attributes, attributing a woman's idea to a man, and labelling women students as "overly aggressive" for behavior that in a man would be considered "forceful" or "strong." Microinequities, Bickel has written, "describe aspects of the work environment that are legally nonactionable and that may even escape conscious attention, but that are inappropriate, unfair, painful, destructive" and that "interfere with the professional development of women physicians."[79]

At the level of house staff training, gender bias also continued. Women did not have the same range of career choices as men. The large majority of women selected residencies in internal medicine, pediatrics, psychiatry, and more recently, family practice and obstetrics and gynecology. The representation of women in surgery and the surgical subspecialties was disproportionately low. In some cases, women were passed over by surgical program directors, who often concluded that women did not have the determination, stamina, or dedication for successful careers in their demanding fields. More commonly, women avoided the surgical specialties, not caring to take on directly the overt prejudices of a program director or department chief. One investigator noted: "Being skillful at their own protection, few contemporary women actually come face-to-face with a door locked against them [in residency selection]. Most veer off into the more acceptable and accepting specialties, without even a wistful look at those fields which might have spurned them."[80]

Lastly, women found it difficult to achieve success in academic medicine. By the mid-1990s, large numbers of women had received medical school appointments, but mainly at the junior levels. Advancement to the senior faculty and to major administrative positions was not easy. In 1995, less than 10 percent of full professors and only 4 percent of department chairs were women—the same proportions as in 1980. Women were promoted more slowly than men of similar accomplishments, and they were frequently paid less than men of comparable rank, seniority, and reputation.[81] Similar obstacles were encountered by women in other scientific and academic fields.[82]

The slow advancement of women within academic medicine should not be interpreted as representing the result of universal hostility among men. Almost all women with successful careers, in academe or in practice, have been assisted by men who were willing to help and teach them. Frances K. Conley, a professor of neurosurgery at Stanford and the victim in a widely publicized case of sexual harassment, wrote how her own life "has been immeasurably enriched by warm relationships with many fine men who, not threatened by my success, and convinced that I had the requisite ability, were willing to respect me and to support and advance my career."[83]

Rather, barriers to the professional advancement of women resulted primarily from the structural organization of medical schools. Reflecting the gender bias of the profession and society, few schools were accommodating to women in terms of providing maternity leave or help with child care. At home, married women faculty typically found that their "second shift" of work began, since few husbands participated equally in child rearing or household chores.[84] Yet, promotion and tenure at medical schools remained geared to those who work 60- or 70-hour weeks. Married men could often work with such single-minded dedication because they, unlike most women faculty members, had full-time backup at home from their spouses. In addition, "microinequities" hindered the advancement of women faculty. Examples here include the lack of mentoring provided junior women faculty by senior professors, the tendency of others to take credit for the work of women instructors, the frequency with which women faculty are asked to do time-consuming administrative or teaching chores not in their career interests, and the withholding—consciously or unconsciously—of institutional resources and opportunities for collaboration.

Advancement of women faculty, in short, depended on the presence of a supportive working environment. Their academic success was impeded by structural problems and "microinequities," not overt discrimination. For this reason the barriers to the promotion of women faculty have been described as resulting from a "sticky floor," not a "glass ceiling."[85] As with racial minorities, full equality in the medical school ultimately depended on constructing an environment that welcomed individuals on their own merits, not merely on breaking down the barriers to appointment.

In recent years some medical schools have begun efforts to correct the organizational dilemmas and "microinequities" that have hindered women. More liberal policies pertaining to pregnancy leave, split residencies in which two individuals cover a single residency position on a part-time basis to allow greater time at home, the provision of on-site child care, lengthening the tenure clock for faculty needing additional time because of family responsibilities, and providing gender sensitivity training for administrators and senior faculty are among the responses medical schools have made to overcome institutional sexism and provide more accommodating environments for women students, house officers, and faculty.[86] The AAMC has established a Women in Medicine program to encourage medical schools to continue in these efforts. The results await to be seen.

14

Academic Health Centers Under Stress: External Pressures

WITH THE END OF THE VIETNAM WAR, domestic tranquility returned quickly to the United States. Nevertheless, in the 1970s and 1980s, academic health centers came under new external pressures. Other aspects of the outside environment began to turn sour, as social and demographic trends, new government policies, and changing public attitudes started to work to their disadvantage. Medical schools and teaching hospitals were increasingly perceived as stressed institutions, and a dispirited mood developed among them. Their confidence and sense of autonomy, so prominent before World War II and during the mythic "golden age" of the 1950s and 1960s, dwindled. Always dependent upon external funding, medical schools had never been as truly autonomous as it once seemed. Nevertheless, it now appeared that they were vulnerable to every jolt on an increasingly bumpy road.

The Decline of the Cities

The urban location of most academic health centers had long made sense, for that had enabled an abundant supply of patients. By the 1970s, however, the location of many academic health centers was creating unexpected new problems for them. These problems arose from the economic and social decline that occurred in many older industrial cities following World War II. During the war years, nearly a million African-Americans migrated from the South to the large, industrial Northeast cities, where opportunities for employment and a better life seemed more likely. Between 1950 and 1970, the black population in the 40 largest cities increased by another two million.[1] As African-Americans, as well as Puerto Ricans and Mexicans, moved to the cities, many businesses and much of the white middle class left for the suburbs. Inner cities, once heterogeneous with respect to race and class, increasingly came to consist of homogeneous, racially segregated ghettos. The tax base eroded, unemployment and poverty rose, essential municipal services sometimes went unprovided, housing stock deteriorated, and crime escalated. In many older industrial cities vast expanses of neighborhoods were left without adequate schools, public transportation, police and fire protection, street lights, garbage collection, and recreational areas. These changes directly affected many academic health centers, for more than half in the 1970s were in the nation's 40 largest cities and more than one-quarter (including many of the most prestigious) were in decaying inner-city neighborhoods.[2]

The evolution of the neighborhood surrounding the Columbia-Presbyterian Medical Center was typical in this regard. When planning for the new medical center took place in the 1920s, the Washington Heights section of upper Manhattan, where the new center was to be located, was primarily middle class and white. The Irish, Jews, and Greeks who lived there had moved from slums in lower Manhattan. The subway system did not serve all of the area, which still had undeveloped sections. Washington Heights was abundantly populated with private medical practitioners as well as with community hospitals—Harlem and Sydenham Hospitals to the south and Jewish Memorial and St. Elizabeth's Hospitals to the north. The number of beds in Presbyterian Hospital was thus established by educational concerns and not by anticipated community needs.

In the next ten years, the subway system was completed, and the population of Washington Heights swelled. After World War II, major ethnic changes began to occur, as many whites departed and growing numbers of blacks and Hispanics moved into the area. The medical center began to seem like a stranger in its own neighborhood. With the influx of Spanish-speaking inhabitants, the professional staff could not communicate easily with many of the patients from the area, and the center began offering crash courses in medical Spanish. Over time many businesses departed, doctors and community hospitals left, the mean income of area residents fell, and crime soared. In 1978, though middle class enclaves could still be found, Washington Heights was officially declared a poverty area.[3]

Academic health centers in deteriorating neighborhoods encountered many problems. One was the personal safety of patients, students, and staff. Records of academic health centers in inner cities from the 1960s onward regularly reported students, staff, employees, patients, and visitors victimized by rapes, assaults, armed robberies, and even a few murders. In 1987, New York's 34th Police Precinct, which included the area of the Columbia-Presbyterian Medical Center, had the highest homicide rate in the city and suffered from one of the worst crack cocaine problems.[4] Many attending physicians and house officers at Presbyterian Hospital were afraid to wear their name tags in the emergency room because of frequent threats from patients.[5]

Students, nurses, and house staff, who often lived in the immediate vicinity of their medical center, were affected by more than the high prevalence of crime. With the development of urban blight, there was a collapse of the structures that formerly had created a sense of community in those neighborhoods. Gone were the theaters, restaurants, coffee houses, shopping areas, and recreational facilities. For house officers and others with young children, the lack of good nearby schools was a particularly distressing problem. Local schools were usually deteriorating, and few house officers could afford to send their children to private schools.

Academic health centers in inner cities took important steps to combat these problems: tighter security measures, closer patrol of the neighborhood by the local police department, tuition subsidies for house officers who wished to send their children to private schools, and abandonment of the requirement that house officers live close to the hospital. Recognizing that their fate and that of the neighborhood were intertwined, many academic health centers became involved in the redevelopment of their community. For instance, though the Washington University Medical Center was situated in a relatively safe neighborhood, transitional areas were not far away. In 1975 the Washington University Redevelopment Corporation was established to coordinate the rehabilitation of homes in the neighborhood. Nevertheless, no inner-city medical school could fully overcome the burden of its environment. For example, concern about safety was the major reason that students accepted at Johns Hopkins and Columbia decided to attend other medical schools.[6]

Academic health centers in inner cities also feared for their own safety. Academic health centers were towering complexes that dominated the urban landscape—symbols, to many, of white imperialism and racism in increasingly African-American and Hispanic neighborhoods. Expansion of an academic health center often meant tearing down nearby minority-owned homes and businesses. To many area citizens, academic health centers projected the racism of society—professional and administrative staffs that were mainly white; laundry, food service, housekeeping, and janitorial workers who were primarily black or Hispanic. In the late 1960s, some academic health centers had found themselves perilously close to sites of urban rioting. Memories lingered. Inner-city academic health centers often continued to be viewed by their community with hostility and resentment, and some centers were frightened for their very survival.

Perhaps no academic health center in the late 1960s was more threatened by its neighborhood than the Johns Hopkins Medical Institutions. The East Baltimore area, the site of Johns Hopkins, had been a middle class area when the school and hospital were constructed, but during and after World War II the area was affected by demographic trends typical of older inner cities. By the 1960s the area around Johns Hopkins had deteriorated into one of the nation's most notorious slums, largely African-American, with one of the highest poverty, unemployment, and crime rates in the country. Relations between the medical center and the community had long been sour, with both sides misunderstanding the other.

The community resented the perceived imperialistic expansion of the medical center, yet school and hospital officials knew that they had to enlarge their facilities to remain competitive with other premier academic health centers. The community deeply resented a fence that surrounded the "compound" (a living area for house officers across the street from the hospital), yet Hopkins officials were reluctant to remove the fence because of the dangerous conditions in the area and the strong protest of the house staff, who feared for their safety if the fence was taken down. In April 1968, following the assassination of Martin Luther King Jr., several days of rioting broke out in East Baltimore. The riots came so close to the compound that house staff and their families had to be evacuated. That entire spring and summer the hospital operated on a semi-emergency basis. Though no further civil disturbances occurred, crime and vandalism in the area remained higher than usual, and the hospital received a number of anonymous bomb threats.[7] A study by Johns Hopkins two years later revealed intense ill feeling toward the medical center still remaining among many residents of the community.[8]

In the 1970s, and continuing in the 1980s and 1990s, many urban academic health centers took steps to become better neighbors. Academic health centers undertook a host of new projects: alcohol and drug abuse programs, methadone clinics, neighborhood health centers and mental health clinics, prenatal screening and comprehensive child care programs, job preference for those living in the local community, and renewed efforts to recruit minorities to the student body and professional staffs. As the University of Maryland put it, "The Medical School exists in a Black community and much of the teaching, service, and clinical research revolves around Black patients of this community; therefore, it is encumbant [*sic*] on the Medical School to be concerned with the problems of this community and develop positive programs to aid in the solution of these problems."[9] Many programs went beyond ordinary medical needs: underwriting summer camp attendance for underprivileged children, providing tickets for sporting or cultural events, donating food and money to homeless shelters, offering job experience for promising high school students, and establishing educational enrichment programs, either independently or in conjunction with local schools.[10] A few academic health centers gave neighborhood residents an effective voice in some of the center's planning efforts; others became more sensitive to the local impact of their plans for expansion. For all the cynicism toward them among local residents, academic health centers stayed the course. Whether from altruism or the practical difficulties of leaving, academic health centers did not abandon their neighborhoods, unlike many banks, supermarkets, department stores, and other businesses that did. Academic health centers remained and worked hard to make their neighborhoods better.

For most urban academic health centers, such community programs were not easy to implement. In general, medical schools, with their decentralized governance, had never been particularly good managers, and they had been unaccustomed to administering community programs. Shared decision-making by consensus-formation—the academic style—was poorly adaptable to nonacademic matters requiring quick, efficient actions and tough, hard-nosed business skills. Moreover, dealing with the "community" could be a confusing matter. Who represented the community? Typically, many community groups—churches, social groups, neighborhood organizations—claimed to speak for a large segment of the population, and it was often bewildering for an inexperienced academic administrator to determine just which section of the community to work with on a particular project. The Columbia-Presbyterian Medical Center found that there were between 200 and 300 community organizations it needed to reach in its efforts to improve community relationships.[11]

In promoting good relations with the community, academic health centers sometimes encountered a dilemma: what was desired by the neighborhood occasionally placed the staff and employees of the institution at risk. This was illustrated by the controversy that arose concerning the use of a Johns Hopkins–owned swimming pool (the Reed Hall swimming pool) in 1970. This pool, located in the "compound" residential area of the Johns Hopkins Hospital and used by students, house officers, and their families, was readily visible to residents of the neighborhood standing on the other side of the wire fence that protected the "compound." A movement arose within the Johns Hopkins Medical Institutions to allow neighborhood youngsters to use the pool at certain times during the week. House staff morale immediately fell. On the wards, house officers were great advocates of the poor, often battling hospital administrators to keep patients in the hospital even if uninsured. Outside the hospital, house officers feared for their families' safety by making their pool available to "the neighborhood." The house staff prevailed, and the program was discontinued. Afterwards, some concerned house officers raised scholarship money for a nearby high school, but to many area residents that response represented another example of tokenism, another rebuff from "whitey."[12]

Serious as the above problems were, the greatest problem academic health centers encountered from the decline of the cities was the economic burden of providing charity care to uninsured and indigent patients. Teaching centers had always provided disproportionately large amounts of free care, but now the volume of that work increased. Medicare and Medicaid had lessened but not eliminated medical indigency. With urban decay, most of the paying patients had moved to the suburbs, while huge numbers of poor and uninsured patients remained in the inner cities. Left with major responsibility for providing medical care for those who could not pay were the academic health centers. By the early 1980s, teaching hospitals, with 5.6 percent of the acute care beds, were providing 47.2 percent of the free care in the country.[13]

It was not the economic decline of the cities alone that left academic health centers with increased responsibility for indigent patients. Rather, it was the change of the inner-city neighborhoods that resulted in so many doctors and community hospitals departing for the suburbs. By default, in city after city, virtually no one was left to care for the inhabitants of the inner cities but the physicians and staffs of the teaching hospitals. For instance, between 1968 and 1988 six hospitals in northern Manhattan closed, leaving Presbyterian Hospital as the sole provider of care in the area.[14]

As many older cities experienced fiscal woes, their municipal hospital systems deteriorated, creating a vacuum of care that placed even greater stress on many academic health centers, including centers not situated immediately in the inner cities. Victims of neglect for decades, municipal hospitals encountered still harder times after 1960, the consequence of rising costs, declining admissions, an inadequate tax base from which to cover deficits, and a pernicious civil service system that led to bloated, inefficient staffing and administration. The plight of municipal hospitals grew worse after the passage of Medicare and Medicaid in 1965, owing to the mistaken belief among many city officials that the federal government would turn all indigent patients into middle class consumers who would be free to choose their own hospital. Municipal hospitals found themselves with fewer resources than before, since state and local budgets for Medicaid drew from money that otherwise would have gone to municipal hospitals. Many municipal hospitals scaled back their operations; others closed.[15] As this happened, academic health centers found themselves with larger numbers of indigent patients. Thus, when Philadelphia General Hospital, once an important teaching hospital, closed in 1977, Temple University Hospital (and to lesser degrees, the other Philadelphia teaching hospitals) inherited the responsibility for caring for the hospital's large indigent patient population.[16]

As inner-city neighborhoods changed, teaching hospitals were inundated with patients. Between 1955 and 1975, the number of outpatient visits to teaching hospitals rose by nearly 700 percent.[17] Emergency rooms of many urban teaching hospitals began to resemble 24-hour family walk-in clinics, overrun by patients seeking routine ambulatory care because there was nowhere else for them to go. "Triage officers" began appearing in emergency rooms, canvassing the hordes of patients in an effort to identify the emergent or urgent cases from the masses of patients with ordinary complaints. The demands on the outpatient and emergency departments made the scheduling of elective admissions difficult. Thus the University of Arkansas Hospital found that its scheduled private patients often could not get in because their beds had been taken by indigent patients who appeared unexpectedly in the emergency room or clinics.[18] Discharge of hospitalized clinic patients could also be difficult because often they had no funds and nowhere to go. The label "disposition problem" appeared with increasing frequency on hospital charts as

professional staff, social workers, and administrators found that the perplexing problems of society had been dropped on their doorstep. How
could they discharge a penniless, incapacitated patient without family or
friends when there were no nursing home beds available that would
accept Medicaid? (This problem became worse in 1981, when Medicaid
decided to limit reimbursement for inpatient care to 20 days.)

For teaching hospitals, the economic consequences of providing care
to the community were profound. Costs were rapidly rising, many
patients in the area remained uninsured despite Medicare and Medicaid,
and the Medicaid program was notorious for late payments and for reim-
bursing hospitals less than the costs incurred. Many teaching hospitals
began to suffer fiscal hemorrhage, as losses from indigent care soared.
For example, the New England Medical Center in the late 1970s lost
between $7,000,000 and $10,000,000 a year from bad debt and free care,
while Presbyterian Hospital in 1989 sustained a staggering $50,000,000
loss, which followed years of smaller but still substantial losses from
uncompensated care.[19] A study in the early 1980s on financially distressed hospitals found that "there is a strong relation between the probability of incurring deficits on the one hand, and caring for the poor and
being situated in a fiscally stressed city, on the other." The study found
that the problem was not one of operating inefficiencies of the hospitals
but of the lack of an adequate financing mechanism for indigent patients.
"The solution to the problem of financial distress lies largely outside the
individual hospital. The question of who pays for the care that the hospital provides seems to be much more important for fiscal health than of
how resources are organized to deliver that care."[20]

Despite this growing financial burden, through the late 1980s most
teaching hospitals, particularly voluntary and state-owned hospitals,
managed to stay financially afloat. Revenues from private patients,
which reimbursed teaching hospitals for "community service" and teaching costs, could be used to offset losses from uninsured patients, as could
gifts, endowment income, and as a last resort, endowment principal. In
addition, many teaching hospitals no longer felt that they had to provide
care to everyone who appeared at their doorstep. Though acutely ill individuals were virtually never denied care, admission for routine matters
was not guaranteed. At many teaching hospitals, uninsured patients who
were not acutely ill or who did not provide particular teaching interest
(especially patients who lived outside the hospital's natural geographic
zone, or "catchment area") were sent to a municipal or veterans hospital.
Through these mechanisms most teaching hospitals were able to provide
vast amounts of free care without becoming insolvent, though some in
the 1970s and 1980s lost many millions of dollars in one year or another.

By the 1980s, academic health centers could no longer be considered
charitable institutions. Many had incomes and budgets of hundreds of
millions of dollars, and most managed to remain consistently profitable
despite the large amounts of free care they provided. They increasingly

demonstrated a corporate ethos, and they had become vendors of services rather than traditional eleemosynary institutions. Nevertheless, in a culture increasingly characterized by self-interest and greed, academic health centers continued to be the keeper of medicine's soul. They remained committed to their neighborhoods and communities even after other doctors and hospitals, along with businesses and the middle class, had retreated to the suburbs. The amount of free care they provided was huge, even if only a small part of their total operations. They were the court of last resort for the seriously ill and for the forsaken and underserved of society. Their problem was that poverty and racism were tough enemies—and few others, including hospitals and doctors, joined them to do battle.

Competition for Patients

Though academic health centers in the 1970s and 1980s continued to provide huge amounts of charity care, the great majority of their patients by that time were private patients. Both public and private third-party payers reimbursed doctors and hospitals generously, especially for tertiary (superspecialized) care, the traditional forte of academic health centers. Clinical revenue, for most academic health centers, represented the largest source of income and was regularly used to cross-subsidize education, research, charity care, and certain essential but money-losing clinical services. Accordingly, virtually no teaching hospital (with the exception of municipal and veterans hospitals that were also major teaching institutions) could escape the need of keeping its beds filled with paying patients.

In the 1970s and 1980s, many academic health centers found it more difficult to attract paying patients for referral and specialty care. Private patients, who once automatically went to teaching hospitals for such care, now became a commodity in scarcer supply. The dean of the University of Colorado School of Medicine described the problem in 1972: "We [university medical centers] must compete, for we are no longer the 'Mecca' that can sit back complacently and expect patients to flock to our doors."[21] The irony of a declining referral base was lost on no one, for it was at academic health centers that specialty medicine had been developed and refined.

Several factors accounted for the new difficulties teaching hospitals encountered in attracting referral patients. One was the traditional tension at teaching hospitals between educational and patient needs. All century long medical educators had praised the value of clinical clerkships and house staff responsibility to good patient care, but in actuality medical education had brought into conflict the need of learners to gain experience and the need of patients for rest and privacy. Always, at teaching hospitals, there was an endless procession of strangers surrounding patients—probing, questioning, examining, measuring, and sticking with needles. In the 1960s and 1970s, these traditional problems grew more severe. The expansion of residency and fellowship programs increased the numbers of physicians who needed to see a particular patient, making patients more uncertain than ever exactly who was in charge. In the consumer era of the 1970s and 1980s, patients complained with increasing frequency about being used as "teaching material." The Patient Bill of Rights, an important symbol of the growing consumerism in health care that was adoped by the American Hospital Association in 1973, asserted that patients had the right "to considerate and respectful care."[22] Assuring that in a teaching hospital was not always easy.

In addition, patients were increasingly using consumer standards in choosing among doctors and hospitals. Few laypersons had the expertise to assess the professional quality of their medical care, but everyone could judge the ease and safety of parking, the quality of the food, the cleanliness of the environment, the presence of amenities like televisions and carpeting, the adequacy of the toilets and showers, the degree of privacy, and the attitudes of the people they encountered during a hospital stay or medical visit. By these standards teaching hospitals frequently fell short. For instance, patients at the Johns Hopkins Hospital complained of the lack of cleanliness, comfort, and privacy as well as of long delays in being escorted to their rooms on admission or after procedures, noisiness, and lack of warmth and attentiveness among the hospital staff.[23] In the 1970s, teaching hospitals began to work hard to foster a caring attitude and improve the comfort of their surroundings, but they had formidable obstacles to overcome in these areas.

Most important of all, patients now had a choice as to where they could go for specialized care. Throughout the century, advanced technology and tertiary care had been concentrated in the teaching hospitals. Since World War II, however, academic health centers had been producing more and more specialists and subspecialists through the expansion of their residency and clinical fellowship programs. Though residency and fellowship in theory were designed to produce academic leaders, in actuality, as noted earlier, the overwhelming majority of specialists entered private practice. Most established bases at urban or suburban community hospitals, but in the 1960s and 1970s even small towns became populated with increasing numbers of specialists.[24] As a result, many community hospitals could now offer most of the specialty services that not many years before had been available only at academic health centers. In essence, academic health centers had trained their competition.

In the 1960s, academic health centers began to notice the increased clinical competition. By the 1970s and 1980s, that competition had become intense. Numerous teaching hospitals reported declines in occupancy as patients with specialized or complicated medical problems were being referred to nearby community hospitals. The University of Colorado was losing gynecological patients to a local hospital that had opened a women's center offering tertiary care in women's health, including high risk obstetrics, genetics, and breast care.[25] A community competitor of the University of Michigan Hospital was performing 50 percent more open heart surgery, led by the defection of six Michigan faculty to the hospital and the more aggressive approach of these surgeons to doing surgery.[26] The University of Arkansas Hospital worried about the increased competition for specialty patients from community doctors and hospitals, as did the Johns Hopkins Hospital, which noted that in Baltimore specialty care "is no longer exclusively an area for teaching hospitals."[27] In St. Louis, the development of open-heart surgical capability at seven suburban hospitals in 1982 and 1983 threatened the financial solvency of the city's three adult teaching hospitals, Barnes, Jewish, and St. Louis University Hospitals. The competing programs, staffed primarily by surgeons who had been trained at the three teaching hospitals and approved only because of a series of procedural blunders by the Missouri Health Facilities Review Committee, seriously eroded one of the most important revenue sources for the teaching hospitals, compromising their ability to support education, research, and charity care. Quality concerns were also raised since the proliferation of programs diluted the prospect that each surgical team at each of the programs would be able to perform enough open-heart procedures to maintain the highest level of proficiency.[28]

Federal and state governments looked upon the spread of tertiary care to community hospitals with misgivings. From their perspective, this was desirable for allowing greater accessibility to those services, but this advantage was offset by the higher costs arising from the duplication of equipment and facilities. To try to contain health care costs, 23 states and the District of Columbia between 1964 and 1972 adopted certificate-of-need laws requiring state approval for the construction of new facilities or the acquisition of expensive equipment. In 1974, federal legislation established new health systems agencies (HSAs) to regulate in a similar fashion construction and the purchase of new equipment by hospitals in 205 designated health-service areas.

These regulatory agencies, however, proved ineffectual in reducing the spread of medical technology and specialized care. The political skill of many community hospitals allowed them to receive approvals from regulators, even in many instances where they did not meet formal regulatory guidelines. Moreover, such regulations did not apply to doctors in private offices, where expensive equipment like ultrasound machines and brain scanners could be purchased without regard to community need. Perhaps the most conspicuous regulatory failure was the inability of HSAs to limit the supply of computed tomographic (CT) scanners, a major improvement in diagnostic radiological technology that first appeared in the United States in 1973. By 1978, the ratio of CT scanners in the U.S. population was 10 times higher than in Canada and 20 times higher than in Great Britain. Rosemary Stevens described the undermining of HSA efforts to limit the spread of CT scanners by community hospitals and doctors. "Groups of doctors, who, like the hospitals, were effective entrepreneurs in the 1970s, readily subverted the planning system by buying CT scanners outside hospitals, where they were not subject to HSA regulation. Canny hospital administrators contracted for CT with a group of radiologists, sometimes leasing them hospital facilities."[29] In the mid-1980s, teaching hospitals in only three states (New York, Maryland, and Massachusetts) were experiencing higher than normal occupancy. Not coincidentally, these were the three states that exercised the highest degree of regulatory control over the spread of new technology outside of teaching hospitals.[30]

Through the 1980s, most academic health centers managed to survive the competition from community hospitals and practitioners, just as they managed to stay financially afloat despite the growing economic burden of providing charity care. The amount of dollars to compete for was large and rapidly growing, and most third party payers still reimbursed doctors and hospitals on a liberal fee-for-service basis. Nevertheless, because of growing competition, academic health centers were in a more vulnerable position than they had been a decade or two before. In the eyes of the public, the distinction between teaching and nonteaching hospitals was beginning to blur. Tertiary care could be obtained at both, and the educational mission of academic health centers seemed less apparent in an era of rapidly escalating faculty practice. In actuality, the nation's academic health centers were just as invaluable a national resource as ever. However, it was becoming more and more difficult for the public, the business community, and government to appreciate that fact. The generous payment environment allowed teaching hospitals to survive—indeed, to prosper—but few stopped to consider how academic health centers would fare in a more competitive environment if the rules for clinical reimbursement were to change.

The New Adversarial Relationship with Government

Medical schools, like their parent universities, had always fiercely defended their rights as educational institutions to determine their academic policies.[31] In the 1970s, however, the academic freedom of medical schools came under attack. The federal government—and state legislatures as well—assumed a historically unprecedented role in determining the internal environment of medical schools. To medical educators, the intrusiveness of government into their internal educational affairs represented a painful loss of the sense of friendship and advocacy that Congress and state legislatures had shown toward medical schools since the beginning of the post–World War II era.

The primary mechanism by which the federal government prescribed educational policies was through its spending power. By the 1960s, the federal influence in medical schools was all-pervasive. "Practically every activity of the College receives some Federal support,"[32] one medical school dean observed in 1967. In the mid-1960s, however, federal appropriations for medical schools began to come with strings attached. Congress—and soon, state legislatures—made their support of medical schools conditional on specific requirements being met. In this way, lawmakers believed that medical education could be enlisted to help achieve social goals that Congress or the legislatures deemed important.

The first incursion of government into the internal affairs of medical schools occurred with the Health Professions Educational Assistance Act of 1963. As discussed earlier, this bill, and additional bills passed in 1965, 1968, and 1971, was intended to increase the output of physicians. The federal government provided a substantial share of the construction costs of new educational facilities as well as student loan funds and a small amount of scholarship support (1965, 1968, and 1971 bills). The availability of federal matching funds for construction and renovation stimulated state and local governments and private philanthropy to increase their aid to medical schools. In addition, beginning with the 1965 legislation, the federal bills provided medical schools funds for operating expenses (called "capitation" grants because the amount of money a school received was tied to its enrollment).[33] These funds were enticing to schools because they could be used for any purpose considered by the dean important to the institution, in contrast to most grants, which were restricted to specific uses such as a faculty member's research.

Among existing schools, these various bills caused considerable consternation. Some of the state schools, restricted by law to admitting state residents, wondered where the new students would come from. The University of Arkansas, for example, felt that it could not enlarge class size without significantly relaxing admission standards.[34] Other schools worried that educational quality might deteriorate with too many students. Medical schools knew that even with new teaching facilities, large classes could lead to overcrowding, insufficient amounts of "clinical material," and inadequate faculty supervision and attention. Thus, the faculty at the Columbia University College of Physicians and Surgeons feared that capitation pressures may "threaten academic standards of the University."[35]

On the other hand, the lure of funds that could be used in an unrestricted fashion was too great. No school turned down the opportunity, whatever misgivings about enlarging class size it may have had. Thus, under the formula from the 1968 bill, Duke increased enrollment for the class entering in the fall of 1970 from 86 to 104 places for a projected windfall of $560,000; the University of Michigan, under the 1971 bill, increased its freshman class size for the 1972–73 academic year from 225 to 237 for an extra $1,664,000 in federal support.[36] Small, financially strapped independent schools sometimes jumped at the opportunity. For instance, Hahnemann Medical College considered doubling its class size to get as much capitation funding as possible.[37]

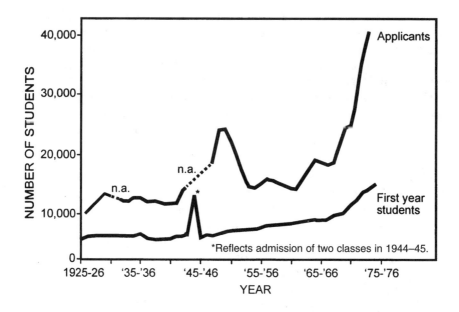

Figure 7   *Applicants and entrants to U.S. Medical Schools, 1925–1974*

In the 1970s Congress became more insistent in its efforts to use capitation grants to promote specific educational practices. With each new health manpower bill, additional conditions were placed on the schools as a requirement for receiving support. The focus of Congress shifted from the use of capitation payments to increase the number of students to their use as a tool to attempt to modify the geographic and specialty distribution of physicians. For instance, the Health Professions Educational Assistance Act of 1976 made capitation payments conditional upon at least 50 percent of a school's graduates selecting certain primary care fields (internal medicine, pediatrics, and family medicine) for their residency training. The bill also provided scholarship assistance to participating schools on the condition that students receiving scholarships agree in writing to practice for one year in a medically underserved area for each year of scholarship assistance.

In the 1970s, state legislatures also began to place restrictions of their own on medical schools. Especially irksome to medical educators was the intrusion of state governments into the medical curriculum. For instance, California passed a bill requiring medical schools in the state to offer a course in human sexuality.[38] Medical school officials chafed at state-mandated curricula since these actions infringed on their right to establish instructional guidelines using professional criteria and represented the substitution of legislative for educational judgment on matters that were academic in character.

No legislative action was more upsetting to medical educators than the interference of Congress with admissions policies. The Health Professions Educational Assistance Act of 1976 contained a provision that made federal financial assistance to medical schools contingent upon acceptance of a government-set quota of Americans studying medicine abroad who wanted to complete their training in this country. Under this law, students who had completed two years of study at a foreign medical school and had passed Part I of the National Board of Medical Examiners examination would be deemed by the Secretary of Health, Education, and Welfare as eligible for admission to a U.S. medical school. No other academic or personal qualifications were to be considered. Students would be apportioned out in an approximately equal number to the various schools accepting capitation funding. It was expected that as many as 1,500 students each year would be involved.

This issue had been forced to a head by the presence of a rapidly growing number of U.S. citizens studying medicine abroad. Before 1970, the number of such individuals had been small. By 1975, however, there were approximately 6,000 Americans enrolled at foreign medical schools, and by 1980, 12,000.[39] This increase was a consequence of stiffening competition for admission to U.S. medical schools. In the early 1960s, there were 1.7 applicants for each available first-year position; by the mid-1970s, that ratio had risen to 2.8 to 1, an increase all the more notable because the number of positions in American medical schools had also grown (*see Figure 7*).[40]

Historically, Americans who studied medicine abroad attended established schools, primarily in Western Europe. As overflow from the United States increased, these schools became overcrowded, and access for Americans was restricted. Accordingly, by the early 1970s the overwhelming majority enrolled in the so-called "offshore" medical schools in Mexico and the Caribbean. The largest American contingent was at the Autonomous University of Guadalajara in Mexico, which enjoyed some small standing among American medical educators. The other schools were nonaccredited profit-making institutions, most of which had been organized in the late 1960s or early 1970s to cater to U.S. citizens rejected by American medical schools.

The training at all the offshore institutions was extremely poor. Admission requirements were far below American standards, classes were unlimited in size, and laboratories, hospital facilities, and faculty were few. Like correspondence schools, many offshore medical schools depended on newspaper advertising to recruit students. Some were frankly fraudulent. For example, they would misrepresent the credentials of their faculty, or they would invite American professors and their families for lavish expense-paid vacations in exchange for a few guest lectures, and then, unbeknownst to their guests, list these persons as regular faculty members of the school. Many of the schools exploited students.

Hefty, nonrefundable full-year tuition payments were often demanded in advance, yet only a small proportion of students completed the course of study. Those who did encountered considerable difficulty in obtaining further clinical training and a license to practice in the United States.[41]

In the early 1970s, the plight of these students received considerable public support. The country was suffering from a perceived doctor shortage, while many community hospitals were desperate for "ANY kind of a 'young doctor in a white suit'"[42] to serve as house officers. The families of the students organized an intense lobbying campaign in their behalf, and all could sympathize with the poignant stories of capable students denied places in medical school. Medical schools were highly reluctant to accept many of these students in transfer because of the inadequacy of their training, but under political pressure, they and the accrediting agencies developed mechanisms to correct the educational deficiencies of the students and facilitate their entry into the profession.

One route, the "Fifth Pathway" program, was established in 1971. Under this program, students who had completed the full curriculum in a foreign medical school could enroll in a special one-year clinical program at participating schools, at the completion of which they would be eligible for a state licensing examination and admission to an accredited internship or residency. In 1973, 12 medical schools participated in this program. A more popular route was the Coordinated Transfer Application System (COTRANS), established and administered by the AAMC in 1970. Under this system, students who had completed the two years of basic science instruction abroad and had passed Part I of the National Board of Medical Examiners examination were eligible to apply for admission to advanced standing at an American medical school. In 1973–74, 153 students were admitted to 49 American medical schools under the COTRANS program. The large American contingent at the Guadalajara school favored this route because Mexico required a period of social service for the M.D. degree. Transfer to a U.S. school allowed them to receive an M.D. degree from an American school without fulfilling the Mexican social service requirement. The COTRANS program provided the model for the provision on U.S. foreign medical students contained in the 1976 legislation, which became widely known as the "Guadalajara clause."[43]

Medical schools found the "Guadalajara clause" to be repugnant, for the law prohibited them from applying their own standards of admission. Medical schools conscientiously tried to take personal factors into account in the admissions process, but the law permitted no such deliberations. One educator pointed out in an extreme example that a person who had committed a felony would automatically be disqualified if applying from the U.S., but the Health Professions Educational Assistance Act of 1976 did not make provisions for such circumstances.[44] In many cases schools were forced to accept students with inferior academic records. The mean college grade point average (GPA) and score on the

Medical College Admissions Test (MCAT) was far lower for COTRANS students than for their undergraduate classmates who had been accepted by medical schools.[45] Medical educators were not swayed when lawmakers pointed out that the legislation applied only to COTRANS students who had passed Part I of the National Board examination (about 30 percent of those taking the test[46]). Students could be coached through a licensing examination, and successful passage did not assure that they had a good grasp of theoretical or practical medicine. On the whole, most graduates of offshore medical schools performed poorly on return to the United States, even after acquiring additional clinical experience in American hospitals. One study found that only 17 percent of U.S. foreign medical school graduates passed their board certification examination in internal medicine after three years of training in U.S. hospitals, whereas 80 percent of American and Canadian graduates were successful.[47] Medical schools sought—unsuccessfully—to maintain their right to individualize admission decisions so that they could accept transfer students with the maximum potential (for instance, students who had been waitlisted when applying to American medical schools from college) and not be forced to expend precious space and resources on students unlikely to perform well.

The passage of the 1976 bill precipitated a rebellion among some medical schools. The federal requirement that schools admit foreign-trained medical students in exchange for capitation payments "invades the academic integrity of the university," Steven Muller, the president of the Johns Hopkins University, and Richard Ross, the medical school dean, declared in a joint statement. Johns Hopkins "is not prepared to abdicate to the Government the right to select its students, nor, for that matter, its faculty, courses of study, and degree requirements."[48] Eighteen schools announced that they would rather forfeit federal assistance, estimated at approximately $500,000 per school, than comply with the order to accept foreign-trained American transfer students.[49] Ultimately, the lure of financial assistance was too strong, and only four schools elected to forgo federal capitation payments. However, the schools that capitulated continued to fume, as did many others that never threatened a boycott.

Equally upsetting to medical educators was the federal government's efforts to direct the internal direction of biomedical research, not just medical education. In the 1970s, federal biomedical research policy became heavily politicized. Powerful lay lobbies, based in voluntary health organizations like the American Cancer Society and American Heart Association, campaigned effectively to influence Congress to increase appropriations for programs "targeted" against specific diseases. This Congress did, despite intense misgivings among most members of the scientific establishment, and at the cost of diminished support for more fundamental biomedical research. The prototype of this approach was the National Cancer Act of 1971 (the "war against cancer"); many other legislative mandates similarly targeting specific diseases (for instance, heart disease, sickle cell anemia, arthritis, and epilepsy) for research support were also passed. The eradication of disease, of course, had always been the goal of the National Institutes of Health (NIH), but its traditional policy of "mission-oriented basic research" had allowed researchers the freedom to pursue basic investigations from which fundamental discoveries of wide and often unforeseen applicability frequently came. Now, in the opinion of most scientists, the country's biomedical research policy was becoming dangerously unbalanced between basic and applied research, and investigators were losing the freedom to follow their intellectual curiosity without having to pass a test of practicality to receive federal funds. "Targeted" research, in the words of Donald S. Fredrickson, director of the NIH, represents "an unfortunate subordination of technical to political judgment or to emotion in the orchestration of major biomedical research efforts."[50]

In the 1970s, and continuing into the 1980s and 1990s, medical schools chafed not only at money that came with strings attached but also at the increased regulatory burden they faced. By the mid-1970s, the federal influence was felt throughout higher education, as the government during the preceding decade had greatly expanded its regulation of colleges and universities along with its funding of them. Universities had to comply with federal regulations concerning student aid, the hiring and firing of employees, affirmative action, the prohibition of sex and age discrimination, the rights of the handicapped, environmental protection, radiation safety, and the directives of the Occupational Safety and Health Act. At least 70 subcommittees of the U.S. Senate had some jurisdiction over the 439 statutory authorities affecting higher education. Compliance with federal regulations cost the typical university 1 to 4 percent of its operating budget, and the task was complex as well as costly because different federal agencies sometimes had conflicting goals.[51] Medical schools were just as subject to the avalanche of federal rules and regulations as any other branch of the university. New layers of administration had to be added to assure compliance, and time, money, and energy was deflected away from the schools' academic mission.

In addition, as the sites where most animal and almost all human research was conducted, medical schools faced other regulations as well. In 1966, new rules from the NIH mandated the establishment of institutional review boards and human studies committees to review all grant applications involving human subjects. Funding of these applications required that federally defined standards of informed consent be met and documented.[52] A revitalized animal rights movement in the late 1970s and 1980s lobbied successfully for costly federal regulations pertaining to animal care. It was estimated in 1988 that revised Office of Management and Budget guidelines for animal facilities would add an extra $1 billion cost to research institutions nationwide.[53] New laws of an egalitarian society providing for the burial of indigents made it more difficult and expensive for medical schools to acquire cadavers for anatomical dissection. And the process of applying for grant support from the medical schools' old friend, the NIH, became more complicated and cumbersome than ever. It was not uncommon for 20 percent or more of the time of a productive biomedical scientist to be consumed by the process of grant application, renewal, and reporting.[54]

Academic health centers were besieged not only by the rules and regulations pertaining to the university but also by those applying to the hospital system. By the mid-1970s, the era of "cost containment" had begun—the result of soaring medical costs in a nation suffering from the severe recession of 1973–74 and the economic stagnation and runaway inflation that followed. To try to hold down Medicare and Medicaid costs, federal and state governments implemented a host of regulations that made hospitals among the most regulation-burdened industries in the country.[55] As a condition for receiving Medicare and Medicaid funds, hospitals were required to establish various "utilization review" and "quality assurance" committees. Independent review organizations were also mandated, such as Professional Standards Review Organizations (PSROs), organizations expensively staffed with doctors who were assigned the task of reviewing decisions from the records of hospitalized patients on matters that affected hospital costs, such as whether a heart operation was necessary. "Certificate of need" regulations required hospitals to prove they needed a new piece of equipment or facility before acquiring it. Teaching hospitals typically experienced the most inconvenience and longest delays from the cumbersome regulations, even as physicians in private practice were free to install expensive equipment without having to receive regulatory approval. None of these measures succeeded in halting rising medical costs, though all contributed to the rising administrative costs of the U.S. health care system.

At this time, Medicare and Medicaid (and some private third party payers, following the government's lead) began to reimburse hospitals for fewer services. Increasingly, preoperative days that did not involve acute care, convalescent days deemed by a reviewer as unnecessary, and hospital admissions for diagnostic evaluations that could have been performed on an outpatient basis were disallowed. Third party payers also became less generous in the price they would pay for certain procedures, and hospitals often experienced lengthy delays before receiving payment. Moreover, for a hospital to be reimbursed, the paperwork in charts had to be complete. All notes had to be signed, and discharge summaries had to be dictated and signed as well. If the paperwork was not completed within a certain time, payment to the hospitals would be disallowed—no matter how necessary or expensive the hospitalization. Often this resulted in excessive efforts to treat patient records rather than patients. Many attending physicians, whose signatures were necessary for billing, found that their attention was diverted away from patient care and teaching to record keeping.[56]

The onerous burden of regulation arose not only from federal but also from state and local authorities. In no state were hospitals subject to more intense regulatory review than New York, where state regulations escalated dramatically to encompass virtually every aspect of hospital activity. A catalog of responsibilities imposed on hospitals included rules regarding the limitation of emergency room waiting time, the requirement that an interpreter be available within 10 to 20 minutes if more than 1 percent of the patient population spoke a foreign language, and a discharge appeal process that allowed a 24-hour delay to any patient objecting to the timing of his or her discharge. Often the requirements of one state agency conflicted with those of another. Reimbursement rates from all third party payers except Medicare were controlled by the state. Typically, the increases in reimbursement rates authorized by the state were inadequate to cover the costs imposed by the latest set of state regulations.[57]

In the last analysis, the learning environment of academic health centers remained strong despite capitation pressures and government mandates and regulations. The administration of academic health centers became more complex and costly, but the quality of education, investigation, and clinical work was seemingly unaffected. Nevertheless, medical faculties were deeply disturbed by the demands that government was now placing on them. The primary problem, from their viewpoint, was that financial support of the schools and clinical reimbursement of the teaching hospitals were increasingly dependent on various social mandates being met, yet political views and fashions were notorious for changing frequently. Like any large, complex organization, academic health centers, after gearing up for a particular mandate, could not reverse directions quickly. Rational planning was made difficult when funding and reimbursement were dependent on the whimsy of politicians and on the flavor of this year's social cause.

Yet, if medical educators were disturbed, so were political leaders. In their view, academic health centers were increasingly unresponsive to national concerns. As perceived geographic and specialty maldistributions in the physician workforce accelerated and as medical costs soared, the intellectual leaders of medicine—the medical school faculties—seemed uninterested in making any sustained effort to address the problems. To many political officials, academic medicine was very good at receiving money, but not at giving back anything in return, particularly in regard to helping make health care delivery more equitable and efficient. Economist Victor Fuchs, addressing the annual meeting of the Association of American Medical Colleges in 1978, spoke to that point:

> Even a sympathetic, friendly observer can't help but get the impression that academic medicine's interest in health policy begins and ends with two commandments:
>   First, 'give us money,'
>   Second, 'leave us alone.'[58]

In the main, academic health centers had served society well, but as problems continued to grow in the health care delivery system, the relevance of academic medicine to the nation's health began to seem less obvious than before. Increasingly, policy experts and public officials viewed academic health centers as cost-generators, as producers of expensive technologies and high-priced specialists, and as scientific institutions where intellectual curiosity surpassed public service or concern for national problems. Government officials had once considered academic health centers the solution to assuring the nation's health, but now many political leaders began to regard academic health centers as part of the problem.

The Dawn of the Age of Limits

Since the beginning of the twentieth century, the main assumption underlying health care policy in the United States had been that the health of the nation depended on the quality and quantity of doctors. This assumption had been clearly apparent after World War II in the growth of the National Institutes of Health (NIH), the spread of private medical insurance, the enactment of Medicare and Medicaid, and the various bills that encouraged the production of more doctors. In this view, more and better medical care translated into a healthier people. Medical schools, as the generators of medical knowledge and producers of doctors, occupied a special position as guardians of the nation's health. Attitudes toward medicine were analogous to popular attitudes toward science: both were perceived as positive forces that could be harnessed for society's benefit. There was relatively little popular appreciation of any limitation or downside to either medicine or science.

After World War II, as discussed earlier, a few eminent critics warned against unrealistic expectations of medicine. René Dubos had pointed out that human beings, like all organisms, are in equilibrium with their environment. Control one disease, and another disease will take its place. Alfred N. Richards had cautioned that quick, definitive advances against disease could not be taken for granted. In the 1970s, sociologist Renée Fox warned against the "medicalization" of social problems. Crime, substance abuse, poverty, teenage pregnancy, marital difficulties, physical violence, and illiteracy, she wrote, were social problems with medical complications, not purely medical problems that doctors should be expected to "cure."[59] Nevertheless, such warnings generally went unheeded. Few citizens—and even fewer policy makers and legislators—doubted that the nation's health depended upon the continued generation of medical knowledge and availability of well-trained doctors.

In the 1970s, the dominant assumption for the first time came under widespread attack. The idea that medical care was only one factor influencing the health of the population was hardly new, but recognition of this idea became much more widespread than before, and it struck policy makers and intellectuals with the power of an epiphany. One prominent spokesman, Aaron Wildavsky, president of the Russell Sage Foundation, wrote in 1977 of the diminishing returns to be expected from more medical care. "According to the Great Equation, Medical Care equals Health. But the Great Equation is wrong. More available medical care does not equal better health." Health, Wildavsky pointed out, is primarily determined not by medical care but by "factors over which doctors have little or no control, from individual lifestyle (smoking, exercise, worry), to social conditions (income, eating habits, physiological inheritance), to the physical environment (air and water quality)." Medical care, he argued, had definite limits to its effectiveness. "No one is saying that medicine is good for nothing, only that it is not good for everything."[60]

In the 1970s and 1980s, several factors led to these more modest expectations of medicine. One was the growing concern over rapidly spiraling medical costs. By the 1970s medical care was increasingly viewed as deleterious to the country's economic competitiveness, as more and more resources were consumed with seemingly less and less to show for it. Automobile manufacturers, who once spoke of the importance of medical care to their industry for enabling workers to be healthy and productive, by the end of the decade were complaining that the cost of health care in each automobile exceeded the cost of the steel.[61]

In addition, the period witnessed a decline in the moral authority of physicians. News stories regularly reported abuses by doctors, hospitals, and nursing homes, such as fraudulent billing. In an age of consumerism and civil rights, there were loud protests against the excesses of some doctors, such as patronizing attitudes toward patients or the custom of asking patients to address medical students by the title "doctor." The ability or willingness of physicians and other health professionals to act in their patients' best interests came into question. Thus arose the "right-to-die" movement, the "patient bill of rights" manifestos, and new ethical guidelines for informed consent in human experimentation. Scholars in medical history and medical sociology, who once viewed doctors as heroic, increasingly saw them as flawed human actors and began writing of their foibles and greed. The common denominator to these movements was the challenge they posed to professional authority.[62]

Another important factor contributing to the lower expectations of medicine was the rise in incidence of chronic diseases. Most serious conditions affecting Americans in the 1970s represented ironies of earlier medical and public health successes: people were living long enough to develop cancer or suffer a heart attack or stroke. From the standpoint of research, these conditions were proving more difficult to understand and control than many infectious and nutritional diseases. From the standpoint of prevention, a large body of research demonstrated that the majority of responsibility for maintaining health lay with the individual rather than the physician. One widely quoted study showed that health and life expectancy in adults were related to common sense health habits such as eating three balanced meals a day without snacking, obtaining adequate sleep, exercising three times a week, avoiding smoking, using alcohol in moderation or not at all, and maintaining proper weight.[63] Good health in adults depended less on regular medical checkups than on the individual's assuming responsibility for the promotion of his own health.

As the limits of medicine were being recognized, the country was becoming aware of its own limits as a nation. The ebullience and optimism of the 1950s and 1960s were replaced by diminished expectations and a much more guarded outlook toward the future. Faith in America's industrial might was severely shaken, as oil embargoes, soaring inflation, high unemployment, and a stagnant economy made it clear that the country did not have the economic capacity to provide everyone with everything. Economist Lester C. Thurow, in an influential book, described America as a "zero-sum society," where generalized growth and expansion should not be expected because, as in poker, the losses of one group will equal the winnings of others.[64] The social fabric was deteriorating, as manifested by an upsurge in illiteracy, drug addiction, crime, divorce, and teenage pregnancy. A permanent "underclass" appeared to be developing, and the educational, welfare, and justice systems appeared to be incapable of reversing the tide. The image of science became tarnished amid widespread concerns about toxic waste, the destruction of the ozone layer, and the potential for biological catastrophe from certain types of genetic research. Confidence in the political system to provide solutions to those problems, in the wake of Watergate and the Vietnam War, was far from great.[65]

As the nation became more conscious of its own limits, many became increasingly vocal about the limits of investing in medical care. One consequence was the cessation of federal aid to medical schools for undergraduate medical education. Even before the last of the new medical schools had opened, a doctor-surplus had been officially declared. The report of the Graduate Medical Education National Advisory Committee (GMENAC report) in 1980 predicted a surplus in the United States of 70,000 physicians by 1990 and 140,000 physicians by 2000.[66] The Health Professions Educational Assistance Act of 1976 elapsed in 1980, and the following year Congress terminated all capitation payments for medical schools. School officials did not miss the government mandates that had accompanied the capitation payments—particularly the "Guadalajara clause" of the 1976 bill—but they did miss the extra $500,000 to $1,000,000 that they received each year for general operating expenses. (This, of course, represented a classic example of politicians changing their minds, ending support for a cause they had championed only a few years before.)

A more substantial blow to medical schools arose from the slowing of federal support for biomedical research. In the late 1960s government appropriations for the NIH leveled off after two decades of double-digit growth, as funds were diverted from domestic programs to help pay for the Vietnam War. In subsequent years, the vicissitudes of federal research funding were many, depending on competing political aims, the state of the economy, and the size of the federal budget deficit. Nevertheless, the general trend was toward a reduced rate of growth. During the Nixon administration there were rescissions of grants for Ph.D. training programs, specialty fellowships, and the construction of research facilities, and throughout the 1970s the overall growth rate of NIH funding in inflation-adjusted dollars remained low. Beginning in 1982, as the economy recovered from a severe recession, there was renewed growth, though at slower rates than in the 1950s and 1960s. In the early 1990s, as a result of soaring federal budget deficits, the growth rate of NIH appropriations again began to fall precipitously in real dollars, and a disturbingly small percentage of grant applications were funded.[67] Moreover, a series of "zero-sum" funding decisions aggravated the plight of some biomedical investigators. For instance, federal decisions to increase the percentage of overhead reimbursement to schools and teaching hospitals were often paid for by decreasing the amount of direct support to individual investigators.

When the NIH budget began to level off, many medical educators found the government's change in attitude incomprehensible and frightening. "For the first time in the memory of most of us, we can expect to see schools being confronted with the necessity of dropping faculty members and staff from the roster,"[68] one leading medical school dean declared in 1969. In fact, downsizing did not occur, but many schools in the early 1970s were forced to cut back on activities, discontinue programs, and suspend plans for hiring new faculty. This did not surprise a few academic leaders (Milton Eisenhower being a prominent example cited earlier), who had warned of the dangers of overdependence on "soft" money from government grants. Now, their predictions came true. The autonomy most medical schools had naively assumed they enjoyed from the federal patron was finally seen to be an illusion.

In reality, it can hardly be said that the federal government stopped supporting the NIH. As *Table 10* indicates, NIH appropriations continued to increase, even allowing for inflation. As *Table 10* also indicates, medical schools continued to prosper, as measured by a variety of indicators of growth.[69] The problems academic medicine encountered resulted less from a penurious government than from the fact that it had expanded to a size that made it more difficult to sustain. As the number of full-time faculty grew, competition for grant support became more intense. The supply of new funds did not keep pace with the even more rapid growth in demand from the ever-increasing number of investigators. Thus, whether there was a "crisis" in research funding depended in part on one's point of view. To the federal government, appropriating ever more money to biomedical research, the accusation of underfunding seemed

Table 10 Growth of academic medicine, 1960–92*

	1960	1970	1980	1992
Support from NIH (millions of $)	1,320	3,028	5,419	8,407
Average medical school budget (millions of $)	24.1	64.6	91.9	200.4
Full-time medical school faculty (no.)				
Basic science	4,023	8,283	12,816	15,579
Clinical	7,201	19,256	37,716	65,913
Average base compensation (thousands of $)†				
Basic science faculty	NA	81.8‡	75.4	86.4
Clinical faculty	NA	140.2‡	132.6	177.0
Revenues from faculty-practice plans (millions of $)	61.0	398.9	1,704.7	8,291.0
Matriculated medical students (no.)	30,288	40,487	65,189	66,142
House staff (no.)	37,562	51,015	61,819	88,602

* Financial data are in 1992 dollars. NIH denotes National Institutes of Health, and NA not available. Data are from the AAMC.

† Average compensation, in 1993 dollars, for a professor.

‡ Data are for 1978.

petulant. To medical schools and individual investigators finding support much more difficult to obtain, the crisis was very real.

Beginning in the 1970s, medical schools, ever entrepreneurial, began seeking research support from sources besides the NIH (and state legislatures, for eligible institutions). Here, the schools enjoyed some major successes, which partially offset the growing difficulty of receiving NIH grants. The pharmaceutical industry was growing stronger, and relations between that industry and the university were continually improving. Private foundations, most notable the Howard Hughes Medical Institute and the Lucille P. Markey Charitable Trust, generously supported fundamental biomedical research. Most important, income from clinical practice began to support research at many schools, as virtually every school used a portion of professional fees to subsidize education and research.

Though NIH revenues grew, and though other sources of research support were found, it became clear that American society during the age of limits was funding biomedical research less generously than it had during the period of abundance that had followed World War II. As a percentage of the total amount of money the nation spent on medical care, the amount of resources directed to research steadily fell. In 1960, 6 percent of the nation's expenditures on health care were directed to research and construction; by 1990, that amount had fallen to 3 percent.[70] In the 1960s, large increases in the NIH budget occurred as a matter of course; by the 1990s, processions of scientific leaders had to march to Washington each year to cajole Congress merely not to reduce the budget. During the period of abundance, it was federal policy that all meritorious research proposals to the NIH should be funded.[71] (As a practical matter, at least 50 percent of applications were funded.) By fiscal years 1993 and 1994, the success rate of new grant applications had fallen to 11.7 percent (an all-time low) and 12.3 percent, respectively. Ninety percent of applications in a typical year would be judged by peer review to be deserving of support, leading to the designation "approved but not funded" for the many worthwhile applications that were rejected. Two of three renewal applications from established investigators were also turned down.[72] Established scientists and young investigators alike were disillusioned and demoralized, and a younger generation of high school, college, and medical students was becoming skeptical that medical research was a viable career choice.

By the 1990s a few ominous signs were appearing of erosion in America's leadership in biomedical research. For instance, in 1985, 72 percent of the scientific reports submitted to the prestigious *New England Journal of Medicine* came from the United States; by 1994, that number had dropped to 50 percent. The editor of the journal observed that Europe was rapidly catching up to the United States. "As Europe has increased its support of clinical research (and the United States, unfortunately, has decreased its support), any claim that the quality of European research is not of the highest standard has long since been disproved."[73] A study of four major clinical research journals in 1990 similarly found a declining representation of U.S. papers relative to Western Europe and Japan, a phenomenon the authors also correlated with a slowed growth of funding from the NIH.[74] These were not cheerful trends for a knowledge-based industry that wanted to retain world leadership. In the declining support of biomedical research, the country appeared to be losing its future-directedness.

Ironically, the slowing support for biomedical research occurred precisely when medicine could offer more than ever before. In earlier eras, medicine received much credit for improvements in the nation's health that more accurately were the results of better public health and nutrition. In the age of limits, medicine was not receiving credit for many things that it did do. In 1977, David E. Rogers and Robert J. Blendon documented reductions of both mortality and morbidity in the American population during the preceding 15 years that resulted from better and more available medical care. "While there remains an important agenda for the future, there seems room for cautious optimism about the abilities of American society to make forward progress."[75] Six years later Blendon and Rogers reviewed additional evidence linking further reductions in mortality in the United States to increased expenditures for health. At the time of a severe recession and growing national concern about health care costs, they pointed out that "more health expenditures do result in less morbidity and mortality" and warned that "reductions in medical care expenditures must be made with particular caution to avoid any untoward future effect on the nation's health."[76]

Even more ironic, in the age of limits the promise of fundamental biomedical research to make genuine inroads against vascular disease, cancer, neurological disease, arthritis, diabetes, and other chronic conditions was greater than ever. A molecular revolution was creating the vision of a direct attack on many chronic diseases. Already by the 1980s, new genetic technologies had resulted in the commercial production of clinically useful compounds—tissue-plasminogen activator (t-PA, an agent to dissolve blood clots), a human form of insulin with minimal allergenic effects, and erythropoietin (a drug used in certain types of anemia); furthermore, a fledgling biotechnology industry had started. The drug cimetidine, whose development was an offshoot of fundamental researches into the physiological influences affecting acid secretion in the stomach, within a few years virtually eliminated the need for surgery for peptic ulcer disease. The application of the computer and principles of theoretical physics to radiology had resulted in important new diagnostic technologies, such as computed tomography (CT scans) and magnetic resonance imaging (MRI), which offered great safety and diagnostic power.

The most prominent spokesman for biomedical research during the age of limits was Lewis Thomas, director of the Memorial Sloan-Kettering Cancer Center and one of the eminent medical statesmen of his age. Thomas continually pointed out that fundamental research was the route to what he called "true medical technologies" (the prevention or definitive treatment of diseases) to replace the current "half-way technologies" that dominated so much of medical practice (for instance, hemodialysis for kidney failure). Thomas pointed out that "true technologies" offered not only curative treatments but also significant cost-savings. He offered as examples the experience with earlier "true technologies" like vaccines and many antibiotics.[77] Thomas and other defenders of biomedical research were not denying the importance of prevention and health promotion. Rather, they were articulating the dangers to the public of decreasing the country's investment in biomedical research.

As furious debate and lobbying raged each year over the NIH budget, larger questions about a rational federal science policy usually went unaddressed. Little attention was given to the question of the optimal size or rate of growth of the NIH. Clearly, double-digit growth as experienced in the 1950s and 1960s could not continue indefinitely; at those rates, a point would be reached where every citizen would be a medical scientist and every federal dollar allocated to medical research. On the other hand, if only one of eight new research applications was being funded, biomedical research had room to grow before the supply of talented investigators and good ideas would be exhausted. To what indicator might the size of the NIH budget best be pegged: the total national expenditures for health? the Medicare and Medicaid budgets? the size of the federal budget deficit or rate of growth of the economy? at some level to assure that a certain percentage (20 percent? 30 percent?) of meritorious applications would be funded? What should be the proper balance between federal and nonfederal support of biomedical research? How might stable, long-term support be provided that would allow medical schools to engage in rational planning, yet provide the public protection against complacency and a sense of entitlement among grant recipients? These and other questions generally went undiscussed. So did the fact that the health needs of the future are likely to be different from those of the present, posing challenges that can be met only by having a strong biomedical research enterprise already in place. The arrival of the acquired immunodeficiency syndrome (AIDS) epidemic in the 1980s stood as a poignant reminder of that point.

In addition, recognition of medicine's legitimate limits during the 1970s, 1980s, and 1990s did not result in a rational health policy in the United States, any more than it resulted in a rational science policy. With Medicare and Medicaid, federal interest clearly shifted from research to service programs. Year by year the country continued to spend more and more on health care, even while decrying health care costs and reducing the relative proportion spent on education and research. There was little evidence that Americans were taking health promotion seriously or assuming adequate responsibility for their own health (despite significant reductions in cigarette consumption and a preoccupation in some circles with cholesterol levels). The problems of tobacco use, excessive alcohol consumption, drug abuse, reckless driving, unprotected sexual activity, obesity, physical inactivity, stress, and heavy tranquilizer use continued unabated. Efforts to invest in social programs such as urban renewal, education, job training, crime prevention, a cleaner and safer environment, and gun control were half-hearted and ineffective. There were few efforts to accommodate the health care delivery system to chronic diseases. As Daniel M. Fox has discussed, in the era of chronic diseases, the system of health care financing and delivery remained based on an acute disease model. Thus, third party payers would often pay for renal dialysis but not for the outpatient treatment of high blood pressure that could have prevented the kidneys from failing in the first place.[78]

Stated another way, though many during the age of limits became more pessimistic about the ability of medical research and care to influence the nation's health, and though many worried about the rising costs of health care, the greatest limit in health care was the lack of vision, leadership, and national will to forge a sensible health care policy. The promise of medical research was bright, and the prospect of "true" cost-saving technologies for chronic diseases was real, but federal support of biomedical research became increasingly erratic. Many of the determinants of good health—not to mention cost-effective care—were already known, but the nation's public and private leadership seemed unwilling or unable to develop, implement, and support policies that would further those goals. The country's academic health centers suffered from these limits of political vision and leadership—but so did the rest of the nation.

15

Academic Health Centers Under Stress: Internal Dilemmas

THROUGHOUT ITS HISTORY, the American medical school, like the rest of the country's system of higher education, had been shaped by social, economic, and political developments in the larger society. Thus it was hardly a surprise that many of the pressures experienced by academic health centers in the 1970s and 1980s arose from outside events. Yet, academic health centers encountered additional dilemmas that could not so clearly be related to external pressures. A number of traditional challenges to medical education grew more intense: the problem of teaching bedside medicine as biomedical research became increasingly molecular, the perpetual difficulty of achieving a suitable institutional balance between teaching and research, and the ongoing dilemmas of residency and fellowship training. These frustrating problems arose mainly from the evolution of medical knowledge and the institutional development of academic health centers rather than from the challenges imposed by a hostile external environment.

Molecular Medicine and the Disappearance of Teachers

In the 1970s and 1980s, the molecular revolution transforming biomedical research continued to gain momentum. The gaze of investigators focused on ever smaller particles, such as genes, proteins, viruses, antibodies, and membrane receptors. By the 1990s, the molecular complexities of the human organism in health and disease were far from fully understood. However, a profound transformation in the nature of biomedical knowledge had already taken place, and the implications for a new molecular medicine were becoming apparent.

Throughout the basic science fields, discoveries of elegance, profundity, and beauty were made.[1] However, four areas of investigation were especially important to creating a new theoretical underpinning of medical knowledge. One was molecular biology and the emerging concept of molecular disease. The precise chemical structure and organization of the gene became known, as did the specific molecular mechanisms by which genes direct the functions of humans and other living organisms. Methods of genetic recombination and techniques for rapidly determining the sequential structure of genes were developed, as were techniques to determine the chromosomal location of genes. A host of new disorders resulting from defective gene products were identified—over 1,000 by 1980, compared with 15 in 1960. By the 1990s, molecular biology had gained the capacity to relate disease processes and biological processes to the functioning of specific genes, to isolate the genes in pure form, to characterize the genes in specific molecular detail, to redesign the gene according to predetermined specifications, and to reintroduce the modified genes into bacterial or mammalian cells growing in culture (or, in a few cases, even into intact organisms).

A second area was cell biology—the study of the cell and its constituent components. The structure of the organizing units of cells, such as membranes, nuclei, lysosomes, and mitochondria, became understood at a molecular level, as did their mode of functioning and regulation. Membrane receptors were studied in minute detail; it was found that configurational changes of a single polypeptide on the cell surface could turn a particular cellular function on or off. Within the cell, "second messenger" systems were discovered that carried out the instructions of hormones and other external stimuli. These discoveries were applicable to the study of abnormal conditions, such as the molecular transformations of the cell that occurred in the malignant process.

The third area was immunobiology, the modern study of immunology made possible by the merging of classical immunobiology with genetics, molecular biology, and biochemistry. New investigations elucidated the complex molecular structure of antibodies and defined the role of lymphocytes and other scavenger cells in the organism's defense system. Immunological reactions were found to be regulated by a genetically determined structure on the surface of these cells. These observations contained enormous implications for the understanding and control of cancer, graft rejection, susceptibility to infection, multiple sclerosis, diabetes, rheumatic diseases, and other illnesses. The monoclonal antibody technique—a method of transforming a malignant plasma cell into an uncontrollable producer of a single immunoglobulin—had a major theoretical impact on immunobiology and provided a powerful tool for the production and isolation of hormones, enzymes, and other molecules of pharmacological importance.

The fourth area was the neurosciences. In the 1970s and 1980s, a series of separate discoveries came together to provide a molecular view of the structure and functioning of the brain. Various classes of chemical neurotransmitters were detected and studied with great specificity. This work enabled the identification of the mechanism of action of various psychotropic drugs like lithium and certain tranquilizers. It also offered the possibility of designing new drugs to help control the wrenching mood disturbances of the affective disorders, particularly those with a genetically determined component. The modern neurosciences even offered the possibility of developing drugs to lessen the permanent neurological consequences of stroke.

If any one aspect of the molecular revolution demonstrated that a new era in basic biomedical research had begun, it was the coalescence of the once separate "preclinical sciences" into a single field speaking a single molecular language. Teaching and research in all the basic science subjects became interrelated and sometimes indistinguishable from each other. Techniques such as recombinant-DNA methodology were used by investigators in all the scientific departments, while areas such as molecular genetics belonged to each of the biomedical fields. Intellectually, the confluence of the basic science subjects had been proceeding for several decades. Now, that process appeared to be nearing completion.

In the clinical departments, research remained more variegated. The observational approach to clinical investigation continued, whether through case reports, observations of the natural history of an illness, or the conduct of drug trials. More sophisticated clinical research—the experimental study of clinical phenomena, using patients in some fashion as the focus of the inquiry—also continued. Epidemiological research remained important—witness the important discoveries concerning the methods of transmission of the human immunodeficiency virus (HIV), which resulted in practical guidelines on how to prevent the spread of the acquired immunodeficiency syndrome (AIDS). Prompted initially by private foundations, some physicians began to study nonbiological issues pertaining to health care: the financing and delivery of health care services, the proper design and statistical analysis of clinical trials, outcomes research, technology assessment, medical ethics, the history of medicine, sociology, and medical informatics (the application of computer technologies and the information sciences to medicine). This latter approach became particularly popular among academic physicians whose clinical interests lay in a general rather than a specialty medical field.

Nevertheless, the forefront of clinical investigation also became molecular, as physician-scientists in clinical departments increasingly adopted the same "reductionist" approaches as workers in the basic science departments. For instance, the pathogenesis of pneumococcal infection began to be investigated at the molecular level. Researchers studied the specific mechanisms by which the cell wall of the organism induced inflammation, and their discoveries created the prospect of developing therapeutic agents to block the ability of the organism to traverse mucosal barriers in the nasopharynx, target specific body sites, or activate inflammatory cells.[2] Similarly, the mysteries of high cholesterol also began to be understood at the molecular level. One major discovery was that certain cells of the human body have receptors on their surfaces that trap and absorb bloodstream particles that contain cholesterol. For this discovery, Michael Brown and Joseph Goldstein—two internists at University of Texas Health Science Center at Dallas—received the Nobel Prize in 1985.[3]

A glance at the literature of clinical investigation shows how fully the scientific forefront of the field had moved from the patient to the laboratory. For instance, by the 1980s and 1990s, only an occasional paper in the *Journal of Clinical Investigation*, the most important journal in the field, focused upon patients. Rather, the majority of articles now employed the techniques of molecular or cellular biology. In 1990 the table of contents of the journal began grouping the articles into thematic sections, such as molecular medicine/genetic disorders, hormones/cytokines/signalling, and cell growth and differentiation. It became difficult to distinguish many of the articles from those appearing in basic science publications.

There were other important signs of the transformation of clinical research. At many academic health centers, clinical research centers (special hospital units where patients of scientific interest were studied) were habitually underutilized.[4] In the 1970s, the submission of abstracts to the major clinical research meeting—the jointly held gathering of the Association of American Physicians, the American Society for Clinical Investigation, and the American Federation for Clinical Research—declined relative to the submission of papers to clinical subspecialty or basic science meetings.[5] In the 1980s and 1990s, new laboratory facilities for clinical investigation (for instance, the Clinical Sciences Research Building at Washington University and the Richard D. Ross Research Building at Johns Hopkins) were built in buildings physically separate from the teaching hospital itself—an architectural embodiment of the shift of clinical investigation from a patient focus to a laboratory focus. By the 1980s, the term "physician-scientist" was replacing the earlier term "clinical investigator" to emphasize that the cutting edge of clinical research now lay squarely in the laboratory.

Though much remained to be learned, the molecular approach resulted in a bold new conception of the human body in health and disease. Moreover, by the 1990s, clinically important benefits had already occurred, and the prospect of a major transformation of medical practice in the decades ahead was real. Knowledgeable students of the health care system knew that the primary determinants of the nation's health would continue to lie in the environment, social conditions, and prevention. On the other hand, as long as human beings remained mortal, everyone eventually would be afflicted with illness, suffering, and death. Many of the most common adult scourges—Alzheimer's disease, schizophrenia, most cancer, high blood pressure, stroke, multiple sclerosis, diabetes, rheumatoid arthritis, kidney failure, and many types of cirrhosis—seemed to appear independently of known environmental causes and defied prevention by jogging, dieting, avoiding tobacco, and other life style changes. Indeed, few preventive strategies in adults were foolproof. Thin, physically active nonsmokers with low cholesterol levels continued to have heart attacks (and other individuals with many risk factors for coronary artery disease suffered no problems). For those who were ill, the capacity of medicine to help was greater than ever, and fundamental biomedical research offered the single brightest hope for understanding and controlling chronic diseases.

Nevertheless, medical faculties discovered that the molecular revolution created new educational dilemmas. For all the theoretical and practical power of molecular medicine, physicians dealing with real patients still had to think in terms of symptoms, physical signs, organ physiology, and classical pharmacology and surgery—that is, they had to respond to illness as traditional doctors. The intellectual integration of the molecular aberrations of disease with physiological disturbances and clinical symptoms had hardly begun. In earlier eras, a distinctive feature of medical education had been the integration of medical research with education and patient care—that is, teachers taught students what they themselves were investigating. Now, biomedical research was far more removed from clinical teaching and care. Accordingly, the intellectual cohesiveness of medical schools was threatened. These trends had been underway since the 1940s, but in the era of molecular medicine the separation of research from education and practice (that is, the "bench-bedside gap") became more pronounced than ever before.

This tension was very clear in the basic science fields, where the research interests of most faculty no longer directly related to much of the subject matter still taught to medical students. As a result, basic science departments around the country began changing their names to reflect their investigative as well as their teaching programs. In 1978 the Department of Physiology at the University of Southern California School of Medicine became the Department of Physiology and Biophysics to acknowledge the significant number of faculty doing work in membrane physiology and to aid the department in recruiting graduate students and applying for research funding.[6] Similarly, the University of Maryland School of Medicine in 1986 voted to change the name of the Department of Anatomy to the Department of Anatomy and Cell Biology.[7] (The complete transformation of the names of the basic science departments during the molecular era at one medical school is illustrated in *Table 11*.) Implicit in these name changes was the fact that faculty members were in the antithetical position of studying fundamental molecular and cellular biology while teaching clinically necessary subjects such as gross and microscopic anatomy, fluid and electrolyte metabolism, and classical organ physiology to medical students.

In some fields, it became difficult to find faculty who could still teach classical subject matter. Gross anatomy was the prime example. Anatomy

Table 11   Basic science departments, Washington University School of
            Medicine

1965	1995
Anatomy	Anatomy and Neurobiology
Biological Chemistry	Biochemistry and Molecular Biophysics
	Genetics
Microbiology	Molecular Microbiology
Pathology	Pathology
Pharmacology	Molecular Biology and Pharmacology
Physiology	Cell Biology and Physiology

departments depended heavily on surgeons, radiologists, anthropologists, and dentists for help in teaching, since the field was virtually dead as an area of active investigation among anatomy faculty. However, to a lesser extent this problem affected instruction in biochemistry, physiology, microbiology, and pharmacology as well. "Who will teach the basic medical sciences?"[8] one medical school dean asked as early as 1964. At many schools, internists, pediatricians, or clinical pharmacologists began to assume major roles in teaching the basic science subjects. At some schools, officials acknowledged the possibility that the basic science faculty might be forced to split into separate research and teaching faculties.

Similar developments occurred in the clinical departments, where the traditional cohesiveness among research, patient care, and education began to erode. Traditionally, the defining characteristic of clinical research had been its focus upon patients, which meant that clinical research had always gone hand-in-hand with patient care and clinical instruction. In the molecular era, patients were bypassed. Molecular biology enabled the fruitful study of many medical problems without the need for contact with patients. As one reflection of this change, more and more clinical research came to be undertaken by Ph.D.s. Indeed, by 1990, over 8,000 nonphysician Ph.D.s held full-time academic positions in the clinical departments of U.S. medical schools.[9]

The results of this approach were gratifying in terms of medical discovery, but for the first time a conspicuous separation of functions occurred betwen clinical research on one hand and patient care and clinical education on the other. Physician-scientists found themselves at the center of the highly competitive universe of biomedical science, forced to compete for funding and recognition with Ph.D. scientists from all the biomedical fields. By most estimates, success in clinical research demanded that investigators spend at least 90 to 95 percent of their professional time in the laboratory. As one prominent investigator explained,

"The physician-scientist trained both in medicine and basic research is going to find it increasingly hard to stay at the forefront of such basic research if he or she continues to care for patients more than a minimum amount of time."[10]

Accordingly, most successful clinical investigators started spending less and less time in patient care and clinical teaching. At George Washington, it was observed that "senior faculty in Medicine haven't paid attention to House Staff, with the exception of fellows."[11] At Jefferson, a school with a long tradition of excellence in clinical teaching, it was now felt that senior faculty had to be "encouraged to play a greater role in bedside teaching."[12] In an account of his experience as a student at Harvard Medical School in the early 1980s, Melvin Konner portrayed the nearly total absence of senior physicians during his clinical clerkships. "Where on earth were these people in Konner's Harvard?" Lewis Thomas asked in his review of Konner's book. When Thomas had been a student at Harvard several decades before, senior clinical faculty "were always near at hand, in and out of the wards, making rounds at all hours, displaying for the students' benefit the complete repertoire of seasoned, highly skilled doctors." In Konner's Harvard, "The real instructors [of students] were the interns and residents, and the professors were off somewhere else."[13]

Beginning in the 1970s, and accelerating in the 1980s and 1990s, medical schools responded to the circumstances that were causing physician-scientists to disappear from the wards. Many clinical departments established two discrete faculty tracks: an academic track, pursued by physician-scientists; and a clinician-teacher or clinical scholar track, pursued by those whose primary interests lay in teaching and patient care. Faculty members in the academic track typically devoted 90 to 95 percent of their time to research. Those in the clinician-teacher track customarily spent 20 to 50 percent of their time in research (doing things like patient-oriented studies, drug trials, and clinical reports) and the rest of their time in patient care and teaching. The criteria for appointment to the clinical track were "excellence in teaching and clinical service" and "some scholarly activity."[14] In the appointment of clinical scholars to the faculty, Abraham Flexner would have approved. In 1910 he had written that there is room in the modern medical school for the "non-productive, assimilative teacher of wide learning, continuous receptivity, critical sense and responsive interest."[15] What was necessary was for departments and medical schools to have a balance between teaching and research, not for there to be an equal balance in each faculty member.

Flexner's viewpoint notwithstanding, members of the new clinician-teacher track encountered difficulties—including the stigma of being considered second-class citizens in departments and schools where research had always been the top faculty priority. "The new ranks will describe the faculty who do not have the qualifications for the regular academic track,"[16] one medical school put it. Nevertheless, those appointed to the clinician track were hardly ordinary practitioners. Though their emphasis was on patient care and teaching, they were creative, thoughtful, and engaged in research and writing—in short, doing all the scholarly work that was necessary for good teaching to be facilitated. They were too busy to roam the wards as clinical teachers once did, since they now had large responsibilities for private patient care that earlier generations of faculty did not. However, they provided excellent teaching and clinical role models and did much to foster the educational mission of their departments.

Nevertheless, the creation of the clinician-teacher track underscored the fundamental intellectual challenge medical schools faced during the molecular era: the growing estrangement between medical science and medical practice. The creation of a separate teaching faculty in the clinical departments and the prospect of such a faculty in the basic science departments ran counter to the traditional notion that teaching and research should be interrelated. The fundamental principle of the university medical school was that the majority of teachers should be engaged in original scientific activity. Yet now, teaching was increasingly divorced from cutting-edge investigation. Similarly, the molecular revolution also made it more difficult than ever to identify which scientific facts and principles students needed to know. Many in the molecular era wrestled with the question of how to define and teach the scientific basis of practice,[17] and many also struggled with the problem of how to keep the medical school whole—that is, of not having the research faculty split into a separate research institute apart from the rest of the school. No one, however, had the answers to these vexing issues.

Reform Without Change

After the passage of Medicare, the popularity of medicine as a career continued to fluctuate (*see Figure 8*). From the late 1960s through the late 1970s, the competition to gain admission to medical school was intense, peaking in 1974 with 42,624 total applicants, or a ratio of 2.9 applicants for each available position. From the late 1970s through the late 1980s, the number of applicants dramatically fell, as did the overall quality of applicants, as measured by average college grade point averages (GPAs) and scores on the Medical College Admissions Test (MCAT). In 1988, the applicant pool to medical schools again began to grow, reaching a ratio of about 2.8 applicants per available position by 1995, while the average GPA and MCAT scores also increased substantially. No one knew why the attractiveness of medicine as a career should have fluctuated so widely in the course of a generation—though informed opinion held that the military draft deferments received by medical students helped account for medicine's popularity during the Vietnam War, and that the decline and subsequent growth in size of the applicant pool related primarily to the changing attractiveness of other careers rather than to the perceptions college students held about medicine.[18]

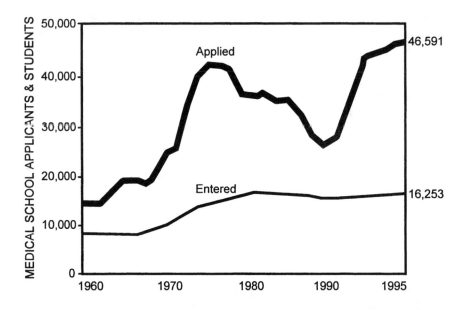

Figure 8   *Medical school applicants and students, 1960–1995*

From Medicare and Medicaid through managed care, the demo-graphic composition of the student body also changed significantly. As noted earlier, the proportion of underrepresented minorities plateaued in the late 1970s, while the percentage of women steadily rose. The propor-tion of white males dropped, while the percentage of Asians (who were not considered an underrepresented minority group) grew. In 1995, the entering class at U.S. medical schools consisted of 57.3 percent men, 42.7 percent women, 17.9 percent Asians, and 14.9 percent underrepresented Americans.[19]

After the passage of Medicare, medicine continued its evolution toward becoming a profession accessible mainly to the well-to-do. This phenomenon resulted primarily from rocketing tuition and the scarcity of scholarship funds. Private medical schools with small endowments—places like Georgetown, George Washington, and Tufts—charged the steepest tuitions, but no school could keep tuition down in the face of high inflation levels, soaring costs, and (in the 1980s) the end of federal education subsidies. As a result, debt among medical graduates became widespread. The decade of the 1980s was particularly devastating in this regard, as tuition and debt load soared at both private and public med-ical schools (*see Figure 9*). Among graduates of the class of 1992, the median indebtedness was $50,000 ($68,000 and $45,000 at private and public medical schools, respectively). Only 20.1 percent of students grad-uating that year had no debt.[20]

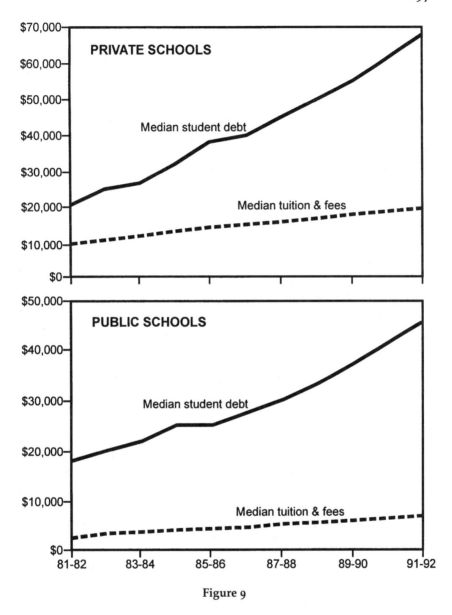

Figure 9

Medical schools worried about soaring debt and tuition. Would this encourage graduates to enter remunerative specialty fields instead of primary care or research? Would this influence physicians to seek the highest possible fees? Despite such concerns, no evidence could be found to substantiate them. For instance, numerous studies failed to find a correlation between debt load and specialty choice (though many educators continued to suspect that such a relationship existed).[21] The one consis-

tently demonstrable effect of rising tuition was that the proportion of students from affluent backgrounds increased still further. By 1989, the
median income of parents of first-year students was $60,000. That year
only 22.1 percent of incoming students came from homes where the parents' combined gross income was less than $40,000, and only 5.1 percent
from families with gross incomes less than $20,000.[22]

Medical faculties repeatedly expressed their consternation over the
prospect of medicine becoming a preserve of the rich—especially when
the country was clamoring for greater opportunities for all racial, ethnic,
and socioeconomic groups. Nevertheless, as had been the case all century
long, private and federal sources failed to show much interest in contributing scholarship funds. Even strong advocates of medical schools
felt uneasy about supporting another person's private business. As the
faculty of one medical school observed, "Congress has a dislike for supporting educational costs for individuals who will be high wage earners."[23] Medical schools viewed scholarship applicants as needy students;
Congress and the public regarded them as tomorrow's rich doctors.

Who were the new medical students? No one knew the answer. Much
quantitative information was available about the students, such as their
sex, age, race, economic status, parents' occupations, college majors, and
aggregate GPAs and MCAT scores. However, little was known about the
students in a qualitative sense—that is, their values, beliefs, attitudes,
aspirations, and reasons for choosing medicine as a career. For instance,
it was often stated that the presence of greater numbers of women in
the profession would have a humanizing effect on medical care. However, empirical studies of the issue were unavailable. In the materialistic
1980s, the interest of college freshmen in obtaining a general education
declined sharply, while their interest in earning a high salary markedly
increased.[24] The consequences of this value shift on premedical and
medical students was similarly unknown. What were the implications of
having more Asians and women enter medicine, or fewer white males
and members of lower income families—in terms of the experience of
learning medicine, the doctor-patient relationship, the prospects for
medical research, or the responsiveness of the profession to problems of
the health care delivery system? The sociological data to resolve these
and many other important questions were lacking.[25]

The question of who the medical students were became especially relevant in view of two contradictory images of the "new" medical student
that were projected in the 1970s. One was of socially committed students
interested in fields like community medicine, public health, family medicine, psychiatry, and pediatrics. Such students were often committed to
broad humanitarian goals like peace, civil rights, the reduction of poverty,
the protection of the environment, and the elimination of nuclear
weapons. Such students also tended to engage in a variety of extracurricular projects, such as sheltering and feeding the homeless, and often

clamored for more community-based fieldwork outside the ivory walls of the academic health center.[26]

The second, more sinister view was that the "new" medical students were afflicted with the "premedical syndrome," which presumably arose from the extreme competitive pressures to gain admission to medical school. Typical symptoms included narrow-mindedness, cynicism, high anxiety levels, ferocious competitiveness, and an overwhelming concern to earn good grades rather than to acquire a broad, liberal education. What made the premedical syndrome so worrisome was the alleged frequency of academic dishonesty, including cheating on examinations, sabotaging experiments of other students, and tearing critical pages out of library books. Many medical educators were disturbed that such behavior seemed not to end in college. As one faculty observed, "Our medical students come from colleges and universities where grade competition was extremely fierce and the undesirable effects of this competition were carried over into professional school."[27] Data were scarce, but grade-grubbing and cheating in medical school seemed to increase in frequency in the 1970s and 1980s—an impression that was supported by two widely discussed studies based on questionnaire data.[28] Dishonesty among medical students even extended to theft of the questions and answers from licensing examinations, copies of which were bought and sold in the 1980s for prices of up to $50,000.[29] Many worried about the ominous implications of such behavior for the future practice of medicine: that cut-throat or dishonest medical students would become cutthroat or dishonest physicians.

The prevalence of either syndrome among medical students was unknown. Nevertheless, the existence of these stereotypes reminded medical educators of the importance of the attitudes, values, and ideas about medicine that medical students brought with them to the training process. The quality of medical education and practice, as always, depended heavily on the characteristics of the individuals who chose medicine as a career.

The responsibility for selecting the best candidates continued to fall to the admissions committees. As before, admissions committees used college GPAs and scores on the MCAT, supplemented by letters of recommendation, personal interviews, and consideration of extracurricular interests and activities. However, these criteria were as imperfect as ever. Medical schools consistently sought students with desirable personal characteristics, but these subjective qualities continued to prove difficult to recognize. College GPAs became increasingly nondiscriminatory as a screening device owing to the diversity among colleges in grading standards and to an overall tendency toward grade inflation. Scores on the MCAT examination, as from the beginning, correlated with performance during the basic science years in medical school but did not serve as good predictors for performance during the clinical years or in subsequent medical practice.[30] This remained true despite changes in the format and scoring of the examination in 1977 and 1991 that were intended to place greater weight on breadth of academic background, reasoning skills, and writing ability. "If the MCAT were a laboratory test . . . its sensitivity, specificity, and predictive value are so poorly known that it would be discarded as useless,"[31] one critic wrote.

The greatest limitation of the admissions process was in the evaluation of minority students with low college grades and MCAT scores, since some of these students performed perfectly well in medical school. The University of Michigan had a typical experience: "Minority students are often admitted with lower grades and MCAT scores than are other students, but experience has indicated that they may well perform at an acceptable level with grades and MCATs which would surely predict disaster if they had been obtained by white middle class students."[32] Conversely, academic failure in medical school could not easily be predicted from minority students' college records. For instance, Howard University carefully reexamined the application records of students who had to be dismissed for academic reasons over one three-year period and found "no correlation between MCAT, GPA and academic performance which would prevent the same admission decision."[33]

In the admissions process, influence rarely helped. Admissions committees by and large were independent lots doing their job honorably and conscientiously. The records of medical schools are replete with letters of rejection to friends and relatives of trustees, major donors, and school officials. As the dean of one medical school remarked, "I have not interfered in the cases of children of my own closest friends and relatives."[34] At many schools, some students had advantages in making the cutoff for interviews: racial minorities or women here; in-state residents or children of alumni there; potential medical scientists somewhere else. However, in the final selection, the rules were almost always followed—despite occasional threats of lawsuits, civil rights complaints, or the withholding of contributions to the school. In the rare cases where they were not, newspaper headlines were made.[35]

The admissions process was nerve-wracking for medical schools as well as for students, since it represented an opportunity to recruit students, not merely to select a student body. Schools took that opportunity seriously. At the University of Southern California, the faculty knew that "the top schools in the country make a fuss over the good applicants." Accordingly, the school instructed its interviewers to work hard at "selling the school to prospective medical students."[36] Many schools studied the reasons why students they accepted decided to attend other schools, hoping to learn something that would improve their competitiveness the next year.[37] After bad recruitment years schools often worked even harder to attract better applicants, as the University of Maryland did in 1986, when it implemented plans to market itself to colleges more effectively and to improve its interviewing procedures.[38] As always, premedical students—at least those competitive enough to be admitted to more than one school—had more power than they sometimes realized.

☙ · ☙ · ☙

For students, the experience of medical school continued to be much the same as it had been all century long. The exhilaration and thrill of gaining competence in the profession should not be underestimated. Nor should the hard work, long hours, demanding routine, total immersion in the institutional culture, and profound anxiety associated with the fear of failure. Students survived in no small part because of the various formal and informal coping mechanisms that had been devised: the advice and guidance of certain instructors, the camaraderie among classmates, and the class plays, ritualistic pranks, and extracurricular class projects.

After 1970, students continued to make their voices heard, which faculty and administrators who had been through the protest era knew that they ignored at their peril. Everywhere, students could be found sitting on official school committees, speaking out about the curriculum or quality of student life, and expressing themselves widely on the strengths and weaknesses of the institution. Even though student opinion could be fickle, and even though students frequently disagreed with each other, the faculties listened. "There has been only one criterion for evaluation of teaching, and that is the student,"[39] a faculty member at Columbia observed. If nothing else, faculties knew that contented students were more likely to become loyal alumni—a crucial source of financial and political support for a school.

In the 1980s reports of extreme stress, including harassment and abuse, began to appear. Some worried that student abuse—defined in one report as "unnecessary or avoidable acts or words of a negative nature inflicted by one person on another person or persons"—was reaching large-scale proportions. A study at one medical school revealed that 80.6 percent of seniors reported being abused (as so defined) during medical school, with the greatest incidence of episodes occurring during the third-year clinical clerkships. House officers were the main offenders in every category of offense, being cited by the students far more often than faculty, nurses, or peers. The perception of students and investigators was that many of these episodes had long-lasting psychological consequences. Striking parallels were pointed out between medical students and abused children, who both exhibited "alterations in attitude and behavior that might be the result of avoidable, unnecessary, and harmful abuse."[40]

Despite such reports, it was not clear whether undergraduate medical education was in fact more stressful or dehumanizing than before. Personal fortitude had always been necessary for success in medical school, which, like the military, involved a hierarchical system based in part on submission to higher authority (however much students were encouraged to develop independence and critical power). The extreme time demands of medical study, the exploitation of students as cheap labor, the use of fear as a means of motivation by house officers and faculty, and the lack of interest of some faculty in the educational and emotional needs of students had occurred at most medical schools all century long. No one knew whether the problem had grown more severe or whether in a consumer era perceptions and outrage had merely been intensified. Moreover, studies of medical student abuse relied on data from student questionnaires. Any reported verbal slight, however unintended or inconsequential, was included as an instance of abuse. This led some to wonder whether the "new" medical students were overly sensitive, perhaps too wrapped up in the era's glorification of the self, or whether the investigators were too cavalier in their use of the emotionally charged term "abuse."

Nevertheless, it could not be denied that medical education was stressful and at times dehumanizing. The long-term effects of this aspect of medical education were unknown. This issue troubled many educators, who had long been aware of the power of the "hidden curriculum" to shape attitudes and behavior. Were medical students permanently scarred from the ordeal, or did compassionate qualities reemerge after the stresses of medical education had ended? Did students who survived the ordeal feel that society now owed them something in return? Many educators asked, as one did, "How can students learn to care for patients as individuals if no one is caring about them as individuals?"[41] However, the sociological data to answer these questions were not available.

One problem that now caused little anxiety among students was the fear of flunking out. Since World War I attrition rates had been steadily falling, but by the 1970s academic dismissal had become rare. In part this reflected the high quality of the applicants; in part, the extensive efforts faculties now took to assist borderline students to remain in school. Moreover, students did not worry about finding work as physicians. In these respects, medical schools differed markedly from other professional and graduate schools, where attrition rates remained high and where even talented graduates had no assurance of finding a job in their chosen field.

On the other hand, a new anxiety arose among medical students: obtaining a residency. Competition for leading university programs in the popular specialty fields had always been intense. However, in the 1970s and 1980s the number of residency positions leveled off, while the number of U.S. and foreign medical graduates seeking positions increased. In the mid-1970s, the ratio of total residency positions to U.S. medical graduates was 2 to 1; a decade later that ratio had fallen to 1.3 to 1. The decline in the availability of positions was not uniform among the clinical fields. Some of the most popular specialties, particularly in the surgical areas, limited the number of positions they offered. In several fields, such as orthopedic surgery, neurosurgery, radiology, and ophthalmology, the number of applicants exceeded the number of positions.

The result of this new competitive environment was a mania among students seeking residencies in certain fields and a disruption of the fourth year of medical school that was termed the "preresidency syndrome." Residency program directors would engender fear among students by announcing that only applicants who had taken electives at the director's institution would be considered. Accordingly, senior students interested in those fields would spend much of the fourth year in a series of "audition electives," exhibiting themselves at various hospitals where they were applying for a position. Instead of concentrating on completing their general professional education, they would travel from hospital to hospital, taking the same elective at each one.[42]

One could understand this behavior of program directors, for it was in their interest to recruit and select the best house officers. Performance in clinical clerkships had long been the best predictor of performance during internship and residency, and deans' letters and faculty recommendations had lost much of their credibility because of their custom of describing almost all candidates in a chorus of superlatives.[43] On the other hand, as residency program directors looked out for their own programs, the preresidency syndrome was intensified, to the detriment of the educational quality of the fourth year. No one considered this situation healthy for medical study, though opinion varied as to how to address it. Many believed that the fourth year should be "recaptured." Some, however, argued that the fourth year should be eliminated, becoming instead the first year of residency.

🍎 · 🍎 · 🍎

After the passage of Medicare and Medicaid, medical faculties continued to wrestle with the many pedagogic issues of medical education—a task more difficult now because of the molecular revolution. In addition, faculties continued to engage in regular curricular reform. The most conspicuous trends were the reduction in the amount of time devoted to the basic sciences and the earlier presentation of clinical teaching.[44] In addition, a number of major curricular experiments were undertaken. Notable departures of this era included the development of a program with a strong emphasis on the humanities at the Pennsylvania State University (Hershey) College of Medicine, the creation of a primary care curriculum at the University of New Mexico School of Medicine, and the establishment of the "New Pathway" program at Harvard Medical School, which featured the division of students into several 40-member societies, each with its own facilities and core faculty, in an effort to replace lectures with tutorial instruction and enhance personal interactions between students and faculty.[45]

No school ever felt that it had achieved an ideal curriculum, and a successful experiment at one school was not necessarily easily exported to another, owing to differing missions, resources, and local traditions. The objective of Harvard's New Pathway curriculum, wrote Daniel C. Toste-son, dean of the medical school and the prime mover behind the development of the program, was not to establish it as a universal model but to encourage other medical schools "to seek their own new pathways in general medical education."[46] In curriculum reform, schools as institutions continued to learn about medical education, in much the same way that doctors as individuals were always learning about medicine. Truth and renewal lay in the ongoing search for the ideal curriculum, not in any momentary product.

Schools undertook experiments not only in the organization and presentation of material but in the use of new teaching and evaluative techniques. For instance, many schools began employing standardized patients (nonphysicians trained to play the role of a patient) in clinical teaching and evaluation.[47] A number of schools adopted "problem-based learning" as an instructional method in the basic science courses. This technique, developed by medical educators at McMaster University in the late 1960s, involved the use of patient problems as a means of introducing basic science concepts. Clinical cases would be presented, and students would learn the pertinent scientific facts and principles to solve the clinical problems.[48] Medical education also entered the computer age, as a variety of new educational tools and devices came into use: computer-assisted literature searches, computer-based interactive learning modalities, computer-generated graphics, and computer-based testing. In some areas, computer technology arrived just in time, as in anatomy, where computer modalities could provide three-dimensional images of parts of the body, just as cadavers and trained instructors of gross anatomy were running short. Particularly in the 1980s and 1990s, medical libraries evolved into information centers, and medical informatics emerged as an important discipline.[49]

Could caring and compassion be taught? It was plausible to assume that formal instruction could help. A number of important concepts from the social sciences were central to understanding the whole patient: the important distinction between disease and illness, the notion of the social construction of clinical reality, and the concept of suffering and its relation to organic illness.[50] Communication skills could be improved with coaching and feedback, particularly in encounters with patients from socioeconomic backgrounds different from those of the interviewing physician.[51] Tools of the behavioral sciences could be used to improve patient compliance with medical prescriptions—for instance, by teaching students to prescribe a drug once a day when possible, rather than several times a day. Most important, empathy involved the ability to understand things from another person's point of view. That provided a cogent argument for courses in college or medical school in the social sciences and humanities, whose fundamental intellectual skills involved the displacement of the self into another perspective: history, into an earlier time; sociology, into another group identity; anthropology, into different cultures; literature, into another's imagination. For this reason, medical schools since World War II had incorporated one or another of these fields into the curriculum: the behavioral sciences and medical history in the 1950s and 1960s, and the medical humanities (including literature, art, and music) and bioethics in the 1970s, 1980s, and 1990s.

On the other hand, empirical evidence that instruction in the medical humanities produced caring doctors was lacking. After 1970, public charges that doctors were impersonal, self-serving, greedy, and dishonest increased despite greater amounts of teaching in the medical humanities. (In a similar fashion, there was no evidence that the introduction of ethics courses in business schools in the 1980s and 1990s produced more ethical behavior among business executives.) Indeed, there was some empirical data that biology majors as a group were more caring, sensitive, and humanitarian than students who had majored in the humanities in college.[52] One writer criticized medical educators—and educators in general—for their conceit that formal course work could serve as "intellectual magic bullets" to shape human attitudes and behavior.[53] Another writer discussed the ecology of medical students—who they were and the cultural and environmental forces acting upon them. "To increase the number of humanistic physicians, the best strategy may be to alter medical school recruitment and selection policies."[54] The rationale for formal instruction in the medical humanities remained cogent—as long as medical educators did not mistakenly conclude that such an approach obviated the need to admit caring individuals to the student body and provide them empathetic role models.

Could the efforts to produce caring physicians be overdone? Literally, of course, the answer was no, since that was one of the prime qualities of good physicianship. However, some educators began to worry that the growing emphasis on the art of medicine, together with early and more extensive clinical instruction, was coming at the sacrifice of providing a sufficient understanding of medical science. One such individual was Walsh McDermott, an internist and infectious diseases authority at Cornell, who repeatedly pointed out that medicine involves science just as much as compassion. "If I were terribly ill it would be all right to get me a physician who knew all about the 'whole man,' but I wished to be damn sure he 'knew about my parts.'"[55] McDermott, like some others, decried the steady reduction in teaching time allotted to the basic sciences at a time of unprecedented growth in the scientific foundation of medical practice. It was easy, in his view, to train individuals "to behave like physicians to handle the run-of-the-mill medical problems of the here and now," and he cited the success of the physician assistant movement as proof of that point. However, the distinguishing quality of properly educated physicians was the "capability to absorb the new developments in medicine as they occur during the four decades or so of their professional lives," and this was made possible only by sufficient "science-based clinical training."[56] To McDermott, the deemphasis of the basic sciences smacked of anti-intellectualism and vocationalism.

What made McDermott's concerns so significant was his stature as a humanitarian. He was a towering figure in internal medicine (he coedited one of the important textbooks in the field) and clinical investigation (he was a member of the National Academy of Sciences and recipient of the Lasker Award for his work on developing effective drug regimens for the treatment of tuberculosis). However, he was equally renowned for his socially responsible approach to medicine, as manifested by his many contributions to public health, his description and defense of what he termed "Samaritanism" in medicine, his passionate efforts to redress inequities in the financing and delivery of medical care, his instrumental part in the organization of the Institute of Medicine, and his seminal role as adviser and confidant to senior officers of the Robert Wood Johnson Foundation.[57] McDermott was hardly an academic hawk or scientific reactionary.

Perhaps the thorniest problem of all in curricular development was evaluating the success of a new teaching method or curricular change. No one was able to document scientifically the advantage of one approach over another—however strong the theoretical rationale for a change or the subjective impressions that a change was making a difference. The variables were simply too many. Arthur Kaufman, an eminent medical educator who had spearheaded New Mexico's innovative primary care curriculum, addressed this point while speaking of the difficulties of evaluating problem-based learning:

> Can we show that graduates of problem-based learning programs are 'better'? While I think almost all students who go through such a program have received a broader, more relevant education than had they gone the traditional route, I suspect that this assertion is virtually impossible to prove. We do not have the instruments to test the hypothesis, and the students are far too complex and unpredictable to ascribe results to any particular variables.
>
> It is difficult to know which results are attributable to personality, which to prior experience, which to extracurricular influences, and which to problem-based learning itself.[58]

On the other hand, throughout the history of American education it had been virtually impossible to judge satisfactorily the success of any major intervention, whether it be the establishment of early childhood enrichment programs, the reduction of class size to small student-teacher ratios, or the creation of separate junior high schools for adolescents.[59] In the dilemma of evaluation, medical educators were not alone.

Who controlled the medical curriculum? In theory, it was the medical schools, each of which established its own course of instruction and criteria for evaluation. In practice, many felt that it was the National Board of

Medical Examiners, since students had to pass all three parts of the board examination for a license. Critics contended that this forced schools to teach to the boards and stifled the ability of schools to innovate and experiment. Indeed, in the early 1990s, at least 73 schools had made passage of Part I of the examination (and at least 53 schools, Part II) a condition for graduation. Representatives of the board denied any coercive intention or effect on the undergraduate curriculum, and they reiterated that responsibility for determining the course of study and criteria for graduation remained solely the province of the schools. Through the late 1990s the debate continued.[60]

As always, considerable diversity continued to exist among medical schools—in terms of their specific educational missions and objectives, their curriculum, and their methods of teaching and evaluation. "If you have seen one medical school, you have seen one medical school," medical educators were fond of saying, referring to the conspicuous differences among the research-intensive schools, the typical state medical schools, the small independent private medical colleges, and the new community-based medical schools, not to mention the fact that each school had its own personality and traditions. On the other hand, schools remained in agreement, as they had all century long, on broad educational goals. Faculties everywhere reiterated the importance of mastering principles, acquiring a genuine understanding of biological phenomena, and cultivating the habits of critical thought and independent learning. After 1970, this educational philosophy seemed more valid than ever. Not only was a profound molecular revolution underway in biological science, but the diseases afflicting the population were changing as well. Many classic diseases declined in epidemiological importance, while new diseases appeared—most conspicuously the acquired immunodeficiency syndrome (AIDS).[61] The problems of the future were unpredictable, and doctors needed to be intellectually prepared to handle any or all contingencies. The commitment to producing doctors who could think critically, absorb new knowledge, and learn independently was shared by medical schools of diverse missions and educational styles.

❦ · ❦ · ❦

Ironically, for all the talk of making medical education an invigorating intellectual experience, that objective was seldom achieved. Almost everywhere, the curriculum suffered from rigidity, overcrowding, too many lectures, and an excessive emphasis on rote memorization. From 1982 to 1993, nine official reports from foundations, educational bodies, and professional task forces criticized medical education for these defects (as had ten earlier reports from 1910 to 1972, beginning with the Flexner report).[62] A century of curriculum reform had shifted hours of instruction here and modes of instruction there, but schools had yet to introduce a true student-centered educational program that made active, self-directed learning the core of the experience. "There's an enormous gap between talking about educational changes and accomplishing them,"[63] one dean remarked. Sociologist Samuel Bloom referred to this history of endless curricular tinkering without realizing the larger educational objectives of medical education as "reform without change."[64]

The greatest deviation from the ideals of medical education occurred in the basic science teaching. Not only did instruction in these subjects continue to be characterized by an intense schedule of lectures and factual overload, but in the 1970s and 1980s the amount of laboratory instruction was greatly reduced (and at some schools in some subjects, eliminated).[65] With such an approach, the emphasis was on identifying and memorizing the "bottom lines." How these "bottom lines" may have been reached, their significance, their interrelationships, and their use in problem-solving were rarely emphasized. The educational result was closer to a correspondence school format than to a graduate mentality, where scholarship and understanding were encouraged. Students themselves tacitly acknowledged the deficiencies of the lecture-memorization format by frequently skipping classes and studying on their own. At a number of schools this process was formalized by the organization of student note-taking cooperatives that produced written versions of the faculty lectures for the entire class, thereby making it an easy matter for anyone other than the designated note-takers to be absent.[66]

In the clinical subjects the rhetoric of medical education also exceeded the reality. Here the problem was not an excess of lectures, for the clinical clerkship allowed ample opportunity for students to learn by doing. Rather, the problem was a dearth of faculty teachers and role models, which left students to fend for themselves in an unstructured, sometimes poorly supervised environment. The primary teachers of students were now the house officers, themselves burdened with their own learning needs and heavy responsibilities for patient care. The role of house officers became similar to that of graduate teaching assistants in arts and sciences faculties, who regularly assumed major responsibilities for undergraduate instruction. However, house officers, unlike graduate students, received little guidance in their teaching. Dialogues with clinical faculty about the content, organization, objectives, methods, and tools of evaluation rarely occurred. Moreover, students and house officers both needed exposure to experienced, mature physicians in the actual work of caring for patients. Such exposure had previously served as an important vehicle for teaching bedside medicine and instilling high professional standards to all who were learning medicine.

The century-long history of reform without change resulted mainly from the fact that medical schools had evolved in a faculty-centered, not a student-centered, manner. In the basic science subjects, the domination of lectures and deemphasis of laboratories and individualized instruction represented a much more efficient use of faculty time. In the clinical subjects, the use of house officers as teaching assistants served a similar purpose. These devices freed faculty to pursue their other interests, such as graduate instruction, patient care, and research. One study in 1982 estimated that 60 percent of full-time faculty spent less than five hours a week in undergraduate teaching.[67] Students, as learners, needed a large amount of time and personal contact with their instructors. However, in a medical school environment driven primarily by the needs of faculty, students often did not receive enough of those opportunities.

In the 1970s and 1980s, the primary distraction of faculty from teaching, as it had been all century long, was research. In the faculty-driven value system of the medical school, as throughout the multiversity, teaching was subordinate to research. Appointments, promotions, pay raises, greater office and laboratory space, and an assortment of other rewards and honors were determined primarily by success at publication and winning research grants—however much lip service might have been paid to the importance of teaching. Faculty with heavy teaching and clinical loads found it much more difficult to get promoted, even if their teaching was superb. "Our system is geared to rewards, and if salary and promotion are based solely on research, that's what people will do,"[68] a faculty member at one school observed.

The incentives (some would say pressures) to concentrate on research were enormous, especially for junior faculty trying to develop their careers. This situation was acknowledged by a former student council president at the University of Maryland School of Medicine who had joined the school's faculty after completing his training. As a student, he and classmates had "antagonistically" expressed their unhappiness that the faculty seemed uninterested in their education and well-being. Now that he had been appointed to the faculty, he could "understand the tremendous pressures and time constraints" that militated against teaching, particularly the pressures of research and publishing.[69]

Some teachers, of course, were promoted, but their rewards usually came more slowly. Faculty on the new "clinician-teacher" tracks, for instance, encountered longer waits and more obstacles in the promotion process than those on conventional academic tracks.[70] Teachers were sometimes promoted for providing necessary but unglamorous services, such as heading the physical examination course or serving as this or that assistant dean. At Michigan, for instance, promotions for teaching and administrative service were common, but those positions were considered "not attractive enough to recruit individuals with better scholarly records."[71] In general, only the scholarship of discovery, and not the scholarship of teaching, integration, and application, was considered the appropriate standard for faculty advancement. This was true throughout the research university, not just at the medical school.[72]

The tension between teaching and research, as readers of this book will recognize, was long-standing at medical schools. However, in the 1970s and 1980s the tension became more severe. In part this resulted from economic factors: the now-entrenched financial incentives to do research in a grants economy in which research awards provided salaries for the investigators and staff as well as overhead monies (indirect costs) for the medical school. In part this resulted from intellectual factors: the growing "bench-bedside gap" during the molecular era. Indeed, among many faculty, enthusiasm for teaching was not so much lost as it was displaced upward to advanced students like Ph.D. candidates and postdoctoral clinical and research fellows who could better understand the subtleties of the instructor's work. An illustration of this phenomenon was a comment made to this writer by a respected cardiologist: "The best part of my day is the time I spend with my fellows."

Many medical school leaders argued that the difficulty in defining and measuring good teaching was what resulted in its subordination to research. In their view research was more objective and amenable to measurement. Certainly, the difficulties of evaluating teaching, as any other educational activity, were real. Student and peer evaluations, though useful, were both subjective and imprecise. Objective "measures" of a teacher's performance were yet to be developed.

However, it was not clear that objective measures of research existed either. As an illustration, some medical schools abandoned efforts to determine the quality of an investigator's work. Instead, they made decisions about promotion strictly on the basis of the number of publications. At Jefferson, for instance, promotion to associate professor in the early 1980s required eight papers in peer-reviewed journals for basic science faculty and six for clinical faculty.[73] Not surprisingly, the century-long devaluation of the academic currency—the published paper—continued, as illustrated by an accentuation of the trends toward multiauthorship and publication of the smallest publishable unit. New evidence in the 1990s confirmed what was long known: that a majority of published papers made negligible contributions to knowledge. From 1981 to 1985, 80 percent of published scientific papers were never cited more than once, including by their own authors.[74] (Self-citation was estimated to account for 5 to 20 percent of all citations.) Of one especially prominent figure in academic medicine, who shall remain anonymous, it was widely said: "Dr. 'X' has never had an unpublished thought." Such a rush to publish, though understandable in view of the reward system, ran contrary to the values of creators of the research system such as Abraham Flexner, who, as noted earlier, had adopted the motto: "Work much; publish little." The emphasis on maximizing the quantity of publications hardly suggested that research "quality" was always as objective and easily measured as some suggested.

Since the end of World War II the education of medical students had increasingly become a by-product of the academic health center, if measured in relation to the many other duties of graduate teaching, research, and patient care that medical faculties had assumed. This in itself was not harmful for medical education, provided that faculties took students and student teaching seriously. However, at medical schools everywhere, instructors demonstrated by their actions and inactions that student teaching was a low priority to them. Medical school records from prestigious and nonprestigious schools alike demonstrated a widespread lack of concern for student matters: the difficulty in recruiting faculty to serve on admissions committees or to help with interviews, repeated complaints from students that they were neglected, reports of the inavailability of faculty advisers, the behavior of faculty who resented their lecture duties (for instance, delivering their lectures without introducing themselves to the class), the refusal of departmental chairpersons to sit on curriculum committees, the conversion of student teaching laboratories into faculty research laboratories, the unwillingness of some faculty to write letters of recommendation for students, and poor faculty turnouts at commencement exercises.

Repeatedly there were reports that faculty did not know their students well. At one school, a student was granted his request to have his grade changed because the faculty preceptor had confused him with another student in the tutorial group.[75] Discouragingly few faculty, particularly in positions of power and influence, seemed to care about students. Even the medical students' best friend—the Association of American Medical Colleges—abandoned its learner-centered outlook for a faculty-centered outlook. For decades the organization had defined its purpose as "the advance of medical education and the nation's health." In 1988 it redefined its mission as "the advancement of academic medicine and the nation's health."[76] The following year the organization's publication, the *Journal of Medical Education*, was renamed *Academic Medicine*.

Of course, in a heterogeneous system of medical schools that drew strength from its diversity, not all schools pursued research with the same intensity or success. Nevertheless, even at schools with modest academic reputations, research values predominated. For instance, at Jefferson, traditionally known for its educational and clinical excellence, junior faculty perceived that "the key to promotion is publications and the ability to bring in research money."[77] Even many of the new community-based medical schools, which often had explicit missions to innovate in medical education, rapidly became traditional in their internal value system. One report estimated that of the 38 new medical schools established in the 1960s and 1970s, "only about five have been able to preserve anything like their original vision of [educational] innovation," owing to the departure of charismatic founding deans and the hiring of traditionally trained faculty.[78] A prime example was the State University of New York at Stony Brook, which at the start had an innovative curriculum designed to provide early patient contact and to accommodate the individual needs of students. After the departure of the school's founding dean, Edmund D. Pellegrino, the experimental curriculum was abandoned for a traditional one, and the school began boasting of its success in conventional academic pursuits such as obtaining external research support, hiring full-time investigators, expanding faculty laboratory facilities, and securing a large number of research training grants.[79]

In short, the primary obstacle to establishing a true student-centered curriculum was the deeply ingrained subordination of teaching to research throughout academic medicine. Accordingly, the medical student experience remained deeply resistant to change, even as numerous curricular reforms at one school after another came and went. It was not credible for schools to make a fanfare of a new curriculum, as they regularly did, when the faculty did not know students well, refused to serve on student-related committees, and would not deign to attend commencement ceremonies. True educational reform—reform with change, to borrow Bloom's terminology—could be possible only with a fundamental restructuring and reorganization of the medical school so that education would be valued and teaching would be respected and rewarded.[80]

For all the official and unofficial calls to reform medical education, it is important to note that the criticisms focused mainly on the educational system, not on the products of the system. In no other country were criticisms of medical education so many but the products of the system considered so good. Many presumed that American medical education could and should be more invigorating, exciting, and humane. Nevertheless, even the sharpest critics of the present faculty-centered system could not fail to be impressed with the quality of American medical education and American doctors.

In part this success reflected the efforts of the many faculty who did teach, out of dedication or passion. Many faculty of this era knew what medical teachers had known throughout history: the immense personal and intellectual rewards of discussing scientific ideas or patient problems with inquisitive students, the joy of observing and contributing to the maturation of good physicians, and the satisfaction of working in an environment where learning was the essential ingredient. Though teaching was seldom rewarded by the system, good teaching could still be found—even if present by chance rather than by design. As in other branches of the multiversity, where research was also rewarded much more readily than teaching, innumerable conscientious and gifted instructors continued to provide good teaching year in and year out. Moreover, with medical faculties now so large, it did not take a high percentage of instructors to provide a nucleus of teachers. In this regard the most lasting contribution of Harvard's New Pathway experiment may prove to be the establishment of its societies of students and core faculty, which essentially represented the creation of small medical schools within the school.

In part the quality of American doctors also reflected the quality of the students, who were bright, motivated, and capable of making good use of the learning environment. Good teachers and good teaching were important, but ultimately the responsibility for learning lay with the learner. As Abraham Flexner once stated, "Though medicine can be learned, it cannot be taught."[81] Faculties could guide and inspire, but ultimately there was no substitute for the learner's initiative. Even at medical schools with the stingiest rewards for teaching, students could find helpful lectures, diverse elective opportunities, an invigorating intellectual atmosphere, exposure to the methods and spirit of scientific inquiry, an abundant population of patients, ample time to study the patients in depth, and some teachers who cared—in short, a rich environment for self-learning, the obstacles of a dry, bloated curriculum notwithstanding. Since the nineteenth century the tenets of progressive medical education had held that all learning ultimately was self-learning. In light of the curriculum's many ongoing deficiencies, American medical students demonstrated the validity of that viewpoint. "Self-learning" did not justify the status quo in medical education, nor did it render unnecessary any efforts to make teaching better—but it did explain why students somehow usually came out better than many critics of the system would have predicted.

The Dilemmas of Graduate Medical Education

After 1970, as medical and social fashions changed, various medical specialties continued to rise or fall in favor as career choices among medical students. Obstetrics and gynecology, once perceived as a happy field, lost popularity as it became troubled by such factors as a severe liability crisis, the feminization of poverty, and a number of perplexing ethical issues.[82] Conversely, radiology, once an afterthought among students, became one of the most competitive fields, as new technological breakthroughs elevated the field to a much higher level of scientific sophistication. Internal medicine, traditionally the most sought-after specialty, went through nearly a full cycle. On internship "match day" in 1987, many of the most prestigious programs failed to fill their positions. (That day came to be known as "Black Tuesday" in internal medicine circles.) Presumed reasons for the decline in popularity of internal medicine included a widespread feeling that the practice of internal medicine was no longer satisfying, unfavorable experience with internal medicine during medical school, and a common misperception that internal medicine consisted of the care of only very old or very ill persons. Yet in the mid-1990s, after nearly a decade of being out of favor, internal medicine began to enjoy a resurgence of popularity, especially among the top-ranking students.[83]

Though particular specialties would wax or wane in popularity, one area was consistently undersubscribed: primary care. In the 1960s, a new field, family medicine, had been created to elevate primary care to the status of a specialty. Despite much fanfare, by 1989 only 13.7 percent of students were choosing the field. Two consulting specialties, general internal medicine and general pediatrics, were redefined as primary care fields. Yet by the 1990s, relatively few physicians were entering those fields either. (Most internal medicine and a sizeable minority of pediatric residents followed their residency with subspecialty fellowships, such as adult rheumatology or pediatric cardiology.) In 1989, only 23.6 percent of students chose careers in any of the three primary care disciplines.[84] Instead, students were going into the specialties, which were continuing to proliferate. Between 1974 and 1992, 28 new specialties and subspecialties were recognized by the Accreditation Council for Graduate Medical Education, including fields like emergency medicine and critical care medicine.[85]

The declining interest among American medical school graduates in primary care caused considerable concern. It was widely noted that primary care or generalist physicians could satisfactorily manage the majority of medical matters in everyday practice and that they practiced less expensively than specialists—both by receiving lower fees and by using fewer resources than specialists to diagnose and treat the same problems.[86] Many looked admiringly at other major English-speaking countries, such as Canada, Great Britain, Australia, and New Zealand, where family physicians provided most of the medical care, yet patients seemed satisfied and the country's health bills were lower. Of note, it was not patients or the general public that was complaining about the specialty mix of U.S. physicians. Rather it was those who paid the bills—employers and government—along with many health care policy analysts. As medical inflation continued its inexorable growth, primary care physicians became important to third party payers and policy makers as a proxy for lower national health care costs.

What distribution between generalists and specialists would best serve the needs of the public? Though heated assertions flew far and wide, no one knew the answer. Toward the end of the 1970s a consensus emerged among medical educators and policy analysts—one that has lasted until the present—that the country should have a 50-50 mix. However, no data could be found to document that recommendation. "Why not 40 or 60 or 70 or 51 percent?" the Association of American Medical Colleges (AAMC) asked in protest. The basic problem, as the AAMC pointed out, was that the conventional wisdom that medical education should produce 50 percent generalists was based on "arbitrary and capricious slogans" rather than rigorously derived data. The only thing to commend it was that the recommendation "does not in any egregiously obvious way offend common sense."[87]

Several problems plagued discussions of the proper distribution of physicians across the specialties. Recommendations about specialty mix rarely took into account changes in the epidemiology and treatment of disease. In the early 1970s some were predicting a need for far fewer specialists in infectious diseases—until a few years later, when lyme disease, Legionnaires' disease, an epidemic of multi-drug resistant tuberculosis, and the acquired immunodeficiency syndrome (AIDS) appeared. Recommendations about specialty mix, again reflecting the here and now, generally overlooked the aging of the population and the resultant need for more specialists in areas like geriatrics, oncology, neurology, orthopedic surgery, and rehabilitative medicine. Most recommendations about specialty mix (and the geographic distribution of physicians as well) ignored the potential of the telecommunications revolution to alter medical practice and expand the reach of physicians.[88] Lastly, "workforce" recommendations seldom took into account the fact that specialists could be shown to take better care of patients with complicated but common problems (as opposed to the rare diseases incorrectly thought by many to be the mainstay of most specialists' work). For instance, one study found cardiologists more knowledgeable about important advances in the management of heart attack than general internists, and general internists more knowledgeable than family practitioners.[89]

Though the optimal percentage of generalists and specialists was difficult to determine, there was little doubt that graduate medical education was producing more specialists than the country needed. Perhaps the best evidence for this was the inability of specialists to keep busy practicing their specialty. The subspecialties of internal medicine provided a classic example. Studies showed that nearly three-quarters of internal medicine subspecialists (for instance, endocrinologists and cardiologists) spent more than half their time delivering primary care and that another 15 percent spent 20 to 50 percent of their time in primary care.[90] Nationwide, specialists provided continuing general medical care to one in five Americans.[91] David E. Rogers and Linda H. Aiken called this America's "hidden system" of primary care.[92]

The imbalance between generalists and specialists resulted in part from the traditional streak of individualism in American medical education. Medical education, as the nation as a whole, tended to place greater emphasis on the rights of the individual than on the individual's responsibility to society. Accordingly, students selected fields based on their interests and ambitions, not on the basis of society's needs. Similarly, residency and fellowship programs expanded their sizes to fulfill their own service and academic agendas, with scant concern for the number of specialists currently in the field. (Only surgery and the surgical subspecialties voluntarily limited the number of positions.) If programs could not attract U.S. medical graduates to fill their positions, they actively recruited foreign medical graduates (FMGs) instead.[93] The aggregate consequence of these individual choices was a specialty mix that most analysts felt was not consistent with the public good.

In the United States, unlike most other countries, the number of specialty training positions was not controlled by external authorities. In the absence of such regulation, many had hoped that market forces would bring about a proper distribution of specialties. However, at least prior to the 1990s, that did not happen, mainly because there was no effective feedback loop regulating graduate medical education. That is, the needs of society for more or fewer physicians in a given field had no modulating effect on the number of residency positions in the specialty or on the choices of students regarding which field to pursue. Physicians could always find practice opportunities in their particular specialty, regardless of the number of others already in the field. The result was the perpetuation of the imbalance between the presumed national need for more generalists and the desire of most students to become specialists.

There was much medical schools could do, if they chose, to redress the balance between generalists and specialists. The difficulties medical students experienced in choosing a specialty were well known. Eighty percent of students changed their specialty preferences during medical school.[94] On questionnaires, students reported that the greatest difficulty they encountered in making choices about specialties was the lack of information about the fields.[95] The most common reason for selecting a specialty was the intellectual content of the field.[96] In these regards primary care was at a decided disadvantage, for few medical schools gave it much attention. Most clinical education occurred in tertiary care centers, where patients tended to be extremely ill and where teaching was provided mainly by specialists. Outpatient work, the mainstay of primary care, received scant curricular time and was often poorly taught. Faculty frequently spoke disparagingly of primary care, and at many schools few inspiring generalist role models existed. Recruitment to primary care could only be aided if schools took the effort to improve the amount and quality of teaching in the field.

On the other hand, many studies of career choice, in the tradition of Daniel H. Funkenstein's earlier work, demonstrated that the primary determinants lay outside the medical school. Medical students had minds of their own and values and aspirations shaped by outside experiences. They entered medical school either with or without predilections toward primary care based on a number of personal variables and on the general social climate of the time. Experiences in medical school influenced students in the selection of one specialty over another, but only rarely in the larger decision they had to make of whether to enter a specialty or primary care field in the first place. Studies of the impact of curricular innovations on decisions to enter primary care (for instance, providing preceptorships with family physicians or greater exposure to ambulatory care) indicated that "the curriculum can help maintain primary care interests of students who were admitted having these interests but that new decisions for primary care specialties as a result of special curricular offerings have, for the most part, failed."[97] A number of the community-based medical schools had better track records than most traditional medical schools in producing primary care practitioners, but studies of this phenomenon could not disprove the hypothesis that students with primary care orientations self-selected the schools that were known for emphasizing primary care.[98] The authors of a major review of the literature on career choice among medical students concluded that "admissions decisions are more important than educational programs if the goal is to graduate primary care physicians."[99]

Decisions of students to specialize were also reinforced by the rewards of society: greater prestige and income.[100] It became popular in health policy discussions in the 1980s to call primary care physicians "gatekeep-ers"—which conjured up images of a triage officer rather than a doctor. This was hardly an attractive image to the achievement-oriented individ-uals who chose to enter medicine, since nurses and physician assistants could do the same thing.[101] Reimbursement policies of all federal and private insurers paid much more for the services of specialists than gen-eralists, even when taking care of the same patients.[102] In addition, some specialties required less time on the job and offered more regular hours—a matter of no small concern to many students seeking more time for their personal lives.

In short, though they could help, medical schools by themselves could not increase the interest of students in primary care. In the absence of external controls on the number of specialists, and given that virtually all specialists could find practice opportunities in their field, the production of more generalists depended on the cooperation of medical education and society. If larger numbers of students were to choose careers in pri-mary care, the prevailing cultural attitudes had to be more appreciative of primary care. As always, the kind and quality of doctors produced reflected not medical education alone but also the type of society Amer-ica was as a nation.

❦ · ❦ · ❦

After 1970, graduate medical education became an industry. House staff costs represented nearly one-half of 1 percent of the country's total health care expenditures, reaching $2 billion by 1986. The major source of sup-port for residency and fellowship programs came from patient care rev-enues to hospitals. This reflected the recognition of Medicare, Medicaid, and private insurers that graduate medical education and patient care were fundamentally linked. Other sources included state, local, and Vet-erans Administration appropriations and, for clinical fellows, faculty practice income, federal training grants, and endowment income. By the mid-1970s, house staff salaries represented 3 to 4 percent of the budget of a typical teaching hospital, a proportion that remained constant for the next two decades.[103] This allowed house officers to receive salaries close to the median income level for their geographic region. (Salaries were a bit lower for interns, a bit higher for residents with several years of expe-rience.) In 1989, for instance, the average salary of an intern was $22,433 in the South and $26,287 in the Northeast.[104]

Who controlled graduate medical education? Certainly not the univer-sities. From the 1960s onward, a variety of foundations and special com-missions issued periodic calls for medical schools to assume greater responsibility for graduate medical education. By then it was too late. Medical schools in the 1920s and 1930s had made the decision not to assume such responsibility. Now the universities found that they could not regain much influence on the field, even if they wished to do so.

Graduate medical education after 1970 remained hospital-based rather than university-based, and only a minority of residency programs were located at major university teaching hospitals. The university could exert some influence on its own teaching hospital, but not on training programs at the many hospitals with only a limited university affiliation or no affiliation at all.

Compounding the university's lack of influence on graduate medical education was the complicated system of administering residency and fellowship training. Even at major teaching hospitals, the university's influence was limited. The traditional impetus for the size and nature of residency training programs came from the clinical service chiefs. Disproportionately large amounts of resources went to the "strong" chairpersons who could triumph in hospital turf battles, even if other training programs at the hospital were left at a decided disadvantage. Hospital administrators controlled the patient care revenues that paid for graduate medical education. Accordingly, they, too, exercised considerable control over the number of trainees a residency program could accept and over the quality of the training programs themselves. Further diluting the university's influence was the complicated system of control of graduate medical education. A plethora of national residency review committees (one for each specialty) controlled the duration and content of training programs and were vested with the power to approve individual programs. Autonomous specialty and subspecialty boards, empowered to certify individual physicians as specialists in a particular area of practice, exercised an indirect but not insignificant degree of control over the programs that trained physicians in their specialty. Governmental and private insurance carriers played a role by virtue of their increasing tendency to specify which services performed by residents and fellows would qualify for reimbursement. Responsibility for graduate medical education was thus highly fragmented, and the influence of the university in all of this was small.

After 1970, the experience of being a house officer reflected a continuation or accentuation of trends that had been developing since World War II. One was the vanishing academic emphasis. Research virtually disappeared from the residency experience, even at the university programs, particularly in the nonsurgical fields. Instead, clinical learning became the exclusive focus. A research component was still present in some surgical residencies and in fellowship training, but this was generally insufficient to prepare mature, independent clinical investigators during the molecular era. One prominent investigator spoke of the research component of clinical fellowships as "scientific dilettantism."[105] Aspiring physician-scientists who needed the heavy dose of basic science training necessary to conduct contemporary clinical research had to acquire that experience elsewhere.

Second, the sense house officers once had of belonging to a metaphorical family for all practical purposes ended. In part this was because the number of residents and clinical fellows grew too large, especially at the large teaching hospitals. In 1979, for instance, the Columbia-Presbyterian Medical Center had 300 residents and 400 clinical fellows.[106] The decline of community also resulted from the disappearance of faculty from the wards. Faculty were around for morning rounds, and they were usually promptly available when needed for help. However, after rounds they were off, with full schedules of private patients to see in the faculty offices or an important experiment to conduct in the laboratory. Most professors had little time to get to know house officers on a personal level or to serve as bedside role models. Accordingly, few house officers spoke any longer of heroes in the profession or described their training in terms of the individuals under whom they worked. Even fewer spoke of any spiritual uplift they might have derived from the experience of being a member of the resident staff.

Third, graduate education (and undergraduate as well) remained primarily an inpatient experience, despite the fact that technological developments were allowing many more conditions to be managed effectively on an outpatient basis. With the exception of family practice and some pediatric programs, outpatient education was rarely emphasized, in part because the financing of graduate medical education was linked to inpatient care, and in part because of the traditional disdain of medical faculty toward outpatient instruction. Additional diversity in medical education was provided by increasing the use of carefully chosen community hospitals to provide greater exposure to primary and secondary care (especially in pediatrics and obstetrics) and municipal and veterans hospitals to allow additional contact with ward patients at a time when the ward census of most major teaching hospitals was decreasing.

Lastly, on the wards, the pace of house staff life grew ever more frenetic, as patients became sicker, technologies more sophisticated, and nights on call busier. This was illustrated by the remarkable expansion of intensive care units. By the 1970s, medical, surgical, coronary, respiratory, and neonatal intensive care units, among others, accounted for a significant part of the work at every teaching hospital. Time was not a luxury in the intensive care unit since clinically unstable patients could decompensate at any moment. Mastery was required of a host of sophisticated technologies: arterial lines, Swan-Ganz catheters, Holter monitors, mechanical ventilators, dialysis machines, electrical cardioverters, pacemakers, new classes of antibiotics, and intravenous pharmacologic agents to raise or drop a person's blood pressure in seconds. Elsewhere in the hospital the pace was also hectic. Organ transplantation was becoming routine, cancer chemotherapy was advancing rapidly, and the diagnosis of "end-stage" disease of any kind often carried the possibility of another treatment rather than resignation to death. For house officers this meant busier days and nights, less time to read and sleep, and greater stress, tension, and fatigue.

Adding to the demands on house officers were the many extraneous duties they had to perform, such as drawing blood and inserting intravenous lines. At a number of teaching hospitals, it was estimated that house officers spent roughly one-quarter of their time at these activities.[107] In the 1970s, most teaching hospitals began to provide house officers greater assistance with such tasks. More phlebotomists and technicians were hired, and nurses were given greater authority to perform certain procedures. However, these steps provided house officers little relief from "scut work," for telephone calls, scheduling chores, dictations, and time spent charting increased even as the time consumed by manual procedures decreased.[108]

Overwork and exhaustion did perverse things to caring individuals who entered medicine to serve. At one teaching hospital there were frequent squabbles between emergency room and floor physicians over whether the admission of a patient was indicated, and calls to the emergency room sometimes went unanswered. House officers there would fight among themselves over who would answer the next call or be stuck with a new patient who happened to arrive within a few minutes of a change of duty.[109] Not surprisingly, stress-related depression, emotional impairment, and alcohol and substance abuse were well-documented phenomena among house officers.[110]

As the work demands on house officers increased, the perpetual tension of graduate medical education was exacerbated. Was graduate medical education an educational or service activity? Were house officers students or hospital employees? As with other dualisms, the answer was "both," for confidence and independence came by assuming graded responsibility for the patient's total care. However, the amount of service actually required for learning was far less than that which hospitals typically extracted from house officers. The tradition of the economic exploitation of house officers persisted, as hospitals continued to rely on trainees for an extraordinary range and amount of ancillary responsibilities.[111]

The dilemmas of residency training were thrust into the public spotlight in 1984, following the death of 18-year-old Libby Zion at the New York Hospital. Ms. Zion had presented to the hospital with the seemingly minor complaints of fever and an earache; eight hours later she was dead. Her family alleged that her death was the result of overwork and under-supervision of the medical house officers who cared for her, and the district attorney of Manhattan convened a grand jury to investigate those charges. Since the turn of the twentieth century a central tenet among medical educators had been that medical education leads to better patient care. Now that article of faith was challenged.

Despite years of review by various medical and legal groups, the cause of Libby Zion's death was never determined. The house officers in the main acted appropriately. They were not fatigued, and they were in communication by telephone with the attending physician, in this case Libby Zion's private physician. The grand jury refused to indict the doctors on criminal charges, and the state medical board did not revoke their licenses.[112]

Nevertheless, the grand jury did indict the system of residency training in the United States, and the case became a cause célèbre for reforming graduate medical education. The grand jury report led to the creation of a special commission, headed by Bertrand N. Bell, professor of medicine at the Albert Einstein College of Medicine. After 19 months of deliberation, the commission issued a series of recommendations on the working hours and supervision of residents that was incorporated into the New York State Health Code, which took effect in July 1989. New York was the only state to pass such legislation, but similar regulations were voluntarily enacted by most of the residency review committees (RRCs) that governed residency training in the various specialties. Specifics varied from one field to another, but in general the new regulations called for a restriction of the resident work week to 80 hours, the mandatory provision of one day off per week, limitations on the length of shifts in the emergency room, similar limitations on the frequency of nights on call in the hospital, and the requirement of greater direct supervision by attending physicians. Only the RRCs in surgery and the surgical subspecialties did not pass such regulations.

From the broad perspective, these events were not surprising. Society had always granted doctors considerable leeway in determining the conditions of medical education, but never total freedom. Medical education always had to meet the burden of proof of reasonableness, and now graduate medical education failed to pass that test. In an age of consumerism, the public demanded more evidence that the house officers caring for them were rested and supervised—even if that meant tilting the delicate balance in graduate medical education away from the educational needs of learners and toward the needs of patients who did not wish doctors to learn at their expense. The grand jury and Bell commission represented the voice of the consumer.

Initially, many medical educators opposed the establishment of regulations governing the working hours and supervision of house officers. Concerns ranged from the added expense necessary to implement the regulations to worries that patient care and house staff education would suffer because of the loss of continuity that would result. A particularly major concern was that the regulations would undermine the principle that house officers should receive graded levels of responsibility in patient care. House officers were also concerned about the effects of the new rules. One survey of chief residents in New York found that only 35 percent felt that the recommendations of the Bell commission would improve the ability of residents to deliver high quality patient care and that only 27 percent thought that the educational experience of residents would be improved.[113] Ironically, in the 1970s, in their efforts to stave off house staff unionization, medical educators had argued that house officers were students. Now, that same argument was used by the RRCs to impose regulations on training programs, particularly the regulations requiring greater supervision, that most medical educators opposed.

There was little doubt that graduate medical education needed reform. The residency had been created in an era when stable patients lingered in the hospital for long periods of time. By the 1980s, hospitalized patients were much sicker, the turnover of patients was much greater, and there was much more for house officers to do during a night on call. These circumstances demanded a reexamination of the issues of workload, autonomy, and supervision. Robert G. Petersdorf, president of the Association of American Medical Colleges, later expressed his regret that "long-overdue changes in structuring residency training were not initiated within our community prior to the serendipitous stimulus of the Zion case." My wish, he said, would be "that the profession had been more perceptive in recognizing the issue and making appropriate changes in training prior to its becoming a cause célèbre."[114]

On the other hand, the new RRC regulations represented a bureaucratic solution to the problems of residency training. As such, they failed to address fully—and might have aggravated—the problems they were intended to correct. One problem with the regulations was that the arbitrary limitation of hours did not resolve the issue of house staff stress. House officers now had more time off, but nights on call were still arduous and long, and the amount of work was even greater since there were fewer house officers in the hospital to share in the duties. Moreover, most hospitals did not add sufficient ancillary staff to protect residents from institutional service needs. Bertrand Bell himself pointed out that New York's new regulations on hours were "being widely flouted" because interns and residents were still "too frequently exploited as cheap labor."[115] The new rules did not guarantee adequate amenities while on duty, a faculty that knew and cared about the house staff, the ready availability of advisers and mentors, counseling services for anxiety and depression, a fair policy regarding parental leave, the immediate accessibility of help, and a strong sense of camaraderie in a department or program. The limitation of working hours, in short, said nothing about the larger issue of working conditions.

Second, it was not clear that the regulations promoted the goals of improving house staff education and patient care. Data on these issues were scarce, but many conscientious educators worried about the educational implications of fewer hours in the hospital: less opportunity to observe the natural history of illness and treatment and the development of a shift mentality among trainees that could undermine their professionalism and dedication to patients.[116] Many also worried that the increased turnover of house officers would increase the chance of mistakes in patient care. From internal medicine came a study suggesting that the restriction of resident working hours was associated with a delay in ordering tests and an increase in hospital complications; from obstetrics and gynecology came another indicating that the restriction of resident hours did not improve the quality of care and adversely affected continuity of care.[117] These studies could hardly be considered conclusive, but they did suggest that the effects of restricting resident work hours were far from understood and not easily predicted.

Third, the new mandates on resident hours did not address the issue of moonlighting, which in the 1980s and 1990s continued to be an important extracurricular activity for many house officers. In theory, as resident work schedules were reduced from every second or third to every fourth or fifth night on call, house officers were supposed to spend their newfound leisure time in rest, reading, and personal affairs. In practice, many of them merely increased their moonlighting, and reports appeared regularly in training program records of house officers whose excessive moonlighting interfered with their responsibilities as residents.[118]

Lastly, the new regulations could not avoid the day of reckoning when a doctor for the first time practiced medicine independently. The cardinal tenet of graduate medical education in the United States had been that this should be done in the controlled setting of teaching hospitals, where someone more senior was always available for help, and where mature physicians were prepared to come in immediately if necessary. To medical educators, this approach was superior to that of allowing a physician independence for the first time when alone in practice. The principle of graded responsibility represented a considered response of medical educators to the fact that ultimately the safety of all patients in all clinical settings was their responsibility and that the quality of care in the community could not be assured unless physicians first demonstrated their ability to practice independently while still under observation as house officers. In view of this, the ultimate language of the RRCs was much softer on the requirements for direct supervision than that of the grand jury and Bell commission, even as the balance nonetheless shifted toward closer supervision.

Ultimately, the responsibility for assuring the quality of education and patient care in graduate medical education lay elsewhere than with official regulations. Part of the responsibility rested with the medical faculties, which had the capacity to humanize graduate medical education in ways that might improve house staff morale, education, and patient care. Faculty members had choices regarding how to approach their teaching responsibilities. They could actively engage themselves in house staff education, or they could fulfill their duties in a perfunctory manner. Attending physicians could drop by in the afternoon, or they could limit discussions to officially designated teaching times. Instructors could establish genuine relationships with the house staff, or they could remain aloof. Faculty could, if they chose, help protect residents from stress and depression through adviser programs, counseling, retreats, luncheons, dinners, cultural or sporting events, outings, and other devices. Such steps represented a large request to make of faculty who placed a low priority on teaching. Nevertheless, the capacity to take such measures lay in their hands.

However, even the most dedicated faculties could not improve graduate medical education alone. A reduction of the workload of house officers was needed, not merely fewer nights on call or greater faculty attentiveness to their emotional needs. This required the provision of more nurses, technicians, clerks, transporters, and other supportive staff—hardly inexpensive budget items. No hospital, however willing, could provide such support unless third party payments were sufficient to make that allowable. Yet, in the managed care era of the 1990s, third party payments to hospitals became more restrictive, forcing institutions everywhere to retrench. Academic health centers were in the paradoxical position of being criticized by the public for working their house officers too hard yet being denied sufficient reimbursement to lessen the workload of residents appreciably. Once again, the quality of medical education—and patient care—reflected not the actions of academic health centers alone but the attitudes and values of American society.

❦ · ❦ · ❦

Many dilemmas of graduate medical education illustrated the interaction of internal and external factors. Yet in one important area, medical faculties had much more influence over the outcome: the test-ordering behavior that they instilled among residents and fellows. After 1970, faculties generally followed the same approach they had all century long: encouraging house officers to order more, not less—to do everything that was available, not just what was needed. The result was the perpetuation of a profligate practice style in American medicine that benefited neither patients nor those who paid the bills.

Test-ordering represented a complex behavior that was influenced by many social, economic, and personal factors. Fear of a malpractice suit, the demands of a patient or family, the convenience of tests, and financial incentives (hospital administrators seldom complained about excessive testing in the fee-for-service era, when more tests meant more revenue) were among the many factors that resulted in excessive testing.[119] In addition, in individual cases it could be extremely difficult to define what constituted an "unnecessary" test. There was often benefit from negative results, such as the peace of mind from knowing that a major problem was probably not present. In the hospital, the ordering of several tests together rather than in a strictly logical sequence could often save money by shortening the length of stay.

Nevertheless, a large body of research clearly indicated that the country suffered from excessive test-ordering zeal by its physicians. Roughly 25 percent of the average hospital bill was accounted for by laboratory tests and radiological studies,[120] yet only 5 percent of laboratory information was actually used in diagnosis and treatment.[121] False-positive tests often resulted in costly and sometimes harmful interventions. Excessive dependence on laboratory information may have fostered the deterioration of bedside skills, the tendency to deal with patients as objects, and the temptation to treat the laboratory numbers rather than the patient.

Excessive testing was not a new phenomenon. What was new after 1970 was the extraordinary proliferation of diagnostic procedures and the high cost of many of them. Excessive testing was hardly the only cause of rising health care costs in the United States. However, it was not an insignificant factor, and it was one that individual physicians could directly influence. "With even a small change in physician test ordering there is an opportunity for a major impact on costs,"[122] one study concluded.

An important cause of excessive testing was the century-long defect in medical education: the failure of medical education to prepare learners to deal with uncertainty. Properly, testing was done when it in some way would influence patient management. In practice, most attending physicians urged their house officers to do every test possible, to strive for completeness, to push toward the asymptote of certainty. Few instructors involved themselves in their residents' reasoning process or asked why something was done. Such "inordinate zeal for certainty,"[123] in the words of Jerome P. Kassirer, a leading student of clinical decision-making, made it difficult for house officers to learn how to use clinical reasoning and observations over time to make sense of a patient's problem.

The misguided quest for certainty resulted in diagnostic profligacy. For instance, some physicians approached patients as if time were not their ally. Rather than waiting a few days to see whether an apparent viral syndrome would resolve, they would immediately test for rheumatologic conditions, unusual infections, and hidden malignancies. Another common behavior was the ordering of duplicate tests when the diagnosis was already established. (Kassirer likened duplicate testing to wearing a belt and suspenders at the same time.[124]) A third widespread practice was laboring to make a diagnosis that had no therapeutic or management implications—for instance, obtaining studies to document the spread of a tumor in a patient with known metastatic cancer when no new treatment would be offered regardless of the results. Unnecessary tests were not only costly but they also added considerable risk: the risk of some of the procedures themselves, and the risk of delaying therapy for an obvious diagnosis while additional information was being gathered.

All century long, medical faculties had done poorly at teaching learners how to manage uncertainty. Yet, with hard work, the goal was achievable. In clinical departments where cost-effectiveness was emphasized, and where attending physicians took the time to review their house officers' reasoning process in detail, much could be accomplished. To aid in the process, there were new tools available to assist faculty in teaching effective clinical problem-solving. Clinical epidemiology had made significant strides as a discipline, much had been learned about decision analysis and the nature of diagnostic reasoning, and the concepts of sensitivity, specificity, and the predictive value of tests had been widely applied to clinical medicine.[125] In addition, other strategies could be employed, such as providing house officers information on the costs of tests or feedback on how their test-ordering practices might be improved. Of course, to ask faculty to engage themselves with house staff in this way represented a large request of instructors who did not like to teach or whose time was already consumed by other activities. Effective training for uncertainty could be accomplished only where bedside teaching was not a lost art and where faculty took the time to provide individualized instruction. Nevertheless, academic health centers had in their grasp the potential to do better—and in the process to strike a major blow for lower costs and better care.

16

Internal Malaise

I N THE 1970S AND 1980S a distinct malaise pervaded many medical
schools. As they increased their role in patient care, and as they grew
ever larger in size, they struggled to maintain their institutional cohesiveness and clear focus on academic work. In addition, medical schools,
long a symbol of public service, began to appear self-serving and unconcerned with the public good. To many, the once-clear distinction between
a university teaching hospital and a large community hospital began to
blur, as did the formerly clear differences between a university medical
school dedicated to serving the public and a scientific corporation seeking to maximize markets and profits.

Rudderless Ships

After the passage of Medicare and Medicaid, medical schools continued
to grow at an extraordinary pace. Most schools developed vast, sprawl-
ing campuses. The number of full-time faculty increased nationwide
from 17,118 in 1965 to 74,621 in 1990; the total revenues of U.S. medical
schools grew during that time from $882 million to nearly $21 billion.[1]
Single departments became huge, complex enterprises in their own right.
Between 1972 and 1992, for instance, the Department of Medicine of
Washington University grew from 50 to more than 150 full-time faculty
members, and its annual budget increased from $5 million to $125 million.[2] A research-intensive medical school in 1965 would have had an
annual operating budget of perhaps $20 million; by 1990 its budget
would have increased nearly 20-fold.

The main driving force for this growth was clinical practice. In 1965,
clinical service provided less than 6 percent of total medical school revenues. After the enactment of Medicare and Medicaid, clinical revenue
quickly became the most important source of income for medical schools.
By 1980 clinical income had surpassed federal research dollars as the

Table 12   Full-time faculty tracks in the Department of Internal
Medicine, University of Michigan Medical Center, 1988

	Physician Scientist	Clinician Scholar	Clinical
Title	Professorial	Professorial	Clinical
Tenure-seeking	Yes	Yes	No
Site of Activity	Campus	Campus	Off-Campus
Research Space	Yes	No	No
Personal Patient Care	5%	50%	95%
Research & Teaching	95%	50%	5%
Guaranteed Salary	100%	50%	25%
Incentive Salary	0%	50%	75%

major source of medical school revenue, and by the 1990s medical service accounted for nearly half of all medical school income. From 1965 to 1990 income from medical practice rose nearly 200-fold at U.S. medical schools, compared with an 11-fold increase in NIH funding (*see Table 8*).

Not surprisingly, the growth of medical schools during this period occurred disproportionately in the clinical departments. From 1965 to 1990, the number of full-time basic science faculty in U.S. medical schools rose from 5,671 to 15,432, whereas the number of full-time clinical faculty increased from 11,447 to 59,189.[3] Within the clinical departments, the majority of new faculty were appointed to the clinician-scholar track rather than the traditional physician-scientist track. Although many clinician-scholars had research agendas, their patient duties were large, and many were hired to do primarily clinical work. In some departments, a third faculty track, the "clinical track," was established to formalize the fact that many full-time faculty were hired to take care of patients, not to engage in academic activities (*see Table 12*).[4] Before World War II, education had been the dominant activity at American medical schools, and during the era of the multiversity, research. Now, the age of clinical practice had begun.

As medical schools grew, trends that had been evolving since World War II were accentuated. Only a memory was the earlier sense of the medical school as a close, tightly knit community. Schools were now large and impersonal. Few faculty members had wide acquaintance throughout the institution—or even in their own department. By the late 1970s, the annual picnic of the Washington University Department of Medicine—which at the time spanned four major teaching hospitals and contained 13 subspecialty divisions and several autonomous research centers—had given way to 15 or so smaller events because the logistics of the departmental picnic had become too unwieldy.[5] Schools everywhere tried to preserve the former feeling of unity in the faculty—here a spouses' club, there a school newsletter or faculty tea. However, the faculties had grown too large for these efforts to enjoy much success. Most faculty members focused on their own work, reserving their loyalty for immediate coworkers and direct supervisors. Departments and divisions functioned as independent units rather than as parts of a cohesive whole.

Also only a memory was the earlier gentility of academic life. The demands of conducting modern biological research were great; so were those of providing personal medical care, even when assisted by residents and fellows. Many faculty were too consumed by these activities to attend departmental conferences, talk with colleagues, or teach. Faculty members were continually under pressure—to publish another paper, to see another patient—a pressure intensified by the expectation that they would generate their own salary and support through research grants or clinical fees. The pressure was especially great for faculty members on academic tracks since research grants were becoming more difficult to obtain. At one medical school the high level of faculty anxiety concerning promotions and tenure was described as "a subculture of fear."[6] No one at a medical school could be totally secure. Even powerful deans and department chairmen, who were subject to periodic institutional review, could be deposed. Academic life continued to offer many rewards—but leisure, genteel collegiality, and security were not among them.

As medical schools grew, internal rivalries also increased. Departments, divisions, and individuals competed fiercely with each other for space and resources. Traditional tensions between the basic science and clinical departments became more intense as the clinical departments grew in size and influence. Within clinical departments, new tensions arose between those on academic and clinical tracks. Physician-scientists resented the generally higher salaries of the clinicians; clinician-teachers were unhappy that they were not promoted as readily as the researchers. Clinical departments also had to contend with the unrest of faculty assigned to one or another of the affiliated hospitals, who sometimes received lower salaries and often felt they had been relegated to the "second string."[7] Departments continued to battle with each other over clinical turf, time in the curriculum, and standards of promotion (for instance, whether standards should be relaxed for departments such as anesthesiology, where the pool of productive investigators was relatively small). A particularly divisive issue was the disposition of clinical income. How much should be used for salaries and how much for the academic activities of the school? How much should be retained by the individual, division, or department that generated the income and how much should be distributed more widely, and according to what formula? At some schools, the lack of collegiality among or within departments was severe enough to cause talented faculty to leave the institution.

In the individualistic medical school of the post-Medicare era, the balkanization of disciplines continued. This process proceeded the furthest in surgery, where most of the subspecialties, such as anesthesiology, orthopedic surgery, and otolaryngology, seceded from the surgery department to become departments of their own. Of note, this occurred primarily for political rather than for scientific reasons. Departmental status for the surgical subspecialties allowed the chief more direct contact with the dean, greater institutional power, more control over clinical revenues, greater ego satisfaction, and more visibility within the field nationally.[8] Internal medicine, the other major clinical field, successfully resisted balkanization. However, in the 1990s its unity was weakening as well. At most schools dermatology had left internal medicine to become a department of its own, and the subspecialty of cardiology was also beginning to demand departmental status—in no small measure because as a department it could retain much more of its bountiful clinical earnings.[9]

As medical schools grew larger, the interests of the school frequently conflicted with those of the departments and faculty. For instance, deans typically imposed a tax, customarily between 5 and 10 percent, on the professional earnings of clinical departments—one that was always paid, but often grudgingly and with endless battles over the proper amount of the tax. Another issue that frequently polarized the faculty and central administration was overhead payments on research grants. Funding agencies, without spending any more money, could increase the amount of direct support to investigators if they decreased overhead payments to the institution—an approach favored by most faculty members but opposed by most deans.

As centrifugal forces in the medical school increased, the role of the dean continued to be weakened. Deans headed medical schools but did not truly run them. Researchers were empowered by their external grants, clinicians and clinician-teachers by their professional earnings. Both groups of faculty tended to feel less and less loyalty to the institution as a whole or to the dean, whose responsibility greatly exceeded his authority. One study found that the "anarchy index" at medical schools increased in proportion to the amount of external research support and patient care revenue an institution received—that is, the more that faculty were self-supporting, the less likely they were to think of the common good.[10] Many deans continued to be effective, but their success resulted mainly from persuasion, force of personality, and consensus-building rather than direct decision-making power.

Most of the administrative control continued to devolve to department chairs, who had considerable control over the research and clinical revenues brought in by their faculty members. Nevertheless, power did not carry with it serenity. In the era of megamedicine, the administrative and fiscal challenges of running a corporate-sized department proved innumerable and nerve-wracking. Many of the pressures and frustrations of the dean's office spilled over to the department chairs, few of whom had much time left for professional or academic work. Time that chairs had once spent in teaching, research, or patient care was now devoured by the administration of practice plans, worry about bed occupancy and the collection of professional fees, and seemingly endless conferences with lawyers and accountants. In 1930 Francis Peabody had described the idealized internal medicine chairman as the clinical, intellectual, and academic leader of the department; it was a position to which most academic internists aspired.[11] In 1975 Eugene Braunwald found that internal medicine department chairmen were in fact harried, exhausted, and overworked. Few perceived themselves as professionally successful, and most were so bedraggled and frustrated that they were contemplating early retirement.[12]

Everywhere in the 1970s and 1980s, the management of medical schools grew exceedingly complex. The fiscal and administrative issues pertaining to their large budgets, sizeable faculties, and broad scope of educational, investigative, and patient care activities became immense. Resources, though large, came from multiple sources that were less stable and predictable than traditional sources of revenue to the university— sources that were not controlled by the institution but dependent on the behavior and actions of those outside the academic health center. This circumstance required that planning be sophisticated and exact. Maintaining good relations with teaching hospitals, which also had grown in complexity, became correspondingly more challenging. Medical schools were no longer isolated academic enclaves concentrating on teaching and research but parts of complex medical centers delivering large volumes of patient services and engaging in a variety of community outreach programs from drug and alcohol rehabilitation to educational enrichment programs for local schools. The academic health center had become one of the largest employers in the city, one of the major tax-exempt landowners and businesses, and home to many complex minisocieties. The task of dealing with government regulatory agencies had also become exasperating. Thus, medical schools, like other large institutions, had to follow a bewildering set of rules for environmental protection, occupational safety, hiring and firing practices, wages, overtime and fringe benefits, workers' compensation, and affirmative action—not to mention sensitive and time-consuming negotiations with community planning boards and local citizen groups. As David E. Rogers and Robert J. Blendon wrote, this new order of managerial effort was "a large order for a collection of doctor scholars."[13]

In the post-Medicare years, schools everywhere adopted new tactics to cope with the growing managerial challenges. Many deans and department chairs took courses on health policy and educational administration, most commonly at the Harvard School of Public Health or the Association of American Medical Colleges. The size of academic administration grew dramatically. At the University of Michigan in 1988, for instance, 169 faculty members received additional pay for assuming an administrative task.[14] The size of the administrative staffs at most teaching hospitals increased even more strikingly, in part to handle the quality assurance requirements of Medicare. (At some teaching hospitals, entire floors were converted from patient rooms to offices to accommodate the quality assurance staff—a tangible manifestation of how the increasing bureaucratic demands of the American health care system were diverting hospitals from patient care to paperwork.) Full-time business managers were hired for the dean's office, most departments, and many clinical divisions. Outside business consultants were regularly brought in to provide guidance on computerization, billing, collecting, the optimal design of faculty practice plans, investing, the management of the payroll and fringe benefits, accounting, reporting, cost-cutting, and the development of more efficient administrative procedures. Schools became skilled at negotiating better construction contracts, and many schools and teaching hospitals aggressively combatted third party payers by suing them (usually successfully) to raise reimbursement rates or to make good on payments that were being withheld. Schools also professionalized their fund-raising (now called "development") activities, which remained an important source of income even in the clinical era. For both medical schools and teaching hospitals, which poured their revenues into the improvement of the institution, gifts sometimes meant the difference between an operating surplus or deficit for any given fiscal year.

Nevertheless, the managerial revolution was far from complete in American medical schools. Medical schools, like the rest of the university, clung to the tradition of governance by consensus. Small committees of powerful department chairs or senior faculty would regularly be formed to address specific issues, but seldom would broad planning for the institution as a whole be undertaken. Major decisions typically occurred in a haphazard fashion, not as part of a larger, coherent plan. Departments and powerful clinical divisions tended to act as a consortium of special interest groups—powerful fiefdoms thinking of their own best interest, not the needs or welfare of the school as a whole. Achieving a consensus among powerful individualists on a major issue often proved to be a slow, cumbersome process. In addition, as medical schools grew larger, the component parts frequently did not communicate with each other. This often led to duplication in purchasing equipment and hiring personnel and to internal competition among programs with similar goals. It was often difficult to know who, if anyone, was in charge.

This management style could work well on narrow academic matters. Ad hoc committees could effectively select the head of a cancer center or basic science department or decide how to allocate space in a new research building among the various departments. However, university mechanisms of governance were not so well suited to deal with the issues of defining and clarifying institutional goals in a complex, rapidly changing world. Nor were they well suited to treat matters of high finance, shifting sources of support, complex organizational structure, intricate government regulations, and rapidly rising social expectations and societal demands of medical schools.

Through the late 1980s, the university management style posed relatively few problems for medical schools. Since there was so much clinical income, hard discussions about missions, goals, and priorities could be avoided. Medical schools grew fat and affluent, not lean and hungry. They were seldom forced to ask whether bigger is better or whether the maximal size is the optimal size. Enough income from clinical practice usually came in to allow them to pursue every academic path, purchase every piece of equipment, and provide every clinical service—without having to ask what were the returns or whether the money and resources could be better used in another fashion. If a program or piece of technology was considered good, most schools felt they had to have it, regardless of cost. For the moment, medical schools could get away with such practices, for the environment was still relatively friendly and clinical revenues flowing. It remained to be seen how suitable such methods of management would be in an environment in which adversity reigned.

As medical schools grew large and unwieldy, so did academic medicine as a whole. The spring "clinical meetings"—the jointly held meeting of the Association of American Physicians, the American Society for Clinical Investigation, and the American Federation for Clinical Research—outgrew the facilities in Atlantic City. In 1976 the societies met there for the last time; in subsequent years the meetings rotated among a handful of cities with major convention facilities, where they lost the informality and personal quality of the Atlantic City era. Even larger were some of the subspecialty society meetings, which now received more abstracts than the "clinical meetings."[15] With the opening of the community-based medical schools, the heterogeneity among medical schools became greater than ever before. Similarly, the number and types of hospitals that participated in medical education also increased, a response to the reliance of the community-based schools on smaller community hospitals and to the greater use of affiliated hospitals by established schools. Of course, diversity constituted a great strength of American medical education, as did the fact that no one institution had a monopoly on excellence. On the other hand, as academic medicine grew in size and heterogeneity, no one group or organization could speak for it. The Association of American Medical Colleges (AAMC), the official "voice" of academic medicine, in fact now represented a diverse and often warring constituency of medical schools, academic societies, and teaching hospitals.

As its size and complexity grew, academic medicine no longer evoked the metaphors of family. As one sign of that change, students and faculty did not remember their professional ancestors. For instance, no figure had more influenced medicine nationally during the age of the multiversity than Eugene Stead, chairman of internal medicine at Duke from 1947 to 1967. To his contemporaries, Stead assumed near-Oslerian proportions. His seminal discoveries in cardiovascular research reshaped understanding of the pathogenesis of congestive heart failure, he was a clinician-teacher of legendary skill, he pioneered the Physician Assistant

Training Program, he helped foster the development of computerized medical records and outcomes research, his department generated 33 department heads, and his name was known by medical students everywhere in the country. A generation later, one writer observed that Stead's name "draws a blank from today's medical students and residents."[16] Yet, for the new generation of students, house officers, and faculty, few new heroes had arisen to replace the many that had existed the generation before. The disappearance of heroes from medicine reflected in part the cynicism of an American society that had been through the trauma of the Watergate affair and the Vietnam War. However, it also reflected the fact that academic medicine had grown too large and fragmented for "heroes" to emerge.

The growth of faculty practice accomplished much good for medical schools. In particular, it allowed education and research to flourish at a time when federal support for biomedical research slackened. With the slowdown in growth of NIH funding in the 1970s and 1980s, and with the end of congressional capitation subsidies to medical schools in the 1980s, clinical revenue became a major source of funds to cross-subsidize the academic mission of medical schools. A typical example was Jefferson Medical College, where clinical dollars came to the rescue when research dollars decreased. In 1984–85, the school suffered a 5 percent drop in sponsored research, but a $700,000 increase in faculty practice income covered the shortfall.[17] As medical schools began using faculty practice income to subsidize the basic science departments, those departments thrived as well. In the 1970s and 1980s, the slowdown in growth of federal research support (in all fields, not just biomedical science) led to considerable retrenchment at America's research universities. Medical schools were spared that fate because they, unlike the rest of the university, had clinical revenue as well.

Nevertheless, faculty practice was not without problems for medical schools. As faculty practice grew in importance, medical schools became dependent on it. Just as the academic mission in the age of the multiversity had depended primarily on federal research support, the academic mission during the clinical era came to depend heavily on cross-subsidies from faculty practice, which were used for salaries, start-up funds for new instructors, seed money for established investigators, holdover funds for faculty between grants, and for the construction and renovation of facilities, the purchase of equipment and supplies, and the support of educational and training programs. If clinical revenues declined, research and education could be hard hit. This lesson was illustrated at Stanford Medical School in 1978, when the school suffered a fiscal crisis because of a substantial shortfall of clinical revenues. As a consequence, the school's research programs were jeopardized—even though Stanford was fifth in the nation among medical schools in the amount of NIH money received.[18] Medical practice, in short, had come to control medical education. Now that the academic mission of medical schools had become economically dependent on clinical practice, education and research could thrive only as long as the financing of health care permitted.

In addition, the growing economic dependence of medical schools on clinical practice blurred their university identity. Clinical faculty were spending more and more time in patient care, at the expense of teaching and research. Such patterns occurred even at the most academically distinguished schools. At Johns Hopkins, the dean conceded that "in building up the clinical practice plan, we found the demands on faculty time increased to the detriment of research."[19] At the Columbia-Presbyterian Medical Center, a faculty report concluded that "the clinical part of the institution is driven by practice patterns that frequently operate to inhibit rather than foster clinical research."[20] At the University of Maryland, which developed into an important research school in the 1980s, senior faculty worried that the "pressures to generate patient care revenues" were having a negative impact on the ability of the faculty "to teach and conduct research."[21] Nationwide, a study by the AAMC in 1985 reported that "the increasing dependence medical schools have on practice income is creating fears that the academic mission is being diverted."[22] According to the president of the AAMC, the practice of medicine "now dominates many medical schools," creating an environment where teaching and research have taken "a back seat to practice."[23]

The tension between academic pursuits and patient care, of course, had been long-standing at American medical schools. Before the passage of Medicare and Medicaid, schools had sought to resolve that tension by trying to restrict the amount of patient care they provided to that necessary to invigorate teaching and research. Though it was never easy, medical schools could usually do that because they were not financially dependent on patient care. If the full-time faculty allowed patients to go to the voluntary staff or returned patients to community doctors after a referral, a school suffered little economic consequence. Now, the opposite situation had developed. Because of their growing financial dependence on patient care, medical schools felt obligated to see as many patients as possible. For most of the twentieth century, appointment to the full-time faculty of a medical school had required demonstration of a serious interest in teaching or research. After 1965, the only reason for the employment of many full-time faculty members was to provide patient care.

Since the end of World War II, when large sums of money began flowing to medical schools, medical faculties had shown themselves to be extremely adept at responding to financial incentives. In the age of the multiversity, research grew enormously, and in the clinical era, faculty practice. Yet in the process something was lost. Medical schools were no longer setting their own agendas. Medical educators were asking fewer and fewer questions about their mission and goals and about how those objectives needed to evolve in a changing society. Competent academic managers were present to run medical schools, but there was a scarcity of academic leaders and educational visionaries. Schools drifted along without a coherent articulation of their purpose or a clear definition of ways they could contribute to the larger good. Increasingly, the schools were content to go where the money was, doing whatever was asked of them along the way. In the era of clinical practice, that meant seeing ever-increasing numbers of patients, even as the growing volume of clinical service eroded the rationale of the medical school and made medical school hospitals and clinics look more and more like those in nonteaching settings. The main solace that could be taken was that, in the fee-for-service era, clinical compensation was sufficiently generous to allow good academic work to continue.

It would be a mistake to be overly harsh on medical schools for allowing faculty practice to grow. After the passage of Medicare and Medicaid, practice income was there for the taking. It would have been foolish for medical schools not to have expanded their clinical roles, especially as research support became more difficult to obtain and as the public increasingly demanded the clinical expertise available at academic health centers. Nevertheless, few schools knew where or how to draw the line between their university work and patient care. Like "morphine," Walsh McDermott wrote to a friend in 1980, there was nothing wrong with practice plans per se. "It is just that they are very tricky things, and the temptation to over-use them can become uncontrollable."[24] That is precisely what happened. Faculty practice plans were originally developed as carefully constructed responses to the economic and social circumstances of the 1960s and 1970s. Soon they came to be considered panaceas, and schools began to engage in the relentless pursuit of all practice opportunities and all possible clinical income. Along the way, the rationale of the medical school as part of the university was forgotten. Medical schools grew rich, but they lost connection with their roots.

From the time America's system of medical education had been created, the American medical school had found itself with two homes: one in the university, the other in the health care delivery system. Of the two, the ties to the university had traditionally been far stronger. The intellectual and social origins of the modern American medical school lay primarily in the creation of the modern American university, and for most of the twentieth century, medical schools had tried to limit their clinical service to that which was needed to promote teaching and research. As faculty practice plans grew, the university ideal in medical education became weaker. More and more the academic mission was undermined by the demands of providing patient care. Medical schools gradually drifted from the core of the university to the periphery, and their ties to the health care delivery system correspondingly increased. In the fee-for-service era, quality teaching and research survived—indeed, thrived. However, the clear identity of the medical school as a core part of the university was lost, and the fate of medical education became dependent on the friendliness of the health care delivery system.

The Decline of Academic
Health Centers as Public Trusts

Historians have long cautioned against romanticizing the past—glorifying an earlier time while overlooking the imperfections and blemishes of that era. Such warnings, of course, apply to the history of American medical education. As earlier chapters have indicated, American medical schools and teaching hospitals were never perfect places. Until the 1950s, full-time positions at medical schools were few in number, salaries were low, and support for research was limited. For many decades both schools and hospitals engaged in racial, religious, ethnic, and gender discrimination. Charity patients were often treated callously, and patients' rights were frequently subordinated to the needs of education and research. All century long, medical schools evolved in a faculty-directed fashion, placing less emphasis on the educational needs of students and house officers than on the academic and professional interests of the faculty.

Nevertheless, the achievements of academic health centers greatly outweighed their blemishes: their emphasis on quality in the production of the nation's doctors, their positive response to the national demand for more doctors in the 1960s and 1970s, the extraordinary successes of medical research, which allowed individuals of each successive generation the opportunity for healthier and longer lives than their parents had enjoyed, the high standards of medical practice they established for the profession as a whole, the generous amounts of free care they provided, and their growing concern for the health conditions of their local communities. Moreover, medical faculties for the first two-thirds of the century had clearly functioned as public trusts. The above good work, together with the relatively low levels of faculty compensation, the disdain toward commercialism, the prevalent attitudes toward commercial patents, and adherence to high standards of intellectual honesty, reinforced public notions that medical schools were dedicated servants of society. It was this image of medical schools as necessary social instruments that had justified the public's deference and financial support all century long.

Beginning in the 1970s, and increasing in the 1980s and 1990s, the behavior of medical faculties no longer so clearly demonstrated a commitment to advancing the public good. Their gaze turned inward, as they increasingly focused on their own rights and entitlements and spoke less of the ways they could continue to act as guardians of the nation's health. In addition, medical schools seemed to fall prey to unprecedented levels of greed, commercialism, and intellectual dishonesty. In the post-Medicare era, as medical schools lost touch with their intellectual roots in the university, they also lost touch with their moral roots as a public trust.

The growing preoccupation of medical faculties with their own well-being was clearly seen in the rising importance given to salary. If funds were tight, the preservation of salaries was typically a faculty's first priority. When research grants to the Department of Biological Chemistry at the University of Michigan were cut in the 1970s, the department elected "to cannibalize graduate student stipends for faculty salaries."[25] Because of the growth of faculty practice, such extreme measures were seldom necessary. Faculty salaries rose sharply in the 1970s, 1980s, and 1990s, particularly in the clinical departments, where little remained of the traditional income disparities with private practice (*see Table 13*).[26] Traditionally, the ethos of academic medicine had been the pursuit of glory, not gold. Now many faculty members expected to have both the benefits of academic life and personal riches.

What constituted proper academic pay? No one could say with authority since such assessments were highly subjective. Certainly it would have been unrealistic not to have expected medical school salaries to rise in the clinical era. Faculty salaries reflected market forces, and the large salaries commanded by high-volume clinical producers were a marketplace phenomenon. Many faculty on clinical tracks were doing work similar to that of their nonacademic counterparts. Without a high salary, large clinical producers could easily be wooed into private practice or to a competing medical school willing to pay what they asked. Nevertheless, for some faculty, especially those in procedural disciplines like surgery, the rise of income was staggering. By the late 1980s, highly compensated clinical faculty commonly received many hundreds of thousands of dollars a year.[27] The highest paid instructors at some schools had incomes approaching or exceeding $1 million a year. In an extreme example, for the fiscal year that ended June 30, 1994, a professor of cardiothoracic surgery at Cornell received a salary of $1.7 million.[28] It was the granting of corporate levels of compensation that led Carleton Chapman, a former medical school dean and foundation president, to speak of the "mammoth personal incomes" of some contemporary medical professors.[29]

The escalation of faculty salaries reflected a new ambience at medical schools, not merely the presence of greater revenues. Although clinical income was widely used to subsidize education and research, the "biggest single reason" for the escalation of faculty practice was the desire for high salaries.[30] The drive to see more patients was particularly great in procedural-oriented specialties, especially when the compensation formula was tied to a professor's individual earnings rather than to the earnings of the division or department as a whole. In surgery and the surgical subspecialties, for instance, many instructors began operating as much as possible. One surgeon pointed out, "With a little operating, one can make a lot of money," which tempted even academically renowned surgeons "to operate a lot and make even more money."[31] Such behavior represented a marked change from Alfred Blalock's renowned department of surgery at Johns Hopkins (1941–1964), where faculty were encouraged to operate no more than once a day so that they could have more time in the laboratory.

Table 13 Mean faculty salaries (base and supplemental compensation), 1997–98

Department	Instructor	Assistant Professor	Associate Professor	Professor	Chairman
Basic Science	38,200	57,300	71,000	103,000	153,100
Anesthesiology	119,500	155,700	186,100	201,400	322,500
Dermatology	57,700	120,600	156,200	174,200	269,000
Family Practice	94,800	110,500	120,300	132,800	199,500
General Surgery	76,400	161,200	210,400	250,600	382,100
Medicine	83,400	111,800	134,700	166,700	277,000
Neurology	59,900	96,900	121,200	150,500	233,600
Neurosurgery	94,800	188,500	251,500	283,800	516,000
Obs–Gynecology	94,500	148,300	178,400	197,400	308,100
Ophthalmology	59,300	134,700	170,400	192,600	324,400
Orthopedic Surgery	84,300	197,600	240,900	262,800	406,800
Otolaryngology	50,800	146,000	188,500	198,500	385,100
Pathology	59,200	93,700	117,400	149,200	259,600
Pediatrics	69,800	99,700	123,400	147,700	254,200
Plastic Surgery	101,400	173,300	250,600	267,900	511,000
Preventive Medicine	69,200	74,900	86,600	111,100	174,600
Psychiatry	69,000	90,100	103,700	138,900	246,000
Radiology	87,400	145,800	172,900	199,200	329,700
Thoracic & Cardiovascular Surgery	111,500	249,800	306,600	412,100	649,100
Urology	78,900	141,500	200,300	238,000	305,200

If changing faculty attitudes toward compensation suggested a more commercial spirit in medical education, so did changing attitudes toward patents and the development of new ventures with industry. Traditionally, medical schools had been known for their altruism, disdain of commercialism, and philanthropic spirit. Through the 1950s and 1960s, Harvard Medical School, the mark of most things medical during the twentieth century, would infuriate the pharmaceutical industry by continuing to dedicate its patents to the public, including patents derived from industry-funded research. In the 1970s, medical schools' attitudes on the matter began to change. In 1974 Harvard entered a relationship with the Monsanto Company in which Monsanto agreed to give the school $23 million for research support over 12 years in exchange for the right to secure a worldwide license for all discoveries and inventions made in connection with company-funded work. The following year Harvard abandoned its long-standing policy requiring medical patents to be dedicated to the public and adopted a new policy that allowed the school to grant licenses to industrial corporations in exchange for remuneration. Other medical schools took note, and in the 1980s a large number and variety of university–industrial arrangements began to appear: research contracts, licensing agreements, collaborative research institutes, biotechnology companies staffed and owned by university scientists, and start-up biotechnology firms in which a university had taken a major equity position. A new image of medical school and university biomedical science began to emerge in the public eye: the academic scientist as entrepreneur, the university as a commercial institution.[32]

There were compelling reasons for medical schools to seek new liaisons with the corporate sector. With the prospect of declining federal support for biomedical research, the idea of corporate sponsorship became more attractive. The growing respectability of industrial research in the 1970s and 1980s, particularly at the pharmaceutical companies, softened many traditional concerns about fostering relationships with industry. In addition, the federal government encouraged the establishment of closer ties with industry as a way to promote "technology transfer" (that is, the development of commercially useful products from federally funded basic research). The Patent and Trademarks Amendments Act of 1980 allowed universities and other nonprofit institutions to retain ownership of inventions that resulted from federally supported research. Another law in 1986 gave universities the right to own start-up companies based on their professors' work, either through direct stock ownership or through university-funded venture-capital firms. By 1990, more than 100 medical schools or universities had started financing new companies to exploit their professors' discoveries.

Though the verdict on these programs is still out, university–corporate arrangements have so far worked well in terms of their primary goals: promoting technology transfer and providing medical schools an additional source of income through royalties, licensing fees, and the direct underwriting of research. It was estimated that industry in 1994 provided universities $1.5 billion for research in the life sciences, or 11.7 percent of the total university research and development funds in the life sciences that year. No one expected that industry would ever replace the federal government as the main source of support for fundamental research, but partnerships between medical schools and industry seemed to be proving durable.[33]

Nevertheless, the commercialization of biomedical research created many dilemmas for medical schools. As with faculty practice plans, the primary problem was that a large amount of money ended up in the hands of faculty members as personal income rather than in the medical school treasury to underwrite teaching and research, as many proponents of these arrangements had originally argued should be the case. The biggest financial winners were entrepreneurial basic scientists whose discoveries led to the creation of a biotechnology company in which they had taken an ownership position. As covered widely in the popular press, many fortunes were made by investigators when their companies went public, resulting in their becoming instant multimillionaires. Other financial winners included the large number of investigators who reaped lucrative consulting fees from industrial concerns, whether or not they held an equity position in those firms. Relatively unpublicized but hardly insignificant were the earnings of medical school workers whose patented discoveries led to successful commercial products. Royalties received by the medical school would be disbursed according to the school's formula of the moment, but typically the investigator would receive up to 50 percent of the royalties, which often could be taken as income. (The remainder would be divided among the dean, the investigator's laboratory, and the investigator's department.) Thus, a number of medical schools found themselves in the ironic predicament that some faculty would be receiving personal royalties from their university work of tens or hundreds of thousands of dollars a year, while the medical school library would be cutting back on books, journals, and services for lack of funds.

In addition, the lure of personal profit created many potential conflicts of interest for biomedical investigators. A variety of concerns were frequently raised: that the prospect of large financial rewards might influence an investigator's choice of problems, that graduate students or postdoctoral research fellows would be directed into narrow projects for the sake of their adviser's economic interests, that the establishment of a set of proprietary relationships would exact heavy tolls on the openness of exchange of scientific information, and that the profit motive might divert an investigator from fulfilling institutional responsibilities. Deans particularly worried about potentially deleterious effects on university citizenship, for it was already difficult enough to persuade some faculty members to spend much time teaching or serving on essential medical school committees. It was not unknown for full-time faculty to spend more hours a week on commercial consulting than on university work, even at schools that tried to limit the amount of outside consulting. Most disconcerting of all, a number of highly publicized scandals occurred in which investigators in clinical trials were found to have a financial interest in the result, such as owning stock or options in the company that made the experimental drug or device they were testing.[34]

The extent and significance of these and other problems pertaining to conflict of interest were impossible to determine. Emotions ran high; empirical data to answer the questions were scarce. Nevertheless, the issue of conflict of interest needed to be taken seriously—if for no other reason than to address public concerns. As one medical faculty observed, inserting a profit motive into a faculty member's research tends "to lower the individual investigator's objectivity and the confidence of the public."[35] Reports of conflict of interest were highly disturbing to the public, even if the perceptions of malfeasance might have exceeded the reality.

By the 1990s, the commercialization of biomedical research had become one of the thorniest issues facing medical schools. It was much easier, perhaps, for biomedical scientists in the past to speak disdainfully of industrial entanglements because they did not have anything to sell as valuable as the revolution in molecular biology. Indeed, other branches of the university—chemistry, physics, the computer sciences, and economics—had preceded the medical school in developing long-standing relations with industry. Academic values are continually in evolution, and it is not surprising that they became more commercial in a commercial age. Those today who question the legitimacy of corporate ties to biomedical research might find it instructive to remember the opposition that greeted foundations as patrons of research during World War I and the federal government after World War II—an opposition that soon dissipated as those novel arrangements proved successful.

Nevertheless, many thoughtful individuals continued to worry about the consequences of the commercialization of biomedical research. One was Derek Bok, whose presidency of Harvard University in the 1970s and 1980s coincided with the commercialization of biomedical science at the university. Though Bok himself supported that transformation—he drew the line only at having the university take an equity stake in biotechnology companies started by faculty members—he never stopped worrying that the desire of a medical school or university to increase profits would conflict with its academic mission. He discussed this problem in his last annual report in 1991. "It will take very strong leadership to keep the profit motive from gradually eroding the values on which the welfare and reputation of universities ultimately depend." The basic issue, in Bok's view, was the challenge medical schools and universities faced in maintaining their position as public trusts if the profit motive at the individual or institutional level was allowed to coexist with the search for truth and the free dissemination of knowledge. As schools increase their pursuit of profit, "they appear less and less as charitable institutions seeking truth and serving students and more and more as a huge commercial operation that differs from corporations only because there are no shareholders and no dividends."[36]

If commercialism became more prevalent among medical schools after 1970, so did signs of a lower sense of academic integrity. Evidence of this appeared throughout the medical school: frequent reports of student cheating, faculty and student violations of the rules of the internship matching program, and the misrepresentation of academic credentials by applicants for fellowships.[37] What most captured the public eye, however, were a number of highly publicized cases of scientific fraud involving plagiarism, the misrepresentation of results, or the fabrication of data. Several of these episodes occurred in large, prolific laboratories at prestigious universities. These cases aroused the interest and concern of the press, in part because of the importance and high visibility of some of those implicated, and in part because of the perceived indecisive response of the academic community. The public image of physicians and biomedical science took a beating, and an underlying tone of distrust of the scientific establishment appeared among funding agencies and Congress. The public worried whether biomedical research was changing in a negative way—whether the structure of medical research was crumbling and whether there was a massive cover-up of wrongdoing. The cover of one issue of *The New Republic* featured a group of leering, evil-looking medical researchers under the caption, "The Science Mob."[38]

The extent of fraud in biomedical research was difficult to determine. Certainly, various forms of deception in many fields had occurred throughout the history of science, and it was popular (and undoubtedly correct) to assume that scientific misconduct represented the deviant behavior of a small number of perpetrators.[39] Nevertheless, from the perspective of history, the appearance of so many documented episodes of scientific misconduct represented the culmination of the century-long trend in which the search for knowledge had become secondary to the quest for academic success and survival. Since World War I the pressures of "publish or perish" had been growing, and medical schools had consistently emphasized the quantity rather than the quality of publications. Accordingly, multiauthorship and the search for the least publishable unit increased. By the 1980s, medical editors were complaining of various abuses of authorship that had become embarrassingly prevalent over the recent past: "salami slicing" (inappropriately dividing the results of a single study into two or more papers), redundant publication (publishing the same results in minimally modified form in different journals), and the widespread custom in which senior professors would list their names among the authors of a paper even if they had contributed little to the work or even had not read the manuscript.[40] This latter practice represented a deterioration of traditional standards of mentorship in which faculty supervised students and junior colleagues closely—not to prevent fraud directly, but to teach good laboratory practices, provide inspiration and support, and instill a proper ethic about scientific research. A high official at Johns Hopkins called it indicative of a "developing amorality in science."[41]

To many, the abuses of authorship represented a more worrisome indication of a declining integrity in biomedical research than the handful of cases of scientific fraud. Overt fraud seemed to be an aberration. Authorship abuse, in contrast, was commonplace and more directly reflected the prevailing culture of academic medicine. The editor of the *Annals of Internal Medicine* wrote that the irony of scientific fraud "is that far more frequent though less dramatic abuses of authorship draw little notice in the scientific community, let alone public concern. This unconcern is no surprise; a murder gets more attention than a mugging."[42] Outright fraud was presumably rare, but not the intense pressure to publish, the widespread decay in the standards for authorship, and the continued devaluation of the academic currency, the published paper. These trends indicated that the culture of academic medicine had evolved to a point where the search for truth was sometimes less important than achieving individual success. Scientists often appeared to be competing against each other rather than against disease and suffering.

Lastly, after 1965 a growing discrepancy developed between society's health care needs and the intellectual interests of medical faculties. In earlier periods, the two had harmonized well. Acute diseases took their toll on all strata of society, life expectancy was much shorter, and medical costs were not considered a major problem. In studying acute illnesses, medical researchers were confronting the major health problems of the nation. In the era of chronic diseases, however, the public increasingly worried about the expense or availability of care rather than the technical capacity of medicine. In 1979, 65 percent of the public considered the cost of care as the most important problem facing medicine, compared with only 10 percent who listed quality first.[43] Most people now feared disease less than the expense or inaccessibility of medical care, were they to be seriously ill.

As the public became increasingly concerned with the system of health care delivery, the attention of medical faculties remained biologically focused. Medical scientists continued to pursue the biological issues of disease and treatment; relatively few faculty became interested in the social and economic problems of delivering health care equitably and inexpensively. One can readily understand the reluctance of biomedical investigators to abandon their traditional interests, given their scientific backgrounds, the relative "softness" of the new field of health services research, and the power, fascination, and genuine potential of the molecular revolution to make an impact on chronic diseases. But the formerly close fit between what society defined as critical to its prosperity and what medical faculty wanted to investigate began to widen. Medical schools for the first time since World War I began to be perceived as insular—as isolated enclaves or ivory towers unresponsive to society's most pressing health care concerns.

The narrow gaze of most medical faculties should not mask the considerable good work they did in fulfilling the service mission of academic health centers. Education and research in and of themselves represented a significant discharge of public duties. It was to every patient's benefit to have well-trained doctors, new medical knowledge, and a continual upgrading of the standards of practice. Academic health centers continued to dispense large amounts of free care, a major contribution in view of the ever-rising costs of care. Many academic health centers also began to take greater responsibility for the overall health of their local communities—for instance, by reorganizing their outpatient services or establishing neighborhood health centers.[44] By the late 1970s, the traditional view that the clinical responsibilities of a medical school consisted only of those arising from the requirements for teaching and research seemed quaint and arcadian, in view of prevailing social forces beyond the control of medical educators: the definition of health care as a right, the growing demands of private patients for care at academic health centers, the new economic dependence of medical schools on clinical income, and the reliance of many urban communities on academic health centers for basic health care. In accommodating to these powerful forces, academic health centers showed they were never so insular or unresponsive as some modern critics contended.

Nevertheless, providing direct clinical services or assuming comprehensive medical responsibility for a defined population was different from addressing the social, political, economic, and organizational problems of a costly and inefficient health care system. Some wondered whether this was the responsibility of medical schools. A fundamental question arose: What was the proper role of the medical school (or that of the university as a whole) as an instrument of social change?

Historically, the university has been much more a reactor to external forces than an agent of social change. The major changes in the Western university have generally been initiated from outside, such as the Revolution in France, the Communist Party in Russia, the various royal commissions in Great Britain, and the land grant movement, foundations, and federal government in the United States. In contrast, the university's role in social change has been indirect and conservative. The ideas and writings of individual members of the university have often been a stimulus to change, but as an institution the university has rarely served as a revolutionary force. A country's system of health care delivery reflects the values, hopes, and aspirations of the society at large and not technical medical knowledge or the wishes of the medical profession alone. This observation explains the existence of different delivery systems in different Western countries, each adapting "scientific medicine" to its peculiar culture and traditions. To look to academic medicine or the medical profession alone to effect a revolution in the delivery system would be naive.

Nevertheless, it could be argued that medical schools had the obligation to lead the debate about health care delivery. As medical schools became more and more economically dependent on providing patient care, they had a direct stake in the fate of the health care delivery system in a way that no other branch of the university had in the outcome of any other social issue. Moreover, if schools were to continue serving as guardians of the nation's health, then it behooved them to address the problems of cost and access so that all might continue to enjoy the fruits of what medicine had to offer. Society itself was looking to medical schools for leadership in solving these problems—in part because of its high regard for medical schools, and in part because of the expectation that medical faculties could mobilize all the intellectual forces of the university—the specialists in economics, political science, sociology, law, ethics, public administration, and other fields—to join them in addressing the mounting crisis in health care delivery. For such reasons, banking and automobile executives in Michigan in 1977 believed that "the University should lead the way in solving health care cost problems."[45]

Some leaders of academic medicine agreed. The AAMC proclaimed as early as 1968, "The medical schools must now assume a responsibility for education and research in the organization and delivery of health services."[46] The establishment of the Institute of Medicine, chartered in 1970 as a semi-independent branch of the National Academy of Sciences, stood as another sign of the commitment of some leaders in academic medicine to confront the social, economic, ethical, and political issues of the health care system. No one was suggesting that medical schools should stop studying disease from the perspective of biology and the individual patient. However, many hoped that the study of health care delivery would be added to the medical school's traditional work.

That did not happen. Many schools began small programs in health services research, but throughout the 1970s, 1980s, and 1990s the field was generally considered a fringe activity—located in a department of public health or community medicine here, a program of general internal medicine there. Faculty who studied the cost, efficiency, and equity of the health care system were frequently considered renegades or second-class citizens—too eccentric or just not smart enough to tackle issues of real biology and medicine. Promotions and academic recognition for workers in the field came slowly and grudgingly. Few schools created an environment in which the problems of health care delivery could be examined as critically or enthusiastically as the problems of human biology. Most schools continued to regard scientific achievement as more important than social effectiveness. Leadership to help patients and the nation cope with the deficiencies of health care financing and delivery was seldom forthcoming.

Of course, there remained considerable room for debate about what medical schools' exact role in reshaping health care delivery should be. Was their proper contribution through study and investigation, the organization of demonstration programs that might serve as models, or direct political leadership and action? However, with few exceptions, medical schools embraced none of those approaches. Rather, they behaved as if there were no crisis at all in health care delivery. Considerable change was effected in health care delivery after 1965, but these changes, as other major developments in the delivery system since World War II, reflected primarily the voices of government, labor, business, consumers, and certain social scientists and not the input of medical professionals. In the late 1980s and 1990s, after a generation of ever-increasing public worry and frustration about the problems of cost and access, socially concerned physicians were still criticizing academic medicine for its narrow definition of its task and pleading with the schools to begin placing a high priority on health services research.[47]

In their growing commercialism, abuses of authorship, and relative lack of interest in the study or improvement of the American health care system, medical faculties were indicating a preoccupation with their own security and interests and an indifference to the needs and wishes of students and the larger society they were expected to serve. In this behavior they reflected many of the prevalent cultural values of the period. Many writers have pointed out that the 1970s and 1980s could be characterized as the era of the "Me generation," a time of ferocious materialism, and an age in which individual rights were emphasized while individual responsibilities to the community were ignored.[48] The spirit of the time was encapsulated in the title of the 1977 best-seller, *Looking Out for Number One*, and in the attitude of Wall Street in the 1980s that "greed is good." If academic medicine—or the practicing profession—appeared to be embracing an attitude that emphasized personal benefit while deemphasizing obligations to others, so did much of the rest of American society.

Yet, for academic medicine, there was something novel in this course of events. Since the beginning of the century, the nation's medical faculties had acted as a public trust, as evidenced by their behavior in the effort to create quality systems of undergraduate and graduate medical education, their leadership in public health and other reform movements during the progressive era, their many sacrifices during World War II, and their traditional commitment to bringing the fruits of medical research to the public without concern for personal financial profit. Now, something seemed to be missing—namely, that clear sense that medical faculties served first and foremost the public and not themselves. In the materialistic 1980s, many entrepreneurial physicians argued that economic incentives were necessary for basic and clinical research to proceed—that without such incentives few investigators would be motivated to develop new products or test their effectiveness. To this, Arnold Relman, then the editor of the *New England Journal of Medicine*, responded that "until very recently, intellectual fulfillment, professional recognition, and the satisfaction of contributing to medical progress were sufficient incentives."[49] In the 1960s, no one would have dared imagine that academic (or practicing) physicians would do anything but act in behalf of their patients and the people. By the 1980s academic physicians were being compared with corporate executives, stockbrokers, and financial scoundrels in their greed and self-serving behavior. Academic medicine was hardly alone in American society in placing personal gain above the welfare of others, but unlike many others, it had traditionally chosen to behave according to a different standard.

For many decades the justification for the privileged position of academic medicine—respect, autonomy to determine the course of medical education and standards of medical practice, support for teaching and research, and a respectable income for faculty who were given the freedom to do exactly what they wanted to do—resulted from the belief that academic health centers existed to advance the welfare of sick people, not themselves. Ironically, as academic medicine in the 1970s and 1980s demonstrated an increasing concern with its own interests and welfare, its centrality to the health of the American people never diminished. Academic health centers remained the center for teaching medical students, the leading site for graduate medical education, the major home for biomedical research, and the arbiter of clinical practice. The wide availability of well-trained doctors in the community reflected the good work of medical school faculties. So did the improving capabilities of medical practice, which were made possible by developments in medical research. Teaching hospitals, staffed by medical school faculties, continued to serve as the sites where the most complex problems in patient care were figured out. Even if the average patient did not need that level of sophistication, everyone benefited from the security of knowing that it was available. Larger contributions of academic health centers, such as the provision of charity care and the development of closer relationships with their local communities, also continued despite the perturbations noted above.

In short, the core missions of academic health centers were still being met. Academic health centers remained national resources with outstanding records of service and accomplishment. However, in an acquisitive age, academic medicine had lost its vision. More and more faculty were asking what they could get out of being a professor; fewer and fewer were asking why they were there or what they might contribute in return. If few medical professors bothered to explain their centrality for the public good to themselves or to others, it is hardly surprising that the public started to perceive them as just another special interest group. One can scarcely fault the public for losing sight of how essential academic health centers were to the well-being of the nation when medical educators themselves exhibited the same diminished vision.

17

Medical Education in an Era of Cost Containment and Managed Care

THE OVERARCHING CHARACTERISTIC of the environment of medical education during the twentieth century was the abundance of resources made available to it by the public. Particularly following World War II, with the rise of the National Institutes of Health and the enactment of Medicare and Medicaid, academic health centers experienced such profound growth in their income, size, and power that leaders of those institutions sometimes forgot they were not autonomous. In this luxurious and forgiving environment, medical schools could get away with their incessant growth, profligate practice style, inadequate teaching of cost-effectiveness, and reluctance to assume leadership in addressing major problems in health care financing and delivery.

In the mid-1980s, that situation rapidly began to change. A new paradigm became accepted, which emphasized that there were limits to what the country could spend on health care, given the reality of finite resources in the face of a seemingly inexhaustible demand for medical services. Concern about health care costs had been growing for many years, but in the 1980s cost-consciousness finally began to dominate the health care debate. Accordingly, the pass-through era of reimbursement of medical care came to an end. In its place, a competitive marketplace for medical care emerged—one that focused on prospective payment, lower prices, and the restricted use of hospitals and specialized services. No one expected that the country would spend less on health care in the decades ahead, but it was clear that resources would no longer be so freely available for the asking. If the twentieth century had been the age of abundance for medicine, it appeared that the twenty-first would be the era of resource constraints.

These new forces left academic health centers reeling. Both teaching hospitals and medical schools were threatened, even as they undertook major steps to reduce costs and operate more efficiently. Teaching hospitals found it increasingly difficult to attract patients when insurers were no longer so willing to pay the higher costs they incurred from education, research, and charity care. Medical schools during the preceding generation had grown dependent on clinical income as their primary source of revenue. Now that their margins from clinical practice were falling, their ability to cross-subsidize education and research also began to fall. The illusion of autonomy was shattered.

Always entrepreneurial, leaders of medical schools and teaching hospitals reacted in clever ways to the competitive new environment. In the 1980s, effective steps were taken to increase the volume of care they delivered and to find novel sources of income. In the 1990s, these efforts were supplemented by a new wave of mergers, acquisitions, affiliations, and the creation of so-called "integrated delivery systems." By the end of the decade, it appeared that some of the angst among medical educators about managed care had lessened.

Yet, as academic health centers fought for survival, education and research all too often were overlooked. Institutional survival was being accomplished, but in the process the core principles those institutions had been entrusted to preserve were being sacrificed. As the end of the century approached, academic health centers were rapidly losing their academic qualities—even as many medical educators proudly congratulated themselves on their "proactive" behavior in the changed marketplace.

Vassals of the Marketplace

Since the 1960s, the generosity of federal and private third party payers had resulted in a supportive environment for academic health centers. However, the dependence of academic health centers on clinical income represented an unstable situation. The public was becoming increasingly anxious about medical costs, which in many opinion polls was perceived as the most urgent problem of the health care system.[1] The escalating price of health care interfered with the international competitiveness of American corporations and, in the 1980s, aggravated the problem of a soaring federal budget deficit. Tragically, even though the percentage of the gross domestic product spent on health care rose dramatically in the 20 years after Medicare and Medicaid were enacted, millions of employees were afraid to change jobs for fear of losing their health benefits, and millions of other Americans remained uninsured or underinsured.[2]

The traditional professional explanation for rising health care expenditures was on the grounds of quality. Good cut-rate medicine was considered an oxymoron. In the 1980s this viewpoint was challenged. John Wennberg, a health services researcher at Dartmouth, documented the existence of widely divergent practice styles from one geographical region to another with no apparent differences in outcome. He showed, for instance, that physicians in one Vermont town performed tonsillectomies three times as often as physicians in nearby towns, even though there was no evidence that the children in the one town were any sicker.[3] Other health services researchers demonstrated that many common procedures were greatly overused. For example, one study of coronary angiography and coronary artery bypass surgery in community hospitals found that only about one-half were performed for clearly appropriate medical indications.[4] In addition, in an era of selfishness and greed, it became clear that some hospitals and doctors were taking advantage of the fee-for-service system by engaging in abusive billing practices such as "unbundling," "upcoding," and even billing for services not rendered.[5] Such developments did much to undermine the authority of the medical profession and emboldened managers, policy experts, and government officials to challenge professional autonomy and control in ways that once would have been inconceivable.

In the 1980s, with health care costs soaring, professional authority weakening, and third party payers increasingly unhappy, a fundamental transformation of the health care system began. Third party payers revolted by demanding—and receiving—lower prices. In the new (and still evolving) system, there was marked skepticism toward the professional authority of physicians, unprecedented external oversight and review of medical decision-making, intense price-based competition among doctors and hospitals, and unparalleled opportunities for large, profit-seeking corporations in health care. Control shifted from the "providers" (doctors and hospitals) to the "payers" (insurance companies and managed care organizations), whose power resulted from their control of the flow of patients and their skill at exploiting the oversupply of doctors and hospital beds.[6]

The era of cost containment began in earnest in 1983, when the federal government passed legislation establishing the "prospective payment" of hospital bills for Medicare patients. Under this new system, Medicare paid a set fee per case, determined by the patient's diagnosis. Diagnoses were placed in one of 467 diagnosis-related groups (DRGs). If the costs of a patient's care were less than the DRG payment, a hospital could keep the difference as a profit. If the costs ran higher than the DRG payment, the hospital would suffer a loss. Subsequently most private insurers adopted similar payment systems.

Prospective payment immediately changed the rules of hospital economics. Efficiency now mattered. Hospitals received a fixed amount of money per case, regardless of their actual expenses. Financial success depended much more heavily than before on lowering costs, utilizing resources more efficiently, and better management. Most important of all, financial success depended on seeing a greater number of patients more quickly. Hospitals made money under the DRG system not by maintaining a high occupancy per se but by attracting a large volume of patients who were admitted and discharged quickly. The new goal of hospitals became a rapid "throughput" of patients.

For teaching hospitals, the advent of the DRG system intensified an already competitive marketplace. Over the preceding decade, community hospitals—staffed increasingly by well-trained specialists produced by the academic health centers—had been posing stiffer and stiffer competition to the old-line teaching hospitals. With prospective payment, the competition for patients needing specialty care became even more intense. Community and teaching hospitals both needed more patients than ever to keep their beds full—and for the first time the supply of patients did not seem inexhaustible. To attract patients, teaching hospitals began aggressively marketing and advertising their services and worked hard to become more comfortable, convenient, and friendly.[7] They also established new affiliations with smaller hospitals to increase the referral of patients for tertiary care, in some cases developing elaborate referral networks that included hospitals hundreds of miles away.

To make matters more difficult for teaching hospitals, one type of patient came to them without recruitment: uninsured and indigent patients. For-profit hospital chains (like Humana and Hospital Corporation of America), which had grown enormously in size and market share since the passage of Medicare, saw their mission as profits, not the care of the medically needy.[8] Out of economic necessity, most nonprofit community hospitals greatly reduced the amount of charity care they provided—to the point that a few critics began to argue that their tax-exempt status should be revoked. This left teaching hospitals, together with municipal and veterans hospitals, as the primary dispensers of charity care. More distressing still, in the 1980s a new and disturbing development occurred that would have been completely unacceptable a mere few years before: the so-called "economic transfer," or the "dumping" of uninsured patients from a private hospital to a teaching or municipal hospital. We are "like mama," one teaching hospital spokesman observed. "Everyone else will throw you out, but you can always come home to mama."[9]

When prospective payment began, many feared for the future of teaching hospitals. The DRG system did not take into account the severity of illness within a given diagnostic category. Of two patients with congestive heart failure, the sicker patient with a more complicated and costly course was more likely to be treated at a teaching hospital than at a community hospital, placing teaching hospitals at a marked disadvantage financially. Nevertheless, most teaching hospitals were able to grow and thrive in the 1980s. This was because they successfully reduced their costs, developed large referral networks, and improved patient "throughput." In addition, teaching hospitals benefited from additional payments that Medicare's DRG system made for "outlier" (unusually costly) patients and for the expenses of education, research, and charity care (the so-called "indirect" graduate medical education payment). Even most private insurers that adopted the DRG system continued to pay more to teaching hospitals in recognition of their additional costs.

Though academic health centers weathered the new system of prospective payment, the rapid spread of managed care in the 1980s and 1990s proved a more formidable and hostile development. The term managed care referred to a large variety of reimbursement plans in which third party payers attempted to control costs by limiting the utilization of medical services, in contrast to the "hands off" style of traditional indemnity (fee-for-service) health insurance. Managed care organizations used various strategies to exercise strong control over their doctors and hospitals, but they achieved most of their savings by reducing the number of hospitalizations and the use of specialists. The most extreme (or "tightest") form of managed care were the health maintenance organizations (HMOs), which themselves represented a diverse array of organizations. The earliest HMOs, such as Kaiser-Permanente, were nonprofit, but in the 1980s the HMO industry came to be dominated by for-profit corporations. As health care costs continued to soar, enrollment in HMOs and other managed care organizations grew rapidly, with particularly explosive growth occurring after the announcement of President Clinton's health care plan in 1993. By 1995, over 50 million Americans received their health care in HMOs, compared with less than 9 million in 1980, and tens of millions more were in "looser" forms of managed care, such as preferred provider organizations (PPOs) and discounted fee-for-service. Only 26 percent of employees who received their insurance through work in 1996 were enrolled in traditional fee-for-service plans, compared with 71 percent as recently as 1988.[10]

An enormous public controversy erupted in the 1990s over whether managed care organizations were denying needed care, whether the companies were placing profits before patients, and whether the quality of care had suffered. Nevertheless, one fact was indisputable: the adverse impact of managed care on medical education and academic health centers. For instance, in the 1990s HMOs brought about a shift from specialized to general medical care. As large employers or contractors of physicians, they controlled much of the marketplace, and they hired or retained far fewer specialists and subspecialists, compared with the fee-for-service system. Newly trained specialists encountered difficulty finding practice opportunities, and specialists in practice were often unceremoniously dropped by HMOs, including some with sterling professional credentials.[11] Medical students took note of these events. The percentage of students seeking residency in a primary care field finally increased, from a nadir of 14.6 percent in 1992 to 27.7 percent in 1995.[12] Forces external to medical education proved more powerful in influencing students to choose careers in primary care than did a generation of exhortations and special programs by medical faculties.

The rise of HMOs also caused some to reconsider the number of doctors the country's medical schools and residency programs should be producing. In the mid-1990s, there were about 240 doctors per 100,000 people in the United States, while HMOs typically had no more than 100 to 140 doctors per 100,000 enrollees.[13] For the first time since the Great Depression, physicians experienced what those in most other fields had long known: the lack of job security. Even primary care physicians faced the prospect of unemployment or underemployment, as many HMOs began to replace some of them with nurse practitioners and physician assistants. Accordingly, the Pew Health Professions Commission called for a 20 to 25 percent reduction in the number of U.S. medical students and a 20 percent reduction in the number of medical schools.[14] Other educators and organizations called for a reduction in the large number of international medical graduates who continued to do residency training in the United States, most of whom remained in the country afterwards to practice.[15]

Most notably, managed care threatened the financial viability of academic health centers. To the surprise of some, academic health centers had fared well under DRGs because they could respond to lower payments by increasing patient volume. However, managed care plans utilized volume as well as price restrictions. HMOs and other managed care organizations emphasized more ambulatory care, less hospitalization, and the substitution of primary care physicians for specialists whenever possible—trends that directly worked against the strengths of academic health centers. When hospitalization was required, price-sensitive HMOs tried to avoid teaching hospitals because of their higher costs, even though these hospitals typically had the highest reputations for clinical excellence. For example, in the late 1990s HMOs were refusing to send open-heart patients to the University of Arizona Medical Center, despite the fact that the center had midrange charges and the lowest mortality rates for heart surgery in Tucson.[16] Particularly after 1993, when the spread of managed care accelerated, the number of admissions to teaching hospitals fell, occupancy rates plummeted, and many teaching hospitals began closing beds.[17]

To attract patients from managed care organizations, academic health centers had to compete with community hospitals on the basis of price. This was no easy task. Because of education, research, charity care, and a sicker case mix of patients, the costs of teaching hospitals ran approximately 30 percent higher than those of community hospitals.[18] Previously, third party payers were willing to accept higher bills from teaching hospitals to cross-subsidize these socially important activities. Now, insurers were increasingly unwilling to do so, insisting instead on paying only for the costs of hospital care actually incurred by their members. Accordingly, the margins academic health centers depended on for education and research were whittled away. In 1996 in many markets (for instance, Boston), the reputation of a teaching hospital brought it only a

5 to 10 percent premium over community hospitals, while in especially competitive markets (for example, San Diego and San Francisco), academic health centers commanded a premium of at most 3 to 5 percent.[19] Some academic hospitals claimed they were forced to price services below cost.[20] Academic health centers now found themselves in a buyers' market indifferent to their needs—a market where the private sector was rapidly withdrawing from the support of socially valuable functions it had nurtured all century long.

Other sources of income for academic health centers could not compensate for the shortfall from private insurers. Indeed, in the 1990s, most of these revenue streams were stagnant or declining. Federal research dollars were leveling off, while federal reimbursement for the overhead expenses of medical research (indirect costs) was falling. State and local governments were decreasing their support of medical education, Congress was proposing caps on the Medicare and Medicaid budgets, and the federal government was considering a major reduction in Medicare's direct and indirect payments for graduate medical education. The latter, a proxy for the increased costs of teaching hospitals and a particularly important source of revenue for academic health centers, was in danger of being cut by as much as 50 percent. The amount of money at stake was too large to be offset by tuition, philanthropy, endowment income, or corporate research grants and contracts.[21]

In the price-competitive age, the closure or consolidation of hospitals of all types became commonplace as the marketplace began to force excess capacity out of the nation's hospital system. However, teaching hospitals, because of their additional costs, were at particular risk. In 1990, the average operating margin of major teaching hospitals was 1.4 percent, compared with more than 4 percent for other hospitals.[22] By 1994, a dozen academic health centers were already losing money, and many more were in precarious financial positions.[23] Teaching hospitals worked hard to reduce their costs, but with the level of payment so low, greater efficiencies alone were not enough to stave off the specter of insolvency. The average community hospital, without expensive state-of-the-art facilities for the sickest patients, without major educational and research programs, and without a significant burden of charity care, stood the greatest chance of remaining financially viable.

The spread of managed care threatened the economic viability of medical schools as well as teaching hospitals. For nearly a generation, faculty practice had represented the most important source of income for medical schools, and nationwide about 28 percent of clinical income was channeled directly into the support of academic programs. From 1989 to 1995, as the HMO movement spread, total medical school revenues from professional fees increased. This reflected the hiring of new clinical faculty, a greater concentration on providing patient care by existing faculty, and more complete reporting. However, because of deeply discounted payments by insurers and new expenses incurred by the plans, the margins on faculty practice plans significantly fell. As a result, discretionary revenue available to medical schools to support academic programs dropped sharply. Many schools—even institutions of national renown—reported faculty layoffs, salary freezes, and the closure of important academic programs. These changes were most pronounced at schools in areas where the penetration of managed care was the highest.[24]

In the mid-1990s, as managed care became pervasive, a wave of mergers, acquisitions, and divestitures of teaching hospitals and medical schools began—the first such restructuring of the institutions of medical education since the immediate post-Flexner period. For instance, the Brigham and Women's Hospital and the Massachusetts General Hospital in Boston merged, as did Presbyterian Hospital and the New York Hospital, the Mount Sinai and New York University Medical Centers, Barnes and Jewish Hospitals in St. Louis, Hahnemann Medical School and Medical College of Pennsylvania in Philadelphia, and the hospitals of Stanford University and the University of California, San Francisco. The University of Minnesota and Indiana University merged their hospitals with local hospitals, while Tulane, St. Louis University, and George Washington, among others, sold or leased their university-owned hospitals to investor-owned proprietary chains like Columbia/HCA.[25] The dean of Medical College of Pennsylvania, speaking of his institution's merger with Hahnemann, said, "I wish I could tell you we created this new institution out of a sense of altruism, but truly it was out of a sense of fear and survival."[26] His fears were well founded, for in 1998 the Allegheny Health, Education and Research Foundation, a nonprofit hospital chain that had bought both medical schools and organized their merger, declared bankruptcy. (Later that year Tenet Healthcare, a for-profit hospital chain with a scandal-tainted past, took control of the Allegheny system, and Drexel University received responsibility for the medical school.)

One can readily understand the wish of HMOs not to subsidize the public activities of academic health centers. For-profit organizations dominated the field (in the mid-1990s, eight of the ten largest HMOs were investor-owned), and their sole legal responsibility was to increase shareholder value. Money spent on education and research that would benefit society as a whole without bringing immediate benefits to investors or their own panel of patients was not in their best interest. Nonprofit HMOs, smaller and less well capitalized, had to keep premiums low to compete in the hostile marketplace. A few, such as Harvard Community Health Plan, set aside a small portion of their yearly premiums to support educational activities, but by the mid-1990s such examples were rare. In 1995, pressured by its competitors, even Harvard Community Health Plan decreased the amount of money it spent on medical education from 1 percent of revenues to 0.45 percent, and that contribution was expected to be decreased further.[27]

HMOs were in a fortunate position. They could utilize the knowledge and techniques developed at the academic health centers, employ the doctors and other health care professionals trained at the teaching centers, and leave the financial support of medical education and research to someone else.[28] Moreover, they could ask—with considerable merit—whether it was appropriate any longer for academic health centers to use revenues from patient care to help support education and research. Why not pay for education and research totally from sources of funding designated specifically for those purposes?

The problem for academic health centers, however, was that no one in the 1990s had much enthusiasm for helping fund education and research. Universities, philanthropic organizations, and federal, state, and local governments were all under considerable budget-reducing pressures of their own. "What is happening now is a nightmare," a prominent medical dean observed. "Every funding stream we have used to pay for [education and] research is being hacked apart."[29] For the American health care system as a whole, a dangerous situation was beginning to unfold: American medicine was losing its future-directedness. The main research and development unit of the American health care system—the academic health center—was being allowed to wither as cost-containing mechanisms designed for the hospital industry as a whole ignored its special needs and mission. Like many other American industries, the health care industry was engaging in short-term thinking, adopting cost-reducing and profit-maximizing strategies for today that weakened its ability to meet the challenges of the long term. As a result, the prospect of having well-trained doctors and improved health care in the future was starting to diminish.

The Loss of Time and the Erosion of the Learning Environment

Throughout the twentieth century, the strength of clinical education in America had arisen mainly from the exceptional learning opportunities available to students and house officers in the wards and clinics of teaching hospitals. A diverse array of patients was present, students actively participated in their care, and house officers assumed increasing amounts of responsibility for their management under the appropriate supervision of faculty. Time was present for learners and teachers alike. Students and house officers could observe first-hand the natural history of disease and therapeutics, learn the nuances of clinical medicine unencumbered by too many extraneous assignments, and explore in depth issues of particular interest. Faculty were not only well-qualified to teach but had sufficient time to devote to that work.

Since the 1960s, teaching hospitals had been gradually losing some of their earlier educational value. In part this resulted from the increasingly complex nature of the care they provided. In specialties like pediatrics and obstetrics and gynecology, many academic health centers had to establish teaching affiliations with community hospitals to provide students and house officers enough exposure to patients with routine problems. In addition, new technologies played a role. For example, the development in the 1980s of less invasive surgical techniques and the use of new anesthetic agents allowed many operations to be performed safely on an outpatient basis. Most important, inpatient medical teaching had been a response to the educational needs of an era in which acute diseases predominated. Inpatient instruction was less suitable for chronic diseases, which were primarily treated in physicians' offices. Only the unusually severe exacerbation of hypertension, emphysema, or congestive heart failure, for instance, required hospitalization. For the most part such conditions could be satisfactorily managed in outpatient settings, where good care could actually reduce the need for hospitalization. Accordingly, the practice of using mainly inpatient teaching to prepare for an office-based career was no longer so justifiable.[30]

In the 1980s, however, the learning environment of the inpatient wards rapidly began to deteriorate. The implementation of Medicare's DRG system of prospective hospital payment created a new objective for hospital care: speed. Almost immediately, the average length of stay for all patients fell by 25 percent (and for elderly patients, by more than 50 percent).[31] Additional pressures from managed care organizations in the 1990s resulted in even further decreases in the length of stay, so that by the middle of the decade the average length of stay had fallen to 5 or 6 days, compared with 10 or 12 days before prospective payment began.[32] In addition, new regulations of many managed care organizations—often promulgated for economic rather than medical reasons—resulted in the removal of many workups, procedures, and treatments from the hospital to the less expensive ambulatory setting. More and more, the inpatient units of teaching hospitals came to be populated with two types of patients: one group that was desperately ill, requiring intensive care or highly complex procedures; another that was admitted the day of an elective procedure and discharged as soon as possible thereafter, often within 24 hours.

The medical effects of such a dramatic reduction in the length of stay and of moving so many procedures out of the hospital were controversial. Nevertheless, one consequence was clearly apparent: the erosive effects on the learning environment of hospital wards. It became much harder for learners to acquire problem-solving skills when patients were admitted with their diagnoses known and treatment plans already determined. Surgical residents, meeting patients under the drapes of the operating table, could still learn how to remove a gall bladder, but their opportunity to develop the clinical experience and judgmental capacity to decide who might actually need the procedure was severely compromised. In addition, as the "throughput" of patients increased, so did the work of interns and residents, who were now admitting many more patients. This increased workload often came in the face of a decrease in the number of nurses and other support personnel, as low reimbursement rates from managed care organizations forced many hospitals to reduce staffing drastically.

Most pernicious of all from the standpoint of education, house officers to a considerable extent were reduced to work-up machines and disposition-arrangers: admitting patients and planning their discharge, one after another, with much less time than before to examine them, confer with attending physicians, teach medical students, attend conferences, read the literature, and reflect and wonder. They were also deprived of much of the opportunity to follow the course of disease since patients would be so quickly discharged—often before the results of important tests had come back and sometimes before a final diagnosis had been made. Ironically, these changes were occurring at a time that both medical and nonmedical groups were becoming more vocal in calling to restore the primacy of "education" in undergraduate and graduate medical education.

The consequences of abbreviated hospital stays for the education of students and house officers have yet to be systematically analyzed, but anecdotal evidence suggested that the effects were not positive. At Johns Hopkins, for instance, house officers in many cases became "just pairs of hands" and students, "just observers."[33] At the Columbia-Presbyterian Medical Center, many faculty felt that teaching rounds dealt too much with administrative chores and not enough with educational issues.[34] At the University of Iowa College of Medicine, faculty described an increasing tendency of residents "to be too quick to accept admitting diagnoses from referring physicians and to pursue the evaluation of the most likely diagnoses to the exclusion of other pertinent diagnoses." The Iowa faculty also observed a decline in the intellectual quality of attending rounds in response to the overarching pressure on residents and attending physicians for speed and efficiency.[35]

As the educational value of inpatient wards diminished, some faculty began proposing that greater emphasis be given to ambulatory education.[36] Ambulatory rotations provided the opportunity to see a broader range of diseases (including some conditions that were now managed completely on an outpatient basis) as well as more patients with new, undiagnosed conditions. The ambulatory setting seemed especially well suited to teach about chronic diseases, disease prevention, health promotion, population medicine, psychosocial medicine, and many of the social and economic issues pertaining to medical practice. Calls for more ambulatory teaching were not new, but in view of the changes wrought by the new payment system for health care, such pleas began to assume much greater urgency.

From the standpoint of educational theory, such arguments made good sense. The essentials of a rich learning environment were site independent. What mattered from the perspective of education was making certain that a broad patient base, a skilled and accessible teaching faculty, a scholarly intellectual atmosphere, the opportunity for house officers to assume responsibility for key decisions, and, most important, the time to learn and practice medicine effectively were present. John Dewey and Abraham Flexner undoubtedly would have approved of increasing the amount of ambulatory education, as long as an appropriate learner-centered environment was maintained.

Moving clinical education to ambulatory sites was not easy. Traditional medical school attitudes that disparaged outpatient work had to be changed. Considerable upgrading of the physical facilities and data systems in hospital clinics and faculty offices was necessary so that they could serve as model facilities for high quality ambulatory care. In off-campus sites (like private doctors' offices), steps had to be taken to overcome the reluctance of private patients to be used in medical education. (Studies showed a willingness of private patients to allow students and house officers to take histories and perform physical examinations—but not much more.[37]) Significant problems lay in securing adequate financing for outpatient teaching. Medicare reimbursement formulas for graduate medical education included salary support for residents working in hospital clinics, but not for residents working in community health centers or private doctors' offices outside the hospital. Teaching hospitals also faced the financial burden of providing additional medical coverage for inpatients while residents were seeing outpatients.[38] By the 1990s, only a few fields—most notably family practice and pediatrics, and to a lesser extent, primary care internal medicine—had made ambulatory work an important part of their training.

However, managed care imposed additional constraints on all who would teach in ambulatory settings. There, too, the dictate of managed care for speed and high volume undermined the quality of education. Payment plans from managed care organizations varied, but they typically contained strong financial incentives for physicians to see their ambulatory patients as quickly as possible. The pace of care in the fee-for-service system had hardly been slow, but in the 1990s the emphasis of payers on "clinical productivity" (that is, seeing large volumes of patients as quickly as possible) reached unprecedented levels. Academic health centers, with increasing numbers of managed care contracts, were highly vulnerable to these pressures. They now had to provide outpatient teaching in an environment in which their reimbursement depended on how well they maximized the "throughput" of patients.

By the late 1990s, most academic health centers had begun providing students and house officers more exposure to outpatient care. However, few of them had solved the problem of assuring educational quality in the face of managed care's imperative to be clinically "productive." Rigorous systematic studies had not been done, but, as in the case of inpatient education, numerous reports suggested that the quality of education was often compromised because of the pressure to see patients quickly. In particular, students and house officers were frequently relegated to the role of observers, faculty accessibility was often poor (particularly when they were expected to practice while they taught), and teaching tended to be cursory.[39] Moreover, the hurried environment carried negative implications for the all-important latent learning of the "hidden curriculum." Habits of thoroughness, attentiveness to detail, questioning, listening, thinking, and caring were difficult if not impossible to instill when both patient care and teaching were conducted in an eight- or ten-minute office visit. Few learners were likely to conclude that these sacrosanct qualities were important when they failed to observe them in their teachers and role models.

To some medical educators, HMOs represented a possible site to cultivate ambulatory teaching—particularly the group or staff model HMOs, which offered the advantage of being large, centralized group practices. For many years a few nonprofit HMOs had sponsored accredited residency programs, especially in internal medicine, and about 15 percent of HMOs had an agreement with an academic health center to serve as an ambulatory care rotation site (though rotation through an HMO rarely served as an important part of the medical school or residency experience).[40] With so much of medical practice now located in ambulatory settings, and with HMOs enrolling more and more members each year, the potential of HMOs to become vibrant sites for education and research in ambulatory medicine could not be denied. The most forceful spokesman for this concept was Gordon T. Moore, a dedicated medical educator at Harvard Medical School and director of the teaching programs at Harvard Pilgrim Health Care, a large nonprofit HMO in Boston. Moore advanced the concept of the "teaching HMO," which in his view had "the potential to transform academic medicine in the next century, just as the teaching hospital transformed it in this century."[41]

The problem, however, was that sufficient funds to support medical education properly in HMOs had not been found. Academic health centers were financially strapped, and most HMOs did not wish to pay for the costs of medical education. Moreover, under competitive pressures— or the push for still greater profits—HMOs were unable or unwilling to slow the pace of ambulatory care sufficiently to accommodate the needs of medical education. Even at Harvard Community Health Plan, one of the nation's most medically respected HMOs (and the forerunner of Harvard Pilgrim Health Care), staff doctors were under such intense pressure to see more patients that in 1991 they revolted, forcing the resignation of the chief executive.[42] Moore himself acknowledged that one of the most difficult obstacles to realizing the concept of a teaching HMO was "how to eliminate or pay for lost patient care productivity while teaching."[43]

During the late 1980s and the 1990s, the root of the difficulty in maintaining a quality learning environment—both for inpatient and outpatient teaching—was that good medical education, like good education in any field, was expensive. A large part of the expense was the time required. In the fee-for-service era, when pressures from third party payers for quick hospital discharges and rapid-fire outpatient visits were minimal, time was a hidden educational cost. In the era of cost containment, third party payers were no longer willing to pay for educational time. As a result, the historic marriage between medical education and practice was threatened.

This was not the first time in the twentieth century that changes in health care financing threatened the country's system of medical education. The spread of private medical insurance after World War II and the passage of Medicare and Medicaid in 1965 had reduced the size of the ward service, creating major problems for medical education. However, the loss of time was a much more serious threat. More than any other reason, quality in clinical education had depended on the presence of sufficient time in medical practice to allow learners to learn and teachers to teach. Now managed care was taking that time away.

Cost containment, of course, was much needed and long overdue. However, cost containment was implemented during the managed care era in a way that did not take into consideration the needs of medical education. With its mandate for speed and industrial efficiency—seeing the most patients in the least possible time—managed care resulted in a deterioration of the learning environment in both inpatient and outpatient settings. As the twenty-first century approached, these pressures threatened to cause a significant erosion in the quality of medical education in the United States. This was true even at academic health centers that managed to remain financially solvent, something they could now hope to do only by seeing increasing numbers of patients ever more quickly.

Proactive Words; Reactive Behavior

The advent of the era of cost containment brought a new type of challenge to academic health centers. The historic feuding within medical schools and teaching hospitals—powerful interest groups competing with one another for their share of an abundant pool of resources—gave way in importance to the challenge of surviving in an unfriendly marketplace that was diverting patients and clinical revenues away from academic health centers. As a result, fear, low morale, and an overwhelming sense of loss of control spread widely. Yet, academic health centers also responded rapidly to the hostile new environment. Realizing that they could not wait to be rescued from outside, leaders of academic medicine attempted to take their futures into their own hands.

One response was to seek new soures of income. Such efforts began in the 1980s with the previously described attempts of academic health centers to increase their ties to industry. Some medical schools or hospitals also established for-profit subsidiary corporations to run nonmedical businesses, using after-tax income to support the work of the medical center. A typical example was Johns Hopkins's Dome Corporation, established in 1984, which developed and managed real estate for the benefit of the medical institutions and university. By the late 1990s, however, such approaches had not progressed far, and income from these sources hardly began to offset the shrinking margins from clinical practice.

A second response was to seek greater operational efficiencies. For instance, many medical schools redesigned their faculty practice plans so there would be one plan for the entire school rather than separate plans for each department. The presence of a single organizational structure offered the opportunity for considerable cost-savings and proved helpful in negotiating contracts with HMOs and other third party payers. Medical schools also reexamined the way research was paid for and conducted—for instance, by encouraging individual scientists and departments to cooperate in the purchase and use of expensive equipment.

Teaching hospitals, too, scrutinized their management practices. The end of a half century of retrospective reimbursement placed a new emphasis on responsible, skilled management. To combat waste and inefficiency, teaching hospitals aggressively consolidated operations, imposed tighter cost controls, and negotiated more advantageous contracts with vendors. They streamlined the complex processes of patient care by utilizing business techniques such as "continuous quality improvement" and "reengineering." They also developed the ability to track money more precisely through the intricate hospital world. This allowed them to begin identifying the cross-subsidies occurring in the teaching, research, and patient care enterprises.

As academic health centers addressed the issue of cost containment, no cherished program or assumption went unexamined. Because of shrinking clinical margins and threatened cuts in Medicare's payment for graduate medical education, some institutions initiated reductions in their residency size. For instance, Duke announced a cut in the size of its residency program of up to 30 percent.[44] In some cities medical educators developed hospital "consortia" for graduate medical education in which residency programs were spread among multiple sponsoring organizations.[45] Medical faculties made tenure more difficult to obtain by limiting the number of tenured positions they awarded. (This was a response not only to the threat of decreasing resources but also to new federal regulations ending mandatory retirement at age 65.[46]) At long last faculties began reexamining the way they taught and practiced medicine, placing greater emphasis on proper training for clinical uncertainty and the appropriate utilization of medical resources. (How unfortunate, some felt, that it took the jolt of managed care to prod medical schools into doing what many knew they should have been doing all along.)

Nevertheless, prudent management and a rigid cost-containment program did not represent a complete solution, given HMOs and insurance companies that were not only paying much lower prices but diverting patients from academic health centers as well. By now, teaching hospitals had a monopoly only on unusually specialized care (sometimes called quaternary care) like organ transplantation and severe body burns. The small number of patients requiring such care was hardly sufficient to keep a hospital solvent or maintain a teaching program. Teaching hospitals, like all hospitals, had high fixed costs. No amount of operating efficiency could offset the fiscal drain when half or two-thirds of the beds were empty. Accordingly, many academic health centers responded in yet another way: by competing aggressively for a higher market share of patients. As leaders of the Columbia-Presbyterian Medical Center observed, "We must market ourselves to the highest bidder in order to survive and thrive."[47]

Efforts of academic health centers to increase their referral base began in the early 1980s with the networking arrangements mentioned earlier. In response to Medicare's DRG system, one academic center after another established affiliations with primary and secondary care hospitals and individual physician practices to try to increase the referral of patients. The competition for patients became even keener as the HMO movement grew stronger. Referrals from HMOs were dictated by organizational policy and not necessarily by the particular wishes of participating patients or physicians. Accordingly, academic health centers began to participate in managed care initiatives, something some academic leaders had thought they never would do. The only question regarding a relationship with an HMO, one teaching hospital administrator declared in 1985, was "whether to develop your own or affiliate with one already in place."[48]

In the 1990s, many of these loosely organized patient care networks evolved into more tightly organized integrated delivery systems (IDSs). An IDS represented an interlocking bottom-to-top health care system that offered a complete continuum of health care services from primary care to complex surgery to home health care and did so for a defined population at a preset price. An important characteristic of these organizations was their "vertical integration." That is, they contained not only an academic health center but primary and secondary care hospitals, individual medical practices, nursing homes, rehabilitation centers, hospices, psychiatric facilities, and home health care programs. Academic health centers typically built their networks by purchase or joint venture. This provided the teaching centers greater stability than if they were to exist independently as vendors of specialized services to insurers and other health care systems. To assure enough referrals to the teaching hospital in an era of declining hospitalization rates, an academic IDS had to be responsible for a huge number of patient lives—as many as one million or more.

The creation of IDSs began around the time that proposals for health care reform were being made during President Clinton's first term. Because they had a single management structure, IDSs could negotiate as a unit with large purchasers of health care for patient contracts. With the collapse of federal legislative efforts, government purchasing alliances did not appear, but academic health centers that belonged to a health care system found themselves in a better position to deal with the larger and stronger HMOs that did emerge. Just as major differences existed from one academic health center to another, there were also large differences among academic IDSs, particularly in regard to the degree that the medical school was a dominant or subsidiary partner of the larger system.[49]

Regardless of whether a medical school became a formal part of a health care system, all schools in the managed care era began delivering more personal patient care than ever before. The clinical faculty of most medical schools in essence became members of large multispecialty group practices. Most faculties expanded their services to include the provision of large amounts of primary care, not just referral care as before. Some schools hired primary care physicians as full-time staff to deliver care in satellite centers located throughout a broad geographic area; other schools bought existing primary care practices and provided the physicians faculty titles. Administrators applied industrial productivity models to faculty practice. Faculty were regarded as "productive" insofar as they saw large numbers of patients and kept patients and referring doctors satisfied. In a shrinking market, medical center officials viewed aggressive clinical competition as the key to preserving the institution's solvency.

As academic health centers restructured to meet the challenges of managed care, a number of subtle and not-so-subtle changes occurred. Hospitals generally proved more nimble and entrepreneurial than medical schools. Once teaching hospitals had followed the leadership and direction of the medical faculties; now, aided by their access to capital, they often became the dominant partner. Stories circulated in medical circles of hospital mergers, acquisitions, or affiliations initiated by the teaching hospital without the participation or even the knowledge of the medical school dean. The field of hospital administration became much more tightly affiliated with programs of business administration, and hospital administrators increasingly had M.B.A. degrees. The new hospital administrators assumed business titles (president or chief executive officer rather than superintendent or director), demanded and received corporate levels of compensation, and retained hordes of management consultants at fees, by some estimates, of up to 2 or 3 percent of the institution's revenues.[50] A corporate approach began to dominate the institutional culture of the academic health center, at both the teaching hospital and medical school. It became increasingly difficult to distinguish some academic health centers from the for-profit hospital chains and HMOs they so often criticized.

As market forces became stronger and more hostile, it was understandable that academic health centers became more businesslike and adopted corporate strategies. Yet as they did, an extraordinary inversion occurred: they began to lose sight of their mission and raison d'être. Academic health centers had always needed to do well financially so that they could do good work. Now, increasingly, doing well rather than doing good was becoming the end in itself, reflected in the high priority institutional officials gave to market share and financial return and the minimal consideration they gave to how the restructuring was affecting education and research. Administrators focused on financial issues and acquisition strategies; they rarely spoke of the academic health center as a force for good that might increase human knowledge and improve the human condition. Only a few years before, important teaching hospitals like Mount Sinai Hospital had prided themselves on doing much better academic work than hospitals with superior balance sheets.[51] Now, even leading teaching hospitals often seemed preoccupied with market domination and profitability rather than academic work and the quality of patient care.

Throughout the twentieth century, medical school faculties had experienced an unrelenting tension between their academic and clinical duties. Since World War II, the general direction at virtually every school had been toward increasing the amount of faculty practice. Prior to the 1980s, however, a successful balance had usually been struck between scholarly and clinical work. A scholarly environment could be maintained because the income generated by faculty practice was sufficient to underwrite the activities of the large numbers of faculty with more distinctly academic interests. The medical school's university mission of education and research thus flourished, even while its corporate business of providing clinical care grew larger and larger.

In the era of cost containment, however, a decided shift occurred at academic health centers. Clinical faculty, even those with scholarly interests, came under much more intense pressure to engage in patient care to help keep the medical school and teaching hospital afloat. As that happened, the balance between the medical school's academic and clinical missions was lost. Administrators even at leading research institutions like Johns Hopkins and Washington University began listing patient care first among the school's several missions.[52] That had always been expected of teaching hospitals but was novel for medical schools. For most of the twentieth century, medical schools had been anchored in the university, and their struggle was to make teaching hospitals as close to true university hospitals as possible. Now, medical schools were beginning to forsake their university moorings to join teaching hospitals in the new health care delivery system.

The extent of these changes differed from center to center, but the overall thrust was decidedly toward a subordination of the academic to the clinical mission. A study of seven sample academic health centers found that each was placing considerably less emphasis on teaching and research because of market-driven health reforms.[53] Another study of nine representative medical schools concluded that most (but not all) U.S.

schools would be able to secure a large enough patient base for survival, even in a competitive marketplace, but that most would experience a significant decrease in their levels of education and research.[54] A national study conducted by the Association of American Medical Colleges reached similar conclusions.[55] Prominent academicians worried that the term "academic medical center" was "becoming an oxymoron" and that "the bond between A and MC (in the A—MC)" was being stretched to the breaking point.[56]

Equally noteworthy, a few academic health centers in the late 1990s were beginning to avoid the most seriously ill patients, thereby aping the behavior of many competing hospital systems and HMOs that aggressively "cherry picked" the healthiest individuals. For instance, when the University of California, Irvine, Medical Center experienced financial difficulties from caring for too many patients with serious illnesses, the hospital chief told the staff, "[We can] no longer tolerate patients with complex and expensive-to-treat conditions being encouraged to transfer to our [medical] group." The faculty was generally, though reluctantly, supportive.[57] The traditional role of the teaching hospital as the dispenser of cutting edge care and as the medical court of last resort was being forgotten.

Much of the response of academic health centers to managed care was shaped by the corporate vision that had come to dominate those institutions. Encouraged by their management consultants, who typically did not have medical backgrounds, medical school and hospital officials approached academic health centers much as if those institutions were making cars or breakfast cereal. They applied the same management strategies to medical centers that were being widely used in other "industries": "restructuring," "reengineering," "downsizing," "right sizing," and "total quality management." Not to be outdone by their consultants, medical faculty and academic health center administrators began using these terms as glibly as anyone else. By the late 1990s such jargon was widespread not only in health management literature but also in some medical journals. In most businesses, all product lines were expected to be self-supporting. Hence, it was concluded that all product lines of the academic health center should be self-supporting as well. To remain competitive in the 1990s, so the argument went, academic health centers had to strip away research, teaching, and ancillary care costs and begin to make each of those activities pay for itself.

Relatively few medical school officials, hospital executives, or management consultants bothered to remember that business strategies needed to be employed cautiously because academic health centers were not just another business. An automobile company tries to sell customers cars whether they need one or not, and the company certainly would not give away cars for free. A teaching hospital acting properly, however, would not "sell" complex heart surgery to someone who did not need it, nor would the hospital deny a necessary operation to a patient who could not pay. Moreover, many of the most important functions of academic health centers were inherently cost-generating rather than income-producing—something that no amount of internal operating efficiency could overcome.[58] If an academic health center were a business, it could spin off unprofitable product lines, just as a manufacturing company could "downsize" by selling off a division that was losing money. But an academic health center did not have the luxury of spinning off unprofitable activities like education, research, and charity care without sacrificing its mission and selling off its soul.[59]

The irony was that a restructuring of academic health centers had long been needed. As Milton Eisenhower and others had pointed out since the 1950s, unbridled growth could not continue indefinitely, and medical schools and teaching hospitals needed to be prepared for a day when society would no longer be willing to satisfy their every request. To do that, medical schools had to do better at establishing academic priorities, eliminating outmoded or unnecessary programs, and operating efficiently. In addition, important changes were needed in the way faculties taught and studied medicine. Examples of changes that were long overdue included a reaffirmation of the importance of teaching, a true commitment to training learners for clinical uncertainty, greater emphasis on outpatient medicine, the reunification of preventive medicine and public health with clinical medicine, the cultivation of new disciplines like clinical epidemiology and technology assessment, and attention to the problems of the health care delivery system.

Yet, there was another important lesson of history to be considered: academic health centers could not be expected to be self-sufficient. From the time the first-generation medical educators began to create the system, the overriding need was for outside help. Financial support and public goodwill were indispensable if medical faculties were to receive the opportunity to produce well-trained doctors and to increase the capacity of medical care to ameliorate human suffering. One could debate where in society that support should come from, or how much it should be, or whether the size of the academic enterprise had grown dysfunctionally large. However, the principle that education and research required external help was immutable.

Proactive behavior, as exemplified by the creators of the system, involved generating outside sources of support for the university and the humanitarian missions of medical schools. It involved helping shape public health care policy, not merely reacting to policy changes to ensure institutional survival at any cost. As the twentieth century was ending, the organized effort and political will among medical educators to behave proactively did not appear to be great. The main emphasis was on expanding the clinical mission, even if that threatened to undermine the core principles upon which the academic health center was based. Critics who contended that medical education followed the flow of money, not principles, had evidence for that belief. Of course, establishing secure sources of external support for the public mission of medical centers was never easy, especially in periods of retrenchment and during times when the public viewed academic and professional leadership as self-serving. Without external help, however, education, research, and charity care would wither, and the moral and political legitimacy of the academic health center would be lost.

18

A Second Revolutionary Period

AS THE TWENTIETH CENTURY WAS ENDING, a second revolutionary period in American medical education had begun. Major characteristics of this period included the erosion of the clinical learning environment, the diminishing of faculty scholarship, and the reemergence of a proprietary system of medical schools in which the faculties' financial well-being was placed before education and research. Medical schools were beginning to leave the university for the health care delivery system, while hospitals once again had begun to dominate medical schools in establishing directions and policies for the joint institution.

In terms of classic studies of revolutions, it would be most accurate to view events of the 1990s as a "prerevolutionary" stage. Such periods are marked by unrest, turbulence, and the disintegration of existing institutions, but not yet by a new platform or model. It is already clear by the prerevolution that radical changes are in the offing, but it is still not certain what those changes will be.[1] (In contrast, the "Flexnerian revolution," which followed 50 years of reform efforts and espoused a new model of active learning, full-time academic faculty, and university-based medical schools, represented an advanced revolutionary stage.) For educators and physicians of the 1990s, the advantage of being in a "prerevolution" was that nothing was yet fixed. They had the opportunity to help shape the new order, just as they had previously shaped the existing one.

Unlike the first revolution, which arose primarily from within the profession, the immediate events leading to the second revolutionary period lay external to medical education. Strategies of cost containment designed for medicine as a whole did not take into account the public functions of academic health centers, particularly education and research. Market forces demanded lower prices, which increasingly compromised the ability of teaching centers to cross-subsidize education, research, and charity care from clinical revenues. Academic health centers found they were ill-prepared to protect their public missions in a competitive system that was eliminating the clinical cross-subsidies that since the mid-1960s had been their lifeblood.

However, the second revolutionary period also arose from circumstances within academic medicine itself. During the preceding generation medical schools had developed an overreliance on clinical income, and they had come to view perpetual growth as their birthright. They had taken advantage of a permissive, resource-rich environment to operate in a free-wheeling fashion with few restrictions and little accountability. Now that the new era of resource constraints had begun, they were poorly prepared to operate in a climate that no longer permitted them to do what they wished and spend what they wanted.

Many of the changes imposed on medical education and practice in the 1990s represented legitimate responses to long-standing problems, and a large number of physicians and educators welcomed them. Nevertheless, the current transformation of American medical education and practice will ultimately serve the public interest only if the fundamental principle illustrated by a century of history is remembered: that producing good doctors is a responsibility shared between society and medical faculties. The hope for the twenty-first century is that both parties will reaffirm their mutual responsibilities. In this optimistic but not utopian scenario, the public will remember that it must continue to invest properly in medical education and research to have outstanding doctors and medical care in the future, and it will insist on a practice environment that provides a market for the educational and research products of the academic health centers. In turn, a wiser, chastened medical profession will once again remember that its privileges and support must not only be earned but re-earned.

The Reemergence of a Proprietary System

By the late 1990s, it was far from clear what the ultimate effect of the cost containment era on medical schools and medical education would be. The managed care movement was still rapidly evolving, as was the response of each of the schools to it. However, it already appeared likely that the worst fears would not be realized. Only a few years earlier some had forecast the insolvency and closure of many teaching hospitals and medical schools, but by the end of the decade it appeared that most academic institutions would survive. The ability of medical schools and teaching hospitals to adapt to the changing marketplace was, as always, remarkable.

As the twenty-first century approached, however, the American medical school was rapidly becoming a different type of institution. The most conspicuous change was the continued expansion of the clinical enterprise. From 1986 to 1995, the number of full-time clinical faculty members increased by 52 percent at public medical schools and 64 percent at private schools, even as the number of basic science faculty plateaued and the number of medical students remained essentially unchanged.[2] Moreover, as noted in the last chapter, many academic health centers were rapidly evolving into academic health systems. By the late 1990s, the level of private practice by full-time faculty dwarfed that which anyone would have dared predict a mere 10 or 15 years before.

The continued expansion of faculty practice accomplished much good. Clinical income at medical schools continued to grow, coincident with the concerted effort to develop the private practice of the full-time clinical faculties.[3] To attract patients, medical schools became much more responsive to customer needs. Patient priorities, such as convenient parking and reasonable waiting times, became a priority of medical centers. Referring doctors at last found that their phone calls were returned and that discharge summaries were sent to them in a timely fashion. At some schools insurance companies could now deal with one integrated group practice representing the entire institution instead of a different practice plan for each division or department.

On the other hand, the aggressive expansion of faculty practice was a reflection of the deteriorating financial condition of most medical schools under managed care. As noted in the previous chapter, revenues from faculty practice continued to grow, but profit margins fell because of new expenses incurred by the plans and the markedly lower payments received from managed care organizations. There were fewer and fewer dollars available to support the academic mission. Medical schools were running on an ever-quickening treadmill—seeing more and more patients to compensate for continuing drops in profitability per case.

As a result, the atmosphere within medical schools became decidedly less academic. The very adaptations medical schools made to preserve their operating income turned them away from their central purpose of education and research. At many schools, the majority of clinical faculty now existed primarily to see patients, not to study problems or teach. Uncanny similarities began to appear between medical schools and teaching hospitals of the late twentieth century and those of their predecessors a century earlier, when university-based medical education had not yet become the norm in America.

One sign of the eroding scholarly atmosphere at medical schools was a reduction in the level of research.[4] This was a direct result of the decline of clinical dollars available for the cross-subsidy of research. All types of research were affected, but the area of investigation most seriously impacted was clinical research (the translation of basic knowledge into practical applications), since investigators in more fundamental areas could still turn to the National Institutes of Health and certain private foundations. The decline in clinical research was most pronounced at medical schools located in regions of the country with the highest levels of managed care.[5] In those areas, the amount of clinical income available to support research fell by 55 percent between 1991 and 1996.[6]

By the late 1990s, a career in medical research had become far more difficult than at any time in recent memory. It became common to hear academic physicians referred to as "dinosaurs," and even established investigators spoke of the frustrations, uncertainties, and insecurities of academic life.[7] One clinical investigator, who left Harvard for the University of Kansas because of better funding opportunities, said: "I'll never starve. I'll always have my clinical practice to fall back on. But what makes me tick is being an academic researcher. And that's dying on the vine."[8] These developments were not lost on students and house officers, who heard much about the frustrations of research and little about the joys and rewards of medical scholarship. From 1985 to 1993, the number of grant applications to the NIH by scientists 36 years old or younger fell from 3,040 to 1,389, and a study of medical students in 1994 demonstrated a continued decline in the number of students with research intentions.[9] It became worrisome as to where the next generation of clinical scientists would come from.

A second mark of the declining intellectual atmosphere at medical schools was the conversion of a scholarly faculty to a clinical faculty. For years, most medical school clinical departments had utilized a two-tier system of investigator-teachers and clinician-teachers. Now, many schools began to give faculty appointments to clinicians without scholarly credentials whose sole responsibility was to practice medicine. Traditional faculty at one school called such appointees "hired hands rather than true faculty."[10] Some schools (for instance, the University of Pennsylvania) bought private practices and gave the physicians faculty appointments; others (for instance, the University of California, Los Angeles) appointed new full-time physicians to the staff and gave them offices at the medical center or at an outside satellite facility.[11] In either case, the net result was the same: the emergence of a large cadre of clinician-nonteachers on the full-time faculty. Clinical departments, once dominated by medical scholars, were being diluted by the appointment of more and more practitioners without discernible teaching or investigative credentials. This violated the century-long tradition that medical school faculty would possess academic attributes in common with other university faculty.

Not only new faculty but traditional faculty as well were being diverted from scholarly to clinical activities. Encouraged by market forces and by the same small pool of highly paid consultants who sold their business advice to one medical school after another, medical schools concluded that the correct operating approach in the 1990s was to require full-time clinical faculty to generate most of their salary themselves. Schools began to measure the "clinical productivity" of their faculty (defined as the amount of clinical income a faculty member generated) and implement new pay scales that created financial incentives for seeing more patients.[12] Each school had its own plan, but the Association of American Medical Colleges (AAMC) in 1996 began a project to develop physician productivity standards that might be applicable to measuring the clinical productivity of faculty at all schools.[13] "The rules are changing," an AAMC official stated. "We're going to make it explicit that . . . you should be generating money."[14]

The specifics of the new pay plans—absolute salary levels, the amount of base pay, and the level of the clinical incentives—varied from school to school. Some schools also attempted to quantify research "productivity" by assigning a certain number of points or dollars for publications, grants, and academic honors. Very few schools, if any, included educational "productivity" as part of the formula. Of note, clinical productivity referred to the professional income generated, not the quantity or quality of clinical care. A plastic surgeon generating large fees by performing routine cosmetic surgery on well-insured patients would be considered "productive." A general surgeon or neurosurgeon at an urban teaching hospital performing lifesaving operations on young indigent trauma victims would not—even if that surgeon developed new approaches to the understanding and treatment of trauma and earned national acclaim as a leader in the field.

To academic medicine and its business consultants, this approach reflected sound business principles. Teaching and research were cost-generators for a medical school (except for fully funded research); patient care was revenue producing. It made sense to them to encourage faculty to put aside scholarly activities for patient care. That way, a school could at least stay solvent. However, few consultants or school officials stopped to ask whether the generation of professional fees was an appropriate standard for a university to use in judging the productivity of its faculty. Like nonvisionary companies and other organizations that were not "built to last," medical schools were instituting incentives incongruous with the fundamental mission of the organization.[15]

The net effect of the new system was to redirect the efforts of clinical faculty from university work to patient care. At medical schools around the country, traditional clinical faculty complained of being forced to spend more time in medical practice and less time in teaching and research. They found that scholarly activities were simply not encouraged by the new rules of faculty practice that would not tolerate any loss of "clinical productivity." "We don't see how we can be educators and at the same time earn our own salaries [from patient care],"[16] a pediatrics professor at the University of Texas Medical School at Galveston lamented. During most of the twentieth century, medical schools had been an integral part of the university primarily because they provided a haven for some of the best and brightest doctors to devote themselves to education and research, free from the burden of having to earn their salary from private practice. Now that haven was disappearing, and the medical school's claim to being a part of the university was correspondingly weakening. Some schools began to resemble the earlier proprietary schools, where the faculty earned their income primarily from the patient care they provided, and where teaching and research (if any) were typically done on the fly.

No medical school was strong enough fully to resist the "proprietarization" process. At the University of Pittsburgh, the president of the medical center told the faculty that the only way for the institution to survive in the managed care environment was to build its own health care system. The objective was to spread the University of Pittsburgh Medical Center name throughout the general Pittsburgh area by merging with or acquiring other hospitals and medical facilities. There would be so many patients to see that clinical faculty must become as "productive" as private practitioners. Only faculty with external grants covering at least 80 and preferably 100 percent of their salary and expenses should expect to be able to do research, and even these investigators would have to live and breathe by their last funding cycle. Merely a handful of scholarly faculty in all the clinical departments would be able to teach and act as traditional medical professors.[17]

At Washington University, there was a similar displacement of university work by private practice. As the Department of Radiology received lower professional fees for the interpretation of radiographic studies, the department required its faculty to increase the volume of studies they interpreted to keep the dollar flow constant. To permit this, the department greatly reduced the amount of teaching it allowed its faculty to do for other departments. In the 1980s radiologists provided eight hours a month of instruction to internal medicine residents; in the 1990s that fell to one hour per month. The Department of Ophthalmology would not pay for the 10 percent of time for either of two distinguished senior professors and teachers in the department to write board questions in ophthalmology. Similarly, the Department of Radiology would not provide the 25 percent salary coverage necessary to allow a senior professor with international stature to participate on a national oncology commission, despite the medical school's need to gain greater national exposure in that field. Some of the clinical departments found it difficult to persuade faculty to accept teaching assignments as attending physicians because the faculty feared they would be viewed as less "productive" and suffer salary decreases.[18]

A third sign of the declining intellectual atmosphere of the medical school was a marked deterioration in the quality of the learning environment afforded medical students and house officers. If one tenet had helped ensure medicine's place as a university discipline in the twentieth century, it was the importance of conducting medical education within an environment of inquiry and discovery. This principle was being violated by the shift in emphasis from research to patient care and the conversion of a scholarly faculty to an exclusively clinical faculty. In addition, most medical school administrators ignored the harmful effects of conducting medical education in an atmosphere in which the primary mandate for patient care was speed. For instance, there was much talk in the 1980s and 1990s about how to accommodate education to outpatient settings without slowing down the flow of patients; there was little discussion about reducing the number of patients seen in teaching settings so that students and house officers might have a better educational experience. In an episode that undoubtedly made William Osler turn over in his grave, officials at Johns Hopkins, while planning a new ambulatory care center, declared that students and house officers could work in the facility "only with careful orchestration by the clinical chiefs who would be charged to make sure that such education did not interfere with efficient patient care."[19] Some schools even prohibited students and residents from working in faculty ambulatory facilities altogether because educational inefficiencies rendered the practices noncompetitive with private practice.[20] Earlier generations of medical educators, who had made the construction of a learner-centered educational environment their life work, would have felt flabbergasted and betrayed.

If the learning environment at the academic health center was eroding, elsewhere in the academic health system a rich learning environment had yet to be created. Medical school officials spoke often about using the entire integrated delivery system for medical education, particularly to expand opportunities in ambulatory education. However, this could be done effectively only if considerable effort was given to assuring that the education offered in community settings would be of the same high quality as the education traditionally offered at teaching hospitals. The proper objective was not merely to place students and house officers in private medical offices and call that "ambulatory education." Rather, it was to create something of distinct educational value.

As of the late 1990s, that had not often happened. As medical schools began expanding their community teaching, school officials generally showed little concern with pedagogical issues or educational quality control. Once sacred matters like defining educational goals and creating the requisite learning experiences, assuring that teachers were highly qualified, providing exposure to a broad mix of patients, requiring that ambulatory visits be long enough to allow the various learning objectives to be met, assuring that time for teaching and feedback be structured into the daily schedule, and establishing ways for students and house officers working in private offices to attend conferences and group discussions— all these were commonly overlooked. A typical example occurred at one Southern medical school, proud of its new primary care rotation for third-year students in physicians' private offices, but seemingly unconcerned with the problems of teaching and learning that arose when the "supervising" physicians were seeing as many as 60 patients a day.[21] Throughout the twentieth century medical school leaders had cared very much about creating the right conditions of learning, but now all that seemed to have been forgotten in the rush to build integrated delivery systems. In the view of one critic, if these trends were to go unchecked, schools would soon be offering little more than "clinical apprenticeships in the new settings of clinical education."[22]

Indeed, apprenticeship was exactly where clinical education in many new ambulatory settings seemed to be heading. Teaching in private doctors' offices was often justified, as faculty at one prestigious medical school did, on the grounds that it "can show students how medicine is actually practiced in their communities."[23] This was in contradiction to the traditional axiom of medical education that good clinical teaching should illustrate exemplary patient care and thereby provide students a model for how medicine *should* be practiced. Another frequent justification of providing instruction in physicians' offices was to teach "the day-to-day managing of a doctor's office"[24] (things like office staffing, billing, and telephone calls). This was in contradiction to another axiom of medical education that the first year of practice was the appropriate time to learn the practical issues of office management, so that medical school and residency could be devoted to the substantive intellectual issues of a professional education.[25] Throughout the twentieth century the private faculty had been carefully chosen on the basis of their scholarly accomplishments, experience, teaching ability, and willingness to devote substantial time and energy to teaching. Now, it was tacitly assumed that any community practitioner could be a university medical teacher—at least as long as he or she was part of the network and was referring cases to the teaching hospital. In short, as clinical education began to move to community sites, there were surprisingly few defenders of educational quality (though important exceptions could be found[26]). Ironically, the many legitimate educational reasons for increasing the amount of instruction in community sites were generally not the ones cited.

Given the dearth of good quantitative measures of educational outcomes, it is impossible to know how the erosion of the learning environment has been affecting students and house officers. However, it is clear that in the cost containment era medical education has been veering away from a tight focus on the needs of learners, and it is difficult to imagine how that can be good for the education of the nation's future doctors. Students and house officers themselves have been complaining that the changing health care environment has been harmful to their education in the ways described above.[27] Equally unknown, but also a matter of deep concern to some, is how the commercialization of the modern academic health center has been influencing students' attitudes and behavior. As one medical educator explained, "I think the student who learns medicine in an environment where the bottom line is a cash flow will become a different kind of a person than someone educated in an atmosphere where, whether we do it or not, we at least hold out that the bottom line is the satisfaction of the patient's needs."[28]

A fourth mark of the changing intellectual atmosphere at the medical school was a growing tendency of medical educators not to defend the notion that medicine is a university-based profession with its own internal standards. A true professional school maintains a delicate balance between the university and the professional constituency for which the school is responsible. The professional school, unlike the faculty of arts and sciences, must be sensitive to the practical needs of professionals in the field. At the same time, the professional school must set and enforce its own standards, remembering that the greatest contribution it can make is to provide practitioners the intellectual tools to assess information critically, stay abreast with changing knowledge, adapt to continuous change, and reflect on the larger role and responsibilities of the profession in society. In these regards, medical schools throughout the twentieth century had always distinguished themselves from the other professional schools of the university.[29]

In the 1990s this began to change, as medical schools came under attack for not producing doctors prepared to work in managed care settings. In frustration, some managed care organizations established their own "graduate schools" to help their physicians adjust to managed care practices.[30] (Witness, for instance, the Mullikin University of Managed Care and the Managed Care College of the Henry Ford Health System.) There was even speculation that large managed care organizations might try to establish medical schools of their own to train doctors in managed care from the beginning.[31] To stanch such criticisms, medical schools began to try to make their training programs more relevant to managed care. Faculty at Case Western Reserve spoke of the need to "adapt student education to the emerging managed care environment," Duke reexamined its undergraduate and graduate teaching "to ensure that they are relevant to managed-care practices," and a department chairman at Johns Hopkins spoke of the "need to increase and formalize the amount of managed-care training and expertise" residents receive.[32] The teaching of managed care meant different things to different people, but to most educators that meant providing more emphasis on cost-conscious decision-making, the appropriate use of diagnostic tests, preventive medicine, and effective communication with patients. The effort to increase medical teaching in ambulatory community sites, where most managed care was practiced, was also part of medical schools' attempt to begin teaching managed care.

There was no doubt that these changes in medical education were sorely needed. The greatest deficiency of medical education throughout the twentieth century, as readers of this book have seen, was the failure to train learners properly for clinical uncertainty, which led to the systematic overuse in medical practice of tests, procedures, and treatments. This was precisely the criticism that managed care organizations were now hurling at medical education. What most medical educators in the 1990s failed to acknowledge, however, was the importance of problem-solving ability and cost-effective decision-making to all settings of practice—solo and group practice, fee-for-service and managed care, and whatever system of practice might replace managed care in the future. For medical educators to call cost-effective behavior managed care rather than "good medicine" was inaccurate and self-deprecating, as if those skills had never before been a desired part of medicine. It suggested a vision of the American medical school abdicating its position in the university— adapting a relatively narrow job-oriented approach designed to meet the specific needs of corporate employers rather than behaving like a true university professional school.

How far would medical schools go in terms of becoming educational vassals of managed care organizations? In the 1990s this became an important question. Many managed care organizations were demanding that medical schools teach skills and attitudes that primarily served the special needs of those organizations, such as submissiveness and docility so that physicians might be easily managed employees. Some managed care organizations even urged that physicians should be taught to be advocates of the insurance payers as well as the patients they cared for.[33] To critics, this raised the specter of doctors becoming "double agents" who would purportedly serve the patient but in fact limit care for the financial benefit of the employing organization.[34]

At the end of the century there were signs that medical schools were succumbing to these pressures. Some observers feared that medical schools were no longer instilling an adequate sense of professionalism (that is, a fiduciary responsibility to the needs of patients, as opposed to insurance companies, health care systems, or investors) among students and house officers.[35] At least a few schools seemed to express a willingness to do whatever managed care organizations asked of them. At the University of California, Los Angeles, for example, certain members of the faculty argued that it was their responsibility to indoctrinate students who might have misgivings about aspects of managed care. "Medical educators not only need to find creative methods of introducing these content areas [managed care] into medical curricula but should also anticipate the need for strategies to deal with negative attitudes held by students."[36]

The final mark of the changing atmosphere at academic health centers was the blurring distinction between teaching hospitals and community hospitals. For years the clinical differences had been diminishing, largely because academic health centers had been so prolific at producing well-trained specialists who became their clinical competition for specialty care. Now, academic work at teaching hospitals was also decreasing, rendering them even more indistinguishable from community hospitals. As early as 1987, seven major Boston teaching hospitals felt the need to launch a public relations campaign to "differentiate teaching hospitals from other hospitals."[37] A decade later that differentiation had not become easier to make.

It was not clear how much financial help the new academic health sys-

tems would provide education and research. As long as third party payers refused to pay the additional costs specifically associated with those
activities, even the most efficient academic health systems were hard-
pressed to maintain quality educational work at earlier levels. (Clinical
cross-subsidies of education and research, it will be remembered, were of
two types: professional fees used by a school to support academic work,
and a complex web of transfers from hospital revenues.) A new system
involving the University of Cincinnati gained attention for assigning up
to 1.5 percent of gross revenues to support medical education. Yet this
modest support of medical education, called "the hardest thing to sell" in
putting together the academic health system, could be withheld if the
system were not operating profitably, and officials of the system were
uncertain whether payments for education could be sustained in their
highly competitive price-sensitive market.[38]

It was also not clear how much moral support the new academic
health systems would provide medical education, especially those systems where the initiative had come from the hospital side. Consider the
BJC Health System in St. Louis, which is regarded by some as the model
of an academic health care system for the twenty-first century. BJC was
established in 1993, when Barnes and Jewish Hospitals (which merged in
1996 to become Barnes-Jewish Hospital) joined Christian Health Services
(the operator of two large St. Louis community hospitals) to form a
regional network of hospitals, nursing homes, outpatient and urgent care
centers, medical office buildings, home health services, and managed
care initiatives. Subsequently, St. Louis Children's Hospital joined the
system, as did a number of community hospitals in Missouri and southern Illinois. Like other integrated delivery systems, BJC has done much
good by eliminating excess hospital capacity within the system, introducing operating efficiencies and economies of scale, and rationalizing the
delivery of health care to its region. In addition, with shrewd executives,
a board of directors that overlaps with that of Washington University,
and a history of cooperation and goodwill between Barnes-Jewish Hospital and the Washington University School of Medicine, BJC has the
opportunity to become a genuine academic health care system in much
the same way that Barnes Hospital became one of the country's first
teaching hospitals at the beginning of the century.

So far that has not happened. The mission statement of BJC speaks at
length of providing quality, low-cost health care in its region but little of
education and research. Although BJC calls itself an "academic" health
care system, to many observers the Washington University School of
Medicine is just an afterthought to it, something the system views as little more than a marketing device. Many actions taken by BJC have been
injurious to the school of medicine, however useful they may have been
from the standpoint of generating hospital revenues. For instance,
Barnes-Jewish Hospital has become as good as any hospital at making
money by increasing the "throughput" of patients—even though that

practice is deleterious to good medical teaching. The first iteration of a new ambulatory care facility for Barnes-Jewish Hospital included no teaching space (teaching slows down the flow of patients), until a few faculty members finally protested loudly enough. BJC has encouraged a number of Washington University specialty services to leave Barnes-Jewish Hospital for one or another of the system's community hospitals a few miles away. However unimportant this may seem to health care delivery, it matters much to education and research, for the dispersal of academic departments weakens the cross-pollinization of ideas necessary for education and research to be at their best.[39] In planning a physical face-lift for Barnes-Jewish Hospital, BJC officials eliminated large amounts of productive research space utilized by clinical investigators at the school—and the faculty were not even told in advance that they would be moving. Dialogues between medical school and BJC officials have not been regular, and many major BJC decisions affecting the school of medicine have been made unilaterally. Whether BJC—and other "academic" health systems as well—will realize their potential to develop a true academic mission and thereby serve the larger good, or whether they will remain community health care systems of only local significance, remains to be seen.[40]

Such changes in the atmosphere of academic health centers represented the consequence of the reactive responses of medical educators to the managed care environment described in the last chapter. In the world of managed care, scholarship had become more difficult to support. The solution adopted by most medical schools and teaching hospitals was to "reengineer" themselves to be less scholarly. Though some schools, teaching hospitals, and academic health systems were still in financial difficulty, most had successfully improved their financial balance sheets and had become more clinically "competitive." However, the cost was the downgrading of their raison d'être: teaching and research. School officials spoke regularly of the importance of preserving the academic mission, but it was the clinical enterprise that most chose to protect first. Historically, the greatest institutional barrier to medical education at American medical schools had been an excessive emphasis on research. Now, the greatest threat was excessive attention to patient care, to the detriment of both education and research.

As a result, as the twenty-first century drew near, a second revolutionary period in American medical education had started. The university system that had characterized American medical education during the twentieth century was being systematically taken apart, and American medical education was beginning to revert to the corporate form it had occupied before the Flexnerian revolution. The challenge of the first revolution in medical education was to pull medical education from the environment of medical practice into the university. Now, medical educators were raising the question whether medical schools should leave their universities to join integrated delivery systems.[41] A task of the first revolution was to establish research as a major focus of the medical school. In the 1990s, medical educators often found themselves apologizing about research, and some even asked, "Should/will the classic model of the research-intensive medical school persist in the future?"[42] A goal of the first revolution had been to make medical education a true university activity by freeing medical professors from having to practice medicine to make a living. Now, as at the proprietary schools a century before, clinical faculty found themselves increasingly dependent on private practice for their livelihood. A central mission of the first revolution was to create a stimulating learning environment to help assure that medical education would be graduate education rather than vocational training. At the end of the century, the learning environment was eroding, with serious implications for the quality of medical education. During the first revolution, university presidents had taken a deep interest in medical education, and many had helped lead the movement to create a strong system of university-based medical schools. In the 1990s, few university presidents defended the medical schools' goal of education and research, and even fewer seemed to be aware that medical schools were in danger of leaving the university. In the early 1900s, and throughout most of the twentieth century, leaders of academic medicine had frequently expressed the view that academic health centers had a fundamental responsibility beyond their own institutional well-being—namely, to play an important role in changing the whole health care system for the better. At the end of the century, those sentiments were seldom heard.

It is impossible, of course, to know how far these trends will continue in the decades ahead. The future, as historians understand, is one of innumerable contingencies, and predictions about tomorrow are often caricatures of the present. Nevertheless, worst-case scenarios envisioned by some were sobering. In one extreme scenario, the quality of clinical education, particularly in community ambulatory sites, would be so poor that the standards of the accrediting organizations would not be met.[43] In another extreme scenario, the country would be left with only a small number of true academic health centers that concentrate on research, specialty training, and complex care. The great majority of current teaching hospitals would become community hospitals with little research or sophisticated care.[44] It is not an exaggeration to say that some traditionalists in academic medicine feared that medical education could be entering an academic Middle Ages, where only a handful of centers would be keeping civilization alive.

It would be a major mistake to overemphasize the parallels between the present system of American medical education and the proprietary system of a century ago. The starting points are much too different. The century-long university tradition of American medical education, the large existing cadre of talented and dedicated biomedical scientists, the billions of private and public dollars spent each year on biomedical research, the public's appreciation of the benefits of new medical knowledge, and the high quality of the current medical students and house officers represent but a few of the differences between medical education of the present and that of the pre-Flexnerian period.

Nevertheless, it would be an equal mistake to ignore the similarities to the proprietary system that have developed during the managed care era. At academic health centers, a money standard has started to replace a university standard. The financial well-being of academic health centers and the continued generous compensation of medical school faculty have been the winners; education and research, the losers. Americans will not wake up tomorrow to find their teaching hospitals and medical schools gone. However, an insidious process has already begun that has been transforming teaching hospitals into community hospitals and university medical schools into proprietary schools.

The Declining Relevance of Medical Education

During most of the twentieth century, medical schools and teaching hospitals had been the most important determinants of medical practice in America. This resulted not only from the doctors they educated and the new knowledge they produced, but from their role in setting and enforcing the standards of care. The conditions of medical practice during this time allowed physicians the freedom to practice according to the precepts they had been taught.

In the second revolutionary period, medical education started to become more tangential to medical practice. Increasingly, insurance companies, health maintenance organizations (HMOs), and other managed care organizations showed little interest in the type of medical care that the profession had always held as the ideal and that the schools had consistently taught. Instead, HMOs were creating an organizational environment that made it difficult for doctors to practice according to long-established tenets of excellence. For the first time in American history, a conflict appeared between the teachings of medicine and the environment of health care delivery.

To appreciate this point, it is important to recognize the fundamental importance to the physician's work of having sufficient time with patients. Like good teaching and good research, good medical care cannot be provided on the fly. Problem solving—figuring out a diagnosis, or determining the best treatment for the individual patient—requires time for the physician to think and reflect. Similarly, thoroughness and attention to detail require enough time for a physician to listen attentively and examine patients carefully. Fulfilling the Samaritan function of medicine and establishing a strong doctor–patient relationship likewise can occur only when the physician is not rushed. When doctors are in too much of a hurry to talk, they cannot get to know patients, determine individual wishes and preferences, provide education and counseling, teach about ways to prevent illness and promote health, address psychosocial concerns, and provide comfort and compassion.[45] And no matter how skilled the doctor, mistakes of all types are much more likely to be made when patients are seen and treated in haste.

Perhaps the most extraordinary development in medical practice during the age of managed care was that time, in the name of efficiency, was being squeezed out of the doctor–patient relationship. Managed care organizations, with their insistence on maximizing "throughput," were forcing physicians to churn through patients in assembly-line fashion at ever-accelerating rates of speed. In the late 1980s, most physicians felt that 30 patients a day was pushing the limit. By the mid-1990s, 25 to 30 patients a day was common at many HMOs, and stories circulated about primary care physicians treating as many as 70 patients a day.[46] In 1997, doctors on average spent eight minutes talking to each patient, less than half as much time as a decade before.[47] By the late 1990s, the pressure on doctors to see more patients in less time showed no signs of abating, and many doctors were staggering under the load. One expert wrote, "Were Maimonides to pray today, he would undoubtedly ask for time to better understand the total dimensions of a patient's needs."[48]

In the worldview of managed care, brief patient encounters represented a desirable economy, for as physician "productivity" increased, fewer doctors needed to be retained to provide the same volume of services. However, undesirable consequences for patient care soon became apparent, in addition to the adverse effects on education already discussed. A number of studies were published suggesting that shorter office visits were associated with poorer patient outcomes.[49] A large survey of doctors sponsored by the Robert Wood Johnson Foundation found that primary care physicians practicing in HMOs felt that they needed between 30 and 40 percent more time with patients than their organizations allotted to provide quality care.[50] Brief office visits were also found to be a significant factor in causing job dissatisfaction, job burnout, and poor mental health among physicians.[51]

Evidence also began to mount that patients were often dissatisfied with their care when office visits were perceived as too short. A variety of studies reiterated what wise clinicians, humanists, and social scientists have long known: that patient satisfaction depended heavily on good communication, a caring, attentive doctor, and a thorough explanation of the patient's condition and treatment. When physician time was in short supply, these goals were seldom achieved, and patients were often unhappy with their care.[52] Stereotypes began to emerge of doctors greeting patients with their hand on the examining room doorknob, using body language to encourage patients to leave even before the consultation had begun. Advice columnist Ann Landers pointed out that the most frequent complaint she received from her readers about doctors was "the feeling that they are not getting enough of their doctor's time."[53] Frank Davidoff, editor of the *Annals of Internal Medicine*, suggested that the growing popularity of alternative medicine in the 1990s could be explained by the fact that its practitioners, unlike physicians, "have discovered the value of time and give patients the time they need."[54]

With the spread of managed care, a major public controversy erupted about the quality of care delivered by HMOs. Through the late 1990s, the controversy focused almost entirely on the amount of care provided. There were deepening fears about undertreatment, even among responsible individuals who recognized that overtreatment had been the major problem in the past. The popular press in the 1990s was replete with frightening stories of avoidable complications and tragedies that resulted from the barriers to care imposed by many HMOs.[55] The problem of undertreatment seemed most prevalent among those patients who needed medical care the most: vulnerable populations, such as the elderly and individuals with chronic, rare, or serious diseases.[56] Such reports sometimes overshadowed the accomplishments of HMOs, which critics of HMOs frequently ignored.

The issue of time involved a more insidious but more fundamental threat. The organizational structure of most HMOs, with its emphasis on patient "throughput," made quality, caring, respect for the individual, and a strong doctor–patient relationship more difficult to achieve. Roger Bulger, president of the Association of Academic Health Centers, wrote, "Students who may have been taught all of the best techniques for communicating with patients will soon learn to ignore those techniques if their practice environment discourages such behavior by, for example, requiring them to see a different patient every ten minutes."[57] In HMOs there were financial rewards for doctors who had large panels of healthy patients requiring few visits and little time; financial penalties were incurred by doctors treating sicker patients needing more frequent visits and longer appointment times. A family physician at Group Health Cooperative of Puget Sound, one of the finest and most respected HMOs in the country, described the situation at her organization: "A doctor with lots of sympathy or possessing expertise in chronic illnesses like asthma pays a price: attracting sicker patients."[58] Only a few years before, and throughout the history of medicine until the advent of managed care, attracting sick patients needing time and expertise had been considered a compliment to the skills of a good doctor, not a penalty.

It cannot be emphasized too strongly that much more needed to be learned about the effects of the managed care movement on the quality of care. Anecdotes abounded, but there was little empirical evidence to document the relative strengths and weaknesses of managed care and fee-for-service medicine. Studies of the subject found mixed results, and the belief of some that HMOs uniformly provided a poorer quality of care was not supported by the data.[59] Patient surveys revealed that the majority of enrollees in managed care plans were generally satisfied with their care.[60] Yet the lack of evidence that managed care was compromising patient care was not completely reassuring, primarily because of the difficulty in measuring health care quality. A major problem was that it was much harder to measure underutilization than overutilization. In addition, fundamental ingredients of quality, such as the doctor–patient relationship, the scientific value of personal care, the therapeutic power of the laying on of hands, the capacity of a personal relationship to inspire a patient to adopt a healthier lifestyle or comply with a treatment regimen, and the importance of good clinical problem-solving that maximized needed tests and procedures and minimized the rest, remained difficult to quantify.[61]

What was notable for this book on medical education was not the degree to which the quality of care had deteriorated or improved under managed care but the absence of leadership of the nation's medical faculties in the debate over quality, even as managed care organizations were denying some of the most fundamental principles of medical professionalism. Traditionally, it had been academic medicine's responsibility to guard the nation's health by establishing and maintaining the standards of care. Throughout most of the twentieth century, academic medicine had met this responsibility well. The creation of strong systems of undergraduate and graduate medical education, the establishment of standards for medical licensing and for specialty and subspecialty certification, and the development of criteria for the accreditation of hospitals were among the positive actions taken by medical school leaders to assure that medical practice was conducted at the highest possible level. However, in the closing years of the twentieth century, as the public became more and more anxious about the quality of care under managed care, little was heard from medical school leaders on the subject. As Jerome P. Kassirer, editor-in-chief of the *New England Journal of Medicine*, observed, the air was filled with a "strained silence" on the issue.[62]

What were medical school officials speaking up about? Primarily, matters pertaining to their own self-interest. In the 1990s, the Association of American Medical Colleges and its member institutions supported Democratic Party health care proposals (which provided more generous funding of graduate medical education), lobbied for more federal research support, worked hard to expand referral networks and build integrated delivery systems, and searched for new ways to commercialize university-based biomedical research. Rather than challenge the more questionable medical practices of HMOs, most academic health centers reacted to managed care as a fait accompli and worked mainly to position their institutions to survive within the new marketplace—even adopting high physician "productivity" requirements for their own faculty so they could better compete for managed care contracts. Academic medicine continued to speak of its unique altruistic and social mission. However, its actions suggested the primacy of self-interest.

Similarly, the medical profession at large said little about the subject of quality. Instead, turf battles reerupted with more intensity than ever before: generalist physicians doing more specialty care, specialty physicians doing more primary care, specialists of all types competing for sundry body parts, and all physicians concerned about encroachments on medical practice from nurse practitioners and physician assistants. As Medicare reimbursement for cataract surgery and prostatectomies fell, many ophthalmologists began doing more radial keratotomies (an operation to correct nearsightedness) and urologists, penile enlargements—lucrative areas appealing to affluent patients who would pay top dollar even when insurers would not pay at all.[63] Neither academic medicine nor the profession as a whole seemed able to put aside internal differences and self-concern to work for the common professional good and public interest. Jordan Cohen, president of the Association of American Medical Colleges, described the "strong tendency" of academic and practicing physicians alike "to hunker down, circle the wagons, become defensive, and tighten the focus on our self-interest."[64]

Ultimately, academic medicine's reluctance to speak up about the quality of care was something it did at its own risk. If efforts to maximize "throughput" in medical practice were to continue unabated, the best teachings of medicine would have to be cast aside when physicians entered practice, and academic health centers would see the market for their educational products decrease. Similarly, if HMOs refused to pay for needed services, academic health centers would eventually find an erosion in the market for the new knowledge, drugs, and technologies they produced. The entire medical profession would lose its sovereignty as determinations about how medicine should be practiced—the quintessence of a professional issue—would be made by insurance companies rather than academic leaders and professional experts. One business writer has already predicted a future in which "there will be three surviving HMOs that own all hospitals and medical schools" and in which "physicians will be licensed by the HMO (not the state) that employs them."[65] Even in less extreme, more likely scenarios, the lesson was clear: Without leadership from academic medicine in maintaining the quality of clinical practice, not only will the health of the nation potentially suffer, but academic health centers will become more tangential to medical care in America.

Restoring the Social Contract

By the late 1990s, a second revolutionary period in American medical education had begun. Under pressure from HMOs, academic health centers were increasingly unable to use clinical revenues to cross-subsidize education, research, and charity care, and managed care's mandate to treat patients quickly was wreaking havoc on a learning environment whose essential characteristic was time. More subtle but equally pernicious, academic health centers were losing the market for their educational products, as the new managed care environment was making it increasingly difficult for doctors to practice in concordance with many traditional professional teachings and values.

Since World War II, there had been several major perturbations in the external environment of academic health centers, such as the growth of the National Institutes of Health, the spread of private medical insurance, and the enactment of Medicare and Medicaid. These events ultimately provided major new sources of revenue to academic health centers and expanded the market for their products. Under managed care, the opposite was happening. Clinical margins were shrinking, and the demand for the educational products of medical centers was contracting. For the first time in nearly a century, the external environment of academic health centers had become hostile.

In the past, academic health centers had demonstrated remarkable alacrity at responding to changing incentives in their external environment, and in the 1990s they strove valiantly to do so again. However, few, if any, experienced genuine success. Most were managing to survive financially, but at the jeopardy of losing their core institutional mission. At some medical schools it became difficult to discern any deeper purpose beyond that of increasing clinical volume and seeing as many paying patients as possible. Lofty goals that medical educators had set for themselves all century long were being forgotten in the competitive scramble for survival.

It would be a mistake to view the problems of academic health centers in the 1990s as simply having resulted from the rise of managed care. Deeper roots of the second revolutionary period lay in the failure of medical faculties to adjust to the changing social expectations of medicine. The health paradigm since World War II had been the abundance of resources, which allowed academic health centers to grow exponentially, operate inefficiently, and be unconcerned about producing doctors who practiced cost-effectively. This behavior was readily understandable, given an admiring nation and the lucrative financial incentives of the time. However, it left them highly vulnerable—and flabbergasted—when social conditions changed and the era of resource constraints began.

Accordingly, academic health centers found themselves drifting toward the millennium with less self-confidence and a greater sense of loss of control than at any time in nearly a century. Yet, for advocates of quality in medical education, there was reason not to despair. The past, bearing as it always does on the present, harbored the principles by which academic health centers and society could better serve each other so that high standards might be retained. Specific solutions would need to be crafted for the twenty-first century; tactics appropriate for one time, place, and social context typically do not serve as a template for another. However, guiding principles could be derived from an understanding of the past.

For the general public, there was one overarching message: academic health centers were fragile institutions that needed aggressive nurturing, sustained protection, and the unwavering support of those with vision, power, and means. The most important social functions of academic health centers—the education of future generations of medical professionals, the discovery of new medical knowledge, the provision of highly specialized services (such as the care of patients with severe burns, complex trauma, and AIDS), and the care of poor and uninsured persons—were revenue-draining, not income-generating, activities. Insurers and third party payers had traditionally helped pay for these public services, but most managed care organizations were unwilling to do so. If American medicine was to retain its future-directedness and its humanity—its investment in education and research, and its capacity to serve the sickest patients and those who could not afford to pay—specific sources of funding for the public missions of academic health centers would be needed.

Where might the money be found to offset the decline from lower clinical payments? This question requires vigorous debate, but a number of potential sources have already been proposed. Suggestions have included the creation of a federal trust fund for the support of academic health centers, increased use of general tax revenues, and the development of an "all payer" system of financing in which education would be supported by a tax on all health insurance premiums. The common feature of these proposals is the view that the financing of medical education and research should be a shared responsibility because these activities benefit everyone. Advocates of the "all payer" approach have contended that such a system would be fair to managed care companies since each organization would be taxed at the same rate, making the playing field level. Proponents have also maintained that an "all payer" system would help improve the image of HMOs as good citizens.

Other suggestions for financing academic health centers have included the continued development of closer ties with industry and the further commercialization of university-based medical research. Such approaches merit consideration, though extreme care must be taken so as not to undercut the values of academic medicine in the long run. An increase in the budget of the National Institutes of Health, a popular idea in Congress in 1998 and 1999, would benefit medical research, particularly at the most prestigious medical schools. A number of changes in the rules governing funds already designated for medical education would also help. For instance, it would aid the efforts to improve ambulatory education if Medicare regulations were changed to allow graduate medical education payments to be used for the training of residents in non-hospital as well as hospital sites.

In the 1990s, schools experienced the greatest difficulty in receiving payment for time. Yet, time remained the most fundamental ingredient of the rich educational environment that academic health centers had always been expected to provide. Without time, instructors could not properly teach, students and residents could not effectively learn, and investigators could not study problems. The most urgent financial need of medical education was not for new buildings or laboratories but for the funds to allow enough time in the care of patients that a rich intellectual atmosphere could be maintained. Fortunately for medical education, methods were becoming available to identify the exact costs of time. For instance, if the inclusion of house officers and students in a faculty outpatient clinic reduced the volume of patients treated (or "productivity") by 25 percent, a number would be at hand to calculate the necessary educational subsidy that would allow the clinic to compete on equal terms with medical practices where no teaching was conducted.

Academic health centers could take cheer that the new environment of resource constraints imposed relative, not absolute, limits on the nation's health care expenditures. A society that was already spending nearly $1 trillion a year on health care clearly possessed the means to maintain a strong system of medical education and research. Moreover, estimates of waste and unnecessary costs from high administrative expenses, duplicated services, unnecessary tests and procedures, and the profits taken out of the system by investor-owned hospital systems and HMOs amounted to one-third or more of the country's health care bill. It has been suggested that savings in these areas could provide ample funds for medical schools and teaching hospitals, not to mention other socially important health care goals.[66]

How much the United States should invest in medical education and research is primarily a matter of values and social priorities, not economics. There is no "natural" size or configuration for academic health centers; this has always been negotiated with society and is exquisitely dependent on income streams. However, at the end of the twentieth century, it was clear that academic health centers were at substantial risk. This posed a major threat to the nation's health. It was plausible to imagine good medical care being provided in the United States without private practice as the country currently knew it. However, it was inconceivable to imagine high-quality care continuing without well-trained doctors and the ongoing discovery of new medical knowledge. If the public wished its incubators of medical progress to be preserved, secure funding for medical education and research was needed. Society would have to recognize academic health centers for the national resources that they were—and support them amply and wisely.

For medical educators, there was also an overarching message: external support could not be expected without convincing demonstration that academic health centers were serving the needs of the public. Medical schools and teaching hospitals had always existed for the community's well-being, and not vice versa. Yet somehow since the 1970s, many medical faculties had forgotten that fact. The travails of academic health centers during the second revolutionary period had resulted not from their inability to discover but from their failure to serve and lead. If medical educators were to succeed in preserving the vitality of academic health centers, they needed to remember Charles Eliot's admonition from over a century before that "the first step toward getting an endowment was to deserve one."[67]

Academic health centers had a number of issues to address if they were to demonstrate that they were still deserving of generous public support. First, they needed to adjust more fully to the new environment of resource constraints. This entailed becoming leaner, more efficient, more agile, and more cost-effective in the practice of medicine. This also required a far more effective process of long-range planning. Academic health centers could no longer try to be all things to all people; rather, they would finally have to make tough decisions about which academic areas to pursue and which to leave to someone else. They would also have to reevaluate the optimal size of their student enrollments, graduate training programs, and faculty and support staffs. Collectively, they would even have to address the thorny question of whether the nation's medical schools and residency programs were producing too many doctors for the country's needs, and if so, how to correct the problem.

Whether (or how far) academic health centers would have to "downsize" was not clear, but at the minimum they would have to adjust to a steady state or slow growth environment. This would require major changes in their organizational behavior. Individualistic, entrepreneurial departments would have to learn to do a much better job of solving problems communally and working for the common good. Many faculty would have to make sacrifices so that the organization as a whole could prosper. Medical schools, to flourish, would need to change their corporate culture so that they could become organizations based on principles. That is, they would need to introduce incentives consistent with their core values and objectives. For instance, if they truly valued scholarly work, they would need to reward clinical faculty for scholarship and not "clinical productivity."[68] Medical schools and teaching hospitals would need to reaffirm that their mutual interests were inseparable. To this end, medical schools would have to elevate the level of service they provided their teaching hospitals, while hospitals would have to do a better job of utilizing their financial capital for academic, not just clinical, purposes.

One possible test of the commitment of medical schools to university work was the degree to which faculty and administrators would be willing to make personal sacrifices to protect educational programs. For instance, considerable money could be recaptured for education and research if faculty and administrators did not insist on being paid like private practitioners. Similarly, more time could be protected for scholarly pursuits if faculty would accept salaries closer in line with historical norms. Such retrenchment would undoubtedly be unpleasant for those who had grown accustomed to the generous compensation levels of the 1980s and 1990s, but it would clearly illustrate to the public that the schools had a purpose beyond making money.[69]

Second, to demonstrate that they were deserving of public support, academic health centers needed to do a better job of producing the type of doctors that the country needed. There was a distinct need to improve instruction in such areas as cost-consciousness, preventive medicine, health promotion, ambulatory medicine, primary care, the appropriate use of diagnostic tests, and the psychosocial dimensions of patient care. Faculties needed to accelerate the effort to introduce a population perspective into medical education—that is, to teach strategies to maximize the health of a defined population (such as that of an HMO or integrated delivery system) with the resources at hand. Faculties also needed to work on those factors under their control to produce a specialty mix more closely aligned with the health care needs of the country.

In view of the rapidly increasing complexity of the science and delivery of health care, it was more important than ever that medical faculties vigorously promote high standards in medical education. This meant insisting that physicians continue to receive a rigorous education in the knowledge base and cognitive skills of medicine. It required defending the integrity of the learning environment so that physicians would still be able to learn by doing, assume graded responsibility, become comfortable with medical uncertainty, and develop the skills of problem-solving and lifelong learning. It also meant remembering, as a task force of the Association of American Medical Colleges phrased it, "the central importance of an environment of discovery to the core missions of medical schools."[70] The education of medical students was the one unique activity of medical schools. Hence, it behooved them to continue to do this well, even if an unfriendly health care marketplace sometimes made the task more difficult.

Third, medical faculties could demonstrate that they were serving the public interest by regaining the critical initiative in monitoring and maintaining the quality of care. As noted earlier, serious questions about quality had been raised in the 1990s. To some critics, American medicine appeared to be engaged in "a race to the bottom."[71] In their view, incentives aimed at reducing waste, improving efficiency, or maximizing profits resulted in so many corners being cut that patient care was often imperiled. The answer to preserving quality was not open-ended spending. However, the intellectual elite of the profession needed to provide guidance regarding how to control medical expenditures wisely. If academic and professional leaders could speak in a unified voice about what was best for patients, a powerful force for the public good would be released.

Fourth, academic health centers needed to make clear that their research interests were fully concordant with the health concerns of the public. In the era of chronic illnesses and an aging population, this meant integrating the study of the organization, financing, and delivery of health care with their traditional scientific work. All the rich intellectual resources of the university could be called upon to assist in this effort. Of course, something as large and complex as the health care delivery system was not the sole responsibility of academic medicine to fix. However, the problems of promoting health and organizing health care in the

United States had become so pressing that they deserved much more attention from medical schools than they traditionally had received. Certainly, rapid evolution of the country's health care system was going to continue with or without the involvement of medical educators, but without their participation, they and the public were less likely to be satisfied with the results.

Lastly, academic health centers needed to remember their basic institutional value: that they were public trusts accountable to society for the resources they received. Funding from the public was not an entitlement. Rather, it represented public assistance to enable them to carry out public service. The public was not interested in certain recent priorities of academic health centers, such as institutional aggrandizement, the capture of market share, or the desire of faculties to be paid like private practitioners. Rather, the public was concerned with the quality of their academic work and their commitment to the public health. "One imagines the gentle administrators and trustees of nonprofit academic medical centers spending their time engaged in good works that benefit patients, rather than calculating new ways to beat the competition,"[72] a retired medical school administrator wrote wistfully. For a generous level of public support in the future, academic health centers would need to do a much better job of realigning their interests with those of the public. They needed to remember that they must do well to do good—but that doing well was only the means to the higher end.

❦ · ❦ · ❦

From a historical perspective, it was not difficult to imagine academic health centers making the types of adjustments outlined above. As Abraham Flexner had pointed out, for medical education to flourish from one generation to the next, it had to reconfigure itself in response to changing scientific, social, and economic circumstances. This it had done extremely well during most of the twentieth century.

What type of individual was needed to lead medical education into the twenty-first century? To use the terminology of a recent study, academic health centers needed wartime leaders, not peacetime managers.[73] That is, academic medicine needed leaders capable of bold vision and decisive action to cope with an unfriendly, unpredictable, and rapidly changing health care environment. Medical leaders, like all wartime leaders, needed the ability to "think outside the box," the flexibility to act quickly, the courage to act decisively, and the fortitude to make difficult and painful decisions for the sake of the general good. Most important, medical leaders needed the wisdom to know what not to change—namely, the timeless core mission and values of the academic health center.

In the 1990s, some in academic medicine longed for charismatic leaders to emerge who might serve as contemporary counterparts to figures like Charles Eliot and William Welch. Such views, though understandable, reflected a romanticized past and an erroneous assumption about the nature of leaders. As one essay observed: "Leadership is not the private reserve of a few charismatic men and women. It is a process that ordinary people use when they are bringing forth the best from themselves and others."[74] Leaders of one era are frequently glorified by subsequent generations, but most of history's leaders have been ordinary flawed people who were not seen as particularly heroic by their contemporaries.

True leaders are generally notable for their convictions, not for their charisma.[75] They ask how their organization or institution can make a difference, they champion and exemplify worthy values and purposes, and they articulate a mission or cause beyond just making money. There is a great temptation to do what is popular or remunerative rather than what is right. Thus, leaders must have "a clear conviction about values and a steadfastness of purpose in distinguishing between right and wrong, wisdom and foolishness."[76] For medical education this meant one thing: its leaders must remember that institutional survival and financial success are meaningless if the core mission and values are not preserved.

For those who would lead American medical education toward success in the twenty-first century, there were a number of strengths in the environment that could be drawn upon. A nation willing to spend nearly a trillion dollars a year for health care was clearly indicating its faith in medicine and its desire to have the most capable doctors and up-to-date medical knowledge. In public opinion polls conducted in several states in 1996, large majorities of respondents indicated that the national commitment to medical research should be higher; between 60 and 65 percent said they would be more likely to vote for a presidential candidate who strongly supported medical research. (Indeed, in 1998 Congress substantially increased funding for the NIH and even spoke of doubling the NIH budget in five years.) The clinical strengths of academic health centers also did not pass unnoticed among the general public. In polls, approximately 70 percent of respondents felt that hospitals with research and training programs provided better patient care, compared with roughly 11 percent who thought better care was less likely and 13 percent who thought there was no difference.[77] A strong reservoir of public support for academic health centers clearly remained.

In addition, support of academic health centers was consistent with the national goal of achieving better control of medical expenditures. Thoughtful, cost-effective medical practice involved skills that could be taught and learned, which was the responsibility of medical education. Medical research could contribute to lower health care costs. For instance, in the mid-1990s it was estimated that the flu vaccine was saving the country $1.6 billion annually from reduced hospitalization of persons 65 and older, and that if an average delay in the onset of Alzheimer's disease of five years could be achieved, the resultant savings would be at least $50 billion a year.[78] New fields of investigation based mainly at academic health centers, such as technology assessment and outcomes research, also had great potential for helping control health care costs rationally.

Another source of strength was that exceptional altruism and public commitment still existed within the medical profession. This could be seen in the behavior of thousands of medical faculty who remained dedicated to teaching, knowing it would probably not help their academic careers and might hurt them financially. This could also be seen in the behavior of tens of thousands of individual physicians who routinely challenged the rulings of HMOs and insurance companies on behalf of their patients. There were even a few martyrs—individual physicians fired by HMOs for publicly exposing abusive practices of their employers. Clearly, many physicians desired direction and purpose to their professional lives and were still seeking to contribute to their students, patients, and the larger good.

Indeed, despite its more tarnished image in recent years, the medical profession retained a large store of credibility and public goodwill. For instance, several public opinion polls found that personal physicians were still considered the most trustworthy source of medical information.[79] (HMOs, in contrast, were ranked the least trustworthy source.) This reservoir of trust was available to be drawn upon for worthy causes—particularly causes in which the medical profession was perceived as speaking in the public interest rather than its own.

Another source of strength was an existing infrastructure to help protect the public from economic encroachments on the quality of medical education: the various accrediting agencies, licensing bodies, and specialty certifying organizations. These agencies had been created to assure the public that high standards would be present at every stage of the educational process. At the end of the century, as the financial environment of academic health centers became hostile and as fewer voices defended educational quality, these agencies were thrust into a critical role. If, for financial expediency, a medical school compromised its instruction, the Liaison Committee on Medical Education was under no obligation to accredit the school. Similarly, if a residency program allowed its standards to deteriorate, or an HMO established a substandard training program to serve its own organizational interests, the responsible residency review committee was not required to approve the program, and the corresponding specialty board did not have to allow graduates of the program to sit for its examination. Whether these agencies would have the courage to defend high standards against powerful countervailing economic and social forces remained to be seen—but they had the authority to do so if they wished.

Fortunately, signs were appearing of a renewed defense of quality among medical educators. In the 1990s a number of schools introduced major changes in their curriculum to accommodate contemporary educational imperatives, and by the end of the decade many more were planning to do so. Especially notable were the efforts of some schools to upgrade the quality of education in ambulatory sites and to develop the teaching skills of community physicians who participated in educational programs.[80] In 1996 the Association of American Medical Colleges launched the Medical School Objectives Project to help make certain that high standards of professionalism, including altruism and dutifulness, remained at the core of medical education.[81] These efforts in themselves hardly guaranteed that schools would be able to maintain the strength of their educational programs against hostile environmental forces, but they did indicate a renewed interest among medical educators in taking responsibility for their own future.

By the late 1990s, HMOs were losing some of their political clout, and infatuation with managed care as a cure-all for the ills of the American health care system was wearing thin. Throughout the country a consumer backlash against the more egregious practices of HMOs had begun. Federal and state governments passed legislation regulating everything from the length of hospitalization after a mastectomy or normal vaginal delivery of babies to the financial pressures that some HMOs placed on doctors to deny care. There was even a movement to allow patients to sue HMOs for malpractice when injury resulted from a health plan's refusal to pay for needed care. In a national poll of attitudes toward a number of industries in 1997, health insurance companies and managed care organizations were second from the bottom in the public's view of how well they were serving consumers, surpassed in disfavor only by the tobacco industry.[82]

The consumer backlash against managed care was not without its downside. Generalized indignation indiscriminately lumped all HMOs together, ignoring the many differences between responsible and irresponsible health plans as well as the improvements in health care delivery that might not have occurred if not for the managed care movement.[83] In addition, significant dangers to patient care were incurred when governmental bodies became involved in the practice of medicine by legislating complex medical decisions.[84] Nevertheless, the consumer revolt did indicate the desire of the public to have a health care system that retained quality and caring, and it opened the door for greater professional leadership in shaping such a system.[85]

Another emerging voice for quality health care was that of the primary purchasers of health care—employers and governments. Though purchasers were hardly unconcerned about the prices they paid, they also cared about the health and economic productivity of the populations for whom they were responsible. Accordingly, in the 1990s some large purchasers of health care began pushing managed care organizations to become more responsive to consumers and to develop measures of quality and performance. As the benefits manager of Xerox remarked, "We don't mind at all driving low-quality health plans out of business." Herein lay another set of natural allies for leaders of medicine who might wish to stand up for quality.[86]

In the long-term, many changes that would help control medical costs would also potentially strengthen the profession's position in the health care marketplace. The extraordinary rise in power of the health insurance industry in the 1980s and 1990s resulted in no small part from the excess medical capacity that had been created since the 1960s. Reduction of this excess capacity—decreasing the number of doctors produced, restricting the number of international medical graduates allowed to practice in the United States, encouraging a higher percentage of doctors to choose generalist careers, and eliminating the duplication of facilities in oversupplied areas—would ultimately not only help lower costs but, through the law of supply and demand, help restore some of the lost power of "providers." Similarly, the recent efforts of some integrated delivery systems to become insurers as well as providers, thereby bypassing the insurance companies, would, if successful, also strengthen the position of "providers."[87] The return of greater power to "providers" would not automatically result in a better health care system, for physicians and hospitals are as vulnerable to venal behavior as anyone else. However, if professionals were once again in control, the opportunity to create a better system—and the responsibility for doing so—would once again lie more fully in their hands.

Particularly in trying times, it is easy for predictions of the future to be overly gloomy. As the late David Rogers pointed out, this occurs because futuristic predictions often "do not take into account the creativity or basic decency of human beings." In Rogers's view: "History suggests that societies, when faced with trends that look as though they will create negative human consequences, often opt for changes of a more socially responsible nature to avoid such outcomes. Thus people often make adjustments in trends that futurologists find quite impossible to predict."[88] Rogers would have been among the first to admit that a socially desirable outcome is never guaranteed. However, he would also have insisted that over time society tends to reward groups that aspire to improving the human condition, and that American society in the twenty-first century is likely to reward the medical profession if it succeeds at placing the interests of patients and the public first.

In this context, the dilemmas of American medical education were not as daunting as at first they might have seemed. The challenges of maintaining a strong system of medical education were certainly less intimidating than those of creating the system a century before. At the end of the twentieth century the public was already accustomed to supporting medical schools generously, the capacity of medical care and potential of medical research were widely recognized, the public was expressing its belief in medicine by spending nearly a trillion dollars a year on health care, considerable national goodwill toward the medical profession remained, the public was realizing that managed care needed significant improvements, and the majority of physicians retained a conscience and deep-seated sense of service. These represented major advantages not available to the pioneering medical educators. Formidable as the contemporary problems were, they were not so profound as those that faced medical educators a century earlier.

Indeed, for those who could see beneath the surface, extraordinary opportunities existed for medical education. The turbulence of the late twentieth century provided an unprecedented chance for academic medicine to reinvent itself for the new era of resource constraints. Only part of the struggle facing academic health centers was against those aspects of managed care that directly threatened it. Rather, the larger part of the struggle was internal: developing the willingness and ability to do more with less, making the commitment to produce the types of doctors the country needed, having the strength to protect the quality of medical practice, fulfilling long-neglected responsibilities of helping mold a better health care system, and mustering the courage to stand up for principles and values, no matter how tempting the financial incentives to abandon them. Wartime leaders embrace major change because "they see more opportunity than threat in turbulence."[89] For medical education, this observation held true. The risks and dangers were great, but there was a genuine opportunity to imagine and attain new heights of excellence.

The outcome of the current turbulence in American medical education and practice carried implications that extended far beyond health care. In the waning years of the twentieth century, many writers were debating America's position in the next century. Will America remain strong and vital, or will it undergo social and economic decline? The country's health care system represented a prism of this larger concern. The underlying problems that led to turbulence in medicine—the earlier acceptance of the myth of unbridled resources and national capacity, the preoccupation with short-term rather than long-term thinking, the emphasis on immediate gratification, the difficulty of retaining purpose and values in a culture that champions greed and material excess, and the dilemma of providing for public goods and human needs through a private market system beholden only to owners and shareholders—were the same problems that jeopardized other aspects of the country's prosperity. If American medicine becomes mediocre, it will not be because of Japanese or German competition but because of internal failings. Conversely, if American medicine retains its excellence, it is likely that America as a nation will remain strong. At risk was not only the quality of American health care in the twenty-first century but also the strength of America as a nation.

From the perspective of over two and one-half millennia of Western medicine, the perturbations of American medicine in the 1990s will one day be a small chapter, perhaps merely a footnote. There is little doubt that the medical profession, perhaps in response to a new scientific breakthrough, technological development, or heightened social conscience, will one day recapture the public's imagination and goodwill. However, it is an open question when, where, and how this will occur. The history of medicine has demonstrated shifting centers of world leadership. Whether 25 or 50 years from now the United States will still occupy its current position of preeminence in medical education and practice is presently unknown.

If the United States is to retain its leadership in medicine, an understanding of the history of American medical education during the past century reveals the principles that must be followed. The key lies in restoring the tattered social contract between medicine and society. The medical profession must remember that it exists to serve; society must remember that it will not have good health care unless it provides the needed financial and moral support. Fortunately for the United States, the opportunity to retain the world's premier system of medical education, research, and practice still exists. The time left to recapture a constructive course of action is shrinking—but there is still sufficient opportunity for visionaries to dream and leaders to act.

Notes

Chapter 1

1. Walter L. Bierring, "Tendencies of Medical Education," *The Diplomate* [of the National Board of Medical Examiners], April 1931, p. 27.

2. A biography of Flexner remains to be written—a somewhat surprising fact, in view of his importance not only to the history of medicine but to the history of education and history of philanthropy as well. Until then, his two autobiographies may be consulted: *I Remember: The Autobiography of Abraham Flexner* (New York: Simon and Schuster, 1940); and *Abraham Flexner: An Autobiography* (New York: Simon and Schuster, 1960). Also helpful is Steven C. Wheatley's account of Flexner's activities at the General Education Board, *The Politics of Philanthropy: Abraham Flexner and Medical Education* (Madison: The University of Wisconsin Press, 1988).

3. Abraham Flexner, *Medical Education in the United States and Canada* (New York: Carnegie Foundation for the Advancement of Teaching, 1910).

4. David L. Edsall to A. Lawrence Lowell, 31 July 1919, Folder 311 (1917–1919), A. Lawrence Lowell Papers, Harvard University Archives, Pusey Library, Cambridge, MA.

5. Abraham Flexner, *Universities: American English German* (New York: Oxford University Press, 1930), pp. 94, 95.

6. On the creation of modern medical education in the United States, see Kenneth M. Ludmerer, *Learning to Heal: The Development of American Medical Education* (New York: Basic Books, 1985). See also William G. Rothstein, *American Medical Schools and the Practice of Medicine: A History* (New York: Oxford University Press, 1987); and Martin Kaufman, *American Medical Education: The Formative Years, 1765–1910* (Westport, CT: Greenwood Press, 1976).

7. Meeting of 6, 7, and 10 June 1942, Agenda and Minutes of the Business Meetings of the Council on Medical Education and Hospitals, American Medical Association, American Medical Association Archives, Chicago, IL; Harold Rypins, "Americans and Foreigners in Medical Licensing Examinations," *The Diplomate* [of the National Board of Medical Examiners], October 1929, p. 4.

8. Herman M. Somers and Anne R. Somers, *Doctors, Patients, and Health Insur-*

ance: *The Organization and Financing of Medical Care* (Washington, D.C.: Brookings Institution, 1961), p. 136.

9. Francis M. Rackemann, *The Inquisitive Physician: The Life and Times of George Richards Minot* (Cambridge: Harvard University Press, 1956), p. 55.

10. On Flexner's view that medical schools were public trusts, see Ludmerer, *Learning to Heal*, pp. 179–182.

11. William H. Welch, "Present Position of Medical Education, Its Development and Great Needs for the Future," in William H. Welch, *Papers and Addresses*, vol. 3 (Baltimore: The Johns Hopkins University Press, 1920), p. 112.

12. An influential example of this literature is Peter M. Senge, *The Fifth Discipline: The Art and Practice of the Learning Organization* (New York: Doubleday Currency, 1990).

13. Helpful sources on the development of nineteenth-century medical science include Robert P. Hudson, *Disease and Its Control: The Shaping of Modern Thought* (Westport, CT: Greenwood Press, 1983); Richard H. Shryock, *The Development of Modern Medicine: An Interpretation of the Social and Scientific Factors Involved*, 2nd ed. (New York: Alfred A. Knopf, 1947); and John Harley Warner, "Science in Medicine," in Sally Gregory Kohlstedt and Margaret W. Rossiter, eds., *Historical Writing on American Science: Perspective and Prospects* (Baltimore: The Johns Hopkins University Press, 1985), pp. 37–58.

14. William H. Welch, "On Some of the Humane Aspects of Medical Science," in Welch, *Papers and Addresses*, vol. 3, p. 5.

15. John Shaw Billings, "Valedictory Address" (unpublished lecture), n.d., Box 44, John Shaw Billings Papers, New York Public Library, New York, NY.

16. Ludmerer, *Learning to Heal*, pp. 67–68.

17. Abraham Flexner, *Medical Education: A Comparative Study* (New York: The Macmillan Company, 1925), p. 148.

18. *Ibid.*, p. 178.

19. Richard Shryock, *American Medical Research, Past and Present* (New York: Commonwealth Fund, 1947), p. 49.

20. On the economic requirements of medical education and the campaign to raise funds, see Ludmerer, *Learning to Heal*, pp. 139–151, 191–206; Wheatley, *The Politics of Philanthropy*; and E. Richard Brown, *Rockefeller Medicine Men: Medicine and Capitalism in America* (Berkeley: University of California Press, 1979).

21. H. Drinkwater, *Fifty Years of Medical Progress: 1873–1922* (New York: The Macmillan Company, 1924), p. v.

22. Alfred E. Cohn, "The Meaning of Medical Research," *Scientific Monthly*, June 1938, p. 514.

23. Brown, *Rockefeller Medicine Men*, p. 251, n. 40.

24. On philanthropy, see Robert H. Bremner, *American Philanthropy* (Chicago: University of Chicago Press, 1960); Merle Curti and Roderick Nash, *Philanthropy in the Shaping of American Higher Education* (New Brunswick, NJ: Rutgers University Press, 1965); and, for a radical critique, Robert F. Arnove, ed., *Philanthropy and Cultural Imperialism: The Foundations at Home and Abroad* (Boston: G. K. Hall, 1980).

25. Brown, *Rockefeller Medicine Men*; Howard S. Berliner, *A System of Scientific Medicine: Philanthropic Foundations in the Flexner Era* (New York: Tavistock, 1985).

26. Jacob G. Schurman to Nicholas Murray Butler, 27 January 1917, Folder 8, Box 2, Papers, Office of the Dean, Cornell University Medical College, 1903–1934 (Niles), Archives, The New York Hospital–Cornell Medical Center, New York, NY.

27. The term "cultural authority" was used in Paul Starr, *The Social Transforma-*

tion of American Medicine: The Rise of a Sovereign Profession and the Making of a Vast Industry (New York: Basic Books, 1982).

Helping further explain the growing cultural authority of doctors was not only the rise in prestige of medicine but also the decline in influence of traditional authority—religion. As faith in God diminished, alternative sources of faith had to be found. Medicine and science helped fill that emotional void. On the decline of religious faith, see James Turner, *Without God, Without Creed: The Origins of Unbelief in America* (Baltimore: Johns Hopkins University Press, 1985).

28. Donald Fleming, *William H. Welch and the Rise of Modern Medicine* (Boston: Little, Brown, 1954); Simon Flexner and James Thomas Flexner, *William Henry Welch and the Heroic Age of American Medicine* (New York: Viking, 1941).

29. Particularly early during the reform movement, many faculty were primarily concerned with education rather than research. However, by the 1890s leadership of the movement had been captured by medical scientists, who could never forget their desire to improve opportunities for medical research as they fervidly campaigned to improve the teaching of students. See Thomas S. Huddle, "Looking Backward: The 1871 Reforms at Harvard Medical School Reconsidered," *Bulletin of the History of Medicine* 65:340–365, 1991.

30. On the development of higher education in the United States, see Laurence R. Veysey, *The Emergence of the American University* (Chicago: University of Chicago Press, 1965); and Burton J. Bledstein, *The Culture of Professionalism: The Middle Class and the Development of Higher Education in America* (New York: Norton, 1976).

31. Henry K. Beecher and Mark D. Altschule, *Medicine at Harvard: The First 300 Years* (Hanover, NH: University Press of New England, 1977), p. 87.

32. *Ibid.*, pp. 85–172.

33. Meeting of 20 October 1899, Medical Faculty Minutes, Cornell University Medical Center, Archives, The New York Hospital–Cornell Medical Center, New York, NY.

34. Meeting of 19 May 1919, Minutes of the Meetings of the Committee on Administration, College of Physicians and Surgeons of Columbia University, Special Collections, Augustus C. Long Health Sciences Library, Columbia University, New York, NY; meeting of 15 November 1915, Minutes of the Meetings of the Faculty, College of Physicians and Surgeons of Columbia University, Augustus C. Long Health Sciences Library, Columbia University, New York, NY.

35. Flexner, *Universities*, pp. 16–17.

36. Welch, "Present Position of Medical Education," p. 113.

37. Flexner, *Universities*, p. 197.

38. Abraham Flexner, *Medical Education in Europe* (New York: Carnegie Foundation for the Advancement of Teaching, 1912), p. vii.

39. A misperception about the introduction of entrance requirements has been widespread in the history of medicine. Many writers, taking note of the profession's desire to improve its social and economic status at that time, have concluded that entrance requirements were established to keep the "riffraff" out of medicine, thereby elevating the profession's prestige. In fact, medical schools introduced entrance requirements for genuine educational reasons: to allow greater efficiency of the medical curriculum and to reduce the very high dropout and failure rates that plagued even the best schools of the period. Medical educators hardly worried about the income levels of physicians in practice. Nevertheless, there can be no question that entrance requirements made it more difficult for economically or socially disadvantaged youths to attempt to pursue a career

in medicine, and many doctors who wished to see the profession become more exclusive certainly cheered as the requirements were put into effect. See Ludmerer, *Learning to Heal*, pp. 113–122.

40. Many writers have pointed out that equality of opportunity in the educational system has always been more myth than reality. Children of economically or socially disadvantaged families scarcely received the same opportunities as offspring of the wealthy. For a review of this subject, see Laurence Veysey, "The History of Education," *Reviews in American History*, December 1982, pp. 281–291.

41. Meeting of 11 June 1924, Agenda and Minutes of the Business Meetings of the Council on Medical Education and Hospitals.

42. Flexner, *Medical Education: A Comparative Study*, p. 210.

43. For more detail on the antipathy of the nineteenth-century hospital to medical education, see Ludmerer, *Learning to Heal*, pp. 152–165.

44. On the creation of the modern American hospital, see Charles E. Rosenberg, *The Care of Strangers: The Rise of America's Hospital System* (New York: Basic Books, 1987); Morris J. Vogel, *The Invention of the Modern Hospital: Boston, 1870–1930* (Chicago: University of Chicago Press, 1980); and David Rosner, *A Once Charitable Enterprise: Hospitals and Health Care in Brooklyn and New York 1885–1915* (New York: Cambridge University Press, 1982).

45. Francis W. Peabody, "The Care of the Patient," *Journal of the American Medical Association* 88:880, 1927.

46. Francis W. Peabody, "The Function of a Municipal Hospital," *Boston Medical and Surgical Journal* 189:127, 1923.

47. Rackemann, *The Inquisitive Physician*, pp. 162–164.

48. Details on these new affiliations between medical schools and hospitals may be found in Kenneth M. Ludmerer, "The Rise of the Teaching Hospital in America," *Journal of the History of Medicine and Allied Sciences* 38:389–414, 1983.

49. Hugh Cabot to A. S. Begg, 5 December 1927, Folder "B 1927," Box 37, University of Michigan Medical School Records, Michigan Historical Collections, Bentley Historical Library, University of Michigan, Ann Arbor, MI.

50. Victor C. Vaughan to E. J. Mehren, 30 April 1915, Folder "April 1915," Box 32, University of Michigan Medical School Records.

Licensing laws, like entrance requirements (see note 39), have often been misunderstood in the secondary literature, as writers have frequently confused cause and effect. Both served to help elevate the status of physicians, but the primary force for their establishment arose from educational considerations, not from any concern of medical educators about the average practitioner's status or income.

51. Meeting of 19 May 1919, Minutes of the Meetings of the Committee on Administration, College of Physicians and Surgeons of Columbia University.

52. John Ettling, *The Germ of Laziness: Rockefeller Philanthropy and Public Health in the New South* (Cambridge: Harvard University Press, 1981).

53. John Duffy, *The Healers: A History of American Medicine* (New York: McGraw-Hill, 1976), p. 240.

54. Frederick T. Gates, *Chapters in My Life* (New York: Free Press, 1977), p. 182.

55. See, for example, meetings of 19 September 1918 and 14 November 1918, Faculty Minutes, Georgetown University School of Medicine, Georgetown University Archives, Georgetown University, Washington, D.C. Similar examples were found at Harvard, Cornell, Johns Hopkins, Washington University, and Michigan, among others.

56. Saul Benison, A. Clifford Barger, and Elin L. Wolfe, *Walter B. Cannon: The*

Life and Times of a Young Scientist (Cambridge: The Belknap Press of Harvard University Press, 1987), pp. 293–297.

57. See David E. Rogers, "The Early Years: The Medical World in Which Walsh McDermott Trained," *Daedalus*, Spring 1986, p. 3.

58. Flexner, *Medical Education in Europe*, p. xvii.

59. James G. Burrow, *Organized Medicine in the Progressive Era: The Move Toward Monopoly* (Baltimore: Johns Hopkins University Press, 1977); Ronald L. Numbers, *Almost Persuaded: American Physicians and Compulsory Health Insurance, 1912–1920* (Baltimore: Johns Hopkins University Press, 1978).

60. Memorandum of the Joint Committee on the Teaching of Preventive Medicine to Students of the School of Medicine, 23 February 1934, with meeting 2 March 1934, Minutes, Advisory Board of the Medical Faculty, The Johns Hopkins University School of Medicine, The Alan Mason Chesney Medical Archives of The Johns Hopkins Medical Institutions, Baltimore, MD.

61. Meeting of 31 October 1931, Minutes, Advisory Board of the Medical Faculty, The Johns Hopkins University School of Medicine.

62. Flexner, *Medical Education in the United States and Canada*, p. 143.

Chapter 2

1. Remarks of Dr. Bevan, with meeting of 11 June 1924, Agenda and Minutes of the Business Meetings of the Council on Medical Education and Hospitals, American Medical Association Archives, Chicago, IL.

2. Malcolme H. Soule to A. C. Furstenberg, 30 April 1940, Folder "1940 D-E," Box 43, University of Michigan Medical School Records, Michigan Historical Collections, Bentley Historical Library, University of Michigan, Ann Arbor, MI.

3. Meeting of 14 February 1957, Transactions of the Executive Faculty, Cornell University Medical College, Archives, The New York Hospital–Cornell Medical Center, New York, NY.

4. Alan M. Chesney to Joseph S. Ames, 25 September 1933, Folder "Chesney-Ames Jun 12, 1933–Sep 27, 1933," Box 47, Correspondence Files, Office of the Dean of the Medical Faculty, The Johns Hopkins School of Medicine, Record Group 3, Series B, Archives of The Johns Hopkins University School of Medicine, The Alan Mason Chesney Medical Archives of The Johns Hopkins Medical Institutions, Baltimore, MD.

5. George W. Corner, *The Seven Ages of a Medical Scientist: An Autobiography* (Philadelphia: University of Pennsylvania Press, 1981), pp. 201–277.

6. Meeting of 25 February 1942, Harvard University Medical Faculty, Minutes of Meetings, Harvard Medical Archives, Rare Books Department, Countway Library, Harvard Medical School, Boston, MA.

7. David E. Rogers, "The Early Years: The Medical World in Which Walsh McDermott Trained," *Daedalus*, Spring 1986, pp. 2–3; quotation, p. 2. Among those Rogers included on his list of medical heroes were Robert Loeb, David Barr, William McCann, Warfield Longcope, Arthur Bloomfield, Henry Christian, Emmet Holt, Harvey Cushing, George Whipple, and Evarts Graham.

8. H. J. Stander to Frederick C. Holden, 22 January 1934, Folder 1, Box 4, Henricus J. Stander Papers, Archives, The New York Hospital–Cornell Medical Center, New York, NY.

9. "Report of Subcommittee on Medical Personnel," 3 May 1948, Folder "Vice President of University Correspondence 1946–1953," Box 4XY, Correspondence

Files, Office of the Dean of the Medical Faculty, The Johns Hopkins School of Medicine.

10. *Annual Report of the Dean, College of Physicians & Surgeons of Columbia University* (1932), p. 12.

11. *Medical Research: A Midcentury Survey*, vol. 1 (Boston: Little, Brown and Company, 1955), pp. xi–xii.

12. America's long romance with technology as a panacea for social problems is discussed in Howard P. Segal, *Technological Utopianism in American Culture* (Chicago: University of Chicago Press, 1985).

13. *Figure 1* is taken from Joseph Ben-David, "Scientific Productivity and Academic Organization in Nineteenth-Century Medicine," in Bernard Barber and Walter Hirsch, eds., *The Sociology of Science* (New York: The Free Press of Glencoe, 1962), p. 309.

14. Roger L. Geiger, *To Advance Knowledge: The Growth of American Research Universities, 1900–1940* (New York: Oxford University Press, 1986).

15. Francis M. Rackemann, *The Inquisitive Physician: The Life and Times of George Richards Minot* (Cambridge: Harvard University Press, 1956), pp. 232, 270.

16. Richard H. Shryock, *American Medical Research: Past and Present* (New York: The Commonwealth Fund, 1947), p. 114.

17. W. Bruce Fye, "Medical Authorship: Traditions, Trends, and Tribulations," *Annals of Internal Medicine* 113:317–325, 1990.

18. Report of the Surgical Department, 1939–40, p. 3, Office of the Dean, Cornell University Medical Center, Annual Reports of Departments and Offices, Archives, The New York Hospital–Cornell Medical Center, New York, NY; meeting of 17 January 1941, Transactions of the Executive Faculty, Cornell University Medical College.

19. See, for example, the materials in Folder "Graduate Courses," Dean's Office Files, University of Southern California School of Medicine, Norris Medical Library, University of Southern California, Los Angeles, CA.

20. Report of the Dean of the Medical School, 1939–40, Folder 473, Dean's Subject File, Harvard Medical School, Harvard Medical Archives, Rare Books Department, Countway Library, Harvard Medical School, Boston, MA.

21. A. McGehee Harvey, *Science at the Bedside: Clinical Research in American Medicine, 1905–1945* (Baltimore: Johns Hopkins University Press, 1981).

22. A. von Haller, *The Vitamin Hunters* (Philadelphia: Chilton Co., 1962).

23. Jonathan Liebenau, *Medical Science and Medical Industry: The Formation of the American Pharmaceutical Industry* (Baltimore: Johns Hopkins University Press, 1987); John P. Swann, *Academic Scientists and the Pharmaceutical Industry: Cooperative Research in Twentieth-Century America* (Baltimore: Johns Hopkins University Press, 1988); and John Parascandola, "Industrial Research Comes of Age: The American Pharmaceutical Industry, 1920–1940," *Pharmacy in History* 27:12–21, 1985.

24. *Table 1* is taken from The Peter Bent Brigham Hospital, *Annual Report* (1943), p. 26.

25. Shryock, *American Medical Research*, p. 122; Ernst P. Boas, *The Unseen Plague: Chronic Disease* (New York: J. J. Augustin, 1940), p. 3. Recent scholarship has emphasized the importance of social factors like improved sanitation, nutrition, living conditions, and public health, and not just medical care, to the marked increase in human life expectancy that occurred from the mid-nineteenth to the mid-twentieth century. See Thomas McKeown, *The Role of Medicine: Dream,*

Mirage, or Nemesis? (Princeton, NJ: Princeton University Press, 1979); and *idem, The Modern Rise of Population* (New York: Academic Press, 1976).

26. Boas, *The Unseen Plague.* In common parlance, acute diseases are often equated with infections, and chronic diseases, with noninfectious illnesses like cancer. A moment's reflection will demonstrate that this is not totally accurate. Many important infections, such as syphilis, tuberculosis, and acquired immunodeficiency syndrome (AIDS), usually follow a chronic course, whereas some cancers, such as certain leukemias, can lead to death within days. Moreover, it is hardly unusual—tuberculosis again being a case in point—for a disease to take an acute course in one patient, a chronic course in another.

27. For a description of some of the wartime scientific work, see Daniel J. Kevles, *The Physicists: The History of a Scientific Community in America* (New York: Alfred A. Knopf, 1977), pp. 102–138.

28. John C. Burnham, ed., *Science in America: Historical Selections* (New York: Holt, Rinehart and Winston, 1971), pp. 252–253; Shryock, *American Medical Research*, pp. 154–155.

29. Robert C. Olby, *The Path to the Double Helix* (Seattle: University of Washington Press, 1974); and Horace Freeland Judson, *The Eighth Day of Creation: The Makers of the Revolution in Biology* (New York: Simon & Schuster, 1979).

30. Robert E. Kohler, *From Medical Chemistry to Biochemistry: The Making of a Biomedical Discipline* (Cambridge: Cambridge University Press, 1982). For more on the "ecology of knowledge"—that is, how nonintellectual factors can influence the development of academic disciplines—see Alexandra Oleson and John Voss, eds., *The Organization of Knowledge in Modern America, 1860–1920* (Baltimore: Johns Hopkins University Press, 1979).

31. Thomas G. Benedek, "A Century of American Rheumatology," in Russell C. Maulitz and Diana E. Long, eds., *Grand Rounds: One Hundred Years of Internal Medicine* (Philadelphia: University of Pennsylvania Press, 1988), p. 168.

32. The Peter Bent Brigham Hospital, *Annual Report* (1942), p. 75.

33. Sol Sherry, *Reflections and Reminiscences of an Academic Physician* (Philadelphia: Lea & Febiger, 1992), p. 94.

34. Steven J. Peitzman, "Nephrology in America from Thomas Addis to the Artificial Kidney," in Maulitz and Long, eds., *Grand Rounds*, pp. 211–241; Herbert Chasis, "History of the Renal Section, New York University School of Medicine 1926–1986, New York University Medical Center," *Bulletin of the New York Academy of Medicine* 65:879–897, 1989.

35. Alfred E. Cohn, "Medicine and Science," *Journal of Philosophy* 25:412, 1928.

36. "Suggested Principles to Govern Departmental Correlation," with meeting of 5 March 1930, Executive Faculty Minutes, Washington University School of Medicine, Washington University School of Medicine Archives, St. Louis, MO.

37. Interview 37 (Henry Dolger, 1988), Oral History Collection, The Mount Sinai Medical Center, Archives, Mount Sinai Medical Center, New York, NY.

38. The Peter Bent Brigham Hospital, *Annual Report* (1938), p. 106.

39. Harvey, *Science at the Bedside.*

40. *Ibid.*, pp. 199–200.

41. For instance, see Report of the Department of Pathology, 1934–35; and Report of the Department of Physiology, 1943–44; both in Office of the Dean, Cornell University Medical Center, Annual Reports of Departments and Offices.

42. Milton Terris, "The Complex Tasks of the Second Epidemiologic Revolution," *Journal of Public Health Policy* 14:8–24, 1983; Mervyn Susser, "Epidemiology

in the United States after World War II: the Evolution of Technique," *Epidemiologic Reviews* 7:147–177, 1958; and Harry M. Marks, *The Progress of Experiment: Science and Therapeutic Reform in the United States, 1900–1990* (Cambridge: Cambridge University Press, 1997).

43. Richard H. Shryock, "The American Physician in 1846 and in 1946: A Study in Professional Contrasts," *Journal of the American Medical Association* 134:417–424, 1947.

44. Corner, *The Seven Ages of a Medical Scientist*, p. 242.

45. A few medical schools did take patents on discoveries of major commercial importance. In the most notable examples—the University of Wisconsin's patents on Vitamin D and certain anticoagulants, and the University of Toronto's patent on insulin—the royalties were used solely for the support of research at the schools. At the time, even this seemingly small step was taken with trepidation and viewed with suspicion by much of the rest of the medical community.

46. Lewis H. Weed to Alan Gregg, 30 November 1931, Folder "Rockefeller Foundation (General) Dec 1930–Dec 1931," Box 31, Weed Papers, The Alan Mason Chesney Medical Archives of The Johns Hopkins Medical Institutions, Baltimore, MD.

47. "The Johns Hopkins University Patent Policy," with meeting of 10 July 1951, Minutes, The Johns Hopkins Hospital Medical Board, The Alan Mason Chesney Medical Archives of The Johns Hopkins Medical Institutions, Baltimore, MD.

48. Meeting of 4 May 1934, Harvard University Medical Faculty, Minutes of Meetings.

49. George P. Berry, Memorandum "Re Chats with Castle and Max Finland re purported 'coolness' of Eli Lilly (company and foundation) toward HMS," 27 April 1964, Folder "BCH—Harvard Medical Unit—Thorndike 1957–June 1965," Dean's Subject File, Harvard Medical School.

50. Donald Fleming, *William H. Welch and the Rise of Modern Medicine* (Boston: Little Brown, 1954), pp. 179, 178.

51. The "triple threat" represented the ideal of a clinical professor, but few faculty were equally talented in all three areas or divided their time in exact thirds.

52. Paul B. Beeson, "The Changing Role Model, and the Shift in Power," *Daedalus*, Spring 1986, pp. 83–84.

53. David E. Rogers, Obituary of David Preswick Barr, Folder 2, Box 1, David P. Barr Papers, Archives, The New York Hospital–Cornell Medical Center, New York, NY.

54. Edith Gittings Reid, *The Great Physician: A Short Life of Sir William Osler* (London: Oxford University Press, 1931), p. 230.

55. William P. Longmire Jr., *Alfred Blalock: His Life and Times* (privately printed, 1991), p. 198.

56. Lewis H. Weed to James D. Bruce, 19 July 1928, Folder "Bruce, J. D. 1929–1943," Box 5, Weed Papers. Similar amounts of professional fees were generated by full-time clinical faculty at other medical schools. See Abraham Flexner, *Medical Education: A Comparative Study* (New York: The Macmillan Company, 1925), p. 323.

57. Discussion of the evolution of a "system" of higher education is found in Hugh Hawkins, *Banding Together: The Rise of National Associations in American Higher Education, 1887–1950* (Baltimore: Johns Hopkins University Press, 1992), pp. 78–103. The appearance of a system of medical education may be interpreted

as part of the transformation of progressive era American society from a group of isolated local communities into a national network discussed by Robert H. Wiebe in *The Search for Order: 1877–1920* (New York: Hill and Wang, 1967).

58. "Arnold Rice Rich 1893–1968," with meeting of 4 June 1968, Minutes, The Johns Hopkins Hospital Board of Trustees, The Alan Mason Chesney Medical Archives of The Johns Hopkins Medical Institutions, Baltimore, MD.

59. Meeting of 7 January 1942, Harvard University Medical Faculty, Minutes of Meetings.

60. Robert G. Petersdorf, "Academic Medicine: No Longer Threadbare or Genteel," *New England Journal of Medicine* 304:841–843, 1981.

61. Worth Hale to A. Lawrence Lowell, 8 October 1930, Folder 52, Series 1930–1933, A. Lawrence Lowell Papers, Harvard University Archives, Cambridge, MA; meetings of 20–21 November 1937 and 13–17 May 1939, Agenda and Minutes of the Business Meetings of the Council on Medical Education and Hospitals.

62. *Table 2* is taken from Herman G. Weiskotten, Alphonse M. Schwitalla, William D. Cutter, and Hamilton H. Anderson, *Medical Education in the United States 1934–1939* (Chicago: American Medical Association, 1940), p. 58.

63. Francis M. Forster to the Very Reverend Edward B. Bunn, 15 July 1954, Folder "Medical School May–December 1954," Box "Medical School 1950–1954," Medical School Records, Georgetown University Archives, Georgetown University, Washington, D.C.

64. Arthur E. Belt to Lewis H. Weed, 27 March 1920, Folder "Belt, A. E. 1920–1939," Box 4, Weed Papers.

65. For instance, see Petersdorf, "Academic Medicine"; Edwin D. Kilbourne, "The Emergence of the Physician-Basic Scientist in America," *Daedalus*, Spring 1986, pp. 43–54; Rogers, "The Early Years"; and Edward F. Adolph, "Perspectives of the First Faculty," in *To Each His Farthest Star: University of Rochester Medical Center 1925–1975* (Rochester, NY: University of Rochester Medical Center, 1975), pp. 55–69.

66. Quoted in Sharon R. Kaufman, *The Healer's Tale: Transforming Medicine and Culture* (Madison: University of Wisconsin Press, 1993), p. 115.

67. *Annual Report*, The Peter Bent Brigham Hospital (1938), pp. 115–116.

68. Minutes of meetings in Folder "Medical Executive Committee 1948–1953," Dean's Office Files, University of Southern California School of Medicine; Minutes of the Advisory Committee of the Medical Faculty, New York University School of Medicine, Archives, New York University Medical Center, New York, NY; Interview 40 (Asher Winkelstein, 5 October 1965), Oral History Collection, Archives, The Mount Sinai Medical Center.

69. A. McGehee Harvey, *The Interurban Clinical Club (1905–1976): A Record of Achievement in Clinical Science* (Philadelphia: W. B. Saunders for The Interurban Clinical Club, 1978).

70. Grace Deuel Cowgill, "Medical Faculty Wives of USC 1930–1960," November 1964, Folder "Medical Faculty Wives," Dean's Office Files, University of Southern California School of Medicine; Report of the Department of Anatomy, 1941–42, Office of the Dean, Cornell University Medical Center, Annual Reports of Departments and Offices.

71. Gordon N. Gill, "The End of the Physician-Scientist?," *American Scholar* 53:354, 1984.

72. C. Sidney Burrell, Memorandum on Appointment, Promotion, and Tenure

in the Medical School, 31 January 1940, Folder 284, Dean's Subject File, Harvard Medical School.

73. Rackemann, *The Inquisitive Physician*; quotations p. 131 ("food"), p. 134 ("studying blood"), p. 172 ("keeping hands on patients").

74. Corner, *The Seven Ages of a Medical Scientist*, pp. 237–238.

75. Robert G. Petersdorf, "The Pathogenesis of Fraud in Medical Science," *Annals of Internal Medicine* 104:253, 1986.

76. Saul Benison, A. Clifford Barger, and Elin L. Wolfe, *Walter B. Cannon: The Life and Times of a Young Scientist* (Cambridge: The Belknap Press of Harvard University Press, 1987), p. 271.

77. Morris Bishop, *A History of Cornell* (Ithaca, NY: Cornell University Press, 1962), p. 386.

78. Vivien T. Thomas, *Pioneering Research in Surgical Shock and Cardiovascular Surgery: Vivien Thomas and His Work with Alfred Blalock* (Philadelphia: University of Pennsylvania Press, 1985).

79. Margaret W. Rossiter, *Women Scientists in America: Struggles and Strategies to 1940* (Baltimore: Johns Hopkins University Press, 1982); Penina Migdal Glazer and Miriam Slater, *Unequal Colleagues: The Entrance of Women into the Professions, 1890–1940* (New Brunswick, NJ: Rutgers University Press, 1987); Pnina G. Abiram and Dorinda Outram, eds., *Uneasy Careers and Intimate Lives: Women in Science, 1789–1979* (New Brunswick, NJ: Rutgers University Press, 1987); Regina Markell Morantz-Sanchez, *Sympathy and Science: Women Physicians in American Medicine* (New York: Oxford University Press, 1985); Barbara Miller Solomon, *In the Company of Educated Women: A History of Women and Higher Education in America* (New Haven: Yale University Press, 1985).

80. Patricia Spain Ward, "An Experiment in Medical Education; or How the College of Physicians and Surgeons of Chicago Became the University of Illinois College of Medicine," in Edward P. Cohen, ed., *Medicine in Transition: The Centennial of the University of Illinois College of Medicine* (Urbana, IL: Distributed by the University of Illinois Press for the University of Illinois College of Medicine, 1981), p. 50.

81. David L. Edsall to A. Lawrence Lowell, 20 December 1918, Folder 311, Series 1917–1919, Lowell Papers.

82. Barbara Sicherman, *Alice Hamilton: A Life in Letters* (Cambridge: Harvard University Press, 1984), pp. 237, 311.

83. Meeting of 19 October 1955, Minutes of Faculty Meetings, Woman's Medical College of Pennsylvania, Archives and Special Collections on Women in Medicine, MCP Hahnemann University, Philadelphia, PA.

84. Leonard L. Mackall to Joseph S. Ames, n.d., Folder "Presidents February 1931–November 1931," Box 29, Weed Papers; Lewis H. Weed to Homer C. Naffziger, 14 January 1937, Folder "Naffziger, H. C. 1937–1949," Box 25, Weed Papers.

85. Lewis H. Weed to Howard C. Naffziger, 14 January 1937, Folder "Naffziger, H. C. 1937–1949," Box 25, Weed Papers.

86. See, for instance, Abraham Flexner to Simon Flexner, 29 September 1918, Folder "Flexner, Abraham 1918," Simon Flexner Papers, American Philosophical Society Library, Philadelphia, PA; Lewis H. Weed to H. J. Seymour, 29 February 1929, Folder "John Price Jones Corporation February 1928–April 1928," Box 19, Weed Papers.

87. Dan A. Oren, *Joining the Club: A History of Jews and Yale* (New Haven: Yale University Press, 1985), p. 136.

88. *Ibid.*, pp. 136–155.

89. William S. Ladd to Edmund E. Day, 4 December 1937, Folder 8, Box 1,

Papers, Office of the Dean, Cornell University Medical College, 1903–1934 (Niles), Archives, The New York Hospital–Cornell Medical Center, New York, NY.

90. Kenneth Dickrell to Lewis H. Weed, 11 April 1939, Folder "Surgery, Committee on Professorship," Weed Papers.

91. Worth Hale to A. Lawrence Lowell, 8 October 1930, Folder 52, Series 1930–1933, Lowell Papers. See also, David L. Edsall to A. Lawrence Lowell, 22 September 1920, Folder 50, Series 1919–1922, Lowell Papers; and J. L. Bremer et al. to David L. Edsall, 7 January 1929, Folder 763, Dean's Subject File, Harvard Medical School.

92. Flexner, *Medical Education*, p. 282.

93. Alan Gregg, *The Furtherance of Medical Research* (New Haven: Yale University Press, 1941), p. 108.

94. *Ibid.*, p. 82.

95. Charles L. Brown to Henry Ruth, 17 June 1946, with meeting 24 June 1946, Minutes of Meetings of the Board of Trustees of Hahnemann Medical College and Hospital, Archives and Special Collections, Hahnemann Collection, MCP Hahnemann University, Philadelphia, PA; University of Arkansas School of Medicine, Report of the Research Committee, 19 February 1943, Folder 6, Dean's Office Files (Byron L. Robinson, 1941–46), University of Arkansas School of Medicine, ID Number 20DB009, Special Collections Division, University of Arkansas for Health Sciences Library, Little Rock, AR.

96. Meeting of 7 April 1931, Faculty Meeting Minutes, Howard University College of Medicine, Office of the Dean, Howard University College of Medicine, Washington, D.C.

97. S. Bayne-Jones, Problems of Selective Admission and Evaluation, 20 May 1940, Folder 280, Dean's Subject File, Harvard Medical School.

98. The Peter Bent Brigham Hospital, *Annual Report* (1952), p. 9.

99. Biennial Report of the Woman's Medical College of Pennsylvania, 1941–42, with meeting of 24 June 1942, Corporation Minutes, Woman's Medical College of Pennsylvania, Archives and Special Collections on Women in Medicine, MCP Hahnemann University, Philadelphia, PA; General Statement of the Financial Needs of Meharry Medical College, 11 March 1940, with meeting of 9–13 June 1940, Agenda and Minutes of the Business Meetings of the Council on Medical Education and Hospitals.

100. Meeting of 19 November 1947, Minutes of the Meetings of the College Committee of the Board of Trustees, Hahnemann Medical College and Hospital, Archives and Special Collections, Hahnemann Collection, MCP Hahnemann University, Philadelphia, PA.

101. W. B. Summers to George Kober, 16 January 1929, Folder "Medical School—January–May 1929," Box "Medical School 1917–1929," Medical School Records, Georgetown University School of Medicine, Georgetown University Archives, Georgetown University, Washington, D.C.

102. Meeting of 27 May 1926, Faculty Meeting Minutes, Howard University College of Medicine.

103. General Statement of the Financial Needs of Meharry Medical College, 11 March 1940, with meeting of 9–13 June 1940, Agenda and Minutes of the Business Meetings of the Council on Medical Education and Hospitals.

104. Hugh Cabot to William J. Gies, 15 September 1924, Folder "1924 C–D," University of Michigan Medical School Records.

105. Meeting of 10–11 June 1944, Agenda and Minutes of the Business Meetings of the Council on Medical Education and Hospitals; Weiskotten et al., *Medical Education in the United States*, pp. 210–211.

106. The Peter Bent Brigham Hospital, *Annual Report* (1916), pp. 105–106.

107. Geiger, *To Advance Knowledge*, p. 12.

108. See, for instance, Report of the Dean of the Medical Faculty of The Johns Hopkins University (1934–35), p. 5, Reports of the Dean of the Medical Faculty of The Johns Hopkins University, The Alan Mason Chesney Medical Archives of The Johns Hopkins Medical Institutions, Baltimore, MD; and meeting of 28 March 1969, Corporation Minutes, Woman's Medical College of Pennsylvania.

109. Shryock, *American Medical Research*, pp. 130–131; Geiger, *To Advance Knowledge*, p. 253.

110. Weiskotten et al., *Medical Education in the United States*, p. 113.

111. *Final Report of the Commission on Medical Education* (New York: Office of the Director of the Study, 1932), p. 287.

112. Ralph E. Morrow, *Washington University in St. Louis: A History* (St. Louis: Missouri Historical Society Press, 1996), p. 373.

113. David L. Edsall to F. W. Hunnewell, 10 September 1924, Folder 50, Series 1919–1922, Lowell Papers.

114. Report of the School of Medicine, with meeting of 10 May 1926; and meeting of 30 June 1927; both Faculty Meeting Minutes, Howard University College of Medicine.

115. Meeting of 16–17 February 1934, Agenda and Minutes of the Business Meetings of the Council on Medical Education and Hospitals.

116. Weiskotten et al., *Medical Education in the United States*, pp. 30–31, 40–44, 285.

117. David L. Edsall to A. Lawrence Lowell, 16 March 1923, Folder 10A, Series 1922–1925, Lowell Papers; David L. Edsall to A. Lawrence Lowell, 14 May 1929, Box 5, Series 1928–1930, Lowell Papers.

118. Peter Bent Brigham Hospital, *Annual Report* (1926), pp. 73–74.

119. On Johns Hopkins between the world wars, see A. McGehee Harvey, Gert H. Brieger, Susan L. Abrams, and Victor A. McKusick, *A Model of its Kind. Volume I: A Centennial History of Medicine at Johns Hopkins* (Baltimore: Johns Hopkins University Press, 1989); and Thomas B. Turner, *Heritage of Excellence* (Baltimore: Johns Hopkins University Press, 1974).

120. Peter Bent Brigham Hospital, *Annual Report* (1924), p. 73.

121. On Harvard Medical School in the twentieth century, see Henry K. Beecher and Mark D. Altschule, *Medicine at Harvard: The First Three Hundred Years* (Hanover, NH: University Press of New England, 1977); and Reginald Fitz, "The School During the Twentieth Century," *Harvard Medical Alumni Bulletin*, October 1935, pp. 2–9.

122. See, for example, A. Lawrence Lowell to David L. Edsall, 29 January 1925, Folder 10, Series 1922–1925, Lowell Papers.

123. A. Lawrence Lowell to David L. Edsall, 15 May 1929, Folder 5, Series 1928–1930, Lowell Papers.

124. Meeting of 4 April 1930, Harvard University Medical Faculty, Minutes of Meetings; Harvard University, *President's Report* (1930–31), p. 20.

125. Report of the Dean of the Medical School, 1930–31, Folder 474, Dean's Subject File, Harvard Medical School; Harvard University, *President's Report* (1930–31), p. 20.

126. A. Lawrence Lowell to E. H. Bradford, 2 July 1917, Folder 224, Series 1914–1917, Lowell Papers.

127. A. Lawrence Lowell to David L. Edsall, 12 September 1919, Folder 311, Series 1917–1919, Lowell Papers.

128. Charles Eliot to David L. Edsall, 11 November 1919, Folder 53, Dean's Subject File, Harvard Medical School.

129. David L. Edsall to A. Lawrence Lowell, 22 March 1920, Folder 50, Series 1919–1922, Lowell Papers.

130. A. Lawrence Lowell to David L. Edsall, 31 May 1933, Folder 306, Dean's Subject File, Harvard Medical School.

Chapter 3

1. Meeting of 9 June 1935, Executive Council Meetings and Agendas, Association of American Medical Colleges, Association of American Medical Colleges Archives, Washington, D.C.

2. *Final Report of the Commission on Medical Education* (New York: Office of the Director of the Study, 1932), pp. 263–264.

3. David O. Levine, *The American College and the Culture of Aspiration, 1915–1940* (Ithaca: Cornell University Press, 1986).

4. N. P. Colwell, "Medical Education," in U.S. Department of the Interior, Bureau of Education, *Report of the Commissioner of Education* (Washington, D.C.: Government Printing Office, 1915), p. 195; "The Selection of Medical Students," with meeting of 27 October 1934, Agenda and Minutes of the Business Meetings of the Council on Medical Education and Hospitals, American Medical Association Archives, Chicago, IL; Herman G. Weiskotten, Alphonse M. Schwitalla, William D. Cutter, and Hamilton H. Anderson, *Medical Education in the United States 1934–1939* (Chicago: American Medical Association, 1940), pp. 66–67; *Final Report of the Commission on Medical Education*, pp. 278–279.

5. "The Selection of Medical Students," with meeting of 27 October 1934, Agenda and Minutes of the Business Meetings of the Council on Medical Education and Hospitals.

6. *Ibid.*

7. Meetings of 20–21 November 1937 and 12–13 February 1938, Agenda and Minutes of the Business Meetings of the Council on Medical Education and Hospitals.

8. *Final Report of the Commission on Medical Education*, pp. 12–13, 384; Irwin A. Brody, "The Decision to Study Medicine," *New England Journal of Medicine* 252:130–134, 1955.

9. "The Selection of Medical Students," with meeting of 27 October 1934, Agenda and Minutes of the Business Meetings of the Council on Medical Education and Hospitals.

10. Detailed descriptions of entrance requirements of the period are provided in *Final Report of the Commission on Medical Education*, pp. 262–282; and Herman G. Weiskotten et al., *Medical Education in the United States*, pp. 63–71. For more on premedical education see Gert H. Brieger, "'Fit to Study Medicine': Notes for a History of Pre-Medical Education in America," *Bulletin of the History of Medicine* 57:1-21, 1983.

11. A. C. Furstenberg to A. M. Chickening, 17 November 1942, Folder "1942 D," Box 45, University of Michigan Medical School Records, Michigan Historical Collections, Bentley Historical Library, University of Michigan, Ann Arbor, MI.

12. Meeting of 1 December 1938, Executive Faculty Minutes, Folder "1935–1939," Box 128, University of Michigan Medical School Records.

13. James B. Conant, "College Education for the Future Doctor," speech delivered 13 February 1939, Folder 277, Dean's Subject File, Harvard Medical School,

Harvard Medical Archives, Rare Books Department, Countway Library, Harvard Medical School, Boston, MA.

14. Samuel W. Lambert to Nicholas Murray Butler, 14 May 1939 ("infinitely more satisfactory"); and Nicholas Murray Butler to Samuel W. Lambert, 15 May 1939 ("adequately taught"); both Minutes and Correspondence of the Committee on Administration, College of Physicians and Surgeons, Dean's Office Files, College of Physicians and Surgeons of Columbia University, Office of the Dean, College of Physicians and Surgeons of Columbia University, New York, NY.

15. Meeting of 6 March 1931, Minutes of Faculty Meetings, Woman's Medical College of Pennsylvania, Archives and Special Collections on Women in Medicine, MCP Hahnemann University, Philadelphia, PA; Weiskotten et al., *Medical Education in the United States*, p. 70; James B. Erdmann, Dale E. Matson, Jack G. Hutton Jr., and Wimburn L. Wallace, "The Medical College Admission Test: Past, Present, Future," *Journal of Medical Education* 46:937–946, 1971.

The Medical Aptitude Test was a predecessor of the present-day Medical College Admission Test, which became required for admission to an American medical school in the early 1950s. The growing use of the Medical Aptitude Test was part of the movement to employ standardized tests and psychological testing more widely in American education. See Claude M. Fuess, *The College Board: Its First Fifty Years* (New York: Columbia University Press, 1950); Michael M. Sokal, ed., *Psychological Testing and American Society, 1890–1930* (New Brunswick, NJ: Rutgers University Press, 1987); and Paula S. Fass, "The IQ: A Cultural and Historical Framework," *American Journal of Education* 88:431–458, 1980.

16. Worth Hale to Edward M. Holfelner, 22 January 1936, Folder 56; Worth Hale to Francis Parkman, 12 March 1934, Folder 57; and Worth Hale to Charles H. Sampson, 19 March 1935, Folder 50; all Dean's Subject File, Harvard Medical School.

17. See, for instance, Report of the Committee on Admissions, with meeting of 1 February 1937, Faculty Minutes, New York University School of Medicine, Archives, New York University Medical Center, New York, NY.

18. See, for instance, A. Lawrence Lowell to C. Clifford Ruh, 11 April 1928, Folder 751, Series 1925–1928, A. Lawrence Lowell Papers, Harvard University Archives, Cambridge, MA.

19. See, for instance, Report of the Committee on Admissions, with meeting of 1 February 1937, Faculty Minutes, New York University School of Medicine.

20. G. Lombard Kelly to Reginald Fitz, 26 March 1951, Folder 1208, Dean's Subject File, Harvard Medical School; meeting of 5 October 1939, Harvard University Medical Faculty, Administrative Board Records, Harvard Medical Archives, Rare Books Department, Countway Library, Harvard Medical School, Boston, MA.

21. Victor Vaughan to H. G. Brawley, 12 August 1915, Folder "July–August, 1915," Box 32; G. W. Edmunds to George Johnson, 11 July 1921, Folder "Correspondence 1921 J–M," Box 34; A. C. Furstenberg to Charles C. Diggs Jr., 16 September 1953, Folder "N 1953," Box 55; all University of Michigan Medical School Records.

22. Meeting of 2 December 1929, Discussions of the Committee on Administration, College of Physicians and Surgeons of Columbia University, Special Collections, Augustus C. Long Health Sciences Library, Columbia University, New York, NY.

23. Harold Lischner to Burrell O. Raulston, n.d., Folder "Association of American Medical Colleges Correspondence 1948–1955," Dean's Office Files, Univer-

sity of Southern California School of Medicine, Norris Medical Library, University of Southern California, Los Angeles, CA.

24. Some excellent studies have been written on barriers to women in medicine. See Regina Markell Morantz-Sanchez, *Sympathy and Science: Women Physicians in American Medicine* (New York: Oxford University Press, 1985); Mary Roth Walsh, *"Doctors Wanted: No Women Need Apply": Sexual Barriers in the Medical Profession, 1935–1975* (New Haven: Yale University Press, 1977); Barbara J. Harris, *Beyond Her Sphere: Women and the Professions in American History* (Westport, CT: Greenwood Press, 1978); and Thomas N. Bonner, *To the Ends of the Earth: Women's Search for Education in America* (Cambridge: Harvard University Press, 1992).

25. A. C. Furstenberg to Charles G. Mixter, 16 April 1943, Folder "1943 G–I," Box 46, University of Michigan Medical School Records; meeting of 13 November 1944, Minutes of the Meetings of the Faculty, College of Physicians and Surgeons of Columbia University, Special Collections, Augustus C. Long Health Sciences Library, Columbia University, New York, NY.

26. Frances Hannet, "Report on the Survey of Female Physicians Graduating from Medical School between 1925 and 1940," *Journal of the American Medical Women's Association* 13:80–85, 1958; Roscoe A. Dykman and John M. Stalnaker, "Survey of Women Physicians Graduating from Medical School 1925–1940," Part 2, *Journal of Medical Education* 32:3–38, March 1957.

27. Worth Hale to P. M. Palmer, 27 February 1930, Folder 51, Dean's Subject File, Harvard Medical School.

28. Excellent studies of discrimination against Jews in college admissions include Harold S. Wechsler, *The Qualified Student: A History of Selective College Admission in America* (New York: John Wiley & Sons, 1977); Marcia Graham Synnott, *The Half-Opened Door: Discrimination at Harvard, Yale, and Princeton, 1900–1970* (Westport, CT: Greenwood Press, 1979); Dan A. Oren, *Joining the Club: A History of Jews and Yale* (New Haven: Yale University Press, 1985); and Stephen Steinberg, *The Academic Melting Pot: Catholics and Jews in American Higher Education* (New York: McGraw-Hill, 1974). Helpful articles on Jewish quotas in medical school admissions include Leon Sokoloff, "The Rise and Decline of the Jewish Quota in Medical School Admissions," *Bulletin of the New York Academy of Medicine* 68:497–518, 1992; Edward C. Halperin, "Frank Porter Graham, Isaac Hall Manning, and the Jewish Quota at the University of North Carolina Medical School," *North Carolina Historical Review* 67:385–414, 1990; Frank Kingdon, "Discrimination in Medical Colleges," *The American Mercury* LXI:391–399, 1945; Alfred L. Shapiro, "Racial Discrimination in Medicine," *Jewish Social Studies* 10:103–134, 1948; and Jacob A. Goldberg, "Jews in the Medical Profession—A National Survey," *Jewish Social Studies* 1:327–336, 1939.

29. Statistics from Kingdon, "Discrimination in Medical Colleges," pp. 392–393.

30. *Ibid.*, pp. 394–395.

31. Meeting of 11 May 1938, Minutes, Executive Committee of the Board of Corporators, The Woman's Medical College of Pennsylvania, Archives and Special Collections on Women in Medicine, MCP Hahnemann University, Philadelphia, PA.

32. Meeting of 5 October 1936, Minutes of the Advisory Committee of the Medical Faculty, New York University School of Medicine, Archives, New York University Medical Center, New York, NY; meeting of 5 February 1928, Agenda and Business Meetings of the Council on Medical Education and Hospitals.

33. See, for example, Lewis H. Weed to Lawrence H. Baker, 7 January 1927,

Folder "Dr. Lawrence H. Baker Correspondence 1926–1928," Box 3XY, Correspondence Files, Office of the Dean of the Medical Faculty, The Johns Hopkins School of Medicine, Record Group 3, Series B, Archive of the Johns Hopkins University School of Medicine; and George Whipple to Lewis H. Weed, 23 January 1932, Folder "Whipple, George April 1929–November 1939," Box 38, Weed Papers; both the Alan Mason Chesney Medical Archives of The Johns Hopkins Medical Institutions, Baltimore, MD.

34. Kingdon, "Discrimination," pp. 392–395.

35. *Final Report of the Commission on Medical Education*, p. 284.

36. *Ibid.*, p. 286; Vernon W. Lippard, *A Half-Century of American Medical Education: 1920–1970* (New York: Josiah Macy, Jr. Foundation, 1974), p. 32.

37. See, for instance, Interview with Anson Hoyt, 7 October 1970, Folder "Anson P. S. Hoyt M.D.," Dean's Office Files, University of Southern California School of Medicine.

38. William A. Johnson to Paul A. Ferrier, 5 February 1937, Folder "USC History," Dean's Office Files, University of Southern California School of Medicine.

39. Michael B. Katz, *The Irony of Early School Reform; Educational Innovation in Mid-Nineteenth Century Massachusetts* (Cambridge: Harvard University Press, 1968); Samuel Bowles and Herbert Gintis, *Schooling in Capitalist America: Educational Reform and the Contradictions of Economic Life* (New York: Basic Books, 1976); Ira Katznelson and Margaret Weir, *Schooling for All: Class, Race, and the Decline of the Democratic Ideal* (New York: Basic Books, 1985); Levine, *The American College*.

40. Detailed descriptions of the medical school curriculum of this period are provided in *Final Report of the Commission on Medical Education*, pp. 171–261; and Weiskotten et al., *Medical Education in the United States*, pp. 80–207.

41. Weiskotten et al., *Medical Education in the United States*, pp. 140, 157.

42. *Final Report of the Commission on Medical Education*; Weiskotten et al., *Medical Education in the United States*; Abraham Flexner, *Medical Education: A Comparative Study* (New York: The Macmillan Company, 1925). David Levine discusses these issues as they appeared in debates over the college curriculum in *The American College*, pp. 89–112.

43. Lippard, *Half-Century*, p. 32.

44. Dean's Report, 1936–37, Office of the Dean, Cornell University Medical Center, Annual Reports of Departments and Offices, Archives, The New York Hospital–Cornell Medical Center, New York, NY.

45. Report of the Committee on Educational Policies, with meeting of 31 January 1936, Minutes, Advisory Board of the Medical Faculty, The Johns Hopkins University School of Medicine, The Alan Mason Chesney Medical Archives of The Johns Hopkins Medical Institutions, Baltimore, MD.

46. Lippard, *Half-Century*, pp. 16–17.

47. David Edsall to Abraham Flexner, 27 March 1924, Folder 152, Dean's Subject File, Harvard Medical School.

48. David L. Edsall to Alan M. Chesney, 17 March 1930, Folder 153, Dean's Subject File, Harvard Medical School.

49. Renée C. Fox, "Training for Uncertainty," in Robert K. Merton, George G. Reader, and Patricia L. Kendall, eds., *The Student-Physician: Introductory Studies in the Sociology of Medical Education* (Cambridge: Harvard University Press, 1957), pp. 207–241.

50. Francis M. Rackemann, *The Inquisitive Physician: The Life and Times of George Richards Minot* (Cambridge: Harvard University Press, 1956), p. 118.

51. *Ibid.*, p. 117.

52. Flexner, *Medical Education*, p. 148.

53. *Ibid.*, p. 270.

54. Report of Willard C. Rappleye, "The Objectives of Undergraduate Medical Education," with meeting of 27 October 1934, Agenda and Business Meetings of the Council on Medical Education and Hospitals.

55. *Final Report of the Commission on Medical Education*, p. 23.

56. Frederic W. Hafferty and Ronald Franks, "The Hidden Curriculum, Ethics Teaching, and the Structure of Medical Education," *Academic Medicine* 69:861–871, 1994. For a review of the literature on socialization during medical school, see Renée C. Fox, *The Sociology of Medicine: A Participant Observer's View* (Englewood Cliffs, NJ: Prentice Hall, 1989), pp. 72–107.

57. *Final Report of the Commission on Medical Education*, pp. 178, 254.

58. Hugh Cabot to William J. Gies, 21 July 1924, Folder "1924 C–D," Box 35, University of Michigan Medical School Records.

59. Robert K. Merton, "Some Preliminaries to a Sociology of Medical Education," in Merton, Reader, and Kendall, eds., *The Student-Physician*, p. 46.

60. Robert W. Lamson to B. O. Raulston, 11 February 1937, Folder "Raulston—Miscellaneous Correspondence," Dean's Office Files, University of Southern California School of Medicine.

61. Merton, Reader, and Kendall, eds., *The Student-Physician*; Howard S. Becker, Blanche Geer, Everett C. Hughes, and Anselm L. Strauss, *Boys in White: Student Culture in Medical School* (Chicago: University of Chicago Press, 1961).

62. In this discussion of student life, it is understood that no two medical students ever had exactly the same experience and that medical school classes had personalities of their own that varied from school to school and from year to year at the same school.

63. Hugh Cabot to H. P. Agersborg, 3 November 1926, Folder "1926 A," Box 36, University of Michigan Medical School Records.

64. Becker et al., *Boys in White*, pp. 65–187. This classic "participant observer" study was conducted in the 1950s, but it is difficult to imagine that the same dynamics were not operating before World War II as well.

65. Eugene F. DuBois, "Address to Students Entering a Medical College," delivered 30 September 1935, Opening Day Addresses, Cornell University Medical Center, Archives, The New York Hospital–Cornell Medical Center, New York, NY.

66. On college student life, see Levine, *The American College*, pp. 113–135; and Paula S. Fass, *The Damned and the Beautiful: American Youth in the 1920s* (New York: Oxford University Press, 1977).

67. See, for instance, meeting of the Committee on Student Donorship, 8 February 1937, Folder 285, Dean's Subject File, Harvard Medical School.

68. Supplement 8, with meeting of 14 February 1943, Agenda and Business Meetings of the Council on Medical Education and Hospitals.

69. David L. Edsall to Walter W. Palmer, 15 October 1928, Folder 1062, Dean's Subject File, Harvard Medical School.

70. Meeting of 16 January 1922, Discussions of the Committee on Administration, College of Physicians and Surgeons of Columbia University.

71. See, for instance, meeting of 5 April 1948, Medical Faculty Executive Committee Minutes, University of Pennsylvania School of Medicine (UPC 12.2), The University Archives and Record Center, University of Pennsylvania, Philadelphia, PA.

72. Meeting of 25 October 1916, Harvard University Medical Faculty, Administrative Board Records; meeting of 3 November 1932, Surgical Advisory Committee, Binder F C.9, Edward D. Churchill Papers, Harvard Medical Archives, Rare Books Department, Countway Library, Harvard Medical School, Boston, MA.

73. Meeting of 3 November 1932, Surgical Advisory Committee, Binder F C.9, Churchill Papers.

74. Meeting of 20 April 1944, Transactions of the Executive Faculty, Cornell University Medical College, Archives, The New York Hospital–Cornell Medical Center, New York, NY.

75. See, for instance, meeting of 17 April 1936, Minutes of Faculty Meetings, Woman's Medical College of Pennsylvania; Report of Subcommittee on Student Welfare, with meeting of 5 February 1940, Faculty Minutes, New York University School of Medicine.

76. Report of Committee on Student Relations, with meeting of 3 February 1937, Executive Faculty Minutes, Washington University School of Medicine, Washington University School of Medicine Archives, St. Louis, MO.

77. See, for instance, meeting of 15 November 1915, Minutes of the Meetings of the Faculty, College of Physicians and Surgeons of Columbia University; Hugh Cabot to Edward A. Balloch, 1 February 1923, Folder "B—Miscellaneous 1923," Box 35, University of Michigan Medical School Records; and meeting of 24 February 1930, Minutes of the Medical Board, The Presbyterian Hospital in the City of New York, President's Offices, Presbyterian Hospital, New York, NY.

78. See, for instance, meeting of 24 October 1923, Faculty Minutes, University of Maryland School of Medicine, Historical and Special Collections, Health Sciences Library, University of Maryland at Baltimore, Baltimore, MD.

79. Meeting of 7 December 1925, Executive Faculty Minutes, University of Colorado School of Medicine, Denison Memorial Library, University of Colorado Health Sciences Center, Denver, CO.

80. Meeting of 5 January 1926, Faculty Minutes, Tufts University School of Medicine, Tufts University Archives, Medford, MA; materials in Folder "Women's Medical Alumni Association JH," Subject Files, The Alan Mason Chesney Medical Archives of The Johns Hopkins Medical Institutions, Baltimore, MD.

81. Alan M. Kraut, *The Huddled Masses: The Immigrant in American Society, 1880–1921* (Arlington Heights, IL: Harlan Davidson, 1982); Herbert G. Gutman, *Power and Culture: Essays on the American Working Class* (New York: Pantheon, 1987).

82. Meeting of 21 January 1938, Transactions of the Executive Faculty, Cornell University Medical College; meetings of 16 January 1922 and 4 February 1929, Discussions of the Committee on Administration, College of Physicians and Surgeons of Columbia University; meeting of 4 October 1946, Harvard University Medical Faculty, Minutes of Meetings, Harvard University Medical Archives, Rare Books Department, Countway Library, Harvard Medical School, Boston, MA.

83. For instance, see the student reports (covering the years 1909–1948) in Folders 1603–1607, Dean's Subject File, Harvard Medical School.

84. Report of the Department of Anatomy, 1934–35, Office of the Dean, Cornell University Medical Center, Annual Reports of Departments and Offices, Archives, The New York Hospital–Cornell Medical Center, New York, NY.

85. Meeting of 25 February 1924, Discussions of the Committee on Administration, College of Physicians and Surgeons of Columbia University.

86. Robert A. Harrell, "A History of the Pithotomy Club," and Robert C. Sergott and Peter D. Olch, "The Society of Pithotomists, 1897–1980," both in Folder "Pithotomy Club," Records of the Pithotomy Club, The Alan Mason Chesney Archives of The Johns Hopkins Medical Institutions, Baltimore, MD.

87. See, for instance, Hugh Cabot to Wilbur R. Twiss, 29 June 1928, Folder "1928 T–Z," Box 38; and A. C. Furstenberg to Lloyd C. Emmons, 2 September 1936, Folder "1936 M," Box 40; both University of Michigan Medical School Records.

88. See, for instance, Association of American Medical Colleges, Report of the Joint Committee on the Teaching of the Social and Environmental Factors in Medicine, in Folder "A.A.M.C. Meetings, October 1946," Dean's Office Files, University of Southern California School of Medicine.

89. Richard C. Cabot, *Training and Rewards of the Physician* (Philadelphia: J. B. Lippincott Company, 1918), p. 45.

90. Report of Willard C. Rappleye, "The Objectives of Undergraduate Medical Education," with meeting of 27 October 1934, Agenda and Minutes of the Business Meetings of the Council on Medical Education and Hospitals.

91. Lewis Mayers and Leonard V. Harrison, *The Distribution of Physicians in the United States* (New York: General Education Board, 1924).

92. See, for instance, B. Edward McClellan, *Schools and the Shaping of Character: Moral Education in America, 1607–Present* (Bloomington, IN: ERIC Clearinghouse, 1992).

93. Lawrence A. Cremin, *American Education: The Metropolitan Experience 1876–1980* (New York: Harper and Row, 1988).

Chapter 4

1. *Annual Report of the Mount Sinai Hospital* (1924), p. 30.

2. Secondary literature on the history of graduate medical education is scarce. Helpful articles include Rosemary A. Stevens, "Graduate Medical Education: A Continuing History," *Journal of Medical Education* 53:1–18, 1978; J. A. Curran, "Internships and Residencies: Historical Backgrounds and Current Trends," *Journal of Medical Education* 34:873–884, 1959; and Council on Medical Education and Hospitals, "Background and Development of Residency Review and Conference Committees," *Journal of the American Medical Association* 165:60–64, 1957. Much about the process of specialization, particularly from the point of view of medical politics, is found in Rosemary Stevens, *American Medicine and the Public Interest* (New Haven: Yale University Press, 1971). The first national report on graduate medical education—and now a valuable historical reference—was *Graduate Medical Education: Report of the Commission on Graduate Medical Education* (Chicago: University of Chicago Press, 1940).

3. Meetings of 17 March 1913, 15 March 1915, 15 November 1915, and 21 January 1918, Minutes of the Meetings of the Faculty, College of Physicians and Surgeons of Columbia University, Special Collections, Augustus C. Long Health Sciences Library, Columbia University, New York, NY.

4. Curran, "Internships and Residencies," p. 876. The last appearance of the term "house pupil" in the *Annual Reports* of the Massachusetts General Hospital was 1920.

5. Victor Johnson, *A History of the Council on Medical Education and Hospitals of the American Medical Association, 1901–1959* (Chicago: American Medical Association, 1959).

6. Meeting of 1–6 December 1945, Agenda and Minutes of the Business Meetings of the Council on Medical Education and Hospitals, American Medical Association Archives, Chicago, IL.

7. *Graduate Medical Education*, pp. 10, 76–77, 255.

8. Curran, "Internships and Residencies," p. 878.

9. *Ibid.*, p. 878; *Graduate Medical Education*, p. 253.

10. Appendix B, with meeting of 18–20 June 1948, Agenda and Minutes of the Business Meetings of the Council on Medical Education and Hospitals.

11. Detailed descriptions of the pre–World War II internship are found in *Graduate Medical Education*, pp. 30–95; and *Final Report of the Commission on Medical Education* (New York: Office of the Director of the Study, 1932), pp. 141–150.

12. Meeting of 14 June 1932, Minutes, Board of Trustees, The Mount Sinai Hospital, Archives, The Mount Sinai Medical Center, New York, NY.

13. "Medical Education in the United States, 1934–1939," *Journal of the American Medical Association* 114:144, 1940.

14. Meeting of 17 May 1921, Minutes, Medical Board, The Mount Sinai Hospital, Archives, The Mount Sinai Medical Center, New York, NY; meeting of 2 December 1918, Minutes of the Medical Board, The Presbyterian Hospital in the City of New York, President's Offices, Presbyterian Hospital, New York, NY.

15. N. P. Colwell to William D. Cutter, 16 January 1930, Folder "Reports AMA and Assn. of Med. Colleges 1929–1933," Dean's Office Files, University of Southern California School of Medicine, Norris Medical Library, University of Southern California, Los Angeles, CA.

16. "A Consideration of Graduate Medical Education . . . ," with Executive Faculty Meeting of 9 December 1941, Folder "1939–1945," Box 128, University of Michigan Medical School Records, Michigan Historical Collections, Bentley Historical Library, University of Michigan, Ann Arbor, MI.

17. Memorandum on Single Service Internships, 25 August 1934, with meeting of 26–27 October 1934, Agenda and Minutes of the Business Meetings of the Council on Medical Education and Hospitals.

18. *Final Report of the Commission on Medical Education*, p. 143.

19. Kenneth M. Ludmerer, *Learning to Heal: The Development of American Medical Education* (New York: Basic Books, 1985), pp. 16–19.

20. *Final Report of the Commission on Medical Education*, pp. 128, 136.

21. See, for instance, the flow chart, "The Ideal Preparation of the Young Otologist," with Report of the Department of Otology, 1930–31, Folder 1, Box 2, Office of the Dean, Cornell University Medical Center, Annual Reports of Departments and Offices, Archives, The New York Hospital–Cornell Medical Center, New York, NY.

22. Meeting of 5 January 1937, Transactions of the Medical Board of the New York Hospital, Archives, The New York Hospital–Cornell Medical Center, New York, NY.

23. Meeting of 23 June 1930, Agenda and Minutes of the Business Meetings of the Council on Medical Education and Hospitals.

24. Meeting of 15 February 1931, Agenda and Minutes of the Business Meetings of the Council on Medical Education and Hospitals.

25. For a description of a typical program, see "The Program of Graduate Medical Education in Columbia University," with meeting of 1 February 1937, Minutes of the Meetings of the Committee on Administration, College of Physicians and Surgeons of Columbia University, Special Collections, Augustus C. Long Health Sciences Library, Columbia University.

26. College of Physicians and Surgeons of Columbia University, *Annual Report of the Dean* (1939), p. 12.

27. *Graduate Medical Education*, p. 14.

28. *Ibid.*, pp. 97–103.

29. Alan M. Chesney, *The Johns Hopkins Hospital and The Johns Hopkins University School of Medicine: A Chronicle*, vol. 1 (Baltimore: The Johns Hopkins Press, 1943), pp. 161–163; A. McGehee Harvey, Gert H. Brieger, Susan L. Abrams, and Victor A. McKusick, *A Model of Its Kind: A Centennial History of Medicine at Johns Hopkins*, vol. 1 (Baltimore: Johns Hopkins University Press, 1989), pp. 183–187; William Osler to Medical Board, 30 January 1890, with meeting of 30 January 1890, Minutes, The Johns Hopkins Hospital Medical Board, The Alan Mason Chesney Medical Archives of The Johns Hopkins Medical Institutions, Baltimore, MD; William S. Halsted, "The Training of the Surgeon," *Bulletin of The Johns Hopkins Hospital* 15:267–275, 1904.

30. Chesney, *The Johns Hopkins Hospital*, p. 162.

31. Halsted, "The Training of the Surgeon," p. 273.

32. *Graduate Medical Education*, pp. 14, 99.

33. For instance, in 1935 every member of the surgical resident staff at the New York Hospital was engaged in investigative research; in 1929, each of the internal medicine house officers at the Massachusetts General Hospital; in 1939, four of the ophthalmology residents at the Presbyterian Hospital. (Meeting of 1 February 1935, Transactions of the Medical Board of the New York Hospital; The Massachusetts General Hospital, *Annual Report* [1929], pp. 17–18; The Presbyterian Hospital in the City of New York, *Annual Report* [1939], p. 56.)

34. A. McGehee Harvey, *Science at the Bedside: Clinical Research in American Medicine* (Baltimore: Johns Hopkins University Press, 1981); Ludmerer, *Learning to Heal*, pp. 123–138, 207–218.

35. For instance, until 1940 Mount Sinai Hospital (New York) required a minimum of one year of research in a preclinical laboratory, in addition to the completion of an internship, for appointment to the resident staff. (Meeting of 12 March 1940, Minutes, Board of Trustees, The Mount Sinai Hospital.)

36. Meeting of 7 January 1942, Harvard University Medical Faculty, Minutes of Meetings, Harvard Medical Archives, Rare Books Department, Countway Library, Harvard Medical School, Boston, MA.

37. The Peter Bent Brigham Hospital, *Annual Report* (1923), pp. 113–115.

38. *Graduate Medical Education*, p. 101.

39. *Ibid.*, p. 101.

40. Report of the Staff Committee on Professional Services on Residency and Graduate Training, with meeting of 15 October 1952, Minutes, Advisory Board of the Medical Faculty, The Johns Hopkins University School of Medicine, The Alan Mason Chesney Medical Archives of The Johns Hopkins Medical Institutions, Baltimore, MD.

41. Meeting of 19 April 1937, Minutes of the Medical Board, The Presbyterian Hospital in the City of New York.

42. "A Review of the Program at the Medical Center," with meeting of 7 July 1937, Minutes of the Medical Board, The Presbyterian Hospital in the City of New York.

43. *Table 3* is adopted from Council on Medical Education and Hospitals, "Background and Development of Residency Review and Conference Committees," p. 62.

44. *Ibid.*; Stevens, *American Medicine and the Public Interest*, pp. 116–124,

244–266; William D. Holden, "The American Specialty Boards," in Thomas Samph and Bryce Templeton, eds., *Evaluation in Medical Education: Past, Present, Future* (Cambridge, MA: Ballinger Publishing Company, 1979), pp. 165–200.

45. An ample body of scholarship has identified features of "progressive" reform continuing through the administration of Franklin D. Roosevelt. See Barry D. Karl, *The Uneasy State: The United States from 1915 to 1945* (Chicago: University of Chicago Press, 1983); William A. Link, *American Epoch: A History of the United States Since 1900* (New York: McGraw-Hill, 1993); and Clarke A. Chambers, *Seedtime of Reform: American Social Service and Social Action, 1918–1933* (Minneapolis: University of Minnesota Press, 1964).

46. The Massachusetts General Hospital, *Annual Report* (1947), p. 49.

47. Minutes of Hospital Committee Meeting, 29 November 1937, with meeting of 1 December 1937, Executive Faculty Minutes, Washington University School of Medicine, Washington University School of Medicine Archives, St. Louis, MO.

48. J. Stewart Rodman, *History of the American Board of Surgery 1937–1952* (Philadelphia: J. B. Lippincott Company, 1956), pp. 1–10.

49. Report of Intern Committee of American Hospital Association, June 1924, Folder 1064, Dean's Subject File, Harvard Medical School, Harvard Medical Archives, Rare Books Department, Countway Library, Harvard Medical School, Boston, MA.

50. J. H. Means to C. Sidney Burwell, 4 December 1939, Folder 157, Dean's Subject File, Harvard Medical School.

51. Meeting of 4 January 1940, Harvard University Medical Faculty, Administrative Board Records, Harvard Medical Archives, Rare Books Department, Countway Library, Harvard Medical School, Boston, MA.

52. Mark M. Ravitch, "The Surgical Residency: Then, Now, and Future," *The Pharos*, Winter 1987, p. 13.

53. Meeting of 5 January 1937, Transactions of the Medical Board of the New York Hospital.

54. Charles L. Bosk, "Occupational Rituals in Patient Management," *New England Journal of Medicine* 303:71–76, 1980. See also Charles L. Bosk, *Forgive and Remember: Managing Medical Failure* (Chicago: University of Chicago Press, 1979).

55. Report of the Surgical Department, 1 September 1932 to 1 March 1933, Folder 5, Box 2, Papers, Office of the Dean, Cornell University Medical College, 1903–1934 (Niles), Archives, The New York Hospital–Cornell Medical Center, New York, NY.

56. Meeting of 4 December 1944, Transactions of the Medical Board of the New York Hospital.

57. *Final Report of the Commission on Medical Education*, pp. 141–143; *Graduate Medical Education*, pp. 32, 38; Essentials in a Hospital Approved for Residencies in Specialties, with meeting of 12 February 1933, Agenda and Minutes of the Business Meetings of the Council on Medical Education and Hospitals.

58. See, for instance, Minutes of the Hospital Committee Meeting, 11 April 1938, with meeting of 13 April 1938, Executive Faculty Minutes, Washington University School of Medicine.

59. William P. Longmire Jr., *Alfred Blalock: His Life and Times* (privately printed, 1991), pp. 82–83.

60. Curran, "Internships and Residencies," p. 882.

61. Meeting of 4 December 1938, Agenda and Minutes of the Business Meetings of the Council on Medical Education and Hospitals.

The tension between education and service was not unique to medical education. Witness the traditional exploitation of nursing students as a source of cheap labor. See Susan M. Reverby, *Ordered to Care: The Dilemma of American Nursing, 1850–1945* (Cambridge, England: Cambridge University Press, 1987); and Barbara Melosh, *"The Physician's Hand": Work Culture and Conflict in American Nursing* (Philadelphia: Temple University Press, 1982).

62. Eugene F. DuBois, "Address to Students Entering a Medical College," delivered 30 September 1935, Opening Day Addresses, Cornell University Medical Center, Archives, The New York Hospital–Cornell Medical Center, New York, NY.

63. Meeting of 12 February 1933, Agenda and Minutes of the Business Meetings of the Council on Medical Education and Hospitals.

64. Meeting of 20 October 1942, Minutes, Medical Board, The Mount Sinai Hospital.

65. Meeting of 8 December 1925, Board of Managers Minutes, The Presbyterian Hospital in the City of New York, President's Offices, Presbyterian Hospital, New York, NY; Hospital Committee Minutes of 13 February 1919, with meeting of 5 March 1919, Executive Faculty Minutes, Washington University School of Medicine.

66. Meeting of 10 October 1934, Box 3, Minutes of the Board of Managers of the Hospital of the University of Pennsylvania (UPC 12.1), The University Archives and Record Center, University of Pennsylvania, Philadelphia, PA.

67. David L. Edsall to Walter W. Palmer, 15 October 1928, Folder 1062; and David L. Edsall to Channing Frothingham, 14 December 1925, Folder 1063; both Dean's Subject File, Harvard Medical School.

68. William Osler to Medical Board, 30 January 1890, with meeting of 30 January 1890, Minutes, The Johns Hopkins Hospital Medical Board.

69. H. J. Stander to Otto H. Schwarz, 13 September 1940, Folder 6, Box 6, Henricus J. Stander Papers, Archives, The New York Hospital–Cornell Medical Center, New York, NY.

70. Ravitch, "The Surgical Residency," p. 14.

71. The best study of black hospitals is Vanessa Northington Gamble, *Making a Place for Ourselves: The Black Hospital Movement, 1920–1945* (New York: Oxford University Press, 1995).

72. Meeting of 2 May 1941, Minutes, Executive Committee of the Board of Corporators, The Woman's Medical College of Pennsylvania, Archives and Special Collections on Women in Medicine, MCP Hahnemann University, Philadelphia, PA.

73. Meeting of 25 November 1935, Minutes of the Medical Board, The Presbyterian Hospital in the City of New York.

74. Charles E. Ziegler to H. J. Stander, 6 January 1938, Folder 9, Box 7, Stander Papers.

75. Mount Sinai was such an outstanding hospital that non-Jews often applied for positions. Its appointment system was one of the fairest in the country, and in some years as many as one-third of its house officers were Christian. The hospital administered examinations to prospective interns that were identified by numbers rather than names, thereby guaranteeing impartiality in making appointments. (Interview with Percy Klingenstein, 16 March 1967, Oral History Collection, Archives, The Mount Sinai Medical Center, New York, NY; Report of Committee on Examinations, with meeting of 10 January 1933, Minutes, Board of Trustees, The Mount Sinai Hospital.)

76. Supplement 22, with meeting of 8 November 1942, Agenda and Minutes of the Business Meetings of the Council on Medical Education and Hospitals.

77. Winthop Pennock to Worth Hale, 27 November 1929, Folder 1062, Dean's Subject File, Harvard Medical School.

78. *Graduate Medical Education*, pp. 90, 163.

79. Meeting of 20 February 1940, Minutes, Medical Board, The Mount Sinai Hospital.

80. The Peter Bent Brigham Hospital, *Annual Report* (1927), p. 72.

81. The hospital's traditional emphasis on maintaining strict control over its internal environment is discussed in Charles E. Rosenberg, *The Care of Strangers: The Rise of America's Hospital System* (New York: Basic Books, 1987). After World War I, many official rules for house officers, such as not smoking in corridors or socializing with nurses, were frequently ignored.

82. Meeting of 2 August 1926, Executive Faculty Minutes, University of Colorado School of Medicine, Denison Memorial Library, University of Colorado Health Sciences Center, Denver, CO.

83. The Peter Bent Brigham Hospital, *Annual Report* (1927), p. 71.

84. Helen Eastman Martin, *The History of the Los Angeles County Hospital (1878–1968) and the Los Angeles County–University of Southern California Medical Center (1968–1979)* (Los Angeles: University of Southern California Press, 1979), p. 77.

85. Meeting of 4 February 1955, Harvard University Medical Faculty, Minutes of Meetings.

86. Meeting of 9 December 1955, Harvard University Medical Faculty, Minutes of Meetings.

87. George E. Mowry and Blaine A. Brownell, *The Urban Nation 1920–1980*, rev. ed. (New York: Hill and Wang, 1981), p. 16.

88. Longmire, *Alfred Blalock*, p. 215. The support system of internship and residency is also discussed in Robert J. Glaser, "House Officership—Then and Now," *The Pharos*, Winter 1987, p. 45.

89. *Final Report of the Commission on Medical Education*, p. 118.

90. The tension between individualism and community has been widely noted, but an especially insightful treatment is found in Karl, *The Uneasy State*.

91. Paul Starr, *The Social Transformation of American Medicine: The Rise of a Sovereign Profession and the Making of a Vast Industry* (New York: Basic Books, 1982), p. 358.

92. This point is a major theme of *Final Report of the Commission on Medical Education*.

93. *Graduate Medical Education*, p. 39.
Ostensibly, specialty training represented a meritocracy, but economic realities belied that view. Residents received only a token stipend, which undoubtedly discouraged many medical graduates of modest means from trying to enter a specialty. Statistical evidence on this matter was not available, but many medical educators had the distinct impression that the lengthy uncompensated period of specialty training was a significant deterrent. (Report of the Dean of the Medical School, 1939–40, Folder 473, Dean's Subject File, Harvard Medical School.)

94. *Graduate Medical Education*, pp. 39, 139.

95. The Peter Bent Brigham Hospital, *Annual Report* (1938), p. 114.

96. Annual Report, Cardiac Clinic, Cornell Clinics, 1926–27, Folder 1, Box 1, Papers, Office of the Dean, Cornell University Medical College, 1903–1934 (Niles).

97. Paul Reznikoff to Victor Schilling, 1 April 1937, Folder "European Trip Correspondence, 1929–1930," Paul Reznikoff Papers, Archives, The New York Hospital–Cornell Medical Center, New York, NY.

98. Meeting of 1–6 December 1945, Agenda and Minutes of the Business Meetings of the Council on Medical Education and Hospitals.

99. Winford Smith to Members of the Medical Board, 21 October 1931, Folder "Johns Hopkins Hospital—Dr. W. Smith Correspondence 1929–1931," Box 4XY, Correspondence Files, Office of the Dean of the Medical Faculty, The Johns Hopkins School of Medicine, Record Group 3, Series B, Archive of The Johns Hopkins University School of Medicine, The Alan Mason Chesney Medical Archives of The Johns Hopkins Medical Institutions, Baltimore, MD.

100. Report of the Department of Radiology, 1944–45, Office of the Dean, Cornell University Medical Center, Annual Reports of Departments and Offices.

Chapter 5

1. Meeting of 27 November 1928, Board of Managers Minutes, The Presbyterian Hospital in the City of New York, President's Offices, Presbyterian Hospital, New York, NY; Statement of 4 February 1935, with meeting of 9 February 1935, Transactions of the Executive Faculty, Cornell University Medical College, Archives, The New York Hospital–Cornell Medical Center, New York, NY; meeting of 15 December 1925, Minutes, Medical Board, The Mount Sinai Hospital, Archives, The Mount Sinai Medical Center, New York, NY. The Mount Sinai Hospital was one of the few major teaching hospitals that did not serve as a primary clinical facility of a medical school at this time.

2. Meeting of 9 September 1946, Minutes of the Meetings of the Committee on Administration, College of Physicians and Surgeons of Columbia University, Special Collections, Augustus C. Long Health Sciences Library, Columbia University, New York, NY.

3. The Massachusetts General Hospital, *Annual Report* (1936), p. 28.

4. Meeting of 14 November 1939, Minutes of the Board of Governors, The Society of The New York Hospital, Archives, The New York Hospital–Cornell Medical Center, New York, NY. The treasurer and secretary were members of the board of governors, not paid members of the administrative staff.

5. Report of the Department of Medicine, 1939–40, Office of the Dean, Cornell University Medical Center, Annual Reports of Departments and Offices, Archives, The New York Hospital–Cornell Medical Center, New York, NY.

6. Meeting of 28 June 1939, Minutes of the Joint Administrative Board, New York Hospital–Cornell Medical College Center, Archives, New York Hospital–Cornell Medical Center, New York, NY.

7. Edmund E. Day to Henry G. Barbey, 3 February 1938, Folder 8, Box 1, Papers, Office of the Dean, Cornell University Medical College, 1893–1956 (Hinsey), Archives, The New York Hospital–Cornell Medical Center, New York, NY.

8. Outline of agreement by the Medical College to the proposed plan of the Hospital for housing medical students in the Annex, 27 May 1942, Folder 4, Box 5, Henricus J. Stander Papers, Archives, The New York Hospital–Cornell Medical Center, New York, NY.

9. Meeting of 20 June 1936, Minutes of the Executive Committee of the Board of Governors, The Society of The New York Hospital, Archives, The New York Hospital–Cornell Medical Center, New York, NY.

10. Meeting of 7 May 1930, Minutes, The Johns Hopkins Hospital Board of

Trustees, The Alan Mason Chesney Medical Archives of The Johns Hopkins Medical Institutions, Baltimore, MD.

11. Meeting of 3 October 1945, Minutes of the Planning Committee of the Medical Board, The Presbyterian Hospital in the City of New York, President's Office, Presbyterian Hospital, New York, NY.

12. Memorandum of Earl B. McKinley, 24 April 1938, Folder "E. B. McKinley, #1," Box 5, Vincent du Vigneaud Papers, Archives, The New York Hospital–Cornell Medical Center, New York, NY.

13. Throughout the twentieth century all nonprofit hospitals, not just teaching institutions, have been torn between their desire to do good work and the need to keep the books balanced. See Rosemary Stevens, *In Sickness and in Wealth: American Hospitals in the Twentieth Century* (New York: Basic Books, 1989); and David Rosner, "Doing Well or Doing Good: The Ambivalent Focus of Hospital Administration," in Diana E. Long and Janet Golden, eds., *The American General Hospital: Communities and Social Context* (Ithaca, NY: Cornell University Press, 1989), pp. 157–169.

14. George Rosen, *The Structure of American Medical Practice 1875–1941*, ed. Charles E. Rosenberg (Philadelphia: University of Pennsylvania Press, 1983), pp. 39, 44, 48–49.

15. Report of Intern Committee of American Hospital Association, June 1924, Folder 1064, Dean's Subject File, Harvard Medical School, Harvard Medical Archives, Rare Books Department, Countway Library, Harvard Medical School, Boston, MA.

16. The Peter Bent Brigham Hospital, *Annual Report* (1958), p. 23.

17. The Peter Bent Brigham Hospital, *Annual Report* (1925), p. 144.

18. *Annual Report of the Mount Sinai Hospital* (1955), p. 23.
Though many patients took their lengthy hospitalization with good humor, some chafed at the bit. One was Abraham Flexner, irate at the time he lost from work during a several-month hospitalization in 1918–19 for a tendon repair. He had a good surgical result but protested that a lengthy treatment "may be one thing in the case of a monkey or guinea pig and ought to be another thing in the case of a busy person." (Abraham Flexner to Simon Flexner, 27 January 1919, Folder "Flex, Ab 1919," Simon Flexner Papers, American Philosophical Society Library, Philadelphia, PA.)

19. Of course, outpatient medicine involved many important skills that could not be learned from treating emergencies—for instance, the prevention and treatment of foot problems in diabetics.

20. Memorandum "Internes," Folder 326–27, Box "Hospital Records 1894–1931," Hospital Records, Georgetown University Archives, Georgetown University, Washington, D.C.

21. Meeting of 21 April 1925, Minutes, Medical Board, The Mount Sinai Hospital.

22. The Peter Bent Brigham Hospital, *Annual Report* (1923), p. 74.

23. Stanley Joel Reiser, *Medicine and the Reign of Technology* (Cambridge, England: Cambridge University Press, 1978).

24. Annual Report, Cardiac Clinic, Cornell Clinics, 1926–27, Folder 1, Box 1, Papers, Office of the Dean, Cornell University Medical College, 1903–1934 (Niles), Archives, The New York Hospital–Cornell Medical Center, New York, NY.
Many "objective" tests were far more subjective than their proponents realized or admitted. X-rays, for example, may have provided a veneer of objectivity but in fact depended on subjective human faculties for their clinical interpretation.

25. See, for instance, The Peter Bent Brigham Hospital, *Annual Report* (1923), p. 67.

26. See materials in Folder "Medical Apprenticeship 1929," Box 38, University of Michigan Medical School Records, Michigan Historical Collections, Bentley Historical Library, University of Michigan, Ann Arbor, MI.

27. General Faculty Meeting and Dinner, 15 November 1939, Dean's Office Files (Stuart P. Cromer, 1939–41), ID Number 20D008, Special Collections Division, University of Arkansas for Medical Sciences Library, Little Rock, AR; Report of the Inspection of the Woman's Medical College of Pennsylvania, 28 February 1919, with meeting of 19 March 1919, Minutes of Faculty Meetings, Woman's Medical College of Pennsylvania, Archives and Special Collections on Women in Medicine, MCP Hahnemann University, Philadelphia, PA.

28. Minutes of Dispensary Committee Meeting, 20 March 1922, with meeting 5 April 1922, Executive Faculty Minutes, Washington University School of Medicine, Washington University School of Medicine Archives, St. Louis, MO.

29. The Peter Bent Brigham Hospital, *Annual Report* (1928), p. 145.

30. Abraham Flexner, *Medical Education: A Comparative Study* (New York: The Macmillan Company, 1925), pp. 231–232; The Peter Bent Brigham Hospital, *Annual Report* (1925), p. 75; (1926), p. 144; (1928), p. 145.

31. Annual Report, Cardiac Clinic, 1926–27, Cornell Clinics, Folder 1, Box 1, Papers, Office of the Dean, Cornell University Medical College, 1903–1934 (Niles).

32. Annual Report, Neurology Department, Cornell Clinics, 1926–27, Folder 1, Box 1, Papers, Office of the Dean, Cornell University Medical College, 1903–1934 (Niles).

33. The Peter Bent Brigham Hospital, *Annual Report* (1928), p. 145.

34. Methods of Teaching the Clinical Branches in the Medical Curriculum, with meeting of 29 December 1934, Agenda and Minutes of the Business Meetings of the Council on Medical Education and Hospitals, American Medical Association Archives, Chicago, IL.

35. See, for instance, Minutes of the Hospital Committee Meeting, 5 April 1937, with meeting of 7 April 1937, Executive Faculty Minutes, Washington University School of Medicine; and meeting of 18 February 1937, Transactions of the Medical Board of the New York Hospital, Archives, The New York Hospital–Cornell Medical Center, New York, NY.

36. Paul S. Russell, "Surgery in a Time of Change," in John H. Knowles, ed., *The Teaching Hospital: Evolution and Contemporary Issues* (Cambridge: Harvard University Press, 1966), p. 58.

Chapter 6

1. Vernon W. Lippard, *A Half-Century of American Medical Education: 1920–1970* (New York: Josiah Macy, Jr. Foundation, 1974), pp. 61–66.

2. Albert R. Lamb, *The Presbyterian Hospital and the Columbia-Presbyterian Medical Center 1868–1943: A History of a Great Medical Adventure* (New York: Columbia University Press, 1955), pp. 217–256.

3. John E. Deitrick and Robert C. Berson, *Medical Schools in the United States at Mid-Century* (New York: McGraw-Hill, 1953), p. 54.

4. Much has been written about the university's utilitarian mission, but I am especially indebted to Laurence R. Veysey, *The Emergence of the American University* (Chicago: University of Chicago Press, 1965); Jacques Barzun, *The American*

University: How It Runs, Where It Is Going, 2nd ed. (Chicago: University of Chicago Press, 1993); and Jaroslav Pelikan, *The Idea of the University: A Reexamination* (New Haven: Yale University Press, 1992).

5. James D. Bruce, "Postgraduate Education in Michigan," *Journal of the Michigan State Medical Society* 36:373, 1937.

6. Abraham Flexner, *Medical Education in the United States and Canada* (New York: Carnegie Foundation for the Advancement of Teaching, 1910), p. 174.

7. Robert K. Richards, *Continuing Medical Education: Perspectives, Problems, Prognosis* (New Haven: Yale University Press, 1978), pp. 24–36.

8. Report of the Committee on Graduate Medical Education, with meeting of 1 December 1941, Faculty Minutes, New York University School of Medicine, Archives, New York University Medical Center, New York, NY.

9. *Annual Report of the Mount Sinai Hospital* (1939), p. 56.

10. Richards, *Continuing Medical Education,* pp. 8–9. Perhaps the most notable was the Bingham Program, an organized program in which the Tufts-New England Medical Center provided consultation and continuing medical education across state lines to physicians of Maine, which did not have a medical school. See Herbert Black, *Doctor and Teacher, Hospital Chief: Dr. Samuel Proger and the New England Medical Center* (Chester, CT: The Globe Pequot Press, 1982), pp. 61–73, 88–94, 141–151).

11. Veysey, *The Emergence of the American University,* p. 108.

12. The Presbyterian Hospital in the City of New York, *Annual Report* (1941), p. 66.

13. A. C. Furstenberg, Dean's Report, 10 October 1940, Folder "R 1940," Box 43, University of Michigan Medical School Records, Michigan Historical Collections, Bentley Historical Library, University of Michigan, Ann Arbor, MI.

14. The Peter Bent Brigham Hospital, *Annual Report* (1925), p. 144.

15. Meeting of 9–10 June 1934, Agenda and Minutes of the Business Meetings of the Council on Medical Education and Hospitals, American Medical Association Archives, Chicago, IL.

16. Minutes of the Medical Staff Meeting, 20 February 1933, Folder "Medical Staff Meetings University Hospital," Box 3, Medical Faculty Executive Committee Minutes, University of Pennsylvania School of Medicine (UPC 12.2), The University Archives and Record Center, University of Pennsylvania, Philadelphia, PA.

17. J. B. Applegate to Dear Doctor, n.d., Folder "Correspondence," Box 1, Charles E. de M. Sajous Papers, Conwella-Templana Collection, Temple University Library, Philadelphia, PA.

18. Meeting of 2 May 1938, Executive Faculty Minutes, University of Colorado School of Medicine, Denison Memorial Library, University of Colorado Health Sciences Center, Denver, CO.

19. The Peter Bent Brigham Hospital, *Annual Report* (1925), p. 144; (1926), pp. 120–121; (1928), p. 148.

20. Daniel M. Fox, *Health Policies, Health Politics: The British and American Experience, 1911–1965* (Princeton, NJ: Princeton University Press, 1986). Fox used the term "hierarchical regionalism" to describe this relationship of hospitals within a geographical region.

21. The Peter Bent Brigham Hospital, *Annual Report* (1945), p. 20.

22. Hospital Committee Meeting, 12 October 1921, with meeting of 9 November 1921, Executive Faculty Minutes, Washington University School of Medicine, Washington University School of Medicine Archives, St. Louis, MO.

23. Alan Chesney, "The Hospitals of Baltimore and the Indigent Sick," 1932,

Folder "Reprints on Medical Education," Box 5, Longcope Papers; meeting of Budget Committee, 28 February 1948, with meeting of 2 March 1948, Minutes, The Johns Hopkins Hospital Board of Trustees; both in The Alan Mason Chesney Medical Archives of The Johns Hopkins Medical Institutions, Baltimore, MD.

24. Deitrick and Berson, *Medical Schools in the United States at Mid-Century*, pp. 61–62.

25. Meeting of 28 October 1940, Board of Managers Minutes, The Presbyterian Hospital in the City of New York, President's Offices, Presbyterian Hospital, New York, NY.

26. Meeting of 22 February 1933, Corporation Minutes, Woman's Medical College of Pennsylvania, Archives and Special Collections on Women in Medicine, MCP Hahnemann University, Philadelphia, PA.

27. For a typical example of a rating system, see Social Service Report, with meeting of 4 December 1929, Executive Faculty Minutes, Washington University School of Medicine.

28. "Medical Center," *Fortune*, June 1944, p. 216.

29. For instance, one patient requested his bill from Barnes Hospital following a successful operation. The hospital was about to provide it when the referring physician, a general practitioner in rural Missouri, informed the surgeon that the family was nearly destitute and would probably have to mortgage the farm in order to pay. The patient had intentionally withheld that information. With hardly a thought, the hospital and surgeon both dropped their charges. (Hospital Committee Minutes, 20 January 1928, with meeting of 1 February 1928, Executive Faculty Minutes, Washington University School of Medicine.)

30. Medical Board, Recommendations of the Committee on Diets, November 1930, Folder 11, Box 54, Society of The New York Hospital, Secretary/Treasurer Papers (1811–1933), Archives, The New York Hospital–Cornell Medical Center, New York, NY.

31. Harry F. Dowling, *City Hospitals: The Undercare of the Underprivileged* (Cambridge: Harvard University Press, 1982). It should not be assumed that ward patients invariably felt oppressed. For instance, a study of patients at Philadelphia General Hospital found that they were very happy with the care they received. The patients felt that the hospital was one of the few places where they were truly welcome. Their worst complaint was the interminable waits and delays. ("Poor Like PGH Service Despite Dingy Facilities," newspaper clipping, Folder "Philadelphia General Hospital," Box 3, Philadelphia General Hospital Papers [UPC 56.4], The University Archives and Record Center, University of Pennsylvania, Philadelphia, PA.)

32. Anne Beadenkopf to Alan Chesney, 20 March 1946, Folder "Negro Physicians and the JHH," Subject Files, The Alan Mason Chesney Medical Archives of The Johns Hopkins Medical Institutions, Baltimore, MD; meeting of 26 November 1930, Minutes, Executive Committee of the Board of Corporators, The Woman's Medical College of Pennsylvania, Archives and Special Collections on Women in Medicine, MCP Hahnemann University, Philadelphia, PA.

33. Clark Kerr, *The Great Transformation in Higher Education: 1960–1980* (Albany: State University of New York Press, 1991), pp. 5, 69–78.

34. Abraham Flexner, *Universities: American English German* (New York: Oxford University Press, 1930), pp. 44, 152.

35. *Ibid.*, pp. 15–17, 92–93.

36. Joseph C. Hinsey to Winslow Carlton, 1 August 1944, with meeting of 21 September 1944, Transactions of the Executive Faculty, Cornell University Med-

ical College, Archives, The New York Hospital–Cornell Medical Center, New York, NY.

37. Rosemary Stevens, *In Sickness and in Wealth: American Hospitals in the Twentieth Century* (New York: Basic Books, 1989), p. 177.

38. Richard H. Shryock, "The American Physician in 1846 and 1946: A Study in Professional Contrasts," in Richard H. Shryock, *Medicine in America: Historical Essays* (Baltimore: The Johns Hopkins Press, 1966), pp. 149–176.

39. Paul Starr, *The Social Transformation of American Medicine: The Rise of a Sovereign Profession and the Making of a Vast Industry* (New York: Basic Books, 1982), p. 359.

40. *Final Report of the Commission on Medical Education* (New York: Office of the Director of the Study, 1932), p. 54.

41. *Ibid.*, pp. 16, 36.

42. Committee on the Costs of Medical Care, *Medical Care for the American People* (Chicago: University of Chicago Press, 1932), p. 35.

43. College of Physicians and Surgeons of Columbia University, *Annual Report of the Dean* (1947), p. 12.

44. *Final Report of the Commission on Medical Education*, p. 328.

45. *Ibid.*, p. 63. Another important report advancing similar views was Committee on the Costs of Medical Care, *Medical Care for the American People*.

Chapter 7

1. Report of Committee on Preparedness, 26–28 October 1942, Folder "1942–1971 MEND: Selected Bibliography," Box 1, MEND Records, Association of American Medical Colleges Archives, Washington, D.C.

2. A. N. Richards, "The Impact of the War on Medicine," *Science* 103:575–576, 1946.

3. *Ibid.*, p. 575. The peacetime number of military physicians had been 1,200. For a broad overview of medical activities during World War II, see Morris Fishbein, ed., *Doctors at War* (New York: E. P. Dutton, 1945).

4. Meeting of 6 October 1939, Harvard University Medical Faculty, Minutes of Meetings, Harvard Medical Archives, Rare Books Department, Countway Library, Harvard Medical School, Boston, MA.

5. Meeting of 4 October 1940, Harvard University Medical Faculty, Minutes of Meetings.

6. Meeting of 7 March 1941, Harvard University Medical Faculty, Minutes of Meetings.

7. Meeting of 19 December 1941, Transactions of the Executive Faculty, Cornell University Medical College, Archives, The New York Hospital–Cornell Medical Center, New York, NY.

8. *Report of the Dean of the Medical Faculty of The Johns Hopkins University* (1941–42), pp. 3–4; *Ibid.* (1942–43), pp. 1, 3; Winford H. Smith to Alan M. Chesney, 13 March 1942, Folder "Johns Hopkins Hospital—Dr. W. Smith Correspondence 1942–1945," Box 4XY, Correspondence Files, Office of the Dean of the Medical Faculty, The Johns Hopkins School of Medicine, Record Group 3, Series B, Archive of The Johns Hopkins University School of Medicine; meeting of 5 October 1942, Minutes, The Johns Hopkins Hospital Medical Board; all at The Alan Mason Chesney Medical Archives of The Johns Hopkins Medical Institutions, Baltimore, MD.

9. Richards, "The Impact of the War on Medicine," pp. 575–576.

10. A. C. Furstenberg, Dean's Report, 1943–1944, Folder "1942 R," Box 45, University of Michigan Medical School Records, Michigan Historical Collections, Bentley Historical Library, University of Michigan, Ann Arbor, MI.

11. Medical faculties did not submit to every request made of them by the Procurement and Assignment Service, the federal government's mobilization agency. For instance, many schools refused to comply with the agency's request that medical students be assigned to community hospitals not previously used for student teaching. The government preferred the rotating type of internship, but most teaching hospitals continued their "straight" internships in particular fields.

12. Meeting of 13 February 1944, Agenda and Minutes of the Business Meetings of the Council on Medical Education and Hospitals, American Medical Association Archives, Chicago, IL.

13. Richards, "The Impact of the War on Medicine," p. 575.

14. Joseph T. Wearn, "The Declining Standards of Medical Teaching," *Journal of the Association of American Medical Colleges* 19:77, 1944.

15. Report of the Dean of the Medical School, 1944–45, Folder 472, Deans' Subject File, Harvard Medical School, Harvard Medical Archives, Rare Books Department, Countway Library, Harvard Medical School, Boston, MA.

16. Victor Johnson, "Effects of the Accelerated Program of Medical Schools on the Curriculum, Faculty, and Students," *Journal of the Association of American Medical Colleges* 19:70, 1944.

17. See, for instance, the discussion of the administrative problems created by the accelerated curriculum in Report of the Curriculum Committee, 22 October 1943, with meeting of 22 October 1943, Transaction of the Executive Faculty, Cornell University Medical College.

18. Interview with Anson Hoyt, 7 October 1970, Folder "Anson P. S. Hoyt—M.D.," Dean's Office Files, University of Southern California School of Medicine, Norris Medical Library, University of Southern California, Los Angeles, CA.

19. Dean's Report, 1943–44, Office of the Dean, Cornell University Medical Center, Annual Reports of Departments and Offices, Archives, The New York Hospital–Cornell Medical Center, New York, NY.

20. Report of the Department of Radiology, 1943–44, Office of the Dean, Cornell University Medical Center, Annual Reports of Departments and Offices.

21. Richards, "The Impact of the War on Medicine," p. 575.

22. See, for instance, Dean's Report, 1945–46, and Report of Student Health Service, 1943–44, both in Office of the Dean, Cornell University Medical Center, Annual Reports of Departments and Offices.

23. Wearn, "The Declining Standards of Medical Teaching," p. 79; Supplement 2, with meeting of 13–16 February 1943, Agenda and Minutes of the Business Meetings of the Council on Medical Education and Hospitals.

24. Johnson, "Effects of the Accelerated Program of Medical Schools on the Curriculum, Faculty, and Students," p. 71.

25. Meeting of 13 February 1944, Agenda and Minutes of the Business Meetings of the Council on Medical Education and Hospitals.

26. Meeting of 7 November 1943, Agenda and Minutes of the Business Meetings of the Council on Medical Education and Hospitals.

27. Report of the Department of Obstetrics and Gynecology, 1945–46, Office of the Dean, Cornell University Medical Center, Annual Reports of Departments and Offices.

28. Richards, "The Impact of the War on Medicine," p. 575; Vannevar Bush, *Science, The Endless Frontier* (1945; reprint ed., Washington, D.C.: National Science Foundation, 1960), pp. 7–8.

29. Materials on Harvard Medical School's decision to admit women are in Folders 1805–1807, Deans' Subject File, Harvard Medical School; The Massachusetts General Hospital, *Annual Report* (1942), p. 55.

Opportunities for women to enter medicine were not always increased by the war. For instance, in 1941 the University of Arkansas School of Medicine decided not to admit any women on the basis that "a woman can wait a year but a boy who is declined might be drafted and have to give up his medical work." (Report to President Harding, School of Medicine, 1941–42, Folder 5, Dean's Office Files [Byron L. Robinson, 1941–46], ID Number 20DB009, Special Collections Division, University of Arkansas for Medical Sciences Library, Little Rock, AR.)

30. For an example of a faculty coping with the administrative issues raised by deceleration, see meetings of 17 April 1944, 12 November 1945, 10 December 1945, and 11 March 1946, Minutes of the Meetings of the Faculty, College of Physicians and Surgeons of Columbia University, Special Collections, Augustus C. Long Health Sciences Library, Columbia University, New York, NY.

31. William H. Chafe, *The Unfinished Journey: America since World War II*, 2nd ed. (New York: Oxford University Press, 1991), p. 8; Richard Polenberg, *War and Society: The United States 1941–1945* (Philadelphia: J. B. Lippincott Company, 1972), pp. 241–242.

32. George Q. Flynn, "American Medicine and Selective Service in World War II," *Journal of the History of Medicine and Allied Sciences* 42:326, 1987.

33. Chafe, *The Unfinished Journey*, p. 8.

34. Willard C. Rappleye, "Effects to Date of the Wartime Program of Medical Education," *Journal of the Association of American Medical Colleges* 19:48, 1944.

35. Report of the Joint Committee on Medical Education in Time of National Emergency, 31 March 1951, Folder 3, Box 247, Chancellor's Office Administrative Files 1936–1959 (Record Series 359), University Archives, Department of Special Collections, The University Library, University of California, Los Angeles, Los Angeles, CA. See also "Medical Education in Time of National Emergency," *Journal of the American Medical Association* 144:1111–1115, 1951; and Joseph C. Hinsey, "Medical Education in this National Emergency," *Journal of Medical Education* 26:81–90, 1951.

36. Alfred W. Crosby Jr., *Epidemic and Peace, 1918* (Westport, CT: Greenwood Press, 1918).

37. George B. Darling, "How the National Research Council Streamlined Medical Research for War," in Fishbein, *Doctors at War*, pp. 379–380.

38. Wartime medical research was summarized in a series edited by John B. Coates Jr., under the title *Activities of Medical Consultants* (Washington, D.C.: Government Printing Office, 1961). Overviews of the work are provided in Darling, "How the National Research Council Streamlined Medical Research for War," pp. 361–398; Richards, "The Impact of the War on Medicine," pp. 576–578; and Richard H. Shryock, *American Medical Research: Past and Present* (New York: The Commonwealth Fund, 1947), pp. 283–294.

39. Richards, "The Impact of the War on Medicine," p. 577.

40. Shryock, *American Medical Research*, pp. 293–294.

41. Richards, "The Impact of the War on Medicine," p. 576–577.

42. *Ibid.*, p. 578.

43. Bush, *Science, The Endless Frontier*; Stephen P. Strickland, *Politics, Science,*

and Dread Disease: A Short History of United States Medical Research Policy (Cambridge: Harvard University Press, 1972); Bruce L. R. Smith, *American Science Policy Since World War II* (Washington, D.C.: The Brookings Institution, 1990).

44. World War II as a watershed in American history is a theme of such works as Chafe, *The Unfinished Journey*; and Polenberg, *War and Society*.

45. Bush, *Science, The Endless Frontier*, pp. 13–14.

46. *Ibid.*, pp. 13–16; quotations, pp. 13, 14.

47. Faith T. Fitzgerald, "The Tyranny of Health," *New England Journal of Medicine* 331:196, 1994.

48. Shryock, *American Medical Research*, p. 319.

Chapter 8

1. Russell A. Nelson, "Town and Gown in Medicine," address delivered 27 October 1961, Folder "Medical School January–December 1962," Box "Medical School 1961–1964," Medical School Records, Georgetown University School of Medicine, Georgetown University Archives, Georgetown University, Washington, D.C.

2. On post–World War II science policy, see Bruce L. R. Smith, *American Science Policy Since World War II* (Washington, D.C.: The Brookings Institution, 1990); John T. Wilson, *Academic Science, Higher Education, and the Federal Government, 1950–1983* (Chicago: University of Chicago Press, 1983); Michael D. Reagan, *Science and the Federal Patron* (New York: Oxford University Press, 1969); and Nathan Reingold, "Vannevar Bush's New Deal for Research; or, the Triumph of the Old Order," in Nathan Reingold, *Science, American Style* (New Brunswick, NJ: Rutgers University Press, 1991), pp. 284–333.

3. Roger L. Geiger, *Research and Relevant Knowledge: American Research Universities Since World War II* (New York: Oxford University Press, 1993); Richard M. Freeland, *Academia's Golden Age: Universities in Massachusetts, 1945–1970* (New York: Oxford University Press, 1992).

4. Clark Kerr, *The Uses of the University*, 3rd ed. (Cambridge: Harvard University Press, 1982), pp. 52–53.

5. *Ibid.*, pp. 1–45. The term "multiversity" had been used by others but came into popularity after the appearance of the first edition of this book in 1963. In the 1960s Kerr became a symbol of opprobrium to critics who mistook his description of the multiversity for an endorsement of it, particularly its ties with government and the defense industry. Such uses of the university—so popular and appreciated during World War II, the Korean War, the Cold War, and the post-*Sputnik* space race—took on a more ominous note to many during the Vietnam War. In a 1982 postscript to the book, Kerr commented on the strength and resiliency of the multiversity, noting how its detractors had become quiet even though the multiversity had undergone no fundamental change. (*Ibid.*, pp. iii–vi, 127–184.)

6. Dean's Report, 1950–51, Office of the Dean, Cornell University Medical Center, Annual Reports of Departments and Offices, Archives, The New York Hospital–Cornell Medical Center, New York, NY; "University of Southern California School of Medicine—February 23, 1951," in Folder "Tuition-Income-Budget Report—1932–1951," Dean's Office Files, University of Southern California School of Medicine, Norris Medical Library, University of Southern California, Los Angeles, CA.

7. John E. Deitrick and Robert C. Berson, *Medical Schools in the United States at Mid-Century* (New York: McGraw-Hill, 1953), pp. 38–39, 34–35, 16.

8. Helpful accounts of postwar American culture include William H. Chafe, *The Unfinished Journey: America Since World War II*, 2nd ed. (New York: Oxford University Press, 1991); John Diggins, *The Proud Decades: America in War and Peace, 1941–1960* (New York: Norton Press, 1988); William L. O'Neill, *American High: The Years of Confidence, 1945–1960* (New York: Free Press, 1987); and Eric F. Goldman, *The Crucial Decade—and After: America, 1945–1960* (New York: Vintage, 1960).

9. Stephen P. Strickland, *Politics, Science, and Dread Disease: A Short History of United States Medical Research Policy* (Cambridge: Harvard University Press, 1972); Victoria A. Harden, *Inventing the NIH: Federal Biomedical Research Policy, 1887–1937* (Baltimore: Johns Hopkins University Press, 1986); Donald C. Swain, "The Rise of a Research Empire: NIH, 1930 to 1950," *Science* 138:1233–1237, 1972; and Daniel M. Fox, "The Politics of the NIH Extramural Program, 1937–50," *Journal of the History of Medicine and Allied Sciences* 42:447–466, 1987.

10. Robert H. Ebert, "Medical Education at the Peak Era of Experimental Medicine," *Daedalus*, Spring 1986, p. 59.

11. The Presbyterian Hospital in the City of New York, *Annual Report* (1960), p. 53.

12. Philip F. Wagley to Thomas B. Turner, 15 December 1961, with meeting of 18 December 1961, Minutes, Advisory Board of the Medical Faculty, The Johns Hopkins University School of Medicine, The Alan Mason Chesney Medical Archives of The Johns Hopkins Medical Institutions, Baltimore, MD. The journal was discontinued after the 1982 volume.

13. James A. Shannon, "The Advancement of Medical Research: A Twenty-Year View of the Role of the National Institutes of Health," *Journal of Medical Education* 42:97, 1967.

14. John R. Hogness and Gwynn C. Arkin, "Administration of Education Programs in Academic Health Centers," *New England Journal of Medicine* 296:656, 1977.

15. Vernon W. Lippard, *A Half-Century of American Medical Education: 1920–1970* (New York: Josiah Macy, Jr. Foundation, 1974), p. 78.

16. A. McGehee Harvey and Susan L. Abrams, *"For the Welfare of Mankind": The Commonwealth Fund and American Medicine* (Baltimore: Johns Hopkins University Press, 1986).

17. Lippard, *A Half-Century of American Medical Education*, p. 75.

18. "A Note on Princeton and Medical School Affiliation," with meeting of 14 October 1963, College Committee Minutes, Board of Trustees, Thomas Jefferson University, Thomas Jefferson University Archives and Special Collections, Thomas Jefferson University, Philadelphia, PA.

19. Ellen W. Schrecker, *No Ivory Tower: McCarthyism and the Universities* (New York: Oxford University Press, 1986).

20. Medical school faculty were sometimes asked to sign loyalty oaths, but at no campus did this create an uproar, and mention of McCarthyism was nonexistent in the records I examined. A few individuals did protest. For instance, Gordon Meiklejohn, an eminent infectious disease specialist who chaired the Department of Medicine at the University of Colorado from 1951 to 1976, was the only faculty member at the University of California, San Francisco, who would not sign a loyalty oath. His disappointment at having to stand alone was one reason he accepted the chairmanship at Colorado. Meiklejohn had always stood up for what he thought was right. As a young man he won a position on the Olympic hockey team, but he did not participate in the 1936 Olympics because of his belief that participation would enhance the regime of Adolf Hitler. He was the only member

of the team not to compete in Germany. (Robert H. Shikes and Henry N. Claman, *The University of Colorado School of Medicine: A Centennial History 1883–1983* [Denver: University of Colorado School of Medicine, 1983], p. 158; biographical materials on Gordon Meiklejohn provided by William R. Hiatt, 13 October 1994.)

21. See, for instance, Annual Expenditures of the School of Medicine, April 1955, Folder "Information of Historical Nature About USC Medicine," Dean's Office Files, University of Southern California School of Medicine; and meeting of 24 April 1952, Faculty Minutes, New York University School of Medicine, Archives, New York University Medical Center, New York, NY.

22. Dean's Report, 1947–48, Office of the Dean, Cornell University Medical Center, Annual Reports of Departments and Offices.

23. Meeting of 14 September 1954, Minutes of the Board of Governors, The Society of The New York Hospital, Archives, The New York Hospital–Cornell Medical Center, New York, NY; Marion E. Altenderfer and Margaret D. West, "Trends in Medical School Staffing," *Public Health Reports* 79:77–84, 1964.

24. Strickland, *Politics, Science, and Dread Disease*, p. 249.

25. Meeting of 5 February 1960, Harvard University Medical Faculty, Minutes of Meetings, Harvard Medical Archives, Rare Books Department, Countway Library, Harvard Medical School, Boston, MA.

26. Harvard Medical School, *Dean's Report* (1972–73), p. 2.

27. Meeting of 15 February 1963, College Committee Minutes, Board of Trustees, Thomas Jefferson University.

28. Meeting of 11 February 1959, Jesuit Educational Association Conference on Medical Schools, Folder "Medical School January–March 1959," Box "Medical School 1959–1960," Medical School Records, Georgetown University School of Medicine. For more on Catholic universities, see William P. Leahy, *Adapting to America: Catholics, Jesuits, and Higher Education in the Twentieth Century* (Washington, D.C.: Georgetown University Press, 1991).

29. Meeting of 7 November 1960, Corporate Board of Trustees Minutes, Thomas Jefferson University, Thomas Jefferson University Archives and Special Collections, Thomas Jefferson University, Philadelphia, PA.

30. Meeting of 28 April 1967, Corporation Minutes, Woman's Medical College of Pennsylvania, Archives and Special Collections on Women in Medicine, MCP Hahnemann University, Philadelphia, PA.

31. Janet A. Tighe, "Defying All Predictions: A History of the Temple University School of Medicine, 1901–1980," Chapter V, p. 38, Dean's Office, Temple University School of Medicine, Philadelphia, PA.

32. University of Arkansas School of Medicine Annual Report, 1969–1970, Folder "Miscellaneous: Annual Reports," Dean's Office Files (Winston K. Shorey, 1961–1974), ID Number 20DB016, Special Collections Division, University of Arkansas for Health Sciences Library, Little Rock, AR; H. C. Chenault to H. E. Mobley, 18 November 1946, Folder "Office Files—1946," Dean's Office Files (Henry Clay Chenault, 1946–49), ID Number 20DB010, Special Collections Division, University of Arkansas for Medical Sciences Library, Little Rock, AR.

33. Harvard Medical School, *Dean's Report* (1959–60), p. 3.

34. William N. Hubbard Jr. to M. L. Niehuss and R. W. Heyns, 10 January 1964, Folder "Heyns, Roger W., 1962–65," Box 83, University of Michigan Medical School Records, Michigan Historical Collections, Bentley Historical Library, University of Michigan, Ann Arbor, MI.

35. Kenneth M. Ludmerer, "The Origins of Mount Sinai School of Medicine," *Journal of the History of Medicine and Allied Sciences* 45:469–89, 1990.

36. George P. Berry to David A. Thomas, 15 September 1958, Folder "Peter Bent Brigham Hospital 1957–1958," Deans' Subject File, Harvard Medical School, Harvard Medical Archives, Rare Books Department, Countway Library, Harvard Medical School, Boston, MA.

37. Dr. F. to J. Folch-pi, 15 May 1962, Folder 56, Box 6, John H. Knowles Papers, Rockefeller Archive Center, North Tarrytown, NY. I have elected not to disclose the identity of the letter writer.

38. Meeting of 6 April 1949, Executive Faculty Minutes, Washington University School of Medicine, Washington University School of Medicine Archives, St. Louis, MO.

39. At Johns Hopkins, for instance, who had the authority to appoint a new medical school dean? The university president said he did, the medical school said it did, and the medical school won. (Meeting of 30 October 1967, Minutes, Advisory Board of the Medical Faculty, The Johns Hopkins University School of Medicine.)

40. Lippard, *A Half-Century of American Medical Education*, pp. 48–49; William G. Rothstein, *American Medical Schools and the Practice of Medicine: A History* (New York: Oxford University Press, 1987), pp. 264–267.

41. Milton S. Eisenhower to Thomas B. Turner, 12 November 1960, with meeting of 28 November 1960, Minutes, Advisory Board of the Medical Faculty, The Johns Hopkins University School of Medicine.

42. Dale R. Lindsay to John H. Knowles, 1 April 1964, Folder 126, Box 10, Knowles Papers.

43. The most complete history of poliomyelitis is John R. Paul, *A History of Poliomyelitis* (New Haven: Yale University Press, 1971).

44. W. Barry Wood Jr., *From Miasmas to Molecules* (New York: Columbia University Press, 1961), p. 79.

45. Statement of the Council on Academic Societies of the Association of American Medical Colleges on Federal Support of Health Research before the Subcommittee on Labor-Health Education and Welfare of the Committee on Appropriations, U.S. House of Representatives, 26 May 1969, Folder 230, Box 19, Knowles Papers.

46. A. N. Richards, "Advantages and Dangers of Government Support for Medical Research," *Annals of Internal Medicine*, vol. 71, suppl. 8, pp. 74–75, November 1969.

47. René C. Dubos, *Mirage of Health: Utopias, Progress, and Biological Change* (New York: Harper & Brothers, 1959), p. 2.

48. A. J. Carroll to Glen R. Leymaster, 12 July 1967, with meeting of 29 September 1967, Corporation Minutes, Woman's Medical College of Pennsylvania.

49. An overview of these changes, as well as those in clinical research, is found in Lippard, *A Half-Century of American Medical Education*, pp. 12–13, 46–48, and 78–80; and Robert R. Wagner, "The Basic Medical Sciences, the Revolution in Biology and the Future of Medical Education," *Yale Journal of Biology and Medicine* 35:1–11, 1962.

50. Earlier generations of medical educators had used the term "basic" or "fundamental" sciences, but in reference to the university-based disciplines of biology, chemistry, and physics and not to the scientific subjects of the first two years of medical school.

51. Meeting of 5 March 1963, Minutes of the Board of Governors, The Society of The New York Hospital.

52. Meeting of 6–8 October 1966, Executive Committee Minutes, National

Board of Medical Examiners, President's Office, National Board of Medical Examiners, Philadelphia, PA.

53. Gordon N. Gill, "The End of the Physician-Scientist?," *American Scholar* 53:353–68, 1984; Lloyd H. Smith Jr., "Presidential Address," *Transactions of the Association of American Physicians* 89:1–9, 1976.

54. Meeting of 14 February 1957, Transactions of the Executive Faculty, Cornell University Medical College, Archives, The New York Hospital–Cornell Medical Center, New York, NY.

55. See, for instance, the discussions concerning the appointment of a new Jackson Professor of Medicine at Massachusetts General Hospital in Folders 44 and 45, Box 4, Knowles Papers.

56. Meeting of 2 March 1955, Executive Faculty Minutes, Washington University School of Medicine.

57. *Table 4* is taken from Deitrick and Berson, *Medical Schools in the United States at Mid-Century*, p. 197; *Table 5*, from meeting of 18 August 1954, Faculty Minutes, University of Maryland School of Medicine, Historical and Special Collections, Health Sciences Library, University of Maryland at Baltimore; *Table 6*, from the agenda items with meeting of 28–29 October 1965, Executive Council Meetings and Agendas, Association of American Medical Colleges, Association of American Medical Colleges Archives, Washington, D.C. Salaries listed for geographic full-time in *Table 6* represent the amount guaranteed by the school. These instructors could keep some of their fees from clinical practice, typically up to 50 percent of their base salary.

58. Meeting of 14 March 1966, Minutes and Correspondence of the Committee on Administration, College of Physicians and Surgeons Dean's Office Files, Office of the Dean, College of Physicians and Surgeons of Columbia University, New York, NY.

59. Robert J. Glaser, "The Medical Deanship: Its Half-Life and Hard Times," *Journal of Medical Education* 44:1123, 1969.

60. Tentative Report of the *Ad Hoc* Committee Concerning W. Gerald Austen, Folder 34, Box 4, Knowles Papers.

61. Edward H. Kass to Nathan B. Talbot, 20 February 1964, Folder 142, Box 12, Knowles Papers. I have elected not to disclose the identity of "Dr. P."

62. Dean's Report, 1954–55, Office of the Dean, Cornell University Medical Center, Annual Reports of Departments and Offices.

63. See, for instance, Francis M. Forster to Edward B. Bunn, 15 July 1954, Folder "Medical School May–December 1954," Box "Medical School 1950–1954," Medical School Records, Georgetown University School of Medicine; Report to the Board of Corporators by the President, with meeting of 29 June 1962, Corporation Minutes, Woman's Medical College of Pennsylvania.

64. Notes on Interview with Deans Berry and Meadow, 3 April 1961, Folder "HU—Carnegie Report (Price)," Deans' Subject File, Harvard Medical School.

65. Meeting of 18 November 1964, Minutes of the Executive Committee of the Faculty, New York University College of Medicine, Archives, New York University Medical Center, New York, NY.

66. Francis D. Moore, "Harvey Cushing at 100," *Harvard Medical Alumni Bulletin* 43:26, 1969.

67. Faculty Council Meeting of 8 May 1947, Folder "Faculty Council May 8th 1947," Box 4, Medical Faculty Executive Committee Minutes, University of Pennsylvania School of Medicine (UPC 12.2), The University Archives and Record Center, University of Pennsylvania, Philadelphia, PA.

68. Robert F. Loeb to Willard C. Rappleye, 9 December 1957, Minutes and Correspondence of the Committee on Administration, College of Physicians and Surgeons.

69. Statement of Dr. Edward F. Bland, MGH Staff Replies to Letter of April 18, 1961, Folder 115, Box 10, Knowles Papers.

70. Deitrick and Berson, *Medical Schools in the United States at Mid-Century*, p. 136.

71. Glaser, "The Medical Deanship," p. 1115.

72. *Ibid.*, p. 1124.

73. Election of the Dean, with meeting of 1 March 1950, Executive Faculty Minutes, Washington University School of Medicine.

74. Meeting of 14 May 1950, Executive Committee, Folder "Executive Committee 1948–55," Box 6, University of Michigan Medical School Records.

75. George P. Berry to Nathan B. Talbot, 25 May 1962, Folder 48, Box 5, Knowles Papers; Paul B. Beeson, "The Changing Role Model, and the Shift in Power," *Daedalus*, Spring 1986, p. 92.

76. Meeting of 4 November 1959, Minutes of the Faculty Executive Committee, Folder "Faculty Executive Committee 1958–1961," Dean's Office Files, University of Southern California School of Medicine.

77. Meeting of 31 January 1968, Minutes of Meetings of the Board of Trustees of Hahnemann Medical College and Hospital, Archives and Special Collections, Hahnemann Collection, MCP Hahnemann University, Philadelphia, PA.

78. George P. Berry to Charles W. Lloyd, 10 October 1952, Folder "HU—Committee on Patents," Deans' Subject File, Harvard Medical School. Similar statements through 1965 appear in this folder.

Chapter 9

1. Abraham Flexner, *Universities: American English German* (New York: Oxford University Press, 1930).

2. Clark Kerr, *The Uses of the University*, 3rd ed. (Cambridge: Harvard University Press, 1982), quotations pp. 41, 85; Clark Kerr, *The Great Transformation in Higher Education: 1960–1980* (Albany: State University of New York Press, 1991), pp. 69–78.

3. See, for example, Robert H. Ebert, "The Dilemma of Medical Teaching," in John H. Knowles, ed., *The Teaching Hospital: Evolution and Contemporary Issues* (Cambridge: Harvard University Press, 1966), pp. 66–70; and John H. Knowles, "Medical School, Teaching Hospital, and Social Responsibility," in Knowles, ed., *The Teaching Hospital*, p. 96. Ebert and Knowles cited such works as John Kenneth Galbraith, *The Affluent Society* (Boston: Houghton-Mifflin, 1958); and David Riesman, *Abundance for What?* (Garden City, NJ: Doubleday, 1964).

4. On the history of the Blue Cross plans, see Louis S. Reed, *Blue Cross and Medical Service Plans* (Washington, D.C.: Federal Security Agency, U.S. Public Health Service, 1947); Odin W. Anderson, *Blue Cross Since 1929: Accountability and the Public Trust* (Cambridge, MA: Ballinger, 1975); and Sylvia A. Law, *Blue Cross: What Went Wrong?*, 2nd ed. (New Haven: Yale University Press, 1976). On the campaign to achieve compulsory national health insurance, see Monte M. Poen, *Harry S. Truman Versus the Medical Lobby: The Genesis of Medicare* (Columbia: University of Missouri Press, 1979). On early health maintenance organizations, see Rickey Hendricks, *A Model for National Health Care: The History of Kaiser Permanente* (New Brunswick: Rutgers University Press, 1993). Helpful general discus-

sions of health policy during this period include Odin W. Anderson, *The Uneasy Equilibrium: Private and Public Financing of Health Services in the United States, 1875–1965* (New Haven, CT: College & University Press, 1968), pp. 104–193; Odin W. Anderson, *Health Services in the United States: A Growth Enterprise Since 1875* (Ann Arbor, MI: Health Administration Press, 1985), pp. 105–176; and Paul Starr, *The Social Transformation of American Medicine: The Rise of a Sovereign Profession and the Making of a Vast Industry* (New York: Basic Books, 1982), pp. 290–378.

5. Starr, *Social Transformation*, p. 350.

6. Rosemary Stevens, *In Sickness and in Wealth: American Hospitals in the Twentieth Century* (New York: Basic Books, 1989), p. 220.

7. Robert J. Glaser, "The Teaching Hospital and the Medical School," in Knowles, ed., *The Teaching Hospital*, pp. 8–9.

8. John E. Deitrick and Robert C. Berson, *Medical Schools in the United States at Mid-Century* (New York: McGraw-Hill, 1953), pp. 57–62; Daniel M. Fox, *Health Policies, Health Politics: The British and American Experience, 1911–1965* (Princeton, NJ: Princeton University Press, 1986). Fox termed this policy "hierarchical regionalism," in recognition of the hierarchies of academic medical centers, large community hospitals, and small community hospitals in a given geographical region.

9. "Nobody Else Does It," newspaper clipping, Folder 236, Box 20, John H. Knowles Papers, Rockefeller Archive Center, North Tarrytown, NY; Stevens, *In Sickness and in Wealth*, p. 249; Deitrick and Berson, *Medical Schools in the United States at Mid-Century*, p. 147.

10. "Nothing But the Best," newspaper clipping containing Knowles's quotation; Robert B. Keller to John H. Knowles, 5 February 1967; John M. Gould to John H. Knowles, 18 March 1967; all Folder 125, Box 10, Knowles Papers.

11. See, for instance, J. M. Hayman Jr. to Richard J. Condon, 14 December 1953, Binder (P) C.4.2., Edward D. Churchill Papers, Harvard Medical Archives, Rare Books Department, Countway Library, Harvard Medical School, Boston, MA.

12. Policy Memorandum 2, 30 January 1946, University of Colorado Medical Center Reports, Veterans Administration Hospital Background and Development, Denison Medical Library, University of Colorado Health Sciences Center, Denver, CO. See also Deitrick and Berson, *Medical Schools in the United States at Mid-Century*, pp. 58, 150–151; Benjamin J. Lewis, *VA Medical Program in Relation to Medical Schools* (Washington, D.C.: U.S. Government Printing Office, 1970); David M. Worthen, "The Affiliation Partnership Between U.S. Medical Schools and the Veterans Administration," *The Alabama Journal of Medical Sciences* 24:83–89, 1987; and John A. Gronvall, "The VA's Affiliation with Academic Medicine: An Emergency Post-War Strategy Becomes a Permanent Partnership," *Academic Medicine* 64:61–66, 1989. By 1965, 90 Veterans Administration hospitals were affiliated with 77 medical schools.

13. Graph of New York Hospital inpatient services, with agenda items, meeting of 2 April 1968, Agendas and Minutes, Board of Governors, The Society of The New York Hospital, Archives, The New York Hospital–Cornell Medical Center, New York, NY.

14. Meeting of 21 February 1967, Minutes of the Medical Board, The Presbyterian Hospital in the City of New York, President's Offices, Presbyterian Hospital, New York, NY.

15. University of Arkansas School of Medicine, *Annual Report* (1951–52), p. 8; (1950–51), p. 7.

16. For a detailed description of the emergency room of a typical teaching hos-

pital, see Joseph I. Reed and George G. Reader, "Quantitative Survey of New York Hospital Emergency Room, 1965," *New York State Journal of Medicine* 67:1335–1342, 1967.

17. Report of the Committee on the Emergency Unit, 27 April 1962, with meeting of 7 June 1962, Transactions of the Medical Board of the New York Hospital, Archives, The New York Hospital–Cornell Medical Center, New York, NY; meeting of 24 September 1968, Minutes, The Johns Hopkins Hospital Medical Board, The Alan Mason Chesney Medical Archives of The Johns Hopkins Medical Institutions, Baltimore, MD.

18. See, for instance, meetings of 5 March 1964 and 4 March 1965, Transactions of the Medical Board of the New York Hospital.

19. Meeting of 21 November 1968, Minutes of the Executive Committee of the Board of Governors, The Society of The New York Hospital, Archives, The New York Hospital–Cornell Medical Center, New York, NY.

20. Meeting of 23 January 1950, Minutes of the Joint Administrative Board, Columbia-Presbyterian Medical Center, President's Offices, The Presbyterian Hospital in the City of New York, New York, NY: The Presbyterian Hospital in the City of New York, *Annual Report* (1960), p. 10.

21. The Establishment of a Private Clinic in the Medical Center, with meeting of 5 November 1947, Executive Faculty Minutes, Washington University School of Medicine, Washington University School of Medicine Archives, St. Louis, MO; *Table 2*, with meeting of 15 December 1952, Minutes, Advisory Board of the Medical Faculty, The Johns Hopkins University School of Medicine, The Alan Mason Chesney Medical Archives of The Johns Hopkins Medical Institutions, Baltimore, MD. Typically, most of the clinical revenues were used to support research activities of the department or medical school, not to pay for faculty salaries.

22. See, for instance, meetings of 1 October 1947, 1 May 1957, and 2 October 1957, Executive Faculty Minutes, Washington University School of Medicine; and meetings of 29 April 1958 and 25 November 1958, Minutes, The Johns Hopkins Medical Board.

23. George P. Berry, Memorandum Concerning Two-Hour Luncheon at the Harvard Club with Sydney Rabb, 29 March 1956, Folder "Beth Israel Hospital—1949–1956," Deans' Subject File, Harvard Medical School, Harvard Medical Archives, Rare Books Department, Countway Library, Harvard Medical School, Boston, MA.

24. Summary and Analysis of a Study of Attitudes of Patients and Hospital Personnel Towards Mt. Sinai Hospital, January 1960, Folder 3, Box 3, Director's Office Papers (Steinberg Series), The Mount Sinai Hospital, Archives, The Mount Sinai Medical Center, New York, NY.

25. Statement of Dr. Maynard, MGH Staff Replies to Letter of 18 April 1961, Folder 115, Box 10, Knowles Papers.

26. Knowles, "Medical School, Teaching Hospital, and Social Responsibility," pp. 107, 111.

27. *Ibid.*, p. 137.

28. Meeting of 13 March 1979, Minutes, Medical Service Staff Meetings, Columbia-Presbyterian Medical Center, Office of the Chairman, Department of Medicine, College of Physicians and Surgeons of Columbia University, New York, NY.

29. This organization lay dormant for 12 years before it was reincorporated as the Association for Academic Health Centers.

The administration of all hospitals, not just teaching hospitals, was in the process of becoming professionalized. See Duncan Neuhauser, *Coming of Age: A 50-Year History of the American College of Hospital Administrators and the Profession It Serves, 1933–1983* (Chicago: Pluribus Press, 1983).

30. Knowles, "Medical School, Teaching Hospital, and Social Responsibility," pp. 108–109.

31. Meeting of 11 October 1961, Transactions of the Medical Board of the New York Hospital.

32. Allan L. Friedlich to Edward D. Churchill, 30 August 1961, Folder 115, Box 10, Knowles Papers.

33. Quoted in Knowles, "Medical School, Teaching Hospital, and Social Responsibility," p. 86.

34. Harvard Medical School, *Dean's Report* (1964–65), pp. 11–12.

35. Walter Bauer, untitled address, Folder 82, Box 8, Knowles Papers.

36. Thomas H. Brem and Clayton G. Loosli to James Watt, 18 July 1960, Dean's Office Files, University of Southern California School of Medicine, Norris Medical Library, University of Southern California, Los Angeles, CA; meeting of 9 October 1959, Minutes, Board of Trustees, The Mount Sinai Hospital, Archives, The Mount Sinai Medical Center, New York, NY.

37. The Massachusetts General Hospital, *Annual Report* (1955), p. 40.

38. Francis D. Moore to John Knowles, 31 December 1968; and John H. Knowles to Francis D. Moore, 3 January 1969; both Folder 36, Box 4, Knowles Papers.

39. John H. Knowles to Department Heads, 13 February 1963, Folder 170, Box 15, Knowles Papers.

40. John H. Knowles to Dear Doctor, 18 April 1962, Folder 77, Box 7, Knowles Papers.

41. Report of the Scientific Advisory Council of the Massachusetts General Hospital, 5–6 January 1962, Folder "MGH Scientific Advisory Committee," Deans' Subject File, Harvard Medical School; Paul Zamecnik, "A Personalized View of the History of the MGH Research Committee," Folder 144, Box 12, Knowles Papers; Benjamin Castleman, David C. Crockett, and S. B. Sutton, eds., *The Massachusetts General Hospital 1955–1980* (Boston: Little, Brown and Company, 1983), pp. 32–44.

42. Discussion with Mr. Conant—April 13, 1952, Folder "Conant, James B.—Talks with GPB," Deans' Subject File, Harvard Medical School.

43. Discussion with Mr. Conant—April 13, 1952, Folder "Conant, James B.—Talks with GPB," Deans' Subject File, Harvard Medical School; The Massachusetts General Hospital, *Annual Report* (1950), p. 48.

44. George P. Berry to Richard J. Condon, 3 March 1953, Binder (F) C.4.2., Churchill Papers.

45. Massachusetts General Hospital, *Annual Report* (1948), p. 59.

46. Meeting of 29 April 1958, Minutes, The Johns Hopkins Medical Board.

47. George P. Berry to James B. Conant, 29 December 1955, Folder "HU—James B. Conant—1950–1960," Deans' Subject File, Harvard Medical School.

48. Deitrick and Berson, *Medical Schools in the United States at Mid-Century*, p. 139; see also pp. 62–63.

49. Institutional Group Practice by Clinical Faculties of Medical Schools: A Statement of Principles, with agenda items for meeting of 7–8 February 1958, Executive Council Meetings and Agendas, Association of American Medical Colleges, Association of American Medical Colleges Archives, Washington, D.C.

50. Meeting of 18 February 1959, Executive Staff of the University Hospital,

Folder "1945–1959," Box 27, University of Michigan Hospitals Records, Michigan Historical Collections, Bentley Historical Library, University of Michigan, Ann Arbor, MI.

51. A Plan for Operation of the Proposed Clinics of the University of Pennsylvania, 25 January 1947 (UPC 12.3C), The University Archives and Record Center, University of Pennsylvania, Philadelphia, PA.

52. Meeting of 27 March 1956, Minutes, The Johns Hopkins Hospital Medical Board. See also A Statement of the Advisory Board of the Medical Faculty, with meeting of 25 February 1952, Minutes, Advisory Board of the Medical Faculty.

53. Report on the Program to Place the Various Activities of the Medical Center Within Reasonable Balance, 3 October 1945, with meeting of 24 October 1945, Minutes of the Planning Committee of the Medical Board, The Presbyterian Hospital in the City of New York, President's Offices, Presbyterian Hospital, New York, NY.

54. Meeting of 2 October 1957, Executive Faculty Minutes, Washington University School of Medicine.

55. Philip A. Tumulty, Second Annual Report, Staff Committee for the Private Patient Clinic, with meeting of 25 May 1959, Minutes, Advisory Board of the Medical Faculty, The Johns Hopkins University School of Medicine.

56. Meeting of 19 October 1964, Board of Managers Minutes, The Presbyterian Hospital in the City of New York, President's Offices, Presbyterian Hospital, New York, NY.

57. See, for instance, meeting of 8 August 1968, Transactions of the Medical Board of the New York Hospital; Thomas B. Turner, "The Problem of Professional Fees," 29 May 1967, with meeting of 29 May 1967, Minutes, Advisory Board of the Medical Faculty, The Johns Hopkins University School of Medicine; and The Peter Bent Brigham Hospital, *Annual Report* (1970), p. 202. In this vein, John H. Knowles considered many leading medical professors to be poor managers. For instance, he said that Carl Moore, the chairman of the Department of Medicine of Washington University, "knows almost nothing about hospital administration and therefore makes decisions which most professors make which foster the teaching and research role and lets the facilities and management of the hospital go to hell." (John H. Knowles to James Knowles, 10 June 1964, Folder 639, Box 55, Knowles Papers.)

58. Report of Committee on Departmental Affiliations and Regional Hospitals, with meeting of 2 January 1963, Minutes of Meetings of the Departmental Chairmen, New York University School of Medicine, Archives, New York University Medical Center, New York, NY.

59. Summary of Survey of University of Pittsburgh School of Medicine, 9–12 December 1957, with agenda items for meeting of 7–8 February 1958, Executive Council Meetings and Agendas, Association of American Medical Colleges.

60. Dean's Report, 1955–56, Office of the Dean, Cornell University Medical Center, Annual Reports of Departments and Offices, Archives, The New York Hospital–Cornell Medical Center, New York, NY.

61. Annual Report, *The Massachusetts General Hospital* (1958), p. 45.

62. Meetings of 2 March 1948 and 16 April 1948, Minutes, The Johns Hopkins Hospital Board of Trustees, The Alan Mason Chesney Medical Archives of The Johns Hopkins Medical Institutions, Baltimore, MD.

63. The Peter Bent Brigham Hospital, *Annual Report* (1953), pp. 57–64.

64. The Peter Bent Brigham Hospital, *Annual Report* (1952), p. 9.

65. Report of the Department of Surgery, 1957–58, Office of the Dean, Cornell University Medical Center, Annual Reports of Departments and Offices.

66. Meeting of 23 November 1949, Box 3, Minutes of the Board of Managers of the Hospital of the University of Pennsylvania (UPC 12.1), The University Archives and Record Center, The University of Pennsylvania, Philadelphia, PA.

67. Meeting of 9 February 1966, Minutes of the Meetings of the College Committee of the Board of Trustees, Hahnemann Medical College and Hospital, Archives and Special Collections, Hahnemann Collection, MCP Hahnemann University, Philadelphia, PA.

68. Meeting of 14 September 1962, Minutes, Executive Staff Meetings, Georgetown University Hospital, Office of the Medical Director, Georgetown University Hospital, Washington, D.C.

69. Meeting of 29 February 1952, Corporation Minutes, Woman's Medical College of Pennsylvania, Archives and Special Collections on Women in Medicine, MCP Hahnemann University, Philadelphia, PA.

70. Report of Private Patients Committee, 28 November 1962, with meeting of 3 January 1963, Transactions of the Medical Board of the New York Hospital; meeting of 3 May 1962, Transactions of the Medical Board of the New York Hospital.

71. Report of the Staff Committee on Professional Services on Residency and Graduate Training, with meeting of 15 October 1952, Minutes, Advisory Board of the Medical Faculty, The Johns Hopkins University School of Medicine.

72. Dean A. Clark, memorandum on "Teaching Hospitals and Medical Care Insurance," 8 July 1952, Folder 1, Box 10, President, NYH-CMC, Papers, 1945–75 (Bayne, Hinsey, Luckey), Archives, The New York Hospital–Cornell Medical Center, New York, NY.

73. See, for instance, "Teaching Affiliations with Other Hospitals," with meeting of 2 May 1960, Corporate Board of Trustees Minutes, Thomas Jefferson University, Thomas Jefferson University Archives and Special Collections, Thomas Jefferson University, Philadelphia, PA; and meeting of 22 October 1958, Hospital Staff Minutes, Hospital of the Woman's Medical College of Pennsylvania, Archives and Special Collections on Women in Medicine, MCP Hahnemann University, Philadelphia, PA.

74. Meeting of 6 February 1961, Corporate Board of Trustees Minutes, Thomas Jefferson University.

75. See, for instance, meeting of 8 February 1963, Major Faculty Minutes, Temple University School of Medicine and Hospital, Dean's Office, Temple University School of Medicine, Philadelphia, PA; and Provision of Medical Service for Paying Patients by Residents, with agenda items for meeting of 15–16 May 1961, Executive Council Meetings and Agendas, Association of American Medical Colleges.

76. Meeting of 14 June 1954, Board of Managers Minutes, The Presbyterian Hospital in the City of New York.

77. Daniel S. Ellis to John Knowles, 27 December 1967, Folder 301, Box 26, Knowles Papers.

78. James Bordley III and A. McGehee Harvey, *Two Centuries of American Medicine: 1776–1976* (Philadelphia: W. B. Saunders Company, 1976), pp. 756–761. So often, one change required others. Thus, the early ambulation of patients created the need for more bathrooms, nurses, and aides as well as for closer nursing observation.

79. Meeting of 19 December 1963, Executive Committee, Folder "Executive Committee September 1963–July 1965," Box 7, University of Michigan Medical School Records, Michigan Historical Collections, Bentley Historical Library, University of Michigan, Ann Arbor, MI.

80. *Figure 2* is taken from Lowell T. Coggeshall, *Planning for Medical Progress Through Education* (Evanston, IL: Association of American Medical Colleges, 1965), p. 23. This graph reflects the average length of stay at all hospitals. The average length of stay at teaching hospitals tended to be longer than at nonteaching institutions.

81. Meeting of 27 September 1965, Transactions of the Medical Board of the New York Hospital.

82. Report of the Department of Medicine, 1953–54, Office of the Dean, Cornell University Medical Center, Annual Reports of Departments and Offices.

Chapter 10

1. C. P. Snow, "The Two Cultures and the Scientific Revolution" (New York: Cambridge University Press, 1959).

2. On the history of medical specialization, see Rosemary Stevens, *American Medicine and the Public Interest* (New Haven: Yale University Press, 1971). The evolution of internal medicine into various constituent subspecialties is described in Russell C. Maulitz and Diana E. Long, *Grand Rounds: One Hundred Years of Internal Medicine* (Philadelphia: University of Pennsylvania Press, 1988).

3. Diane Ravitch, *The Troubled Crusade: American Education, 1945–1980* (New York: Basic Books, 1983), p. 183.

4. Vernon W. Lippard, *A Half-Century of American Medical Education: 1920–1970* (New York: Josiah Macy, Jr. Foundation, 1974), pp. 94–95; John E. Deitrick and Robert C. Berson, *Medical Schools in the United States at Mid-Century* (New York: McGraw-Hill, 1953), pp. 276–277.

5. Postwar Medical Education, 10 March 1945, Folder "Bulletins, Association of American Medical Colleges, 1945–48," Dean's Office Files, University of Southern California School of Medicine, Norris Medical Library, University of Southern California, Los Angeles, CA.

6. Meeting of 1–6 December 1945, Agenda and Minutes of the Business Meetings of the Council on Medical Education and Hospitals, American Medical Association Archives, Chicago, IL.

7. R.H. Bishop Jr. to Winford H. Smith, 2 November 1945, Folder "Committee Survey of Post Graduate Training Facilities," Subject Files, The Alan Mason Chesney Medical Archives of The Johns Hopkins Medical Institutions, Baltimore, MD; *Report of the Dean of the Medical Faculty of The Johns Hopkins University* (1944–45), p. 3.

8. Charles F. Wilkinson Jr. to A. C. Furstenberg, 7 January 1947, Folder "1947 W-Z," Box 50, University of Michigan Medical School Records, Michigan Historical Collections, Bentley Historical Library, University of Michigan, Ann Arbor, MI.

9. Report of Henry Renfert Jr., 1958–59, Office of the Dean, Cornell University Medical Center, Annual Reports of Departments and Offices, Archives, The New York Hospital–Cornell Medical Center, New York, NY.

10. George Rosen, *The Specialization of Medicine, with Particular Reference to Ophthalmology* (New York: Froben Press, 1944). In addition to the technological factors, the evolution of some specialties had much to do with the desire of physicians to eliminate competition from paramedical professions. The early history of

ophthalmology, for instance, involved bitter territorial disputes between ophthalmologists and optometrists. See Stevens, *American Medicine and the Public Interest*, pp. 98–114.

11. For more on the factors promoting specialization, see Patricia L. Kendall, "Medical Specialization: Trends and Contributing Factors," in Robert H. Coombs and Clark E. Vincent, eds., *Psychosocial Aspects of Medical Training* (Springfield, IL: Charles C Thomas, 1971), pp. 449–497.

12. Lippard, *A Half-Century of American Medical Education*, p. 96.

13. See, for instance, meeting of 11 September 1951, Faculty Minutes, University of Maryland School of Medicine, Historical and Special Collections, Health Sciences Library, University of Maryland at Baltimore; and meeting of 1 May 1950, Folder "Executive Committee 5/1/50," Box 3, Medical Faculty Executive Committee Minutes, University of Pennsylvania School of Medicine (UPC 12.2), The University Archives and Record Center, University of Pennsylvania, Philadelphia, PA.

14. Annual Report of the Residency Committee, with meeting of 16 February 1960, Minutes of the Medical Board, The Presbyterian Hospital in the City of New York, President's Offices, Presbyterian Hospital, New York, NY.

15. Meeting of 3 April 1956, Minutes of the Board of Governors, The Society of The New York Hospital, Archives, The New York Hospital–Cornell Medical Center, New York, NY.

16. Citizens Commission on Graduate Medical Education, *The Graduate Education of Physicians* (Chicago: American Medical Association, 1966), p. 15.

17. For instance, see the discussion of this problem in Allan M. Butler to C. Sidney Burwell, 3 January 1948, Folder 1603, Deans' Subject File, Harvard Medical School, Harvard Medical Archives, Rare Books Department, Countway Library, Harvard Medical School, Boston, MA.

18. J. A. Curran, "Internships and Residencies: Historical Backgrounds and Current Trends," *Journal of Medical Education* 34:883, 1959.

19. Meeting of 11 March 1965, Executive Committee, Folder "Executive Committee Sept. 1963–July 1965," Box 7, University of Michigan Medical School Records.

20. Curran, "Internships and Residencies," p. 879.

21. Russell A. Nelson, "The Hospital and Education," Folder 807, Box 65, John H. Knowles Papers, Rockefeller Archive Center, North Tarrytown, NY.

Of course, foreign medical graduates could be found on the house staffs of even the best teaching hospitals. For instance, approximately 10 percent of the house officers at the Johns Hopkins Hospital from 1958 to 1963 were graduates of recognized medical schools outside of the United States and Canada. (Meeting of 1 October 1963, Minutes, The Johns Hopkins Hospital Medical Board, The Alan Mason Chesney Medical Archives of The Johns Hopkins Medical Institutions, Baltimore, MD.)

By the late 1950s the number of foreign medical graduates had become so great that the American Medical Association and the Association of American Medical Colleges found that they could no longer survey and accredit foreign medical schools, as they did American medical schools. Instead, responsibility for certifying foreign medical schools and graduates devolved to a newly created Educational Council for Foreign Medical Graduates (ECFMG). Effective 1 July 1960, all graduates of foreign medical schools (except Canadian medical schools) serving as house officers in the United States had to be certified by the ECFMG.

22. Lippard, *A Half-Century of American Medical Education*, p. 96.

23. Meeting of 3 September 1959, Transactions of the Medical Board of the New York Hospital, Archives, The New York Hospital–Cornell Medical Center, New York, NY.

24. Graph showing percentages of Cornell graduates by types of internship, with meeting of 18 September 1973, Transactions of the Executive Faculty, Cornell University College of Medicine, Archives, The New York Hospital–Cornell Medical Center, New York, NY. For more on how students selected specialties, see Robert E. Coker Jr., Norman Miller, and Alice Levine, "Study of Choice of Specialties in Medicine," Folder 811, Box 66, Knowles Papers.

25. Citizens Commission on Graduate Medical Education, *The Graduate Education of Physicians*; Lowell T. Coggeshall, *Planning for Medical Progress Through Education* (Evanston, IL: Association of American Medical Colleges, 1966).

26. Max Michael Jr., "Phasing Out the Freestanding Internship," *Journal of the American Medical Association* 218:1690–1691, 1971.

27. Meeting of 3 October 1968, Executive Committee, Folder "Executive Committee Sept. 1968–Feb. 1969," Box 8, University of Michigan Medical School Records.

28. The Massachusetts General Hospital, *Annual Report* (1947), p. 50.

29. Meeting of 17 March 1967, College Committee Minutes, Board of Trustees, Thomas Jefferson University, Thomas Jefferson University Archives and Special Collections, Thomas Jefferson University, Philadelphia, PA. See also Mary D. Overpeck, "Physicians in Family Practice 1931–67," *Public Health Reports* 85:485–494, 1970. The imbalances that occurred in the physician workforce included maldistributions among specialties, not merely an oversupply of specialists. For instance, in the late 1960s it was felt that there were an excessive number of general surgeons and surgical subspecialists, whereas radiologists were considered in short supply. (Lippard, *A Half-Century of Medical Eduction*, p. 96.)

30. "Reassessment of Surgical Subspecialty Training in the United States," *Archives of Surgery* 104:760, 1972.

31. Ravitch, *The Troubled Crusade*, p. 183.

32. *Ibid.*, pp. 324–325.

33. General surgery was the one field that retained a pyramidal residency structure after the war. Thus, although many individuals entered surgical subspecialty residencies by choice, others did so because they had not been promoted in a general surgical residency. Because of their length (five years or more) and exclusivity, residencies in general surgery continued to provide designated time for research, in contrast to other clinical fields, where formal opportunities for research were moved to the fellowship period.

34. Lippard, *A Half-Century of American Medical Education*, p. 45.

35. "Year 64–65," Folder 77, Box 7, Knowles Papers.

36. Meeting of 23 January 1974, Minutes, Faculty Executive Committee, University of Southern California School of Medicine, Dean's Office, University of Southern California School of Medicine, Los Angeles, CA.

37. Meeting of 9 May 1978, Minutes, Medical Service Staff Meeting, Columbia-Presbyterian Medical Center, Office of the Chairman, Department of Medicine, College of Physicians and Surgeons of Columbia University, New York, NY.

38. *Final Report of the Commission on Medical Education* (New York: Office of the Director of the Study, 1932), p. 124.

39. Statement of Dr. Whiting, MGH Staff Replies to Letter of 18 April 1961, Folder 115, Box 10, Knowles Papers.

40. Important sociological studies of internship during this period include Emily Mumford, *Interns: From Students to Physicians* (Cambridge: Harvard University Press, 1970); and Stephen J. Miller, *Prescription for Leadership: Training for the Medical Elite* (Chicago: Aldine Publishing Company, 1970). The major studies of residency are Charles L. Bosk's analysis of surgical residency, *Forgive and Remember: Managing Medical Failure* (Chicago: University of Chicago Press, 1979); and Donald Light's study of psychiatry training, *Becoming Psychiatrists: The Professional Transformation of Self* (New York: W. W. Norton & Co., 1980). For a review of the sociological literature on graduate medical education, see Renée C. Fox, *The Sociology of Medicine: A Participant Observer's View* (Englewood Cliffs, NJ: Prentice-Hall, 1989), pp. 108–141.

41. As house officers began to live outside the hospital, many subdramas occurred. The availability of affordable housing close to the hospital became a factor in the competition among teaching hospitals to attract the best house officers. Here, programs in expensive cities like New York were at a disadvantage. In cities with housing shortages, house officers and other hospital personnel often lived in apartment buildings owned by the hospital or university. The priorities established for allocating apartments and hospital parking spaces said much about the social hierarchy of the academic medical center.

42. Among the important works focusing on the development of a mass-consumption society are George E. Mowry and Blaine A. Brownell, *The Urban Nation: 1920–1980*, rev. ed. (New York: Hill and Wang, 1981); Richard Wightman Fox and T. J. Jackson Lears, eds., *The Culture of Consumption: Critical Essays in American History 1880–1980* (New York: Pantheon Books, 1983); and John Kenneth Galbraith, *The Affluent Society* (Boston: Houghton-Mifflin, 1958).

43. The Massachusetts General Hospital, *Annual Report* (1958), pp. 60–61; Robert S. Palmer to Daniel Ellis, 26 January 1970, Folder 295, Box 25, Knowles Papers; Walter T. St. Goar to M.G.H. Staff Members, 9 February 1970, Folder 295, Box 25, Knowles Papers; Edward B. Benedict to John V. Lawrence, 30 June 1969, Folder 296, Box 25, Knowles Papers.

44. The Massachusetts General Hospital, *Annual Report* (1964), p. 58.

45. L. E. Martin to Dear Doctor, 7 June 1963, Folder 62, Box 6, Knowles Papers; Dean A. Clark to members of Intern and Resident Staff, 21 June 1951, Folder "Johns Hopkins Hospital—Dr. E. L. Crosby Correspondence 1951–1952," Box 4XY, Correspondence Files, Office of the Dean of the Medical Faculty, The Johns Hopkins School of Medicine, Record Group 3, Series B, Archive of The Johns Hopkins University School of Medicine, The Alan Mason Chesney Archives of The Johns Hopkins Medical Institutions, Baltimore, MD.

46. Joel H. Goldberg, "House Officers Are Getting a Living Wage at Last," *Hospital Physician*, March 1970, pp. 59–67.

47. Sherman M. Mellinkoff to F. H. Sherwood and C. E. Young, 10 December 1966; and David H. Solomon and Sherman M. Mellinkoff to Franklin P. Murphy, 26 January 1965; both Folder "Medicine: Interns & Residents (House Staff) 1961–70," Box 11, Series 401, Administrative Subject Files of Franklin Murphy, 1935–71 (Record Series 401), University Archives, Department of Special Collections, The University Library, University of California, Los Angeles, Los Angeles, CA.

48. See, for example, meetings of 4 November 1963 and 8 January 1968, Corporate Board of Trustees Minutes, Thomas Jefferson University, Thomas Jefferson University Archives and Special Collections, Thomas Jefferson University, Philadelphia, PA.

49. Meeting of 23 May 1968, Graduate Staff Training Program Committee,

Medical Board of The New York Hospital, Minutes (May 1968–November 1968), Archives, The New York Hospital–Cornell Medical Center, New York, NY.

50. Goldberg, "House Officers Are Getting a Living Wage at Last," p. 67.

The existence of moonlighting reflected the revolt of this generation of house officers against paternalism and authority. Very few house officers before World War II, even with pressing financial needs, would have dared to defy their department's official sanctions against moonlighting.

51. See, for instance, W. Hardy Hendren to Nathan B. Talbot, 8 January 1965, Folder 141, Box 11, Knowles Papers.

Some older faculty were of the view that the poor attendance of house officers at conferences reflected changes in lifestyle and culture—the desire to get home earlier in the evening—rather than an increase in the amount of work per se.

52. The New York Hospital, Chief Residents' Luncheon, 3 February 1961, Folder 3, Box 5, Associate Director of Professional Services, Society of The New York Hospital (Kady, Carver, Baldridge), Archives, The New York Hospital–Cornell Medical Center, New York, NY.

53. Meeting of 2 November 1961, Transactions of the Medical Board of the New York Hospital.

54. Richard C. Friedman, J. Thomas Bigger, and Donald S. Kornfeld, "The Intern and Sleep Loss," *New England Journal of Medicine* 285:201–203, 1971.

55. Institute of Medicine Social Security Studies Final Report, with agenda items for meeting of 25–26 March 1976, Executive Council Meetings and Agendas, Association of American Medical Colleges, Association of American Medical Colleges Archives, Washington, D.C.

56. Report of the Department of Medicine, 1953–54, Office of the Dean, Cornell University Medical Center, Annual Reports of Departments and Offices.

57. Report of the Committee to Study Present Methods for Periodic Review of Clinical Experience, with meeting of 26 May 1959, Minutes, The Johns Hopkins Medical Board.

58. The Massachusetts General Hospital, *Annual Report* (1964), p. 59.

Chapter 11

1. Clark Kerr, *The Uses of the University*, 3rd ed. (Cambridge: Harvard University Press, 1982).

2. Harvard Medical School, *Dean's Report* (1967–68), pp. 5–6.

3. Quoted in John W. Henderson, "Allocation of the Medical Student's Time in Educational Programs," Folder 16, Box 3, Joseph C. Hinsey Papers, Archives, The New York Hospital–Cornell Medical Center, New York, NY.

4. Reports of the Department of Pharmacology, 1949–50 and 1950–51, Cornell University Medical Center, Annual Reports of Departments and Offices, Archives, The New York Hospital–Cornell Medical Center, New York, NY.

5. University of Southern California Multidisciplinary Laboratories, Folder "Multidisciplinary Laboratories," Dean's Office Files, University of Southern California School of Medicine, Norris Medical Library, University of Southern California, Los Angeles, CA.

6. For more on the NBME, see John P. Hubbard and Edith J. Levit, *The National Board of Medical Examiners: The First Seventy Years* (Philadelphia: National Board of Medical Examiners, 1985); and Bryce Templeton, "The National Board of Medical Examiners and Independent Assessment Agencies," in Thomas Samph and Bryce

Templeton, eds., *Evaluation in Medical Education: Past, Present, Future* (Cambridge, MA: Ballinger Publishing Company, 1979), pp. 121–163.

7. Meeting of 25 May 1956, Harvard University Medical Faculty, Minutes of Meetings, Harvard Medical Archives, Rare Books Department, Countway Library, Harvard Medical School, Boston, MA.

8. Robert H. Ebert, "Medical Education at the Peak of the Era of Experimental Medicine," *Daedalus*, Spring 1986, p. 65.

9. Harriet L. Hardy to John H. Knowles, 19 February 1965, Folder 226, Box 19, John H. Knowles Papers, Rockefeller Archive Center, North Tarrytown, NY.

10. Memorandum to the Executive Faculty, with agenda items for meeting of 21 May 1958, Executive Faculty Minutes, University of Colorado School of Medicine, Office of the Chancellor, University of Colorado Health Sciences Center, Denver, CO.

11. Here, of course, Fox meant by the term "uncertainty" the fact that patients often pose perplexing diagnostic or therapeutic dilemmas. It should be pointed out that her studies also explored other types of uncertainty that occur in medicine, such as the uncertainty practitioners face in making decisions when existing knowledge provides little guidance and the many uncertainties investigators face in exploring the unknown. See Renée Fox, "Training for Uncertainty," in Robert K. Merton, George Reader, and Patricia L. Kendall, eds., *The Student-Physician: Introductory Studies in the Sociology of Medical Education* (Cambridge: Harvard University Press, 1957), pp. 207–241; and Renée C. Fox, *Experiment Perilous: Physicians and Patients Facing the Unknown* (Glencoe, IL: The Free Press, 1959).

12. Meeting of 19 December 1953, Executive Committee Minutes, National Board of Medical Examiners, President's Office, National Board of Medical Examiners, Philadelphia, PA; "Increasing Use of Objective Tests," *The National Board Examiner*, vol. 2, no. 4, January 1955, pp. 1–3 (including quotations).

13. Arlene R. Barro, "Survey and Evaluation of Approaches to Physician Performance Measurement," *Journal of Medical Education* 48:1048–1093, 1973.

14. Helpful sources on curricular reform during this period include Peter V. Lee, *Medical Schools and the Changing Times: Nine Case Reports on Experimentation in Medical Education, 1950–1960* (Evanston, IL: Association of American Medical Colleges, 1962); Margaret Bussigel, Barbara Barzansky, and Gary Grenholm, *Innovative Processes in Medical Education* (New York: Praeger Publishing Company, 1988); Vernon W. Lippard, *A Half-Century of American Medical Education: 1920–1970* (New York: Josiah Macy, Jr. Foundation, 1974), pp. 8–27; and Patricia L. Kendall and George G. Reader, "Innovations in Medical Education of the 1950s Contrasted with Those of the 1970s and 1980s," *Journal of Health and Social Behavior* 29:279–293, 1988.

15. Lee, *Medical Schools and the Changing Times*, pp. 5–28; Lippard, *A Half-Century of American Medical Education*, pp. 22–24; "A Revised Program of Medical Education at Johns Hopkins," *Journal of Medical Education* 33:225–233, 1958; John A. D. Cooper and Moody Prior, "A New Program in Medical Education at Northwestern University," *Journal of Medical Education* 36:80–90, 1961.

16. Lippard, *A Half-Century of American Medical Education*, pp. 21–22; Lyman M. Stowe, "The Stanford Plan: An Educational Continuum for Medicine," *Journal of Medical Education* 34:1059–1069, 1959.

17. Lee, *Medical Schools and the Changing Times*, pp. 29–61; Kendall and Reader, "Innovations in Medical Education," pp. 280–285; Lippard, *A Half-Century of American Medical Education*, pp. 20–21. Temple's program in comprehensive care

emphasized psychosomatic medicine; North Carolina's, preventive medicine; Cornell's, the opportunity for a research team of sociologists to study medical education; and Colorado's, the opportunity for investigators to use psychological techniques to evaluate the results of the educational experiment.

18. The most complete account of the Western Reserve experience is Greer Williams, *Western Reserve's Experiment in Medical Education and Its Outcome* (New York: Oxford University Press, 1980).

19. Lee, *Medical Schools and the Changing Times*, pp. 76–77.

20. A. McGehee Harvey and Susan L. Abrams, *"For the Welfare of Mankind": The Commonwealth Fund and American Medicine* (Baltimore: Johns Hopkins University Press, 1986), pp. 203–337.

21. Lippard, *A Half-Century of American Medical Education*, p. 112.

22. Meeting of 6 March 1959, Harvard University Medical Faculty, Minutes of Meetings.

23. Lee, *Medical Schools and the Changing Times*, p. 77.

24. An account of the development of this field is George E. Miller, *Educating Medical Teachers* (Cambridge: Harvard University Press, 1980). Here, too, the influence of the Commonwealth Fund was conspicuous. Miller wrote (p. viii), "The Commonwealth Fund supported so many pieces of the work described here that it might better be thought of as a partner than as merely a benefactor."

25. Barbara Barzansky, "The Growth and Divergence of the Basic Sciences," in Barbara Barzansky and Norman Gevitz, eds., *Beyond Flexner: Medical Education in the Twentieth Century* (New York: Greenwood Press, 1992), p. 30.

26. Harold Jehgers to Hugh Hussey, 3 February 1962, Folder "Medical School January–December 1962," Box "Medical School 1961–1964," Medical School Records, Georgetown University School of Medicine, Georgetown University Archives, Georgetown University, Washington, D.C.

27. Meeting of 9 March 1967, Executive Council Minutes, Tufts University School of Medicine, Tufts University Archives, Medford, MA.

28. The Department of Human Sciences in the Proposed Mount Sinai Medical School, February 1964, Folder "Blumenkranz: Correspondence; Reports," Mount Sinai School of Medicine, Early Papers, Archives, The Mount Sinai Medical Center, New York, NY.

29. Commentary—Class of 1964, 7 July 1964, Folder "Evaluation by Students," Box 2, University of Michigan Medical School Records, Michigan Historical Collections, Bentley Historical Library, University of Michigan, Ann Arbor, MI.

30. See, for instance, John H. Knowles to Joseph W. Gardella, 3 May 1961, Folder 344, Box 30, Knowles Papers; and meeting of 12 January 1956, Executive Committee, Folder "Executive Committee 1956–59," Box 7, University of Michigan Medical School Records.

31. From 1949 to 1958, the national dropout rate from medical school was 8.28 percent for men and 15.51 percent for women. Each school had its own experience. At Harvard, for instance, the dropout rate during the 1950s was only 3.5 percent, most of which occurred for personal rather than academic reasons. By the junior year, dropout rates at most schools were extremely low—in part because schools had the flexibility to adjust class size in the hospital years, and in part because medical faculties commonly undertook every possible effort to help junior and senior students who were failing. (Davis G. Johnson and Edwin B. Hutchins, "Doctor or Dropout? A Study of Medical School Attrition," *Journal of Medical Education* 41:1116, 1966 [national statistics]; meeting of 2 Octo-

ber 1959, Harvard University Medical Faculty, Minutes of Meetings [Harvard experience].)

32. Report of the Curriculum Committee, with meeting of 30 October 1958, Transactions of the Executive Faculty, Cornell University Medical College, Archives, The New York Hospital–Cornell Medical Center, New York, NY; meeting of 17 January 1956, Executive Faculty, Folder "1956–1959," Box 129, University of Michigan Medical School Records.

33. Report of the Department of Anatomy, 1957–58, Office of the Dean, Cornell University Medical Center, Annual Reports of Departments and Offices; W. J. Nungester to W. N. Hubbard Jr., 13 December 1961, Folder "Student Evaluation Policy 1960–61," Box 82, University of Michigan Medical School Records.

34. University of Arkansas School of Medicine, *Annual Report* (1951–52), p. 13.

35. Some faculty also had misgivings about pass-fail grading. For instance, basic science faculty at Harvard felt that the pass-fail system in their courses removed an important incentive for students to acquire more than a minimal knowledge of the subjects (Harvard Medical School, *Dean's Report* [1971–72], p. 13).

36. Report on Harvard University Medical School Field Visit of 9 December 1966, Folder "INS 2–1 Harvard Medical School 1967," President/Dean's Papers (James Series), Mount Sinai School of Medicine, Archives, The Mount Sinai Medical Center, New York, NY.

37. David Seegal to John A. D. Cooper, 30 December 1963, and John H. Knowles to David Seegal, 29 July 1963, both Folder 303, Box 26, Knowles Papers; Harold I. Lief, Robert C. Lancaster, and Vann Spruiell, "Is Self-Kick the Answer?," *Journal of Medical Education* 38:971, 1963. This controversy was precipitated by David Seegal's editorial, "The Value of a Self-Kick in the Seat of the Pants for the Anxious Medical Student," *Journal of Medical Education* 38:605–606, 1963.

38. Issues of *Borborygmi* are kept at Norris Medical Library, University of Southern California Medical School, Los Angeles, CA.

39. As a typical example, medical students at Boston University were asked whether the essay examinations in gross anatomy were more of a measure of their learning than the objective examinations. Fifty percent of the students replied "yes"; 50 percent, "no." (Report of the Class of 1963 Curriculum Evaluation Committee, with meeting of 2 April 1962, Executive Committee of the Faculty Minutes, Boston University School of Medicine, Dean's Office, Boston University School of Medicine, Boston, MA.)

40. Evidence suggests that medical education was as hard on the spouses and families of students and house officers as on the students and house officers themselves. The demanding call schedules, the perennial exhaustion when finally at home, and time taken away from family because of the need to study wreaked havoc on the marriages of many students and young physicians. See Robert H. Coombs, "The Medical Marriage," in Robert H. Coombs and Clark E. Vincent, eds., *Psychosocial Aspects of Medical Training* (Springfield, IL: Charles C Thomas, 1971), pp. 133–167.

41. F. J. Mullin and John M. Stalnaker, "The Matching Plan for Internship Appointment," *Journal of Medical Education* 26:341–345, 1951; John M. Stalnaker, "The Matching Program for Intern Placement," *Journal of Medical Education* 28:13–19, 1953.

42. Selecting students continued to be challenging because of the lack of correlation between any of the criteria used in the admissions process, including scores

on the Medical College Admissions Test and ultimate performance as a physician. See James W. Bartlett, "Medical School and Career Performances of Medical Students with Low Medical College Admission Test Scores," *Journal of Medical Education* 42:231–237, 1967; and Harrison G. Gough, Wallace B. Hall, and Robert E. Harris, "Admissions Procedures as Forecasters of Performance in Medical Education," *Journal of Medical Education* 38:983–998, 1963.

43. Lippard, *A Half-Century of American Medical Education*, pp. 33–34.

44. AAMC Statement on Financial Assistance to Medical Students, with meeting of 23–24 May 1960, Executive Council Meetings and Agendas, Association of American Medical Colleges, Association of American Medical Colleges Archives, Washington, D.C.

45. The Surgeon General's Consultant Group on Medical Education, *Physicians for a Growing America* (Washington, D.C.: U.S. Government Printing Office, Public Health Service Publication No. 709, 1959), pp. 20–21.

46. *Ibid.*, p. 21.

47. Dean's Report (1954–55), Office of the Dean, Cornell University Medical Center, Annual Reports of Departments and Offices.

48. See, for instance, Dean's Report (1953–54), Office of the Dean, Cornell University Medical Center, Annual Reports of Departments and Offices.

49. See, for instance, Report on Financial Aid and Admissions to Medical School, with meeting of 31 January 1966, Minutes, Advisory Board of the Medical Faculty, The Johns Hopkins University School of Medicine, The Alan Mason Chesney Medical Archives of The Johns Hopkins Medical Institutions, Baltimore, MD.

50. Harvard Medical School, *Dean's Report* (1958–59), pp. 2–3; meeting of 10 November 1961, Harvard University Medical Faculty, Minutes of Meetings.

51. Thomas B. Turner to the Advisory Board, 15 March 1963, with meeting of 25 March 1963, Minutes, Advisory Board of the Medical Faculty, The Johns Hopkins University School of Medicine.

52. In 1962, of applicants accepted at both Harvard and Johns Hopkins, 14 of 16 chose to go to Harvard; in 1963, 23 of 24; in 1964, 14 of 17. (Report of Committee on Admissions, with meeting of 31 January 1966, Minutes, Advisory Board of the Medical Faculty, The Johns Hopkins University School of Medicine.)

53. Winston K. Shorey, Remarks at General Faculty and Hospital Staff Meeting, 14 October 1965, Folder "Miscellaneous: Annual Report," Dean's Office Files (Winston K. Shorey, 1961–1974), ID Number 20DB016, Special Collections Division, University of Arkansas for Health Sciences Library, Little Rock, AR. According to Shorey, the second least competitive school was the University of Tennessee, with 2.9 applications per position, and the third, Louisiana State University, with 3.1 applicants per position.

54. Executive Council Meeting, 8 November 1965, Folder "Executive Council Minutes 1961–1967," Dean's Office Files (Winston K. Shorey, 1961–1974).

55. Meeting of 21 October 1963, Minutes of the Meetings of the Faculty, College of Physicians and Surgeons of Columbia University, Special Collections, Augustus C. Long Health Sciences Library, Columbia University, New York, NY.

56. Daniel H. Funkenstein, *Medical Students, Medical Schools and Society During Five Eras: Factors Affecting the Career Choices of Physicians 1958–1976* (Cambridge, MA: Ballinger Publishing Company, 1978).

57. Agnes G. Rezler, "Attitude Changes During Medical School: A Review of the Literature," *Journal of Medical Education* 49:1023–1030, 1974; quotations, p. 1029.

58. The secondary literature on this subject is vast. A helpful introduction to published works on this topic, as well as other important topics in the history of education, is Laurence R. Veysey, "The History of Education," *Reviews in American History* 10:281–291, 1982.

59. For instance, an important study of medical students in the 1950s found that interest in general practice declined in favor of specialization as students passed from the first to the fourth year of medical school—clear evidence that something happened during medical school to affect attitudes and career choices. (Patricia L. Kendall and Hanan C. Selvin, "Tendencies toward Specialization in Medical Training," in Merton, Reader, and Kendall, eds., *The Student-Physician*, pp. 153–174.)

60. *Figure 3* is taken from Lowell T. Coggeshall, *Planning for Medical Progress Through Education* (Evanston, IL: Association of American Medical Colleges, 1965), p. 7.

61. See, for instance, Report of *Ad Hoc* Committee of Deans, 23 May 1958, Folder "1942–1971 MEND: Selected Bibliography," Box 1, MEND Records, Association of American Medical Colleges Archives, Washington, D.C.; and New and Developing Medical Schools: A Statement of Position, 5 February 1970, with agenda items for meeting of 7 May 1970, Executive Council Meetings and Agendas, Association of American Medical Colleges.

62. Dean F. Smiley, "Some Public Relations Problems in Medical Education, 1950–51," Folder "Association of American Medical Colleges Reports—1948–1952," Dean's Office Files, University of Southern California School of Medicine.

63. The Surgeon General's Consultant Group on Medical Education, *Physicians for a Growing America*.

64. J. R. Schofield, *New and Expanded Medical Schools, Mid-Century to the 1980s* (San Francisco: Josey-Bass, 1984), pp. 16–21; Lippard, *A Half-Century of American Medical Education*, pp. 114–121.

65. On the new medical schools, see Schofield, *New and Expanded Medical Schools*; Vernon W. Lippard and Elizabeth F. Purcell, eds., *Case Histories of Ten New Medical Schools* (New York: The Josiah Macy, Jr. Foundation, 1972); and John Z. Bowers and Elizabeth F. Purcell, eds., *New Medical Schools at Home and Abroad* (New York: Josiah Macy, Jr. Foundation, 1978). *Table 7* and *Figure 4* are adapted from Schofield, *New and Expanded Medical Schools*, pp. 32 and 33, respectively.

In the 1960s and 1970s, existing medical schools that had operated as two-year basic science schools were converted to four-year schools. Most of these schools were located in rural areas, but population growth and improved transportation had resulted in a large enough growth of their hospitals to support clinical teaching. A number of the new medical schools were opened as two-year institutions, but almost all were subsequently converted to four-year schools. By 1981, the University of Minnesota-Duluth was the country's only remaining two-year medical school.

The question of whether to build new schools or enlarge existing ones was often a highly charged political issue. Established institutions felt that they deserved all the help they could get, while universities and communities without schools, hoping to be granted a medical school, competed intensely for the same resources.

66. AAMC Statement on Accreditation, with agenda items for meeting of 5 February 1972; Functions and Structure of a Medical School, with agenda items for meeting of 19 May 1972; Glen R. Leymaster to John R. Proffitt, 13 January

1972, with agenda items for meeting of 5 February 1972; Summary of Information on Medical Schools in Development, with agenda items for meeting of 28–29 April 1965; and statement of Edward L. Turner and Ward Darley, with agenda items for meeting of 6 February 1959; all Executive Council Meetings and Agendas, Association of American Medical Colleges.

67. Materials on the AAMC's reorganization in 1968 are found in Box 3, Ward Darley Papers; and Boxes 1–3, 1968 Reorganization Records; both Association of American Medical Schools Archives, Washington, D.C.

The blueprint for the AAMC's reorganization and move to Washington had been provided by the Coggeshall report of 1965 (Coggeshall, *Planning for Medical Progress through Education*). Though its recommendations for organizational change were followed, the report's call for sweeping reforms of graduate medical education were not. See Joel D. Howell, "Lowell T. Coggeshall and American Medical Education: 1901–1987," *Academic Medicine* 67:711–718, 1992.

68. Meeting of 9–10 February 1956, Executive Council Meetings and Agendas, Association of American Medical Colleges.

69. Meeting of 31 March 1960, Executive Committee, Folder "Executive Committee 1959–61," Box 7, University of Michigan Medical School Records.

70. Eli Ginzberg, *Men, Money, and Medicine* (New York: Columbia University Press, 1969). See also Kenneth B. Castleton, "Are We Building Too Many Medical Schools?," *Journal of the American Medical Association* 216:1989–1992, 1971.

71. See, for instance, George P. Berry to James B. Conant, 18 December 1952, Folder "HU—James B. Conant—1950–1960," Deans' Subject File, Harvard Medical School, Harvard Medical Archives, Rare Books Department, Countway Library, Harvard Medical School, Boston, MA.

72. John E. Deitrick and Robert C. Berson, *Medical Schools in the United States at Mid-Century* (New York: McGraw-Hill, 1953), pp. 319–321; quotations, p. 320.

73. Meeting of 14 February 1957, Transactions of the Medical Faculty, Cornell University Medical College, Archives, The New York Hospital–Cornell Medical Center, New York, NY.

74. Meeting of 18 November 1960, Transactions of the Medical Faculty, Cornell University Medical College.

75. Meeting of 20 January 1964, Minutes of the Executive Committee of the Faculty, New York University College of Medicine, Archives, New York University Medical Center, New York, NY.

76. Minutes of Executive Faculty Meeting of 18 June 1956, Folder 2, Box 104, Series 300, Administrative Files of Stafford Warren, 1925–68 (Record Series 300), University Archives, Department of Special Collections, The University Library, University of California, Los Angeles, Los Angeles, CA.

77. Robert J. Glaser, "The Medical Deanship: Its Half-Life and Hard Times," *Journal of Medical Education* 44:1121, 1969.

78. Augustus S. Rose to Sherman M. Mellinkoff, 27 January 1971, Folder 3, Box 6, Series 255, Administrative Files of Jeanne Williams, 1945–1987 (Record Series 255), University Archives, Department of Special Collections, The University Library, University of California, Los Angeles, Los Angeles, CA.

79. John H. Knowles, "Elephant by the Tail," 6 March 1960, Folder 836, Box 69, Knowles Papers.

80. The Peter Bent Brigham Hospital, *Annual Report* (1958), p. 98.

81. Meeting of 22 October 1958, Hospital Staff Minutes, Hospital of the Woman's Medical College of Pennsylvania, Archives and Special Collections on Women in Medicine, MCP Hahnemann University, Philadelphia, PA.

82. Jonathan R. Cole and James A. Lipton, "The Reputations of American Medical Schools," *Social Forces* 55:662–684, 1977.

83. University of Southern California School of Medicine Department of Medical Microbiology, Comments on Students, First Semester 1960–61, Folder "Committee on Promotions and Academic Standing," Dean's Office Files, University of Southern California School of Medicine.

Of course, even at the most research-intensive schools, only a minority of students ultimately pursued academic careers. For instance, in 1960, 18 percent of Harvard's active graduates were in full-time teaching or research. (Meeting of 4 November 1960, Harvard University Medical Faculty, Minutes of Meetings.)

84. Charles S. Cameron, Message to the Board of Trustees, 29 April 1969, with meeting of 30 April 1969, Minutes of Meetings of the Board of Trustees of Hahnemann Medical College and Hospital, Archives and Special Collections, Hahnemann Collection, MCP Hahnemann University, Philadelphia, PA.

85. On the neglect of undergraduate teaching for research throughout the multiversity, see Kerr, *The Uses of the University*; Page Smith, *Killing the Spirit: Higher Education in America* (New York: Viking, 1990); Ernest L. Boyer, *Scholarship Reconsidered: Priorities of the Professoriate* (Princeton, NJ: The Carnegie Foundation for the Advancement of Teaching, 1990); and Bruce Wilshire, *The Moral Collapse of the University: Professionalism, Purity, and Alienation* (Albany, NY: State University of New York Press, 1990).

86. Memorandum of Meeting of AAMC Executive Committee with HEW Secretary Richardson, 7 January 1971, with agenda items for meeting of 12 February 1971, Executive Council Meetings and Agendas, Association of American Medical Colleges.

87. Franz K. Bauer, Rough Draft of Talk for Trustees Conference, 1971, Folder "Trustees Retreat," Dean's Office Files, University of Southern California School of Medicine.

88. Joseph C. Hinsey, untitled address, 1949, Folder 1, Box 1, Papers, Office of the Dean, Cornell University Medical College, 1893–1956 (Hinsey), Archives, The New York Hospital–Cornell Medical Center, New York, NY; Rashi Fein, "Tensions in Medical Education: The Search for Balance," lecture delivered 29 November 1973, Folder 1051, Box 91, Knowles Papers.

89. Meeting of 26 November 1969, Executive Committee, Folder "Executive Committee September–December 1969," Box 8, University of Michigan Medical School Records.

Chapter 12

1. Table D3, "Revenues for the Programs of U.S. Medical Schools," AAMC Data Book, Association of American Medical Colleges Archives, Washington, D.C.

2. Robert J. Glaser, "The Medical Deanship: Its Half-Life and Hard Times," *Journal of Medical Education* 44:1125, 1969.

3. Many specific political factors, of course, also were pivotal in the passage of this legislation—for instance, the effective lobbying of the American Association of Retired Persons, the landslide Democratic victory in the 1964 elections, Lyndon B. Johnson's prodigious energy and adroit handling of Congress, and the skillful political work of Wilbur Cohen, Wilbur Mills, and other officials and legislators. On the passage and implementation of Medicare and Medicaid, see Judith M. Feder, *Medicare: The Politics of Federal Hospital Insurance* (Lexington, MA: Lexing-

ton Books, 1977); Herman Miles Somers and Anne Ramsay Somers, *Medicare and the Hospitals: Issues and Prospects* (Washington, D.C.: Brookings Institution, 1966); Theodor R. Marmor, *The Politics of Medicare* (Chicago: Aldine Publishing Company, 1970); Robert Stevens and Rosemary Stevens, *Welfare in America: A Case Study of Medicaid* (New York: Free Press, 1974); and Sheri I. David, *With Dignity: The Search for Medicare and Medicaid* (Westport, CT: Greenwood Press, 1985).

4. Rosemary Stevens, *In Sickness and in Wealth: American Hospitals in the Twentieth Century* (New York: Basic Books, 1989), pp. 333, 334.

5. In understanding why Medicare but not Medicaid received such liberal financing, it is important to recognize that the two programs reflected different traditions. "Medicare was buoyed by popular approval and acknowledged dignity of Social Security; Medicaid was burdened by the stigma of public assistance." (Paul Starr, *The Social Transformation of American Medicine: The Rise of a Sovereign Profession and the Making of a Vast Industry* [New York: Basic Books, 1982], p. 370.) Except where mention of Medicaid is specifically made, the remainder of this section will be concerned with Medicare.

6. William C. Hilles and Sharon K. Fagan, *Medical Practice Plans at U.S. Medical Schools: A Review of Current Characteristics and Trends*, 2 vols. (Washington, D.C.: Association of American Medical Colleges, 1977).

7. Meeting of 10 October 1975, Minutes, Advisory Board of the Medical Faculty, The Johns Hopkins University School of Medicine, The Alan Mason Chesney Medical Archives of The Johns Hopkins Medical Institutions, Baltimore, MD (1970–71 and 1974–75 data); meeting of 12 October 1984, Trustee Policy Committee, with agenda items for meeting of 6 November 1984, Minutes, The Johns Hopkins Hospital Board of Trustees, The Alan Mason Chesney Medical Archives of The Johns Hopkins Medical Institutions, Baltimore, MD (1983–84 data).

8. *Table 8* is adopted from Table D3, "Revenues for the Programs of U.S. Medical Schools," AAMC Data Book. The figures in this table represent conservative estimates because they reflect only the income reported on medical school accounting records. At many schools the practice plans did not channel all their earnings through the dean's office. (Hilles and Fagan, *Medical Practice Plans at U.S. Medical Schools*, vol. 1, p. 41.)

9. Institute of Medicine Social Security Studies Final Report, with agenda items for meeting of 25–26 March 1976, Executive Council Meetings and Agendas, Association of American Medical Colleges, Association of American Medical Colleges Archives, Washington, D.C.

10. *Table 9* is adopted from "Report on Medical School Faculty Salaries, 1975–76," Association of American Medical Colleges Archives, Washington, D.C. These figures underestimate the compensation received by clinical faculty, since most had geographic rather than strict full-time appointments. Geographic faculty received lower base salaries than strict full-timers but higher total compensation because of various incentive plans that allowed them to retain a higher fraction of their professional earnings.

11. Meeting of 21 June 1971, Minutes, Advisory Board of the Medical Faculty, The Johns Hopkins University School of Medicine.

12. The liberal educational reimbursements provided by Medicare reflected Congress's belief that teaching significantly improves patient care. See Memorandum on Reimbursement for Part-time Teaching Physicians, 10 December 1968, Folder 295, Box 25, John H. Knowles Papers, Rockefeller Archive Center, North Tarrytown, NY.

13. J. Robert Willson to John A. Gronvall, 17 April 1972, with Executive Com-

mittee meeting of 27 April 1972, Folder "Executive Committee April–May 1972," Box 9, University of Michigan Medical School Records, Michigan Historical Collections, Bentley Historical Library, University of Michigan, Ann Arbor, MI.

14. Meeting of 13 April 1978, Executive Faculty Minutes, University of Colorado School of Medicine, Office of the Chancellor, University of Colorado Health Sciences Center, Denver, CO.

15. Hilles and Fagan, *Medical Practice Plans at U.S. Medical Schools*, vol. 1, pp. 17–21, 41–48.

16. Use of the term "academic health center" was also encouraged by the frequency with which such centers now included other professional schools and schools of allied health as well as a medical school.

17. The Peter Bent Brigham Hospital, *Annual Report* (1970), p. 205.

18. Report of Subcommittee on Renovation of Vanderbilt Clinic, with meeting of 25 May 1960, Minutes of the Planning Committee of the Medical Board, The Presbyterian Hospital in the City of New York, President's Offices, Presbyterian Hospital, New York, NY.

19. Of note, Medicare and Medicaid also brought about the end of segregation in American hospitals. To be eligible for reimbursement from Medicare and Medicaid, hospitals and nursing homes had to integrate patient care in the institution as a whole as well as in the assignment of individual rooms. (Steven Shea and Mindy Thompson Fullilove, "Entry of Black and Other Minority Students into U.S. Medical Schools," *New England Journal of Medicine* 313:934–935, 1985.)

20. For expressions of this view, see Paul S. Russell, "Surgery in a Time of Change," in John H. Knowles, ed., *The Teaching Hospital: Evolution and Contemporary Issues* (Cambridge: Harvard University Press, 1966), pp. 38–65; and Robert H. Ebert, "The Dilemma of Medical Teaching in an Affluent Society," in Knowles, ed., *The Teaching Hospital*, pp. 66–83.

21. Meeting of 29 November 1966, Minutes, The Johns Hopkins Hospital Medical Board, The Alan Mason Chesney Medical Archives of The Johns Hopkins Medical Institutions, Baltimore, MD.

22. Allan L. Friedlich to Edward D. Churchill, 30 August 1961, Folder 115, Box 10, Knowles Papers.

23. For discussion of strategies to make better use of private patients in medical teaching, see Russell, "Surgery in a Time of Change," pp. 55–65; and Ebert, "The Dilemma of Medical Teaching in an Affluent Society," pp. 76–83.

24. Progress Notes on Plans for the *Mount Sinai School of Medicine*, with agenda items for meeting of 11 July 1966, Agendas and Minutes, Board of Trustees, Mount Sinai School of Medicine, Archives, Mount Sinai Medical Center, New York, NY.

25. Executive Committee Meeting, 26 November 1969, Folder "Executive Committee September–December 1969," Box 8, University of Michigan Medical School Records.

26. Summary of LCME Team Observations and Recommendations, with agenda items for meeting of 5 April 1982, Administrative Council Meetings, Georgetown University Medical Center, Office of the Dean, Georgetown University School of Medicine, Washington, D.C.

27. Consultative and Referral Practice Report, with meeting of 25 January 1973, Faculty Meeting Minutes, Howard University College of Medicine, Office of the Dean, Howard University College of Medicine, Washington, D.C.

28. Meeting of 24 January 1972, Minutes, Advisory Board of the Medical Faculty, The Johns Hopkins University School of Medicine.

29. H. Paul Jolly, Leon Taksel, Robert J. Boerner, Janet Bickel, and Charles W. Macenski Jr., "US Medical School Finances," *Journal of the American Medical Association* 248:3261, 1982.

30. Institute of Medicine, *Medicare-Medicaid Reimbursement Policies* (Washington, D.C.: U.S. Government Printing Office, 1976), pp. 128, 130.

31. Meetings of 6 January 1975 ("destructive") and 24 June 1974 ("'second-class'"), Minutes, Advisory Board of the Medical Faculty, The Johns Hopkins University School of Medicine.

32. Meeting of 21 October 1974, Minutes, Advisory Board of the Medical Faculty, The Johns Hopkins University School of Medicine.

33. Hayden C. Nicholson to Paul Schaefer, 19 March 1953, Folder "House Staff Matters," Dean's Office Files (Hayden C. Nicholson, 1950–55), ID Number 20DB014, Special Collections Division, University of Arkansas for Medical Sciences Library, Little Rock, AR.

34. Statement of Policy [circa December 1954], Folder "House Staff Matters," Dean's Office Files (Hayden C. Nicholson, 1950–55).

35. Minutes of the Executive Council, 10 May 1965, Folder "Executive Council Minutes 1961–1967," Dean's Office Files (Winston K. Shorey, 1961–1974), ID Number 20DB016, Special Collections Division, University of Arkansas for Health Sciences Library, Little Rock, AR.

36. Robert H. Ebert, "Medical Education at the Peak of the Era of Experimental Medicine," *Daedalus*, Spring 1986, p. 64.

37. Abraham Flexner, *Universities: American English German* (New York: Oxford University Press, 1930), p. 92.

Chapter 13

1. A vast literature has appeared on student protest, the New Left, and the antiwar movement. Excellent overviews of the period are provided in William L. O'Neill, *Coming Apart: An Informal History of America in the 1960s* (Chicago: Quadrangle Books, 1971); Morris Dickstein, *Gates of Eden: American Culture in the Sixties* (New York: Basic Books, 1977); David M. Chalmers, *And the Crooked Places Made Straight: The Struggle for Social Change in the 1960s* (Baltimore: Johns Hopkins University Press, 1991); and David Farber, *The Age of Great Dreams: America in the 1960s* (New York: Hill and Wang, 1994).

2. The most valuable source on student (and also house staff) activism is Fitzhugh Mullan's autobiographical account, *White Coat, Clenched Fist* (New York: Macmillan, 1976). Other helpful sources include Charles S. Davidson, "Student Revolt and Our Medical Schools," in Hans Popper, ed., *Trends in New Medical Schools* (New York: Grune & Stratton, 1967), pp. 124–128; "Unrest on the Medical Campus," *Medical World News*, 13 October 1967, pp. 63–67; Michael R. McGarvey, Fitzhugh Mullan, and Steven S. Sharfstein, "A Study in Medical Action—The Student Health Organizations," *New England Journal of Medicine* 279:74–79, 1968; Fitzhugh Mullan, "The New Dynamic," *American Journal of Diseases of Children* 116:505–508, 1968; Fitzhugh Mullan, "A House Officer Looks at Medical Student Activism," *American Journal of Psychiatry* 126:1010–1012, 1970; and the October 1969 issue of *The Pharos*, which contains nine articles on student activism.

3. Diane Ravitch, *The Troubled Crusade: American Education, 1945–1980* (New York: Basic Books, 1983), pp. 222–223.

4. Fitzhugh Mullan to author, 14 March 1997.

5. Meeting of 26 October 1970, Transactions of the Faculty Council, Faculty of

Medicine, College of Physicians and Surgeons of Columbia University, Office of the Dean, College of Physicians and Surgeons of Columbia University, New York, NY; meetings of 27 May 1970 and 23 June 1970, Executive Council Minutes, Tufts University School of Medicine, Tufts University Archives, Medford, MA; meeting of 6 May 1970, General Faculty Minutes, Boston University School of Medicine, Dean's Office, Boston University School of Medicine, Boston, MA.

Here it should be noted that a physician draft existed during the Vietnam War, though many doctors entered the military under the "Berry Plan"—a program created in the early 1950s that allowed medical graduates to complete their residencies in exchange for subsequent military service as specialists in their field. During the Vietnam War, many recent medical graduates escaped military service by taking postgraduate research fellowships at the National Institutes of Health. This program was sometimes facetiously called the "Yellow Beret" since the research interests of many fellows waned appreciably after they were no longer vulnerable to the physician draft. The fact that young researchers received deferments—in distinction to World War II, when only "essential teachers" were deferred—represented another manifestation of the newfound power of the scientific ideal on public attitudes and federal policy.

6. Materials on student support of the strike are in Folder "STU 8 Student Demonstrations 1973," President/Dean's Papers (Chalmers Series), Mount Sinai School of Medicine, Archives, The Mount Sinai Medical Center, New York, NY.

7. A Statement of Concern from the First and Second Year Classes, with meeting of 17 November 1969, Minutes and Correspondence of the Executive Committee of the Faculty Council, College of Physicians and Surgeons, Office of the Dean, College of Physicians and Surgeons of Columbia University, New York, NY.

8. Report, "Medicine and Social Responsibility: Towards a New Model of the Physician," 24–25 October 1969, Folder "Medical Resistance Union 1969," Box 104, University of Michigan Medical School Records, Michigan Historical Collections, Bentley Historical Library, University of Michigan, Ann Arbor, MI.

9. Harvard Medical School Dean's Report, 1967–68, p. 14, Harvard Medical Archives, Rare Books Department, Countway Library, Harvard Medical School, Boston, MA.

10. McGarvey, Mullan, and Sharfstein, "A Study in Medical Action"; Mullan, "The New Dynamic"; S. Douglas Frasier, "The Medical Student as Activist," *The Pharos* 32:115–118, 1969.

11. Meeting of 13 June 1972, Executive Committee of the Faculty Minutes, Boston University School of Medicine, Dean's Office, Boston University School of Medicine, Boston, MA.

12. Loyal Davis, "Why the Declining Census in University Hospitals?," *Surgery, Gynecology & Obstetrics* 136:785, 1973.

13. *The Weekly Flatus*, September 1971, p. 1. Issues of *The Weekly Flatus* are kept at Norris Medical Library, University of Southern California School of Medicine, Los Angeles, CA.

14. Donald F. M. Bunce, "Medical Student Participation in Academic Affairs," Folder "Com Student Faculty Council 1969," President/Dean's Papers (James Series), Mount Sinai School of Medicine, Archives, The Mount Sinai Medical Center, New York, NY.

15. George Johnson Jr. to Joseph Hinsey, 1 April 1976, Folder 5, Box 11, Joseph C. Hinsey Papers, Archives, The New York Hospital–Cornell Medical Center, New York, NY.

16. *Figure 5* appeared in the Cornell student publication *Synapse*, Spring 1969, p. 24, Archives, The New York Hospital–Cornell Medical Center, New York, NY.

17. Leonard Scherlis to William S. Stone, 18 December 1968, with Faculty Board meeting of 15 January 1969, Executive Board Minutes, University of Maryland School of Medicine, Dean's Office, University of Maryland School of Medicine, Baltimore, MD.

18. Harvard Medical School Dean's Report, 1973–74, pp. 23–25.

19. John Colombotos and Corinne Kirchner, *Physicians and Social Change* (New York: Oxford University Press, 1986), pp. 115–133.

20. Interns and Residents of the Boston City Hospital to The Honorable John F. Collins, 25 May 1965, Folder "Boston City Hospital—1965 Jan–June," Deans' Subject File, Harvard Medical School, Harvard Medical Archives, Rare Books Department, Countway Library, Harvard Medical School, Boston, MA.

21. Meetings of 10 January 1969 and 18 June 1969, Minutes, Medical Director's House Staff Meetings, The George Washington University Hospital, Office of the Medical Director, The George Washington University Hospital, Washington, D.C.

22. B. Lamar Johnson Jr. to Sherman M. Mellinkoff, 24 July 1964, Folder "Medicine: Interns & Residents (House Staff) 1961–70," Box 11, Series 401, Administrative Subject Files of Franklin Murphy 1935–71 (Record Series 401), University Archives, Department of Special Collections, The University Library, University of California, Los Angeles, Los Angeles, CA.

23. See, for instance, Statement of Position of the House Staff Association of Columbia-Presbyterian Medical Center, with meeting of 19 May 1970, Minutes of the Medical Board, The Presbyterian Hospital in the City of New York, President's Offices, Presbyterian Hospital, New York, NY.

24. Joel H. Goldberg, "Why $12,300–$18,500 Isn't Enough for New York Residents," *Hospital Physician*, June 1971, pp. 33–41.

25. Joel H. Goldberg, "A New Look at House Officers' Incomes," *Hospital Physician*, March 1968, pp. 34–39.

26. Joann S. Lublin, "Interns, Residents Turn to 'Unions' to Improve Wages, Patient Care," *Wall Street Journal*, 6 March 1972, p. A14; Robert G. Harmon, "Intern and Resident Organizations in the United States: 1934–1977," *Milbank Quarterly* 56:500–530, 1978. As Harmon discusses (pp. 501–505), antecedent organizations to the CIR existed in the 1930s and 1940s, most notably the Association of Interns and Medical Students, a national organization that lobbied for higher pay and shorter hours. This organization fell to McCarthyite pressures in the early 1950s.

27. Lublin, "Interns, Residents Turn to 'Unions'," p. A1. Of course, house staff associations rarely represented the views of all interns and residents of the hospital.

28. Meetings of 5 February 1973 and 5 March 1973, Minutes of the Meetings of the Executive Committee of the Medical Staff, Howard University Hospital, Office of the Medical Director, Howard University Hospital, Washington, D.C.

29. Meeting of 23 May 1975, Medical Center Council Minutes, Georgetown University Medical Center, Office of the Dean, Georgetown University School of Medicine, Washington, D.C.; Mark M. Ravitch, "Sequelae of the House Officers' Strike in New York," *Resident & Staff Physician*, August 1975, pp. 87–88.

30. "Resolved: House Staffs Will Unite," *Medical World News*, 2 April 1971, pp. 15–17; National House Staff Conference Task Force on House Staff Economics, with agenda items for meeting of 16 April 1971, Executive Council Meetings and

Agendas, Association of American Medical Colleges, Association of American Medical Colleges Archives, Washington, D.C.

31. Joel H. Goldberg, "Will House Staff Associations Become More than Unions?," *Hospital Physician*, June 1971, pp. 59–60, pp. 60 ("overriding stress"), 59 ("drive toward house staff unity").

32. Lublin, "Interns, Residents Turn to 'Unions'," p. A14.

33. Association of American Medical Colleges, Memorandum #77–28, 1 June 1977, Association of American Medical Colleges Archives, Association of American Medical Colleges, Washington, D.C.

34. A rich collection of newspaper clippings on this strike is found in House Staff Strike—Clippings File, Archives, The Mount Sinai Medical Center, New York, NY.

35. Quoted in David Bird, "The Sleepless-Nights Syndrome," *New York Times*, 18 March 1975.

36. Quoted in *Ibid*.

37. Meeting of April–May 1974, Small Committee, Folder "Small Committee," President/Dean's Papers (Chalmers Series).

38. Robert A. Green to John A. Gronvall, 1 August 1975, Folder "House Officers Association 1973–76," Box 95, University of Michigan Medical School Records.

39. Michael Pietro, "Moonlighting: The View from the Top," *Resident & Staff Physician*, May 1976, p. 95.

40. Roseann Caffaro, "Annual Wage & Education Survey," *Hospital Physician*, January 1978, p. 25.

41. National House Staff Conference Task Force on House Staff Economics, with agenda items for meeting of 16 April 1971, Executive Council Meetings and Agendas, Association of American Medical Colleges.

42. See, for instance, Christopher Lasch, *The Culture of Narcissism: American Life in an Age of Diminishing Expectations* (New York: W. W. Norton & Company, 1979); and Daniel Yankelovich, *New Rules: Searching for Self-Fulfillment in a World Turned Upside Down* (New York: Random House, 1983). The development of a mass-consumption culture has been viewed as a major organizing theme in twentieth-century American history. See, for example, George E. Mowry and Blaine A. Brownell, *The Urban Nation 1920–1980*, rev. ed. (New York: Hill and Wang, 1981); and Richard Wightman Fox and T. J. Jackson Lears, eds., *The Culture of Consumption: Critical Essays in American History, 1880–1980* (New York: Pantheon Books, 1983).

43. Colombotos and Kirchner, *Physicians and Social Change*, pp. 115–133.

44. Ravitch, "Sequelae of the House Officers' Strike in New York," p. 939.

45. Herbert W. Nickens, Timothy P. Ready, and Robert G. Petersdorf, "Project 3000 by 2000—Racial and Ethnic Diversity in U.S. Medical Schools," *New England Journal of Medicine* 331:472–473, 1994; Steven Shea and Mindy Thompson Fullilove, "The Entry of Black and Other Minority Students into U.S. Medical Schools: Historical Perspective and Recent Trends," *New England Journal of Medicine* 313:933–935, 1985.

46. Shea and Fullilove, "The Entry of Black and Other Minority Students," p. 935.

47. Meeting of 20 September 1968, College Committee Minutes, Board of Trustees, Thomas Jefferson University, Thomas Jefferson University Archives and Special Collections, Thomas Jefferson University, Philadelphia, PA.

48. See, for instance, Sterling M. Lloyd Jr., Davis G. Johnson, and Marion Mann, "Survey of Graduates of a Traditionally Black College of Medicine," *Journal of Medical Education* 53: 640–650, 1978.

49. James L. Curtis, *Blacks, Medical Schools, and Society* (Ann Arbor: The University of Michigan Press, 1971), pp. 162–163.

50. Shea and Fullilove, "The Entry of Black and Other Minority Students," p. 939.

51. Meeting of 28 January 1969, Minutes of the Executive Committee of the Faculty, Hahnemann Medical College, Archives and Special Collections, Hahnemann Collection, MCP Hahnemann University, Philadelphia, PA.

52. AAMC data, with meeting of 13 October 1988, Faculty Meeting Minutes, Howard University College of Medicine, Office of the Dean, Howard University College of Medicine, Washington, D.C.

53. Report of the Teaching Proficiency Committee, with meeting of 1 October 1971, Faculty Meeting Minutes, Howard University College of Medicine.

54. See, for instance, Report of the Ad Hoc Committee on Disadvantaged Student Program, with meeting of 12 December 1977, Minutes, Executive Faculty Meetings, Medical College of Pennsylvania, Dean's Office, MCP Hahnemann University, Philadelphia, PA.

55. Meeting of 14 October 1972, Executive Committee, Folder "Executive Committee July–October 1972," Box 10; and meeting of 29 April 1976, Folder "Executive Committee May–June 1976," Box 14; both University of Michigan Medical School Records.

56. *Minority Students in Medical Education: Facts and Figures* (Washington, D.C.: Association of American Medical Colleges, 1983), *Tables 13 and 14*.

57. Executive Committee Meeting, 17 April 1974, Executive Board Minutes, University of Maryland School of Medicine.

58. New York University School of Medicine, Annual Report (1974–75), p. 12, Archives, The New York University Medical Center, New York, NY.

59. Ravitch, *Troubled Crusade*, p. 280.

60. AAMC Statement on Medical Education of Minority Group Students, with agenda items for meeting of 14 June 1987, Executive Council Meetings and Agendas, Association of American Medical Colleges.

61. Summary of LCME Report, with Russell L. Miller to James E. Cheek, 18 March 1985, with meeting of 15 August 1985, Minutes of Meetings of the Executive Committee and Department Chairmen, Howard University College of Medicine, Office of the Dean, Howard University College of Medicine, Washington, D.C.

62. *Figure 6* is taken from Nickens, Ready, and Petersdorf, "Project 3000 by 2000," p. 473.

63. *Ibid.*, p. 473; Shea and Fullilove, "Entry of Black and Other Minority Students," p. 936.

64. Nickens, Ready, and Petersdorf, "Project 3000 by 2000," p. 473.

65. *Ibid.*, p. 473 (quotation); John A. D. Cooper, "The Bakke Decision," *Journal of Medical Education* 53:776–777, 1978. The Bakke case has been extensively studied. See, for instance, Joel Dreyfus and Charles Lawrence, *The Bakke Case: The Politics of Inequality* (New York: Harcourt, Brace, Jovanovich, 1979); and Timothy J. O'Neill, *Bakke and the Politics of Inequality* (Middletown, CT: Wesleyan University Press, 1985).

66. *A Nation at Risk: The Imperative for Educational Reform* (Washington, D.C.: The National Commission on Excellence in Education, 1983).

67. Jonathan Kozol, *Savage Inequalities: Children in America's Schools* (New York: Crown, 1991).

68. Nickens, Ready, and Petersdorf, "Project 3000 by 2000," pp. 472–476; Robert G. Petersdorf, Kathleen S. Turner, Herbert W. Nickens, and Timothy Ready, "Minorities in Medicine: Past, Present, and Future," *Academic Medicine* 65:663–670, 1990; and Robert G. Petersdorf, "Not a Choice, an Obligation," *Academic Medicine* 67:73–79, 1992.

69. See, for instance, Randi Henderson, "Up from Bigotry," *Hopkins Medical News*, Winter 1995, pp. 26–33; and Cheryl S. Rucker, "Wrestling with Ignorance," *Journal of the American Medical Association* 267:2392, 1992.

70. AAMC, *U.S. Medical School Faculty, 1994: Faculty Roster System* (Washington, D.C.: Association of American Medical Colleges, 1994), p. 2.

71. Carol Lopate, *Women in Medicine* (Baltimore: Johns Hopkins Press, 1968), p. 30.

72. *Ibid.*, pp. 79, 94–95.

73. Florence deL. Lowther and Helen R. Downes, "Women in Medicine," *Journal of the American Medical Association* 129:512–514, 1945; Roscoe A. Dykman and John M. Stalnaker, "Survey of Women Physicians Graduating from Medical School 1925–1940," *Journal of Medical Education*, vol. 32, March 1957, Part 2, pp. 3–38.

74. Lopate, *Women in Medicine*, p. 182–185.

75. *Ibid.*, pp. 25–67, 105–144. An extensive literature exists on sexism in education. See, for instance, Susan Bereaud, Judith Stacy, and Joan Daniels, eds., *And Jill Came Tumbling After: Sexism in American Education* (New York: Dell, 1974); and Nancy Frazier and Myra Sadker, *Sexism in School and Society* (New York: Harper & Row, 1983).

76. Janet Bickel, Aarolyn Galbraith, and Renee Quinnie, *Women in U.S. Academic Medicine Statistics* (Washington, D.C.: Association of American Medical Colleges, 1994), *Table 1*.

77. Committee Report on Opportunities for Women in Medicine, with agenda items for meeting of 29 March 1979, Executive Council Meetings and Agendas, Association of American Medical Colleges; Report of the Committee on the Status of Women at Boston University School of Medicine, with meeting of 13 December 1972, General Faculty Minutes, Boston University School of Medicine.

78. Men (in lesser numbers) as well as women were subject to sexual harassment in medical school. However, as one recent study has shown, the harassers of men were typically nurses, while those of women were mainly attending physicians and house officers. This made sexual harassment a more serious professional problem for women than for men. (Miriam Komaromy, Andrew B. Birdman, Richard J. Haber, and Merle A. Sande, "Sexual Harassment in Medical Training," *New England Journal of Medicine* 328:322–326, 1993.)

79. Janet Bickel, "Scenarios for Success—Enhancing Women Physicians' Professional Advancement," *Western Journal of Medicine* 162:165–169, 1995 (quotations, p. 166); Janet Bickel, "Special Needs and Affinities of Women Medical Students," in Ellen Singer More and Maureen A. Milligan, eds., *The Empathetic Practitioner: Empathy, Gender, and Medicine* (New Brunswick, NJ: Rutgers University Press, 1994), pp. 237–249.

80. Lopate, *Women in Medicine*, pp. 119–144 (quotation, p. 129); Report of the Committee on Opportunities for Women in Medicine, with agenda items for meeting of 29 March 1979, Executive Council Meetings and Agendas, Association of American Medical Colleges; Janet Bickel, "Women in Medical Education: A Status Report," *New England Journal of Medicine* 319:1581–1582, 1988.

81. Bickel, "Scenarios for Success," p. 165. See also Bickel, "Women in Medical Education," pp. 1579–1584; and Phyllis L. Carr, Robert H. Friedman, Mark A. Moskowitz, and Lewis E. Kazis, "Comparing the Status of Women and Men in Academic Medicine," *Annals of Internal Medicine* 119:908–913, 1993.

82. Harriet Zuckerman, Jonathan Cole, and John Bruer, *The Outer Circle: Women in the Scientific Community* (New York: W. W. Norton and Company, 1991); Steven G. Brush, "Women in Science and Engineering," *American Scientist* 79:404–419, 1991.

83. Frances K. Conley, "Toward a More Perfect World—Eliminating Sexual Bias in Academic Medicine," *New England Journal of Medicine* 328:352, 1993.

84. Arlie Hochschild with Anne Machung, *The Second Shift* (New York: Avon Books, 1990).

85. Bonnie J. Tesch, Helen M. Wood, Amy L. Helwig, and Ann Butler Nattinger, "Promotion of Women Physicians in Academic Medicine: Glass Ceiling or Sticky Floor?," *Journal of the American Medical Association* 273:1022–1025, 1995.

86. Bickel, "Women Medical Students," pp. 245–247; AAMC, *Building a Stronger Women's Program: Enhancing the Educational and Professional Environment* (Washington, D.C.: Association of American Medical Colleges, 1993).

Chapter 14

1. George E. Mowry and Blaine A. Brownell, *The Urban Nation 1920–1980*, rev. ed. (New York: Hill and Wang, 1981), p. 166; David E. Rogers and Robert J. Blendon, "The Academic Medical Center: A Stressed American Institution," *New England Journal of Medicine* 298:942, 1978.

2. Rogers and Blendon, "The Academic Medical Center," p. 941.

3. Report of the Historical Base Committee for the Goals and Mission Statement of the Presbyterian Hospital in the City of New York, 17 February 1981, Folder "January 1981–June 1981," Records of the Long Range Planning Committee on Missions and Goals, College of Physicians and Surgeons of Columbia University, Office of the Dean, College of Physicians and Surgeons of Columbia University, New York, NY; meeting of 25 November 1970, Minutes of the Planning Committee of the Medical Board, The Presbyterian Hospital in the City of New York, President's Offices, Presbyterian Hospital, New York, NY; meeting of 23 February 1926, Minutes of Meetings of the Joint Administrative Board, Columbia-Presbyterian Medical Center, Special Collections, Augustus C. Long Health Sciences Center, Columbia University, New York, NY.

4. Meeting of 20 April 1987, Transactions of the Faculty Council, Faculty of Medicine, College of Physicians and Surgeons, Office of the Dean, College of Physicians and Surgeons of Columbia University, New York, NY.

5. Meeting of 20 April 1983, Minutes of the Medical Board, The Presbyterian Hospital in the City of New York, President's Offices, Presbyterian Hospital, New York, NY.

6. Meeting of 16 December 1972, Minutes, Advisory Board of the Medical Faculty, The Johns Hopkins University School of Medicine, The Alan Mason Chesney Medical Archives of The Johns Hopkins Medical Institutions, Baltimore, MD; P&S Admissions Questionnaire Preliminary Analysis, September 1978, with meeting of 12 October 1978, Minutes and Correspondence of the Executive Committee of the Faculty Council, College of Physicians and Surgeons, Office of the Dean, College of Physicians and Surgeons of Columbia University, New York, NY.

7. Meetings of 7 May 1968, 4 June 1968, 3 September 1968, and 4 March 1969, Minutes, The Johns Hopkins Hospital Board of Trustees, The Alan Mason Chesney Medical Archives of The Johns Hopkins Medical Institutions, Baltimore, MD.

8. Report of Medical Planning and Redevelopment Committee, Johns Hopkins Medical Institutions, 19 March 1970, with meeting of 2 June 1970, Minutes, The Johns Hopkins Hospital Board of Trustees.

9. Report of the Ad Hoc Committee to the Faculty Board, 21 June 1972, with Faculty Board Meeting of 28 June 1972, Executive Board Minutes, University of Maryland School of Medicine, Dean's Office, University of Maryland School of Medicine, Baltimore, MD.

10. As an example of one medical school's efforts to establish programs for the community, see the materials in Community Relations Records, College of Physicians and Surgeons of Columbia University, Office of the Dean, College of Physicians and Surgeons of Columbia University, New York, NY.

11. Attachment C-II, with meeting of 19 December 1972, Minutes of the Medical Board, The Presbyterian Hospital in the City of New York.

12. Meetings of 31 March 1970 and 28 April 1970, Minutes, The Johns Hopkins Hospital Medical Board, The Alan Mason Chesney Medical Archives of The Johns Hopkins Medical Institutions, Baltimore, MD.

13. David E. Rogers and Robert J. Blendon, "The Academic Medical Center Today," *Annals of Internal Medicine* 100:751, 1984.

14. "Presbyterian Hospital Is a Voluntary Hospital with the Role of a Municipal Hospital," Presentation Prepared for the Mayor of the City of New York, 27 January 1988, with meeting of 3 February 1988, Minutes and Correspondence of the Health Sciences Administrative Committee, College of Physicians and Surgeons of Columbia University, Office of the Dean, College of Physicians and Surgeons of Columbia University, New York, NY.

15. On the problems of municipal hospitals, see Harry F. Dowling, *City Hospitals: The Undercare of the Underprivileged* (Cambridge: Harvard University Press, 1982), pp. 173–189; and Rosemary Stevens, *In Sickness and in Wealth: American Hospitals in the Twentieth Century* (New York: Basic Books, 1989), pp. 310–316.

16. Meeting of 24 October 1989, Executive Faculty Minutes, Temple University School of Medicine, Dean's Office, Temple University School of Medicine, Philadelphia, PA.

17. Rogers and Blendon, "The Academic Medical Center," p. 942.

18. Meeting of 10 May 1989, Council of Departmental Chairmen Minutes, University of Arkansas College of Medicine, Dean's Office, University of Arkansas for Medical Sciences College of Medicine, Little Rock, AR.

19. Memorandum on Bad Debt and Free Care, 14 August 1981, with meeting of 11 September 1981, Medical Board Minutes, New England Medical Center Hospitals, Office of the President, New England Medical Center Hospitals, Boston, MA; Howard W. French, "As a Hospital Grows, Debt Threatens It," *New York Times*, 18 December 1989, p. B1.

20. Jack Hadley, Ross Mullner, and Judith Feder, "The Financially Distressed Hospital," *New England Journal of Medicine* 307:1287, 1982.

21. Meeting of 15 June 1972, Executive Faculty Minutes, University of Colorado School of Medicine, Office of the Chancellor, University of Colorado Health Sciences Center, Denver, CO.

22. David J. Rothman, *Strangers at the Bedside: A History of How Law and Bioethics Transformed Medical Decision Making* (New York: Basic Books, 1991), p. 146.

23. Meeting of 25 May 1971, Minutes, The Johns Hopkins Hospital Medical Board.

24. William B. Schwartz, Joseph P. Newhouse, Bruce W. Bennett, and Albert P. Williams, "The Changing Geographic Distribution of Board-Certified Physicians," *New England Journal of Medicine* 303:1032–1038, 1980.

25. Meeting of 16 May 1985, University of Colorado Health Sciences Center, University Hospital, Medical Board Minutes, Office of the President, University Hospital, Denver, CO.

26. Meeting of 9 November 1973, The University of Michigan Medical Center Board-in-Control, Folder "November 9, 1973," Box 20, University of Michigan Medical School Records, Michigan Historical Collections, Bentley Historical Library, University of Michigan, Ann Arbor, MI.

27. "Mission, Role and Scope of the College of Medicine," with agenda items for meeting of 14 September 1987, Council of Departmental Chairmen Minutes, University of Arkansas College of Medicine; meeting of 4 May 1982, The Johns Hopkins Board of Trustees Executive Session, with agenda items for meeting of 8 June 1982, Minutes, The Johns Hopkins Hospital Board of Trustees.

28. David A. Gee and Lisa A. Rosenfeld, "The Effect on Academic Health Centers of Tertiary Care in Community Hospitals," *Journal of Medical Education* 59:547–552, 1984.

29. Stevens, *In Sickness and in Wealth*, pp. 307–308; quotation, p. 308.

30. Meeting of 3 April 1986, Medical Board Minutes, New England Medical Center Hospitals.

31. Historically, the courts had upheld the independence of universities from government intervention in their internal educational affairs. A Supreme Court decision during the McCarthy era, for instance, declared that there were "four essential freedoms" of a university: "to determine for itself on academic grounds who may teach, what may be taught, how it shall be taught, and who may be admitted to study." (Quoted in Diane Ravitch, *The Troubled Crusade: American Education, 1945–1980* [New York: Basic Books, 1983], p. 303.)

32. Dean's Report to the President of Cornell University, 31 July 1967, Box 6, Office of the Dean, Cornell University Medical College, Annual Reports of the Departments and Offices, Archives, The New York Hospital–Cornell Medical Center, New York, NY.

33. Descriptions of the various congressional bills providing direct aid to medical schools for medical education is found in William G. Rothstein, *American Medical Schools and the Practice of Medicine: A History* (New York: Oxford University Press, 1987), pp. 283–287.

34. Winston K. Shorey, "Remarks at General Faculty and Hospital Staff Meeting," 14 October 1965, Folder "Miscellaneous: Annual Report," Dean's Office Files (Winston K. Shorey, 1961–1974) ID Number 20DB016, Special Collections Division, University of Arkansas for Health Sciences Library, Little Rock, AR.

35. Meeting of 25 October 1971, Transactions of the Faculty Council, Faculty of Medicine, College of Physicians and Surgeons.

36. Thomas D. Kinney to William G. Anlyan, 25 September 1969, Folder 283, Box 23, John H. Knowles Papers, Rockefeller Archive Center, North Tarrytown, NY; meeting of 1 February 1972, Executive Faculty, Folder "July–December 1972," Box 132, University of Michigan Medical School Records.

37. Final Report, Dean's Feasibility Committee on Enrollment Doubling, Hahnemann Medical College and Hospital, with meeting of 8 December 1970, Minutes of Meetings of the College Committee of the Board of Trustees, Hahnemann

Medical College and Hospital, Archives and Special Collections, Hahnemann Collection, MCP Hahnemann University, Philadelphia, PA.

38. Meetings of 16 November 1977 and 3 October 1979, Minutes, Executive Committee, University of Southern California School of Medicine, Dean's Office, University of Southern California School of Medicine, Los Angeles, CA.

39. "U.S. Citizens Studying Medicine Abroad," with agenda items for meeting of 18–19 September 1975, Executive Council Meetings and Agendas, Association of American Medical Colleges, Association of American Medical Colleges Archives, Washington, D.C.; Memorandum on Foreign Medical Schools, with agenda items for meeting of 10 September 1981, Minutes, Advisory Board of the Medical Faculty, The Johns Hopkins University School of Medicine.

40. *Figure 7* is taken from John A. D. Cooper, "Undergraduate Medical Education," in John Z. Bowers and Elizabeth F. Purcell, eds., *Advances in American Medicine: Essays at the Bicentennial* (New York: Josiah Macy, Jr. Foundation, 1976), 1:280. The rising number of applicants reflected the growing prestige of medicine as a career, the larger number of women seeking admission, and the eligibility of medical students for a draft deferment during the height of the Vietnam War.

41. AAMC Statement on Involvement of U.S. Faculty with Foreign Medical Schools, meeting of 23 March 1978, Executive Council Meetings and Agendas, Association of American Medical Colleges; "Policies on U.S. Citizens Studying Medicine Abroad Need Review and Reappraisal," with agenda items for meeting of 29 January 1981, Executive Council Meetings and Agendas, Association of American Medical Colleges; "Warning About Present and Future Proliferation of Spurious Foreign (and Domestic) Medical Schools," Folder "COTRANS," Box 6, Office of the Dean, Thomas H. Meikle Papers (Personal), Archives, The New York Hospital–Cornell Medical Center, New York, NY; John Walsh, "U.S. Foreign Medical Students: After the 'Guadalajara Clause'," *Science* 197:346–348, 1977; Bart Barnes, "Med Schools Balk at Law to Admit Transfer Students," *Washington Post*, 17 August 1977.

42. "American Foreign Medical Graduates," with agenda items for meeting of 17 December 1971, Executive Council Meetings and Agendas, Association of American Medical Colleges.

43. Cooper, "Undergraduate Medical Education," p. 281; Walsh, "U.S. Foreign Medical Students," pp. 346–348.

44. Patricia Bell Williams, "Admission of U.S. Students Trained in Foreign Medical Schools," letter to the editor, *New England Journal of Medicine* 296:765, 1977.

45. Walsh, "U.S. Foreign Medical Students," p. 347. Sixty-two percent of COTRANS examinees in 1975 had applied for admission to medical school in the United States two years before. Their mean undergraduate GPA was 2.79 and MCAT science score 531, compared with a mean GPA of 3.38 and MCAT science score of 592 among successful applicants.

46. W. F. Dubé, "COTRANS and the U.S. Citizen Studying Medicine Abroad," *Journal of Medical Education* 49:395, 1974.

47. John A. Meskauskas, John A. Benson, and Elizabeth Hopkins, "Performance of Graduates of Foreign Medical Schools on the Examinations of the American Board of Internal Medicine," *New England Journal of Medicine* 297:808–810, 1977; and Arnold S. Relman, "USFMG's and Their Board Scores," *New England Journal of Medicine* 297:836–837, 1977.

48. Quoted in Gene I. Maeroff, "Colleges in Conflict over Federal Role," *New York Times*, 6 September 1977.

49. *Ibid.*

50. Donald S. Fredrickson, "Health and the Search for New Knowledge," in John H. Knowles, ed., *Doing Better and Feeling Worse: Health in the United States* (New York: W. W. Norton & Company, 1977), p. 163. See also Robert H. Ebert, "Biomedical Research Policy—A Re-evaluation," *New England Journal of Medicine* 289:348–351, 1973; and Richard A. Rettig, *Cancer Crusade: The Story of the National Cancer Act of 1971* (Princeton, NJ: Princeton University Press, 1977).

51. Ravitch, *The Troubled Crusade*, pp. 312–320; Maeroff, "Colleges in Conflict over Federal Role."

52. Rothman, *Strangers at the Bedside*, pp. 70–100.

53. Constance Holden, "Billion Dollar Price Tag for New Animal Rules," *Science* 242:662–663, 1988.

54. Alexander G. Bearn, "The Washington Paper Chase," *American Journal of Medicine* 65:894–895, 1978; H. S. Gutowsky, "Federal Funding of Basic Research: The Red Tape Mill," *Science* 212:636–641, 1981.

55. The American Hospital Association estimated in 1979 that the Department of Health, Education, and Welfare promulgated 650 to 700 new or revised regulations affecting hospitals each year. ("Sick Hospitals," *Wall Street Journal*, 3 April 1979.)

56. Leighton E. Cluff, "Responsibility, Accountability, Self-discipline: Changing Emphases in Medical Education," *The Pharos*, Winter 1981, p. 5. In the late 1990s, "physician of record" requirements at teaching hospitals grew much more stringent. Before, attending physicians could countersign the notes of house officers. Now, attending physicians had to write their own daily notes if Medicare billing was to be allowed.

57. Thomas Q. Morris, "A Hospital Administrator's Perspective on Regulation," *Bulletin of the New York Academy of Medicine* 66:59–63, 1990.

58. Quoted in Richard A. Knox, "Stanford Medical School Suffers Fiscal Ideological Crises," *Science* 203:152, 1979.

59. Renée C. Fox, "The Medicalization and Demedicalization of American Society," in Knowles, ed., *Doing Better and Feeling Worse*, pp. 9–22.

60. Aaron Wildavsky, "Doing Better and Feeling Worse: The Political Pathology of Health Policy," in Knowles, ed., *Doing Better and Feeling Worse*, pp. 105–123; quotations, p. 105.

61. This theme pervades the essays in Knowles, ed., *Doing Better and Feeling Worse*.

62. Rothman, *Strangers at the Bedside*; Paul Starr, *The Social Transformation of American Medicine: The Rise of a Sovereign Profession and the Making of a Vast Industry* (New York: Basic Books, 1982), pp. 379–419.

63. John H. Knowles, "The Responsibility of the Individual," in Knowles, ed., *Doing Better and Feeling Worse*, pp. 61–63.

64. Lester C. Thurow, *The Zero-Sum Society: Distribution and the Possibilities for Economic Change* (New York: Basic Books, 1980).

65. Peter N. Carroll, *It Seemed Like Nothing Happened: America in the 1970s* (New Brunswick, NJ: Rutgers University Press, 1990); William H. Chafe, *The Unfinished Journey: America Since World War II*, 2nd ed. (New York: Oxford University Press, 1991), pp. 430–469.

66. *Summary Report of the Graduate Medical Education National Advisory Committee* (Washington, D.C.: U.S. Department of Health and Human Services, 1980).

67. Eli Ginzberg and Anna B. Dutka, *The Financing of Biomedical Research* (Baltimore: Johns Hopkins University Press, 1989); Harold Varmus, "Shattuck Lec-

ture—Biomedical Research Enters the Steady State," *New England Journal of Medicine* 333:811–815, 1995. A similar pattern occurred in the federal funding of other sciences. See Bruce L. R. Smith, *American Science Policy Since World War II* (Washington, D.C.: The Brookings Institution, 1990).

68. Robert J. Glaser, "The Medical Deanship: Its Half-Life and Hard Times," *Journal of Medical Education* 44:1123, 1969.

69. *Table 10* is taken from John K. Iglehart, "Rapid Changes for Academic Medical Centers (First of Two Parts)," *New England Journal of Medicine* 331:1394, 1994.

70. John K. Iglehart, "The American Health Care System: Introduction," *New England Journal of Medicine* 326:965, 1992.

71. Fredrickson, "Health and the Search for Knowledge," p. 167.

72. H. George Mandel, "Funding of NIH Grant Applications: Update," letter to the editor, *Science* 269:13–14, 1995. These statistics, representing overall averages, did not reflect the marked heterogeneity in research strength among medical schools. For instance, at the 13 prestigious schools that constituted the country's "research consortium," the success rate at this time among investigators applying for their first NIH grant was 40 to 50 percent, with another 20 percent being successful on resubmission. At many schools, the success rate fell below the national averages. (Remarks of Dean William A. Peck to the faculty and administration of the Washington University School of Medicine, 29 September 1995.)

73. Jerome P. Kassirer, "My Years at the *Journal*—So Far," *New England Journal of Medicine* 333:654–655, 1995; quotation, p. 655.

74. Thomas P. Stossel and Sage C. Stossel, "Declining American Representation in Leading Clinical-Research Journals," *New England Journal of Medicine* 322:739–742, 1990.

75. David E. Rogers and Robert J. Blendon, "The Changing American Health Scene: Sometimes Things Get Better," *Journal of the American Medical Association* 237:1710–1714, 1977; quotation, p. 1710.

76. Robert J. Blendon and David E. Rogers, "Cutting Medical Care Costs: *Primum Non Nocere*," *Journal of the American Medical Association* 250:1880–1885, 1983; quotation, p. 1880.

77. See the classic essay by Lewis Thomas, "The Technology of Medicine," in Lewis Thomas, *The Lives of a Cell: Notes of a Biology Watcher* (New York: The Viking Press, 1974), pp. 35–42.

78. Daniel M. Fox, *Power and Illness: The Failure and Future of American Health Policy* (Berkeley: University of California Press, 1993).

Chapter 15

1. A helpful description of some of the main scientific currents is David Weatherall, *Science and the Quiet Art: The Role of Medical Research in Health Care* (New York: W. W. Norton, 1995), esp. pp. 227–304. An analytic historical account of the molecular revolution in medicine remains to be written.

2. Elaine I. Tuomanen, Robert Austrian, and H. Robert Masure, "Pathogenesis of Pneumococcal Pneumonia," *New England Journal of Medicine* 332:1280–1284, 1995.

3. A. G. Motulsky, "The 1985 Nobel Prize in Physiology or Medicine," *Science* 231:126–129, 1986.

4. See, for instance, meeting of 4 October 1984, Transactions of the Medical

Board of the New York Hospital, Archives, The New York Hospital–Cornell Medical Center, New York, NY.

5. Lloyd H. Smith, "Presidential Address," *Transactions of the Association of American Physicians* 89:1–9, 1976; C. Seth Landefeld, "The Spring Meetings—Are They Dying?," *New England Journal of Medicine* 328:1645–1647, 1993. See also Gordon N. Gill, "The End of the Physician-Scientist," *American Scholar* 53:353–368, 1984.

6. Meeting of 27 September 1978, Minutes, Faculty Executive Committee, University of Southern California School of Medicine, Dean's Office, University of Southern California School of Medicine, Los Angeles, CA.

7. Executive Committee Meeting, 3 December 1986, Executive Board Minutes, University of Maryland School of Medicine, Dean's Office, University of Maryland School of Medicine, Baltimore, MD.

8. John C. Rose, "Who Will Teach the Basic Medical Sciences?," *Science* 185:1022–1027, 1974.

9. Table C2, *AAMC Data Book*, Update November 1991, Association of American Medical Colleges Archives, Washington, D.C.

The growing presence of Ph.D.s in clinical departments created challenges as well as opportunities. How and where would Ph.D.s acquire enough pathophysiological and clinical background to inform their work in clinical investigation? Would Ph.D.s work for or with M.D.s? These and other issues are discussed in Samuel S. Herman and Allen M. Singer, "Basic Scientists in Clinical Departments of Medical Schools," *Clinical Research* 34:149–158, 1986; Alfred P. Fishman and Paul Jolly, "Ph.D.s in Clinical Departments," *Physiologist* 24:17–21, 1981; C. N. Gills, "The Role of the Basic Scientist in an Academic Clinical Setting," *Federation Proceedings* 38:2355–2358, 1979; and Irwin M. Arias, "Training Basic Scientists to Bridge the Gap Between Basic Science and Its Application to Human Disease," *New England Journal of Medicine* 321:972–974, 1989.

10. John W. Littlefield, "On the Difficulty of Combining Basic Research and Patient Care," *American Journal of Human Genetics* 36:731–735, 1984.

11. Meeting of 9 April 1987, Graduate Medical Education Committee Minutes, The George Washington University Hospital, Office of the Medical Director, The George Washington University Hospital, Washington, D.C.

12. Meeting of 7 March 1989, Executive Council Minutes, Jefferson Medical College, Dean's Office, Jefferson Medical College of Thomas Jefferson University, Philadelphia, PA.

13. Melvin Konner, *Becoming a Doctor: A Journey of Initiation in Medical School* (New York: Viking, 1987); and Lewis Thomas, "What Doctors Don't Know," review of Melvin Konner's *Becoming a Doctor*, *New York Review of Books*, 24 September 1987, pp. 6–11.

14. Meeting of 12 April 1989, Executive Faculty Minutes, Temple University School of Medicine, Dean's Office, Temple University School of Medicine, Philadelphia, PA.

15. Abraham Flexner, *Medical Education in the United States and Canada* (New York: Carnegie Foundation for the Advancement of Teaching, 1910), p. 57.

16. Meeting of 5 April 1978, Minutes, Faculty Executive Committee, University of Southern California School of Medicine.

17. See, for instance, Charles P. Friedman and Elizabeth F. Purcell, eds., *The New Biology and Medical Education: Merging the Biological, Information, and Cognitive Sciences* (New York: Josiah Macy, Jr. Foundation, 1983); and Robert Q. Marston and Roseann M. Jones, eds., *Medical Education in Transition. Commission on Medical*

Education: The Sciences of Medical Practice (Princeton, NJ: The Robert Wood Johnson Foundation, 1992).

18. Allen Singer, "The Effect of the Vietnam War on Numbers of Medical School Applicants," *Academic Medicine* 64:567–573, 1989; Donald G. Kassebaum and Philip L. Szenas, "The Decline and Rise of the Medical School Applicant Pool," *Academic Medicine* 70:334–340, 1995. *Figure 8*, courtesy of the Association of American Medical Colleges.

19. Data, courtesy of the Association of American Medical Colleges.

20. Donald G. Kassebaum and Philip L. Szenas, "Relationship between Indebtedness and the Specialty Choices of Graduating Medical Students," *Academic Medicine* 67:699–707, 1992. *Figure 9* is taken from p. 701 of this article.

21. See, for instance, *ibid.*; Gloria J. Bazzoli, "Medical Education Indebtedness: Does It Affect Physician Specialty Choice?," *Health Affairs* 4:98–104, 1985; Gloria J. Bazzoli, "Does Educational Indebtedness Affect Specialty Choice?," *Journal of Health Economics* 4:1–19, 1985; and Thomas H. Dial and Paul R. Elliott, "Relationship of Scholarships and Indebtedness to Medical Students' Career Plans," *Journal of Medical Education* 62:316–324, 1987.

22. 1989 Matriculating Student Questionnaire, Folder 37, Box 2, Students/Miscellaneous Records, Association of American Medical Colleges Archives, Washington, D.C.

23. Meeting of 14 December 1983, Executive Faculty Minutes, Temple University School of Medicine.

24. Kenneth C. Green, "A Profile of Undergraduates in the Sciences," *American Scientist* 77:475–480, 1989.

25. Renée C. Fox, *The Sociology of Medicine: A Participant Observer's View* (Englewood Cliffs, NJ: Prentice-Hall, 1989), pp. 89–103.

26. Renée C. Fox, "Is There a 'New' Medical Student?: A Comparative View of Medical Socialization in the 1950s and 1970s," in Renée C. Fox, *Essays in Medical Sociology: Journeys into the Field* (New York: John Wiley, 1979), pp. 78–101.

27. Meeting of 29 July 1969, Minutes of the Executive Committee of the Faculty, Hahnemann Medical College, Archives and Special Collections, Hahnemann Collection, MCP Hahnemann University, Philadelphia, PA.

28. Frederick Sierles, Ingrid Hendrickx, and Sybil Circle, "Cheating in Medical School," *Journal of Medical Education* 55:124–125, 1980. See also Barry Stimmel and David Yens, "Cheating by Medical Students on Examinations," *American Journal of Medicine* 73:160–164, 1982.

29. Richard D. Lyons, "Cheating on Exams for Doctors Causes Alarm," *New York Times*, 3 April 1984. See also L. Thompson Bowles, "The Illegal Use of NBME Examination Materials," *Academic Medicine* 69:35, 1994.

30. William C. McGaghie, "Perspectives on Medical School Admission," *Academic Medicine* 65:136–139, 1990; Karen J. Mitchell, "Traditional Predictors of Performance in Medical School," *Academic Medicine* 65:149–158, 1990; and James W. Bartlett, "Medical School and Career Performances of Medical Students with Low Medical College Admission Test Scores," *Journal of Medical Education* 42:231–237, 1967.

31. Bruce B. Dan, "MCAT: Desperately Seeking Med School," *Journal of the American Medical Association* 259:407, 1988. For a sense of the controversies surrounding the MCAT, see Folders 5 and 6, Box 38, Walsh McDermott Papers, Archives, The New York Hospital–Cornell Medical Center, New York, NY; Interim Report on the MCAT Essay Pilot Project, with agenda items for meeting of 9–10 September 1987, Executive Council Meetings and Agendas, Association of

American Medical Colleges, Association of American Medical Colleges Archives, Washington, D.C.; Lawrence Biemiller, "Johns Hopkins Medical School Abandons Test," *Chronicle of Higher Education*, 22 May 1985; and the three articles on the MCAT in the 9 February 1984 issue of the *New England Journal of Medicine*. A few schools, most notably Johns Hopkins, abandoned the MCAT as an entrance requirement.

32. Meeting of 9 January 1973, Executive Faculty, Folder "January–February 1973," Box 132, University of Michigan Medical School Records, Michigan Historical Collections, Bentley Historical Library, University of Michigan, Ann Arbor, MI.

33. Meeting of 11 September 1986, Faculty Meeting Minutes, Howard University College of Medicine, Office of the Dean, Howard University College of Medicine, Washington, D.C. For more on this point, see William E. Sedlacek and Dario O. Prieto, "Predicting Minority Students' Success in Medical School," *Academic Medicine* 60:161–166, 1990.

34. Hans Popper to Mrs. Paul Ritchfield, 26 August 1968, Folder "Admissions Committee," Box 1, Hans Popper Files, Early Series, Archives, The Mount Sinai Medical Center, New York, NY.

35. The most notorious admissions scandal occurred in the early 1970s when, according to newspaper reports, a few schools would admit students in exchange for large financial contributions from the families of the candidates. The school most often mentioned in this connection was Chicago Medical College. In 1973, families and friends of 77 of the 91 entering students allegedly pledged an average of $50,000 per student to the institution. (The school's regular tuition that year was about $4,000.) From 1970 to 1974, parents of 270 of the 349 students who matriculated to the school reportedly made almost $11 million in contributions. The school maintained that all matriculants were qualified and that financial considerations were used only as tiebreakers. However, the school changed its admission practices after the story broke. (Jack Anderson, "The Medical School Payola System," *Washington Post*, 6 July 1978; newspaper clipping, "Expert Tells How Many 'Buy' Into Med School," in Box 1, Series II, Office of the Dean, Thomas H. Meikle Papers [Official], Archives, The New York Hospital–Cornell Medical Center, New York, NY; meeting of 22 June 1978, Executive Council Meetings and Agendas, Association of American Medical Colleges.)

36. Meeting of 30 November 1977, Minutes, Faculty Executive Committee, University of Southern California School of Medicine.

37. See, for instance, 1979–1980 Annual Report to the Dean, Office of Admissions, Folder "Dean's Report 1979–80," Box 10, Office of the Dean, Cornell University Medical College, Annual Reports of the Departments and Offices, Archives, The New York Hospital–Cornell Medical Center, New York, NY.

38. Executive Committee Meeting of 9 April 1986, Executive Board Minutes, University of Maryland School of Medicine. As another sign that schools were always competing for students, some schools in the late 1980s temporarily rolled back their tuition, hoping to attract the better students from a declining applicant pool.

39. Meeting of 13 June 1977, Minutes and Correspondence of the Faculty Council, College of Physicians and Surgeons, Office of the Dean, College of Physicians and Surgeons of Columbia University, New York, NY.

40. Henry K. Silver and Anita Duhl Glicken, "Medical Student Abuse: Incidence, Severity, and Significance," *Journal of the American Medical Association*

263:527–532, 1990 (quotations, p. 527). See also K. Harnett Sheehan, David V. Sheehan, Kim White, Alan Leibowitz, and DeWitt C. Baldwin, "A Pilot Study of Medical Student 'Abuse': Student Perceptions of Mistreatment and Misconduct in Medical School," *Journal of the American Medical Association* 263:533–537, 1990; and Jerald Kay, "Traumatic Deidealization and the Future of Medicine," *Journal of the American Medical Association* 263:572–573, 1990.

41. Janet Bickel, "Special Needs and Affinities of Women Medical Students," in Ellen Singer More and Maureen A. Milligan, eds., *The Empathetic Practitioner: Empathy, Gender, and Medicine* (New Brunswick, NJ: Rutgers University Press, 1994), p. 244.

42. Report of the AAMC Officers' Retreat, with agenda items for meeting of 23 June 1985, and Final Report of the Ad Hoc Committee on Graduate Medical Education and the Transition from Medical School to Residency, with agenda items for meeting of 21–22 January 1987, Executive Council Meetings and Agendas, Association of American Medical Colleges; AAMC, The Experiences of Medical Students in Obtaining a Residency, with meeting of 14 November 1986, Minutes, Executive Staff Meetings, Georgetown University Hospital, Office of the Medical Director, Georgetown University Hospital, Washington, D.C.; and August G. Swanson, "The 'Preresidency Syndrome': An Incipient Epidemic of Educational Disruption, " *Journal of Medical Education* 60:201–202, 1985.

43. James M. Richards Jr., Calvin W. Taylor, and Philip B. Price, "The Prediction of Medical Intern Performance," *Journal of Applied Psychology* 46:142–146, 1962; and Richard B. Friedman, "Fantasy Land," *New England Journal of Medicine* 308:651–653, 1983.

44. Barbara Barzansky, "The Growth and Divergence of the Basic Sciences," in Barbara Barzansky and Norman Gevitz, eds., *Beyond Flexner: Medical Education in the Twentieth Century* (New York: Greenwood Press, 1992), pp. 19–34.

45. Patricia L. Kendall and George G. Reader, "Innovations in Medical Education of the 1950s Contrasted with Those of the 1970s and 1980s," *Journal of Health and Social Behavior* 29:279–293, 1988; George T. Harrell, "Experiments in Medical Education," *Pennsylvania Medicine* 89:44–46, 48–49, June 1986; Arthur Kaufman, ed., *Implementing Problem-Based Medical Education: Lessons from Successful Innovations* (New York: Springer Publishing Company, 1985); Daniel C. Tosteson, "New Pathways in General Medical Education," *New England Journal of Medicine* 322:234–238, 1990; and Daniel C. Tosteson, S. James Adelstein, and Susan T. Carver, eds., *New Pathways to Medical Education: Learning to Learn at Harvard Medical School* (Cambridge: Harvard University Press, 1994).

46. Tosteson, "New Pathways in General Medical Education," p. 238.

47. C. P. M. van der Vleuten and David B. Swanson, "Assessment of Clinical Skills with Standardized Patients: State of the Art," *Teaching and Learning in Medicine* 2:58–76, 1990; see also the June 1993 issue of *Academic Medicine*, which contains the proceedings of the AAMC's Consensus Conference on the Use of Standardized Patients in the Teaching and Evaluation of Clinical Skills.

48. Mark A. Albanese and Susan Mitchell, "Problem-Based Learning: A Review of Literature on Its Outcomes and Implementation Issues," *Academic Medicine* 63:52–81, 1993; Robert S. Donner and Harmon Bickley, "Problem-Based Learning in American Medical Education: An Overview," *Bulletin of the Medical Library Association* 81:294–298, 1993.

49. By the 1990s, new computer technologies had proven useful as a way to help students and physicians manage information more effectively, though the

roles for computer-aided instruction were still unclear. See R. Bryan Haynes, Michael Ramsden, K. Ann McKibbon, Cynthia J. Walker, and Nancy C. Ryan, "A Review of Medical Education and Medical Informatics," *Academic Medicine* 64:207–212, 1989.

50. Arthur Kleinman, Leon Eisenberg, and Byron Good, "Culture, Illness, and Care: Clinical Lessons from Anthropologic and Cross-Cultural Research," *Annals of Internal Medicine* 88:251–258, 1978; Eric J. Cassell, "The Nature of Suffering and the Goals of Medicine," *New England Journal of Medicine* 306:639–645, 1982.

51. Dennis H. Novack, Douglas A. Drossman, and Mack Lipkin Jr., "Medical Interviewing and Interpersonal Skills Teaching in US Medical Schools," *Journal of the American Medical Association* 269:2101–2105, 1993; Arnold M. Epstein, William C. Taylor, and George R. Seage III, "Effect of Patients' Socioeconomic Status and Physicians' Training and Practice on Patient-Doctor Communication," *American Journal of Medicine* 78:101–106, 1985.

52. Meeting of 10 November 1989, Scientific and Academic Affairs Committee Minutes, Board of Trustees, Thomas Jefferson University; James Erdmann, "Academic Backgrounds of Those Aspiring to and Accepted into U.S. Medical Schools," *Interdisciplinaria* 2:95–116, 1980.

53. Renée C. Fox, "Training in Caring Competence: The Perennial Problem in North American Medical Education," in Hugh C. Hendrie and Camille Lloyd, eds., *Educating Competent and Humane Physicians* (Bloomington, IN: Indiana University Press, 1990), pp. 199–216, quotation, p. 204.

54. Peter Conrad, "Learning To Doctor: Reflections on Recent Accounts of the Medical School Years," *Journal of Health and Social Behavior* 29:323, 1988.

55. Walsh McDermott to Alexander G. Bearn, 24 January 1979, Folder 8, Box 22, McDermott Papers.

56. Walsh McDermott to Stanley Berger, 15 March 1979, Folder 5, Box 3, McDermott Papers.

57. On McDermott, see Paul B. Beeson, "Walsh McDermott," *Biographical Memoirs of the National Academy of Sciences* 59:283–307, 1990.

58. Arthur Kaufman, "Reflections," in Kaufman, ed., *Implementing Problem-Based Medical Education*, p. 262.

59. David Tyack and Larry Cuban, *Tinkering Toward Utopia: A Century of Public School Reform* (Cambridge: Harvard University Press, 1995).

60. For a sense of the controversy, see Henry M. Seidel, "The Role of National Board Examinations in Medical Education," *The Pharos* 55:12–14, 1992; Robert A. Chase, "Medical Education and the National Boards," *The Pharos* 55:43, 1992; Elizabeth Barrett-Connor, "Whither National Boards?," *New England Journal of Medicine* 303:61–62, 1980; and William D. Holden and Edithe J. Levit, "Medical Education, Licensure, and the National Board of Medical Examiners," *New England Journal of Medicine* 303:1357–1360, 1980.

Traditionally, there were two examinations utilized in the licensing process: the examinations of the National Board of Medical Examiners, and the Federation Licensing Examination (FLEX) of the Federation of State Medical Boards. Most U.S. medical graduates took the National Board examination, but all foreign medical graduates seeking licensure in the United States and about one-quarter of U.S. graduates took the FLEX. In the 1990s, after years of discussion, a single examination program, the United States Medical Licensing Examination (USMLE), replaced the two earlier examinations. The changeover to the USMLE, which was administered by the National Board of Medical Examiners, was initiated in 1992 and completed in 1994.

61. Bennett Lorber, "Changing Patterns of Infectious Diseases," *American Journal of Medicine* 84:569–578, 1988; Alfred Jay Bollet, "The Rise and Fall of Disease," *American Journal of Medicine* 70:12–16, 1981; Paul B. Beeson, "Some Diseases That Have Disappeared," *American Journal of Medicine* 68:806–811, 1980.

62. Nicholas A. Christakis, "The Similarity and Frequency of Proposals to Reform U.S. Medical Education: Constant Concerns," *Journal of the American Medical Association* 274:706–711, 1995. See also Cam Enarson and Frederic D. Burg, "An Overview of Reform Initiatives in Medical Education: 1906 Through 1992," *Journal of the American Medical Association* 268:1141–1143, 1992.

63. Thomas Allen Bruce, "State of the College June 5, 1985," with agenda items for meeting of 6 June 1985, Faculty Meetings, University of Arkansas College of Medicine, Dean's Office, University of Arkansas for Health Sciences College of Medicine, Little Rock, AR.

64. Samuel W. Bloom, "Structure and Ideology in Medical Education: An Analysis of Resistance to Change," *Journal of Health and Social Behavior* 29:294, 1988.

65. Barzansky, "The Growth and Divergence of the Basic Sciences," pp. 30–32.

66. Dorthea Juul, "Medical Student Culture: Note-Taking Cooperatives in Basic Science Curricula," *Teaching and Learning in Medicine* 4:206–209, 1992. It should not be concluded that lectures were unimportant. Rather, the challenge was to achieve the proper balance among lectures, laboratories, and small group instruction.

67. Hilliard Jason and Jane Westberg, *Teachers and Teaching in U.S. Medical Schools* (Norwalk, CT: Appleton-Century-Crofts, 1982), pp. 56–59. These hours included the time of preparation and evaluation.

68. Meeting of 28 May 1987, Executive Committee Minutes, University of Michigan School of Medicine.

69. School of Medicine Council Meeting, 21 October 1987, Executive Board Minutes, University of Maryland School of Medicine.

70. Mark L. Batshaw, Leslie P. Plotnick, Brent G. Petty, Patricia K. Woolf, and E. David Mellits, "Academic Promotion at a Medical School: Experience at Johns Hopkins University School of Medicine," *New England Journal of Medicine* 318:741–747, 1988; Janet Bickel, "The Changing Faces of Promotion and Tenure at U.S. Medical Schools," *Academic Medicine* 66:249–256, 1991.

71. Meeting of 31 December 1985, Executive Committee, Folder "Ex Com Dec 1975," Box 13, University of Michigan Medical School Records.

72. Ernest L. Boyer, *Scholarship Considered: Priorities of the Professoriate* (Princeton, NJ: Carnegie Foundation for the Advancement of Teaching, 1990).

73. Professorial Faculty Meeting, 20 January 1983, with meeting of 7 February 1983, Corporate Board of Trustees Minutes, Thomas Jefferson University, Thomas Jefferson University Archives and Special Collections, Thomas Jefferson University, Philadelphia, PA.

74. David P. Hamilton, "Publishing by—and for?—the Numbers," *Science* 250:1331–1332, 1990. In addition, only a small proportion of journals had a significant "impact factor," as 90 percent of the citations were to 10 percent of the journals. (*Ibid.*, p. 1331.) See also Gordon N. Gill, "Publishing the New Biology," *American Scholar*, Autumn 1991, pp. 584–588.

75. Meeting of 14 October 1981, Minutes, Faculty Executive Committee, University of Southern California School of Medicine.

76. AAMC Mission Statement and Goals, with agenda items for meeting of 22–23 June 1988, Executive Council Meetings and Agendas, Association of American Medical Colleges.

77. Meeting of 6 May 1986, Executive Council Minutes, Jefferson Medical College.

78. *Fullfilling the Mission: Medical Schools and the Education of Medical Students.* The Acadia Institute and Medical College of Pennsylvania Project on Undergraduate Medical Education (Philadelphia: Medical College of Pennsylvania and Hahnemann University, 1996), p. 22.

79. For the early vision of the school, see State University of New York at Stony Brook Health Sciences Center, School of Medicine Preliminary Accreditation, 29 March 1971; and Report of the Subcommittee to Study the Progress in Attaining the Goals of the School of Medicine, 29 March 1971, pp. 1–2, Medical Education Data Base, State University of New York at Stony Brook, 12–15 December 1977; both Office of the Vice President, Health Sciences Center, State University of New York at Stony Brook. On the subsequent transmutation, see Report of the Survey of the State University of New York–Stony Brook School of Medicine, 12–15 December 1977, pp. 8–10, 60–68, and 156–157; and "Objectives," p. 8, Medical Education Data Base, State University of New York at Stony Brook School of Medicine, 23–25 October 1979; both Office of the Vice President, Health Sciences Center, State University of New York at Stony Brook.

80. Bloom, "Structure and Ideology"; and Samuel W. Bloom, "Medical Education in Transition: Paradigm Change and Organizational Stasis," in Marston and Jones, eds., *Medical Education in Transition*, pp. 15–25.

81. Abraham Flexner, *Medical Education: A Comparative Study* (New York: The Macmillan Company, 1925), p. 148.

82. Council on Long Range Planning and Development, American College of Obstetricians and Gynecologists, "The Future of Obstetrics and Gynecology," *Journal of the American Medical Association* 258:3547–3553, 1987.

83. "Black Tuesday" spawned many articles on the plight of internal medicine. A helpful review of this literature is Claire H. Kohrman, Ronald M. Anderson, and Mary Margaret Clements, *Training Physicians: The Case of Internal Medicine* (San Francisco: Jossey-Bass, 1994).

84. AAMC data, courtesy of August G. Swanson.

85. Andre J. Ognibene, "Graduate Medical Education: Projections for the Future," *The Pharos*, Winter 1990, p. 28. As always, the development of new specialties was characterized by political as much as by professional issues. See, for instance, Mark A. Kelley, "Critical Care Medicine—A New Specialty?," *New England Journal of Medicine* 318:1613–1617, 1988.

86. See, for instance, Sheldon Greenfield, Eugene C. Nelson, Michael Zubkoff *et al.*, "Variations in Resource Utilization Among Medical Specialties and Systems of Care: Results from the Medical Outcomes Study," *Journal of the American Medical Association* 267:1624–1630, 1992.

87. Summary of Responses from Administrative Board Members on CCME Report, with agenda items for meeting of 31 March–1 April 1977, Executive Council Meetings and Agendas, Association of American Medical Colleges.

88. Joseph V. Scaletti, "Telecommunications and Rural Health Communities," *Annals of Internal Medicine* 122:379, 1995; Stanley J. Reiser, "The Coming Resurgence of the Generalist in Medicine: Its Technological and Conceptual Basis," *The Pharos*, Winter 1995, pp. 8–11; Jim Grigsby and Jay H. Sanders, "Telemedicine: What It Is and Where It's Going," *Annals of Internal Medicine* 129:123–127, 1998.

89. John Z. Ayanian, Paul J. Hauptman, Edward Guadagnoli, Elliott M.

Antman, Chris L. Pashos, and Barbara J. McNeil, "Knowledge and Practices of Generalist and Specialist Physicians Regarding Drug Therapy for Acute Myocardial Infarction," *New England Journal of Medicine* 331:1136–1142, 1994.

90. See, for instance, Richard J. Reitemeier, John A. Spittell Jr., Richard E. Weeks, Guy W. Daugherty, Fred T. Nobrega, and Robert W. Fleming, "Participation by Internists in Primary Care," *Archives of Internal Medicine* 135:255–257, 1975.

91. Linda H. Aiken, Charles E. Lewis, John Craig, Robert C. Mendenhall, Robert J. Blendon, and David E. Rogers, "The Contribution of Specialists to the Delivery of Primary Care: A New Perspective," *New England Journal of Medicine* 300:1363–1370, 1979.

92. David E. Rogers and Linda H. Aiken, "Yes, but What Do Internists *Really* Do?," *Annals of Internal Medicine* 90:977, 1979.

93. The term "foreign medical graduate" applied to foreign nationals who had graduated from foreign medical schools, in distinction to U.S. citizens who had graduated from foreign medical schools, who were labeled "USFMGs." From 1970 through the 1990s, FMGs continued to account for roughly 30 percent of the interns and residents in U.S. hospitals. In the 1990s the term "international medical graduate" (IMG) began replacing the term "foreign medical graduate."

94. David Babbott, DeWitt C. Baldwin Jr., Paul Jolly, and Donna J. Williams, "The Stability of Early Specialty Preferences Among U.S. Medical School Graduates in 1983," *Journal of the American Medical Association* 259:1970–1975, 1988.

95. Mark L. Savickas, Dale E. Alexander, A. Patrick Jonas, and Fredric M. Wolf, "Difficulties Expressed by Medical Students in Choosing a Specialty," *Journal of Medical Education* 61:467–469, 1986.

96. August G. Swanson, "Presentation on Medical Students' Specialty Choices to the New York State Council on Graduate Medical Education," 22 June 1990, courtesy of author.

97. Wayne K. Davis, Peter A. J. Bouhuijs, W. Dale Dauphinee et al., "Medical Career Choice: Current Status of Research Literature," *Teaching and Learning in Medicine* 2:134, 1990.

98. *Ibid.*, pp. 133–134.

99. *Ibid.*, pp. 135.

100. Michael E. Whitcomb and J. P. Desgroseilliers, "Primary Care Medicine in Canada," *New England Journal of Medicine* 326:1471, 1992.

101. Robert G. Petersdorf, "Primary Care Applicants—They Get No Respect," *New England Journal of Medicine* 326: 408–409, 1992.

102. Income differentials among specialists were also pronounced since reimbursement formulas paid much more to physicians who performed technical procedures than to those who spent time talking with patients or thinking about their problems. Thus, an infectious disease specialist whose choice of antibiotics allowed an infected leg to be saved would be paid modestly, while a surgeon performing an amputation would receive a large fee.

103. The Structure of Graduate Medical Education and Its Financing, with agenda items for meeting of 10 April 1986, Executive Council Meetings and Agendas, Association of American Medical Colleges.

104. Christine Wiebe, "An Overview of Residents' Stipends," *ACP Observer*, September 1989, p. 14.

105. David M. Kipnis, "Clinical Biomedical Research Training: A Challenge for the Medical Subspecialties," *Journal of Laboratory and Clinical Medicine* 93:5, 1979.

106. Meeting of 24 January 1979, Minutes of the Staff Committee of the Medical Board, The Presbyterian Hospital in the City of New York, President's Office, Presbyterian Hospital, New York, NY.

107. See, for instance, meeting of 25 May 1971, Minutes of the Medical Board, the Presbyterian Hospital in the City of New York, President's Offices, Presbyterian Hospital, New York, NY; Executive Committee Meeting, 8 April 1981, Executive Board Minutes, University of Maryland School of Medicine.

108. Nicole Lurie, Brian Rank, Connie Parenti, Tony Woolley, and William Snoke, "How Do House Officers Spend Their Nights? A Time Study of Internal Medicine House Staff on Call," *New England Journal of Medicine* 320:1673–1677, 1989; Mitchell H. Katz and Steven A. Schroeder, "The Sounds of the Hospital: Paging Patterns in Three Teaching Hospitals," *New England Journal of Medicine* 319:1585–1589, 1988.

109. Committee on House Staff Meeting, 3 August 1973, Folder "Committee on House Staff," Box 3, Philadelphia General Hospital Papers (UPC 56.2), The University Archives and Record Center, University of Pennsylvania, Philadelphia, PA. The behavioral depths to which exhausted house officers would sometimes descend in order to avoid "hits" (admissions) has been described in Terry Mizrahi, *Getting Rid of Patients: Contradictions in the Socialization of Physicians* (New Brunswick, NJ: Rutgers University Press, 1986).

110. Jay W. Smith, William F. Denny, and Donald B. Witzke, "Emotional Impairment in Internal Medicine House Staff," *Journal of the American Medical Association* 255:1155–1158, 1986; Resident Services Committee, Association of Program Directors in Internal Medicine, "Stress and Impairment during Residency Training: Strategies for Reduction, Identification, and Management," *Annals of Internal Medicine* 109:154–161, 1988; and Richard D. Aach, Donald E. Girard, Holly Humphrey et al., "Alcohol and Other Substance Abuse and Impairment among Physicians in Residency Training," *Annals of Internal Medicine* 116:245–254, 1992.

111. The dermatology service at the Columbia-Presbyterian Medical Center provided a good illustration of how an educational opportunity for house officers could be quickly transformed into hospital service. When the Psoriasis Unit was established, dermatology residents were made responsible for providing phototherapy to patients on weekends, when no nurse was available. Three or four patients a day were in the unit, and the faculty thought this would be a good learning experience for the dermatology residents. However, to the consternation of the residents, who began pleading for additional nursing support, the number of patients on the service quickly grew to about 20, requiring the residents to spend seven or eight hours a day providing phototherapy on weekends. (Meeting of 23 October 1979, Minutes of the Medical Board, The Presbyterian Hospital in the City of New York.)

112. The Libby Zion affair attracted considerable attention in the medical literature and lay press. See, for example, Norman Spritz, "Oversight of Physicians' Conduct by State Licensing Agencies: Lessons from New York's Libby Zion Case," *Annals of Internal Medicine* 115:219–222, 1991; M. A. Farber, "Who Killed Libby Zion?," *Vanity Fair*, December 1988, pp. 190–195, 214, 216, 218, 220, 222, 224, 226, 228; and Natalie Robins, *The Girl Who Died Twice: The Libby Zion Case and the Hidden Hazards of Hospitals* (New York: Delacorte Press, 1995).

For all the discussion of the Libby Zion case and the question of residency reform, surprisingly little attention was directed to the issue of how house officers cope with mistakes. Anecdotal observations suggested that errors very much shaped house officers' outlooks on their roles in medicine, but the only systematic study of the subject was Charles L. Bosk's analysis of surgical training, *Forgive and Remember: Managing Medical Failure* (Chicago: University of Chicago Press, 1979).

113. Analysis of Bell Committee Recommendations by GNYHA, Folder "New York State Commission on Graduate Medical Education," Graduate Medical Education Records, Dean's Office Files, College of Physicians and Surgeons of Columbia University, New York, NY. Attitudes among house officers toward the new regulations appeared to vary by specialty. For instance, a survey of residents at Johns Hopkins revealed considerable concern about the adverse impact of sleep deprivation on patient care among residents in psychiatry and pediatrics but not general surgery. (Preliminary Report of the Survey on House Staff Hours and Supervision, 5 October 1989, with meeting of 29 November 1989, Minutes, Advisory Board of the Medical Faculty, The Johns Hopkins University School of Medicine, The Alan Mason Chesney Medical Archives of The Johns Hopkins Medical Institutions, Baltimore, MD.)

114. Robert G. Petersdorf, "Regulation of Residency Training," *Bulletin of the New York Academy of Medicine* 67:331, 1991.

115. Bertrand M. Bell, "Greenhorns in White," *Wall Street Journal*, 9 February 1995, p. A15.

116. See, for instance, Department of Medicine Residency Report, 12 May 1989, with meeting of 12 May 1989, Minutes, Executive Staff Meetings, Georgetown University Hospital; and David A. Asch and Ruth M. Parker, "The Libby Zion Case: One Step Forward or Two Steps Backward?," *New England Journal of Medicine* 318:774, 1988.

117. Christine Laine, Lee Goldman, Jane R. Soukup, and Joseph G. Hayes, "The Impact of a Regulation Restricting Medical House Staff Working Hours on the Quality of Patient Care," *Journal of the American Medical Association* 269:374–378, 1993; Amalia Kelly, Frances Marks, Carolyn Westhoff, and Mortimer Rosen, "The Effect of New York State Restrictions on Resident Work Hours," *Obstetrics & Gynecology* 78:468–473, 1991.

118. No one knew the extent of moonlighting or the reasons for it. It was widely said that residents and fellows needed to moonlight to help pay off educational loans, but the importance of that factor vis-à-vis the motivation to live better or to begin accumulating wealth was not known. Anecdotally, it was observed that many heavy moonlighters did not have burdensome educational debts. However, few medical educators would admit publicly that reasons other than educational debt might lead house officers to moonlight.

119. John M. Eisenberg, "Sociologic Influences on Decision-Making by Clinicians," *Annals of Internal Medicine* 90:957–964, 1979; Peter J. Greco and John M. Eisenberg, "Changing Physicians' Practices," *New England Journal of Medicine* 329:1271–1274, 1993; Paul F. Griner and Robert J. Glaser, "Misuse of Laboratory Tests and Diagnostic Procedures," *New England Journal of Medicine* 307:1336–1339, 1982.

120. Paul F. Griner and Benjamin Liptzin, "Use of the Laboratory in a Teaching Hospital: Implications for Patient Care, Education, and Hospital Costs," *Annals of Internal Medicine* 75:157–163, 1971.

121. Richard H. Dixon and John Laszla, "Utilization of Clinical Chemistry Services by Medical House Staff," *Archives of Internal Medicine* 134:1064–1067, 1974.

122. Steven A. Schroeder and Albert R. Martin, "Will Changing How Physicians Order Tests Reduce Medical Costs?," *Annals of Internal Medicine* 94:535, 1981.

480   NOTES TO PAGES 325–331

123. Jerome P. Kassirer, "Our Stubborn Quest for Diagnostic Certainty: A Cause of Excessive Testing," *New England Journal of Medicine* 320:1489, 1989.

124. *Ibid.*, p. 1490.

125. Stephen G. Pauker and Jerome P. Kassirer, "Decision Analysis," *New England Journal of Medicine* 316:250–258, 1987; Jerome P. Kassirer, "Diagnostic Reasoning," *Annals of Internal Medicine* 110:893–900, 1989.

Chapter 16

1. Table C1, AAMC Data Book, Update November 1991, Association of American Medical Colleges Archives, Washington, D.C.

2. C. Seth Landefeld, "The Spring Meetings—Are They Dying?," *New England Journal of Medicine* 328:1646, 1993.

3. Table C1, AAMC Data Book, Update November 1991.

4. *Table 12* is taken from William N. Kelley, "Are We About to Enter the Golden Era of Clinical Investigation?," *Journal of Laboratory and Clinical Medicine* 111:369, 1988.

5. Dorothea Wolfgram, "Megamedicine," *Washington University Magazine*, Spring 1978, p. 24.

6. Meeting of 26 October 1979, Executive Committee Minutes, University of Colorado School of Medicine, Office of the Chancellor, University of Colorado Health Sciences Center, Denver, CO.

7. For a typical example, see the materials on Harbor General Hospital, an important teaching affiliate of the University of California, Los Angeles, School of Medicine, in Folders 4–7, Box 4, and Folders 1–13, Box 5, Series 255, Administrative Files of Jeanne Williams (Record Series 255), University Archives, Department of Special Collections, The University Library, University of California, Los Angeles, Los Angeles, CA.

8. The political forces leading to the balkanization of surgery departments were readily apparent at the University of Colorado. See, for instance, the meetings and attached reports of 15 September 1969, 7 December 1972, 29 March 1973, 15 November 1973, and 17 June 1976, Executive Faculty Minutes, University of Colorado School of Medicine, Office of the Chancellor, University of Colorado Health Sciences Center, Denver, CO.

9. Eugene Braunwald, "Cardiology—Division or Department?," *New England Journal of Medicine* 319:1887–1890, 1993; Barry L. Zaret, William B. Hood Jr., and Robert A. O'Rourke, "Cardiovascular Medicine: Subspecialty or Specialty," *American Journal of Cardiology* 72:968–970, 1993; and William B. Hood Jr., "Subdividing Departments of Medicine," *Annals of Internal Medicine* 119:1225, 1993.

10. Marvin Weisbord, Paul R. Lawrence, and Martin P. Charns, "Three Dilemmas of Academic Medical Centers," *Journal of Applied Behavioral Science* 14:292–293, 1978.

11. Francis W. Peabody, *Doctor and Patient: Papers on the Relationship of the Physician to Men and Institutions* (New York: Macmillan, 1930).

12. Eugene Braunwald, "Can Medical Schools Remain the Optimal Site for the Conduct of Clinical Investigation?," *Journal of Clinical Investigation* 56: i–vi, 1975. For more on the administrative challenges confronting department chairmen, see Paul B. Beeson, "The Ways of Academic Clinical Medicine in America Since World War II," *Man and Medicine* 1:65–79, 1975; and Paul B. Beeson, "The Changing Role Model, and the Shift in Power," *Daedalus*, Spring 1986, pp. 83–97.

13. David E. Rogers and Robert J. Blendon, "The Academic Medical Center: A Stressed American Institution," *New England Journal of Medicine* 298:944, 1978.

14. Meeting of 6 December 1988, Dean's Advisory Council, University of Michigan School of Medicine, Dean's Office, University of Michigan School of Medicine, Ann Arbor, MI.

15. C. Seth Landefeld, "The Spring Meetings—Are They Dying?," *New England Journal of Medicine* 328:1645–1647, 1993; Lloyd H. Smith Jr., "Presidential Address," *Transactions of the Association of American Physicians* 89:1–9, 1976. In 1999, the American Federation for Clinical Research (which three years before had changed its name to the American Federation for Medical Research) for the first time did not meet with the other two organizations.

16. William Parson, review of Barton F. Haynes, ed., *A Way of Thinking*, *The Pharos*, Winter 1996, p. 47.

17. Meeting of 23 July 1984, Corporate Board of Trustees Minutes, Thomas Jefferson University, Thomas Jefferson University Archives and Special Collections, Thomas Jefferson University, Philadelphia, PA.

18. Richard A. Knox, "Stanford Medical School Suffers Fiscal Ideological Crises," *Science* 203:148–152, 1979; AAMC Memorandum on "Top 40" Research Schools: 1985–86, 27 May 1988, Box 4, Section for Operational Studies, IMCIS-IPS, Association of American Medical Colleges Archives, Washington, D.C.

19. Quoted in "The Hopkins Physician Scientist," *Hopkins Medical News*, Spring 1990, p. 30.

20. Executive Summary, CPMC Research Retreat, Folder "Retreat CPMC 1986, Folder 1," CPMC Retreat Records, Office of the Dean, College of Physicians and Surgeons of Columbia University, New York, NY.

21. Executive Committee Meeting of 11 April 1984, Executive Board Minutes, University of Maryland School of Medicine, Dean's Office, University of Maryland School of Medicine, Baltimore, MD.

22. Robert F. Jones, Marcie F. Mirsky, and Joseph A. Keyes Jr., "Clinical Practice of Medical School Faculties: An AAMC Survey of Problems and Issues," *Journal of Medical Education* 60:910, 1985.

23. Robert G. Petersdorf, "The Scylla and Charybdis of Medical Education," *Journal of Medical Education* 63:91, 1988.

24. Walsh McDermott to Eric Cassell, 22 August 1980, Folder 7, Box 24, Walsh McDermott Papers, Archives, The New York Hospital–Cornell Medical Center, New York, NY.

25. Meeting of 12 May 1983, Executive Committee Minutes, University of Michigan School of Medicine, Dean's Office, University of Michigan School of Medicine, Ann Arbor, MI.

26. *Table 13* is adopted from William C. Smith Jr., *Report on Medical School Faculty Salaries 1997–98* (Washington, D.C.: Association of American Medical Colleges, 1998). This table reflects the salaries of all medical school faculty, including those without the M.D. degree. If only M.D. faculty were included, salaries levels would be higher than those shown.

27. Debra E. Blum, "Many Medical Professors at Private Research Universities Earn More Than Presidents," *Chronicle of Higher Education*, 13 September 1989, p. A1.

28. Jonathan Welsh, "Charities Still Raise Salaries of CEOs, to Lure Officers, Used to Corporate Pay," *Wall Street Journal*, 5 September 1995, p. B7A.

29. Carleton B. Chapman, "Education for Medicine in the University," in

Beyond Tomorrow: Trends and Prospects in Medical Science (New York: The Rockefeller University, 1977), p. 47.

30. Robert G. Petersdorf, "The Scylla and Charybdis of Medical Education," *Journal of Medical Education* 63:90–91, 1988.

31. Richard L. Simmons to Dr. Wolf, n.d., with Thomas C. Chalmers to Gustave L. Levy, 28 December 1973, President/Dean's Papers (Chalmers Series), Mount Sinai School of Medicine, Archives, The Mount Sinai Medical Center, New York, NY.

32. Helpful discussions of university-corporate relationships from both favorable and critical perspectives include Martin Kenney, *Biotechnology: The University-Industrial Complex* (New Haven: Yale University Press, 1986); Gary W. Matkin, *Technology Transfer and the University* (New York: Macmillan, 1990); Sheldon Krimsky, *Biotechnics and Society: The Rise of Industrial Genetics* (New York: Praeger, 1991); Arthur Kornberg, *The Golden Helix: Inside Biotech Ventures* (Sausalito, CA: University Science Books, 1995); Gilbert S. Omenn, "Taking University Research into the Marketplace," *New England Journal of Medicine* 307:694–700, 1982; Barbara J. Culliton, "Biomedical Research Enters the Marketplace," *New England Journal of Medicine* 304:1195–1201, 1981; Bernard D. Davis, "Profit Sharing between Professors and the University?," *New England Journal of Medicine* 304:1232–1235, 1981; David Blumenthal, Michael Gluck, Karen S. Louis, and David Wise, "Industrial Support of University Research in Biotechnology," *Science* 231:242–246, 1986; and Udayan Gupta, "Turning University Research into a Profitable Business," *Wall Street Journal*, 12 June 1990, p. B2. This issue, of course, affected biomedical science throughout the university, not just at the medical school.

33. David Blumenthal, Nancyanne Causino, Eric Campbell, and Karen S. Louis, "Relationships between Academic Institutions and Industry in the Life Sciences—An Industry Survey," *New England Journal of Medicine* 334:368–373, 1996 (funding statistics, p. 368).

34. Warren E. Leary, "Business and Scholarship: A New Ethical Quandary," *New York Times*, 12 June 1989, p. A1; Marilyn Chase, "Mixing Science, Stocks Raises Question of Bias in the Testing of Drugs," *Wall Street Journal*, 26 January 1989, p. A1; Arnold S. Relman, "Dealing with Conflicts of Interest," *New England Journal of Medicine* 310:1182–1183, 1984; Arnold S. Relman, "Economic Incentives in Clinical Investigation," *New England Journal of Medicine* 320:933–934, 1989; and Ezekiel J. Emanuel and Daniel Steiner, "Institutional Conflict of Interest," *New England Journal of Medicine* 332:262–267, 1995.

35. Meeting of 3 May 1983, Executive Council Minutes, with meeting of 6 June 1983, Corporate Board of Trustees Minutes, Thomas Jefferson University.

36. Quoted in Susannah Hunnewell, "The Medical-Industrial Complex," *Harvard Magazine*, January–February 1994, p. 37.

37. On the misrepresentation of credentials, see Gail Sekas and William Hutson, "Misrepresentation of Academic Accomplishments by Applicants for Gastroenterology Fellowships," *Annals of Internal Medicine* 123:38–41, 1995; and Harry Kimball, "Credentials Misrepresentation: Another Challenge to Professionalism," *Annals of Internal Medicine* 123:58, 1995. Reports also appeared of falsified credentials among physicians applying for staff privileges. See, for instance, William A. Schaffer, F. David Rollo, and Carol A. Holt, "Falsification of Clinical Credentials by Physicians Applying for Ambulatory-Staff Privileges," *New England Journal of Medicine* 318:356–358, 1988. Faculty and student violations of the

rules of the internship matching program are discussed in Robert G. Petersdorf, "From the President," *Academic Medicine* 64:308, 1989. Student cheating was discussed in Chapter 15.

38. *The New Republic*, 18 May 1992. The most highly publicized case of scientific fraud involved John Darsee, a postdoctoral research fellow working in an eminent cardiovascular laboratory at Harvard Medical School. A thoughtful discussion of the Darsee affair is Barbara J. Culliton, "Coping with Fraud: The Darsee Case," *Science* 220:31–35, 1983.

39. Accounts of the history of fraud in science include William Broad and Nicholas Wade, *Betrayers of the Truth: Fraud and Deceit in the Halls of Science* (New York: Simon & Schuster, 1983); Alexander Kohn, *False Prophets: Fraud and Error in Science and Medicine* (Oxford: Basil Blackwell, 1986), and Marcel C. LaFollette, *Stealing into Print: Fraud, Plagiarism, and Misconduct in Scientific Publishing* (Berkeley: University of California Press, 1992).

40. Edward J. Huth, "Abuses of Authorship," *Annals of Internal Medicine* 100:147–148, 1984; Edward J. Huth, "Abuses and Uses of Authorship," *Annals of Internal Medicine* 104:266–267, 1986; Marcia Angell and Arnold S. Relman, "Redundant Publication," *New England Journal of Medicine* 320:1212–1214, 1989; Jerome P. Kassirer and Marcia Angell, "Redundant Publication: A Reminder," *New England Journal of Medicine* 333:449–450, 1995; Marcia Angell, "Publish or Perish: A Proposal," *Annals of Internal Medicine* 104:261–262, 1986; Thomas P. Stossel, "Volume: Papers and Academic Promotion," *Annals of Internal Medicine* 106:146–149, 1987; and N. Fotion and C. C. Conrad, "Authorship and Other Credits," *Annals of Internal Medicine* 100:592–594, 1984.

41. Meeting of 28 December 1981, Minutes, Advisory Board of the Medical Faculty, The Johns Hopkins University School of Medicine, The Alan Mason Chesney Medical Archives of The Johns Hopkins Medical Institutions, Baltimore, MD.

42. Huth, "Abuses of Authorship," p. 147.

43. Robert J. Blendon, Carl J. Schramm, Thomas W. Maloney, and David E. Rogers, "An Era of Stress for Health Institutions: The 1980s," *Journal of the American Medical Association* 245:1844, 1981.

44. The question of how much community service medical schools should provide was extremely vexing. Some believed that medical faculties had a long way to go in providing such services to their local community. (For a well-known expression of this view, see Irving J. Lewis and Cecil G. Sheps, *The Sick Citadel: The American Academic Medical Center and the Public Interest* [Cambridge, MA: Oelgeschlager, Gunn & Hain, 1983].) On the other hand, one could easily imagine the academic mission being lost amid a swelter of service activities.

45. Meeting of 26 May 1977, Executive Committee, Folder "May–June 1977," Box 138, University of Michigan Medical School Records, Michigan Historical Collections, Bentley Historical Library, University of Michigan, Ann Arbor, MI.

46. Principal Recommendations of the Workshop on Medical School Curriculum, with meeting of 11 November 1968, Minutes, Executive Faculty Meetings, Medical College of Pennsylvania, Dean's Office, MCP Hahnemann University, Philadelphia, PA.

47. John W. Colloton, "Academic Medicine's Changing Covenant with Society," *Academic Medicine* 64:55–60, 1989; Steven A. Schroeder, Jane S. Zones, and Jonathan Showstack, "Academic Medicine as a Public Trust," *Journal of the American Medical Association* 262:803–812, 1989; Samuel Hellman, "The Intellectual Quarantine of American Medicine," *Academic Medicine* 66:245–248, 1991; and

Samuel O. Thier, "Preventing the Decline of Academic Medicine," *Academic Medicine* 67:731–737, 1992.

48. See, for instance, Robert Bellah, Richard Madsen, William M. Sullivan, Ann Swidler, and Steven M. Tipton, *Habits of the Heart: Individualism and Commitment in American Life* (Berkeley: University of California Press, 1985); James Lincoln Collier, *The Rise of Selfishness in America* (New York: Oxford University Press, 1991); Wilfred M. McClay, *The Masterless: Self and Society in Modern America* (Chapel Hill: University of North Carolina Press, 1994); and Christopher Lasch, *The Culture of Narcissism: American Life in an Age of Diminishing Expectations* (New York: W. W. Norton, 1979).

49. Relman, "Economic Incentives in Clinical Investigation," p. 934.

Chapter 17

1. See, for instance, the public opinion poll reported in Robert J. Blendon, Carl J. Schramm, Thomas W. Maloney, and David E. Rogers, "An Era of Stress for Health Institutions: The 1980s," *Journal of the American Medical Association* 245:1844, 1981.

2. The impact of these problems in human terms was portrayed in Erik Eckholm, ed., *Solving America's Health-Care Crisis: A Guide to Understanding the Greatest Threat to Your Family's Security* (New York: Times Books, 1993).

3. John E. Wennberg and Alan Gittelsohn, "Variations in Medical Care among Small Areas," *Scientific American* 246:120–134, 1982.

4. C. M. Winslow, J. Kosecoff, R. H. Brook, M. R. Chassin, and D. E. Kanouse, "The Appropriateness of Use of Coronary Angiography and Coronary Artery Bypass Surgery," *Clinical Research* 34:635A, 1986.

5. The most thorough discussion of this subject is Marc A. Rodwin, *Medicine, Money, and Morals: Physicians' Conflicts of Interest* (New York: Oxford University Press, 1993).

The issue of conflicts of interest is more complex than simple greed. Although there is clear data that some physicians are avaricious, more important is the way in which financial incentives can subconsciously affect the behavior of even well-meaning physicians. (Thomas Gallagher to author, 8 June 1998.)

6. The still-unfolding history of the revolt of the payers remains untold, but helpful analyses include Thomas Bodenheimer and Kevin Grumbach, "The Reconfiguration of U.S. Medicine," *Journal of the American Medical Association* 274:85–90, 1995; John Iglehart, "The American Health Care System: Managed Care," *New England Journal of Medicine* 327:742–747, 1992; John Iglehart, "Physicians and the Growth of Managed Care," *New England Journal of Medicine* 331:1167–1171, 1994; Erik Eckholm, "While Congress Remains Silent, Health Care Transforms Itself," *New York Times*, 18 December 1994, p. A1; Robin Toner, "Harry and Louise Were Right, Sort Of," *New York Times*, 24 November 1996, section 4, p. 1; and Emily Friedman, "The Power of Physicians: Autonomy and Balance in a Changing System," *American Journal of Medicine* 99:579–586, 1995.

7. Robert Fenley, *Advertising & the Academic Medical Center* (Washington, D.C.: Association of American Medical Colleges, 1986).

Traditional professional ethics, of course, prohibited advertising. However, in 1975 the U.S. Supreme Court overturned bar association regulations prohibiting lawyers from advertising. Thereafter, advertising by lawyers, physicians, hospitals, and other professionals spread rapidly. (Elisabeth Rosenthal, "Medicine

Promotes Itself, with Help from Professionals," *New York Times*, 11 December 1991, p. B1.)

8. Dave Lindorff, *Marketplace Medicine: The Rise of For-Profit Hospital Chains* (New York: Bantam Books, 1992).

9. Newspaper clipping, "Welfare Patients Dumped on County," with meeting of 23 September 1981, Minutes, Faculty Executive Committee, University of Southern California School of Medicine, Dean's Office, University of Southern California School of Medicine, Los Angeles, CA. See also, George J. Annas, "Your Money or Your Life: 'Dumping' Uninsured Patients from Hospital Emergency Rooms," *American Journal of Public Health* 76:74–77, 1986. Even teaching hospitals could no longer handle all demands for free care that were placed upon them. In particular, privately owned teaching hospitals began transferring some patients to public facilities, especially clinically stable patients who lived outside the hospital's catchment area.

10. Analysts have described four stages in the evolution of health care markets from fee-for-service into HMOs. See John K. Iglehart, "The American Health Care System: Teaching Hospitals," *New England Journal of Medicine* 329:1054, 1993; and Dennis Murray, "The Four Market Stages, and Where You Fit In," *Medical Economics*, 13 March 1995, pp. 44–57.

11. Kate Ledger, "Specialists for Hire," *Hopkins Medical News*, Spring–Summer 1996, pp. 20–27; Alfred E. Stillman, "Modern Times," *New England Journal of Medicine* 333:1086–1087, 1995.

12. Philip L. Szenas, "Graduates' Interest in Generalist Specialties Nearly Doubles in Three Years," *Academic Physician and Scientist*, November 1995, pp. 2–3.

13. Jordan J. Cohen, "Time to Stanch the Flow of Residents," *Academic Medicine* 69:464, 1994.

14. Pew Health Professions Commission, *Critical Challenges: Revitalizing the Health Professions for the Twenty-first Century* (San Francisco: Pew Health Professions Commission, 1995).

15. See, for instance, Jordan J. Cohen, "Too Many Doctors: A Prescription for Bad Medicine," *Academic Medicine* 71:654, 1996. The issue of international medical graduates (IMGs) was highly charged. Some, like Cohen, argued for a reduction in their number because of the perceived physician glut. However, many residency programs in medically underserved areas depended on IMGs and would have been forced to close without them. Accordingly, strong political support continued to be found in behalf of IMGs.

16. Jane Erikson, "Five UA surgeons resign, head to 'greener pastures'," *Arizona Daily Star*, 22 April 1998, p. 1A.

17. John K. Iglehart, "Rapid Changes for Academic Medical Centers," *New England Journal of Medicine* 331:1391–1395, 1994; 332:407–411, 1995.

18. Alan Dobson, Kevin Coleman, and Robert Mechanic, *Analysis of Teaching Hospital Costs* (Fairfax, VA: Lewin-VHI, 1994).

19. David Blumenthal and Gregg S. Meyer, "Academic Health Centers in a Changing Environment," *Health Affairs*, Summer 1996, pp. 202–204.

20. Jerome P. Kassirer, "Academic Medical Centers Under Siege," *New England Journal of Medicine* 331:1370, 1994.

21. *The Financing of Medical Schools—A Report of the AAMC Task Force on Medical School Financing* (Washington, D.C.: AAMC, 1996). It should be noted that after Congress started to encourage Medicare patients to enroll in HMOs in the mid-

1990s, HMOs began sticking another thorn in teaching hospitals. Many HMOs kept for themselves the portion of the Medicare premium that was intended to subsidize medical education, even though they incurred none of the costs of education.

22. Donald A. Young, "The Prospective Payment Assessment Commission: Responsibilities and Recent Findings," *Academic Medicine* 66:401, 1991.

23. Kassirer, "Academic Medical Centers Under Siege," p. 1370.

24. *The Financing of Medical Schools*.

25. Not surprisingly, hospital chain officials have stated that they will support education and research generously, while many in academic medicine remain extremely skeptical. In the long run, whether the culture of proprietary hospitals will allow academic values to be respected and protected remains to be seen.

26. Quoted in Susan Sanderson, "Faculty Affairs Deans Grapple With Downsizing, Tenure Guarantees, and Increased Accountability," *Academic Physician and Scientist*, November 1995, p. 6.

27. Kenneth I. Shine, "The Future of Academic Health Centers," *Physiologist* 38:51, 1995. In 1995, Harvard Community Health Plan and Pilgrim Health Care merged to become Harvard Pilgrim Health Care.

28. Some executives of investor-owned HMOs argued that their organizations paid taxes in lieu of direct support to medical education. Industry critics rebutted that it had never been shown that this represented their fair share of the cost of maintaining the "medical commons."

29. Quoted in Elisabeth Rosenthal, "Hospital Research Falling Victim to Lean Budgets," *New York Times*, 30 May 1995, p. A1.

30. John F. Steiner, Lawrence E. Feinberg, Andrew M. Kramer, and Richard L. Byyny, "Changing Patterns of Disease on an Inpatient Medical Service: 1961–1962 to 1981–1982," *American Journal of Medicine* 83:331–335, 1987.

31. Robert H. Brook, Caren J. Kamberg, and Elizabeth A. McGlynn, "Health System Reform and Quality," *Journal of the American Medical Association* 276:479, 1996; Lawrence K. Altman, "In Health Care, a Question of Quality: Cost-Control Efforts Raise Concerns," *New York Times*, 2 January 1990, p. C3.

32. For instance, average length of stay at the University of Washington's Harborview Medical Center in 1991 was 5.4 days, and at Barnes Hospital in 1994, 6.6 days. (Richard K. Root and Cathryn L. Nation, "Legislated Limits for Housestaff Training," *Annals of Internal Medicine* 116:695, 1992; Barnes Hospital of St. Louis Average Length of Stay Data, courtesy of BJC Finance Office.)

33. Quoted in Elise Hancock, "The Squeeze is On," *Johns Hopkins Magazine*, November 1995, p. 54.

34. Meeting of 22 September 1986, Minutes and Correspondence of the Executive Committee of the Faculty Council, College of Physicians and Surgeons, Office of the Dean, College of Physicians and Surgeons of Columbia University, New York, NY; and meeting of 18 September 1985, Minutes of the Medical Board, The Presbyterian Hospital in the City of New York, President's Offices, Presbyterian Hospital, New York, NY.

35. Larry S. Schlesinger and Charles M. Helms, "Cost-Conscious Care, Housestaff Training, and the Academic Health Center," *Academic Medicine* 70:561–562, 1995.

36. A particularly influential paper was Gerald T. Perkoff, "Teaching Clinical

Medicine in the Ambulatory Setting: An Idea Whose Time May Have Finally Come," *New England Journal of Medicine* 314:27–31, 1986.

37. See, for instance, Michael J. Reichgott and J. Sanford Schwartz, "Acceptance by Private Patients of Resident Involvement in Their Outpatient Care," *Journal of Medical Education* 58:703–709, 1983.

38. John M. Eisenberg, "How Can We Pay for Graduate Medical Education in Ambulatory Care?," *New England Journal of Medicine* 320:1525–1531, 1989.

39. See, for instance, Christine A. Taylor, Thomas G. Dunn, and Martin S. Lipsky, "Time Spent by Preceptors on Specific Educational Activities in Inpatient and Ambulatory-Care Settings," *Academic Medicine* 66:121, 1991; D. A. Litzelman, "Residents' Perceptions of Patient Volume and Amount of Faculty Precepting in a General Medicine Ambulatory Practice," *Academic Medicine* 70:448, 1995; Joan Feltovich, Terrill A. Mast, and Norman G. Soler, "Teaching Medical Students in Ambulatory Settings in Departments of Internal Medicine," *Academic Medicine* 64:36–41, 1989; and David M. Irby, "Teaching and Learning in Ambulatory Care Settings: A Thematic Review of the Literature," *Academic Medicine* 70:898–931, 1995.

Some disciplines weathered these pressures better than others. For instance, in family practice, faculty were prohibited by the Residency Review Committee from seeing their own patients while they were teaching residents in clinic. (Gerald T. Perkoff to author, 19 January 1998.)

40. Janet M. Corrigan and Laurie M. Thompson, "Involvement of Health Maintenance Organizations in Graduate Medical Education," *Academic Medicine* 66:656–661, 1991. In the late 1960s several medical schools founded HMOs. However, the cost of funding education and research in the HMOs proved formidable, and only two survived into the 1990s in their original form.

41. Gordon T. Moore, Thomas S. Inui, John M. Ludden, and Stephen C. Schoenbaum, "The 'Teaching HMO': A New Academic Partner," *Academic Medicine* 69:595–600, 1994; quotation, p. 595. In the mid-1990s, a number of private foundations, most notably the Pew and Robert Wood Johnson, also began to encourage the formation of "academic partnerships" between HMOs and academic health centers.

42. Richard A. Knox and Charles Stein, "HMO Doctors Want Boss out in Dispute on Patient Load," *Boston Globe*, 21 November 1991, p. 1; Charles Stein, "Compensation Plan Ignited Doctor Revolt," *Boston Globe*, 22 November 1991, p. 75.

43. Moore, Inui, Ludden, and Schoenbaum, "The 'Teaching HMO'," p. 599.

44. Jon Schafer, "Postgraduate Training Feels the Pinch," *Journal of Investigative Medicine* 43:399, 1995. In view of the perceived physician surplus, most medical educators and policy analysists agreed that fewer postgraduate positions were desirable. However, many were concerned that it was outstanding university programs like Duke rather than nonuniversity programs of marginal quality that were contracting.

45. Joyce V. Kelley, Stephen Larned, and Helen L. Smits, "Graduate Medical Education Consortia: Expectations and Experiences," *Academic Medicine* 69:931–943, 1994; Mahendr S. Kochar and Richard A. Cooper, "A Medical School–Based GME Consortium in Milwaukee," *Academic Medicine* 71: 238–242, 1996.

46. Jordan J. Cohen, "Academic Medicine's Tenuous Hold on Tenure," *Academic Medicine* 70:294, 1995.

47. Meeting of 26 November 1985, Minutes of the Planning Committee of the

Medical Board, The Presbyterian Hospital in the City of New York, President's Office, Presbyterian Hospital, New York, NY.

48. Meeting of 7 March 1985, Transactions of the Medical Board of the New York Hospital, Archives, The New York Hospital–Cornell Medical Center, New York, NY.

49. Helpful discussions of these developments include Eli Ginzberg, *Tomorrow's Hospital: A Look to the Twenty-first Century* (New Haven: Yale University Press, 1996); Lee Goldman, "The Academic Health Care System: Preserving the Missions as the Paradigm Shifts," *Journal of the American Medical Association* 273:1549–1552, 1995; and David Blumenthal and Gregg S. Meyer, "The Future of the Academic Medical Center Under Health Care Reform," *New England Journal of Medicine* 329:1812–1814, 1993. A sense of the diversity among academic health care systems is provided in Richard A. Culbertson, Leslie D. Goode, and Robert M. Dickler, "Organizational Models of Medical School Relationships to the Clinical Enterprise," *Academic Medicine* 71:1257–1274, 1996; and Jon Schafer, "Academic Centers Venture Disparately in Approach to Managed Care," *Journal of Investigative Medicine* 44:499–505, 1996.

In the late 1990s, academic IDSs were still evolving. Some observers were predicting the complete organizational merger of the physicians and hospitals in a system into a single ownership group (so-called physician hospital organizations, or PHOs). PHOs could offer insurance companies a set price per patient that included both physician and hospital fees. It was also expected that at least some IDSs would develop the capacity to assume the financial risk of providing health care, thereby allowing them to bypass HMOs and insurance companies and deal directly with primary purchasers of health care like corporations and government. In previous eras, the organization of hospitals, the creation of PHOs, and the assumption of insurance risk by physicians or hospitals would have been prohibited by antitrust regulations. However, in acknowledgment of the need to keep the playing field level between "payers" and "providers," federal antitrust regulations in the late 1990s were interpreted less restrictively. (Robert Kuttner, "Physician-Operated Networks and the New Antitrust Guidelines," *New England Journal of Medicine* 336:386–391, 1997.)

50. Jerome P. Kassirer, "Mergers and Acquisitions—Who Benefits? Who Loses?," *New England Journal of Medicine* 334:722, 1996.

51. Report of a Site Visit to the Rush-Presbyterian-St. Luke's Medical Center in Chicago, 23 April 1979, with meeting of 17 May 1979, Minutes, Board of Trustees, The Mount Sinai Hospital, Archives, The Mount Sinai Medical Center, New York, NY.

52. See, for instance, the circular letter to alumni from the Office of Johns Hopkins Medicine, 9 April 1996; and "Executive Faculty Approves School's Clinical Practice Plan," *Washington University Record*, 12 December 1996, p. 5.

53. Blumenthal and Meyer, "Academic Health Centers in a Changing Environment," pp. 200–215.

54. Alan M. Fogelman, Leslie D. Goode, B. Lyn Behrens et al., "Preserving Medical Schools' Academic Mission in a Competitive Marketplace," *Academic Medicine* 71:1168–1199, 1996.

55. *The Financing of Medical Schools.*

56. Kenneth I. Berns, "Preventing *Academic Medical Center* from Becoming an Oxymoron," *Academic Medicine* 71:117, 1996; David A. Blake, "Whither Academic Values during the Transition from Academic Medical Centers to Integrated Health Delivery Systems?," *Academic Medicine* 71:819, 1996.

57. "Calif. hospital under fire for seeking healthier patients," *Modern Healthcare*, 21 August 1995, p. 172.

58. Some architects of academic integrated delivery systems have argued that those systems are intended to save education and research by allowing such previously unimaginable efficiencies in clinical care to be achieved that surplus income will become available to support the academic enterprise. At present, in an era of cutthroat price-based competition, it is unclear how those surpluses will be generated without jeopardizing the quality of care. Moreover, such surpluses would be tantamount to a clinical cross-subsidy of the academic mission, which managed care organizations have been unwilling to pay. In the present marketplace, it is likely that insurers would try to ratchet down payments in the next go-around of contract talks, were they to learn of such surpluses. It should also be noted that such operating efficiencies would be achievable only with an exceedingly high "throughput" of patients—a feature, as already noted, that is in itself inimical to the education process.

59. A recent discussion of the limitations of popular management strategies and the need for caution in their application is John Micklethwait and Adrian Wooldridge, *The Witch Doctors: Making Sense of the Management Gurus* (New York: Times Books, 1996).

Chapter 18

1. Crane Brinton, *The Anatomy of Revolution*, revised and expanded edition (New York: Vintage Books, 1965).

2. *The Financing of Medical Schools—A Report of the AAMC Task Force on Medical School Financing* (Washington, D.C.: AAMC, 1996), pp. 6–14.

3. *Ibid.*, pp. 8, 10.

4. *The Financing of Medical Schools*; Alan M. Fogelman, Leslie D. Goode, B. Lyn Behrens et al., "Preserving Medical Schools' Academic Mission in a Competitive Marketplace," *Academic Medicine* 71:1168–1199, 1996; and David Blumenthal and Gregg S. Meyer, "Academic Health Centers in a Changing Environment," *Health Affairs*, Summer 1996, pp. 200–215.

Some very important research went unfunded. For instance, pilot studies, which were essential to gathering sufficient information to support an NIH application, and ideas too creative or unusual to receive funding from conventional agencies had always depended heavily on clinical cross-subsidization. In addition, clinical revenues had traditionally been relied on for recruiting new faculty, supporting young investigators at the beginning of their careers, and funding established scientists between grants.

5. *The Financing of Medical Schools*, pp. 34–35; and Eric G. Campbell, Joel S. Weissman, and David Blumenthal, "Relationship Between Market Competition and the Activities and Attitudes of Medical School Faculty," *Journal of the American Medical Association* 278:222–226, 1997.

6. "New Effort Launched to Increase Funding for Academic Centers," *ACP Observer*, February 1997, p. 3.

7. See, for instance, Ab Sadeghi-Nejad and Marion M. Marquardt, "Academic Physicians: Today's Dinosaurs?," *American Journal of Medicine* 90:371–373, 1991.

8. Quoted in Alex Pham, "Medical Brain Drain," *Boston Globe*, 13 July 1996, p. 67.

9. Joseph B. Martin, "Academic Health Centers: Vulnerabilities in 1995 and Beyond," *Archives of Internal Medicine* 155:2047, 1995; Donald G. Kassebaum,

Philip L. Szenas, Alexis L. Ruffin, and Danielle R. Masters, "The Research Interests of Graduating Medical Students," *Academic Medicine* 70:847–852, 1995.

10. Meeting of 25 August 1988, Executive Committee Minutes, University of Michigan School of Medicine, Dean's Office, University of Michigan School of Medicine, Ann Arbor, MI.

11. Fogelman, Goode, Behrens et al., "Preserving Medical Schools' Academic Mission," pp. 1183–1199.

12. Typically, the new salary plans consisted of an "A," "B," and "C" (sometimes labelled "X," "Y," and "Z") component. "A" represented a core salary guaranteed by the medical school; "B," an incentive based on the clinical revenues generated; and "C," an additional bonus for unusually high earning outliers who might bill for $1,000,000 per year or more in professional fees.

13. "MGMA and AAMC to Develop Physician Productivity Standards," *Academic Medicine* 71:161, 1996.

14. Quoted in Katherine S. Mangan, "Medical Schools Are Reining in the Salaries of Faculty Members," *Chronicle of Higher Education*, 26 July 1996, p. A18.

15. James C. Collins and Jerry I. Porras, *Built to Last: Successful Habits of Visionary Companies* (New York: HarperBusiness, 1994), pp. 80–90, 136, 215–216.

16. Quoted in Mangan, "Medical Schools," p. A18. Ironically, this infringement on teaching time occurred at precisely the moment when the role of an attending physician was becoming more demanding. As the mix of hospitalized patients became sicker, and as the average length of hospital stay fell, the need for an attending to supervise the house staff closely had become greater than ever. Volunteer faculty, who traditionally had provided over half the clinical teaching at many schools, often found it difficult to continue contributing to the same degree. Market pressures had made it financially hard for them to take time from their practices to teach without explicit remuneration. (Raymond H. Murray and Vence L. Bonham Jr., "The Threatened Role of Volunteer Faculty Members," *Academic Medicine* 66:455–456, 1991.)

17. Jeffrey A. Romoff, "The Transformation of the AMC: The Managed Care Market Place and the Future of the University of Pittsburgh Medical Center," 1995 (videotape).

18. Conversation with David M. Kipnis, 27 March 1997.

19. The Consensus Statement on Clinical Practice, 20 September 1985, with agenda items for meeting of 1 October 1985, Minutes, The Johns Hopkins Hospital Board of Trustees, The Alan Mason Chesney Medical Archives of The Johns Hopkins Medical Institutions, Baltimore, MD.

20. Thomas L. Delbanco, "Wheeling and Dealing with Graduate Medical Education," *Annals of Internal Medicine* 105:962, 1986.

21. Personal communication to author from members of the school's third-year class.

22. Donald G. Kassebaum, "Heavy Weather Ahead for Clinical Education in Restructured Academic Health Care Systems," *Academic Medicine* 70:860, 1995. See also, Jerome P. Kassirer, "Redesigning Graduate Medical Education—Location and Content," *New England Journal of Medicine* 335:507–509, 1996.

Many faculty, particularly clerkship and residency program directors, still understood and cared about pedagogical issues. However, their viewpoint seldom permeated the upper power echelons of the schools, where the large institutional decisions were made.

23. Marvin C. Rulin, Donald B. Middleton, Steven L. Kanter, and Sheldon Adler, "Undergraduate Course in Ambulatory Care," *Academic Medicine* 70:85, 1995.

24. *Ibid.*, p. 85.

25. Lawrence G. Smith, "First Year of Practice: A Year of Rapid Learning," *Academic Medicine* 71:580–581, 1996.

26. For instance, many schools participating in the Generalist Physician Initiative sponsored by the Robert Wood Johnson Foundation have developed curricular guidelines for ambulatory education and faculty development programs for community faculty. See the supplement to the January 1999 issue of *Academic Medicine*, which discusses the Generalist Physician Initiative.

27. See, for instance, David R. Jones, Denise Dupras, and Alexis L. Ruffin, "Importance of the Perspective of Residents in Defining and Maintaining Quality in GME," *Academic Medicine* 71:820–822, 1996.

28. Julius R. Krevans, "Medicine's Dying Angels," *Johns Hopkins Magazine*, August 1989, p. 40.

29. Many authorities on higher education have discussed this point. See, for instance, Jaroslav Pelikan, *The Idea of the University: A Reexamination* (New Haven: Yale University Press, 1992), pp. 182–184.

30. Theresa Defino, "Educating Physicians in Managed Care," *Health System Leader*, May 1995, pp. 4–11.

31. See, for instance, David Korn, "Reengineering Academic Medical Centers: Reengineering Academic Values?," *Academic Medicine* 71:1041, 1996.

32. David P. Stevens, David C. Leach, Gail L. Warden, and Neil S. Cherniak, "A Strategy for Coping with Change: An Affiliation between a Medical School and a Managed Care Health System," *Academic Medicine* 7:133, 1996; Mark C. Rogers, Ralph Snyderman, and Elizabeth L. Rogers, "Cultural and Organizational Implications of Academic Managed-Care Networks," *New England Journal of Medicine* 331:1377, 1994; and quotation of Edward J. Benz in Janet Farrar Worthington, "In Osler's Footsteps," *Hopkins Medical News*, Summer 1996, p. 19.

33. Louise Kertesz, "Payers start to worry about impact of HMOs' bad press," *Modern Healthcare*, 12 February 1996, p. 125.

34. See, for instance, Marcia Angell, "The Doctor as Double Agent," *Kennedy Institute of Ethics Journal* 3:279–286, 1993.

35. See, for instance, Herbert W. Swick, "Academic Medicine Must Deal with the Clash of Business and Professional Values," *Academic Medicine* 73:751–755, 1998.

36. Michael S. Wilkes, Samuel A. Skootsky, Stuart Slavin, Carol S. Hodgson, and Luann Wilkerson, "Entering First-Year Medical Students' Attitudes toward Managed Care," *Academic Medicine* 69:307, 1994.

37. Meeting of 4 November 1987, Board of Governors Minutes, New England Medical Center Hospitals, Office of the President, New England Medical Center Hospitals, Boston, MA.

38. Fogelman, Goode, Behrens et al., "Preserving Medical Schools' Academic Mission," p. 1191.

39. Though BJC has not publicly stated its reasons, it stands to gain much financially if clinical services are moved from Barnes-Jewish Hospital to other hospitals in the system. By an earlier agreement, operating profits at Barnes-Jewish Hospital are nearly evenly divided between the hospital and the medical school. If those services are moved elsewhere in the system, BJC would be able to retain all the hospital profit for itself, even if the professional services continue to be provided by medical school faculty.

40. These issues were discussed at the business meeting of the Department of Medicine, Washington University School of Medicine, 5 December 1996. See also

Margie Manning, "Case, Peck vie for top post at BJC," *St. Louis Business Journal*, 23–29 November 1998, p. 1.

41. "Setting priorities for topics and papers in 1997," courtesy Mark E. Frisse. This document, an agenda item for the fall 1996 meeting of the editorial board of *Academic Medicine*, served as the focus for a discussion of topics for future articles and issues.

42. *Ibid.*

43. James E. Lewis, "Academic Departments of Internal Medicine in the 1990s," *American Journal of Medicine* 97:ii, 1994.

44. David Blumenthal and Gregg S. Meyer, "The Future of the Academic Medical Center under Health Care Reform," *New England Journal of Medicine* 329:1814, 1993.

45. It should also be noted that patients, particularly when troubled by sensitive issues, may not blurt out their questions or concerns immediately. Time is often required for patients to become sufficiently at ease to bring up what is really bothering them.

46. Robert L. Lowes, "Are You Expected to See Too Many Patients?," *Medical Economics*, 27 March 1995, pp. 52–59.

47. Robert M. Goldberg, "What's Happened to the Healing Process?," *Wall Street Journal*, 18 June 1997, p. A22.

48. Edward J. Stemmler, "Professionalism in Contemporary Medicine: Can It Be Measured?," *Federation of State Medical Societies Bulletin* 80:186, 1993.

49. These studies, with citations to the original papers, were reviewed in Frank Davidoff, "Time," *Annals of Internal Medicine* 127:483–485, 1997.

50. Mark A. Linzer, "The Physician Worklife Study: The Results Are In!," *Society of General Internal Medicine Forum*, October 1998, pp. 2, 9.

51. *Ibid.*, pp. 2, 9.

52. Howard Waitzkin, "Doctor-Patient Communication," *Journal of the American Medical Association* 252:2441–2446, 1984; Christine Laine, Frank Davidoff, Charles E. Lewis et al., "Important Elements of Outpatient Care: A Comparison of Patients' and Physicians' Opinions," *Annals of Internal Medicine* 125:640–645, 1996; Gregory W. Froehlich and H. Gilbert Welch, "Meeting Walk-in Patients' Expectations for Testing," *Journal of General Internal Medicine* 11:470–474, 1996; Haya R. Rubin, Barbara Gandek, William H. Rogers et al., "Patients' Ratings of Outpatient Visits in Different Practice Settings: Results from the Medical Outcomes Study," *Journal of the American Medical Association* 270:835–840, 1993; J.G. Howie, A.M.D. Porter, D. J. Heaney, and J. L. Hopton, "Long to Short Consultation Ratio: A Proxy Measure of Quality of Care for General Practice," *British Journal of General Practice* 41:48–54, 1991; and Leone Ridsdale, Maria Carruthers, Richard Morris, and Jane Ridsdale, "Study of the Effect of Time Availability on the Consultation," *Journal of the Royal College of General Practitioners* 39:488–491, 1989.

53. Ann Landers, "What Patients Want," *Harvard Medical Alumni Bulletin* 67:42–43, Autumn 1993.

54. Davidoff, "Time," p. 485.

55. See, for instance, George Anders, *Health against Wealth: HMOs and the Breakdown of Medical Trust* (Boston: Houghton Mifflin, 1996).

56. See, for instance, John E. Ware Jr., Martha S. Bayliss, William H. Rogers, Mark Kosinski, and Alvin R. Tarlov, "Differences in 4-Year Health Outcomes for Elderly and Poor, Chronically Ill Patients Treated in HMO and Fee-for-Service Systems," *Journal of the American Medical Association* 276:1039–1047, 1996; and

"Sick People in Managed Care Have Difficulty Getting Services and Treatment, New Survey Reports," Robert Wood Johnson Foundation News Release, 28 June 1995.

57. Roger J. Bulger, "Responding to Incentives in Academic Health Centers," *Health Affairs*, Winter 1992, p. 262.

58. Lowes, "Are You Expected To See Too Many Patients?," p. 57.

59. Robert H. Miller and Harold S. Luft, "Does Managed Care Lead to Better or Worse Quality of Care?," *Health Affairs*, September/October 1997, pp. 7–25; Robert H. Miller and Harold S. Luft, "Managed Care Plan Performance Since 1980: A Literature Analysis," *Journal of the American Medical Association* 271:1512–1519, 1994.

60. See, for instance, James R. Knickman, Robert G. Hughes, Humphey Taylor, Katherine Binns, and Marie P. Lyons, "Tracking Consumers' Reactions to the Changing Health Care System: Early Indicators," *Health Affairs*, Summer 1996, pp. 21–32; and Everett C. Ladd, "Health Care Hysteria, Part II," *New York Times*, 23 July 1998, p. A21.

61. Jerome P. Kassirer, "The Quality of Care and the Quality of Measuring It," *New England Journal of Medicine* 329:1263–1265, 1993.

62. Jerome P. Kassirer, "Our Endangered Integrity—It Can Only Get Worse," *New England Journal of Medicine* 336:1667, 1997.

63. Milt Freudenheim, "As Insurers Cut Fees, Doctors Shift to Elective Procedures," *New York Times*, 24 August 1996, p. A1.

64. Jordan J. Cohen, "Forging and Channeling Consensus: The AAMC's Mission," *Academic Medicine* 69:277, 1994.

65. Malcolm Berko, "The Real Story about HMOs," *Des Moines Business Record*, 2 September 1996, p. 17.

66. Jerome P. Kassirer, "Managed Care and the Morality of the Marketplace," *New England Journal of Medicine* 333:51–52, 1995; Arnold S. Relman, "Reforming Our Health Care System: A Physician's Perspective," *The Key Reporter*, Autumn 1992, pp. 1–5.

67. "The Success of the Harvard Medical School," *Boston Medical and Surgical Journal* 88:632, 1873.

68. William C. Steere Jr., "Key Leadership Challenges for Present and Future Executives," in Frances Hesselbein, Marshall Goldsmith, and Richard Beckhard, eds., *The Leader of the Future: New Visions, Strategies, and Practices for the Next Era* (San Francisco: Jossey-Bass, 1996), pp. 267–268.

69. Some have argued that lower salaries would deter capable people from entering academic medicine. However, studies of organizations have found that "the first step to insuring that your organization is committed to its core values is to find the right people." These studies would suggest that physicians who value a high salary above the freedom, privileges, and nonmonetary rewards of academic life are not individuals who would serve the medical school well in the first place. (William N. Plamondon, "Energy and Leadership," in Hesselbein, Goldsmith, and Beckhard, eds., *The Leader of the Future*, p. 277.)

70. Henry J. Ralston III, Diana S. Beattie, Kenneth I. Berns et al., "Capturing the Promise of Science in Medical Schools," *Academic Medicine* 71:1314, 1996.

71. Steffie Woolhandler and David U. Himmelstein, "Extreme Risk—The New Corporate Proposition for Physicians," *New England Journal of Medicine* 333:1706, 1995.

72. Spyros Andreopoulous, "The Folly of Teaching-Hospital Mergers," *New England Journal of Medicine* 336:64, 1997.

73. Judith M. Bardwick, "Peacetime Management and Wartime Leadership," in Hesselbein, Goldsmith, and Beckhard, eds., *The Leader of the Future*, pp. 131–139.

74. James M. Kouzes and Barry Z. Posner, "Seven Lessons for Leading the Voyage to the Future," in Hesselbein, Goldsmith, and Beckhard, eds., *The Leader of the Future*, p. 110.

75. Hesselbein, Goldsmith, and Beckhard, eds., *The Leader of the Future*.

76. Bardwick, "Peacetime Management and Wartime Leadership," p. 137.

77. Mary Woolley and Keri Sperry, "Take off the Stethoscope and Put on a Microphone," *American Journal of Medicine* 101:241–243, 1996.

78. *Ibid.*, p. 241.

79. *Ibid.*, p. 242.

80. Charles O. Hershey, Pamela D. Reed, Paul James, and Thomas Rosenthal, "Experience with Community Academic Practice: Strategies for the Ambulatory Education of Residents," *American Journal of Medicine* 99:530–536, 1995; Carl E. Hunt, Gene A. Kallenberg, and Michael E. Whitcomb, "Ambulatory Care-Based Medical Student Education" (manuscript, submitted for publication). See also the supplement to the January 1999 issue of *Academic Medicine*, which is a special issue on the Generalist Physician Initiative sponsored by the Robert Wood Johnson Foundation.

81. *Medical School Objectives Project. Report I. Learning Objectives for Medical Student Education—Guidelines for Medical Schools* (Washington, D.C.: Association of American Medical Colleges, 1998).

82. Thomas Bodenheimer, "The HMO Backlash—Righteous or Reactionary?," *New England Journal of Medicine* 335:1601–1604, 1996; Jerome P. Kassirer, "Managing Managed Care's Tarnished Image," *New England Journal of Medicine* 337:338–339, 1997 (poll results); and Jane Bryant Quinn, "States, Courts Look at HMO Liabilities," *St. Louis Post-Dispatch*, 9 September 1997, p. 11C.

83. Carolyn M. Claney and Howard Brody, "Managed Care: Jekyll or Hyde?," *Journal of the American Medical Association* 273:338–339, 1995; David M. Lawrence, Patrick H. Mattingly, and John M. Ludden, "Trusting in the Future: The Distinct Advantage of Nonprofit HMOs," *Milbank Quarterly* 75:5–10, 1997.

84. Jerome P. Kassirer, "Practicing Medicine without a License—The New Intrusions by Congress," *New England Journal of Medicine* 336:1747, 1997.

85. In the 1960s, 1970s, and 1980s, a sizeable body of historical and sociological literature described medicine as an authoritarian profession intent on controlling patients and protecting its autonomy. Now that medical practice was so often mandated by insurers, writings about professional dominance suddenly seem dated. In this context, it would be a great irony if doctors were ultimately reempowered in the day-to-day practice of medicine by consumers.

86. John Iglehart, "The National Committee for Quality Assurance," *New England Journal of Medicine* 335:995–999, 1996; quotation, p. 997.

87. This end run around HMOs may be interpreted as part of a major shift in the methods of distribution throughout the U.S. economy, where there has been "a pandemic elimination of the middleman from countless purchasing relationships, whether through catalogue retailing, factory-outlet stores, direct selling of IPO shares or commerce on the Internet." (J. D. Kleinke, "Managed-Care Meltdown," *Barron's*, 22 December 1997, p. 51.)

88. David E. Rogers, "Where Have We Been? Where Are We Going?," *Daedalus*, Spring 1986, p. 225.

89. Bardwick, "Peacetime Management and Wartime Leadership," p. 133.

Index

Academic gentility, decline in, 151–61

Academic health centers: as academic health systems, 372; challenges to, 362–69; commercialization of, 377; vs. community hospitals, 354; decline of, as public trusts, 337–48; dependence of, on clinical income, 350; in deteriorating neighborhoods, 260–67; enlarging responsibilities of, 227; and external pressures, 260–87; failure of, to serve and lead, 390; government, adversarial relationship with, 270–79; internal dilemmas in, 288–326; and loss of future-directedness, 357; loss of vision of, 348; and need for long-range planning, 391; and need for ongoing support, 368–69, 371, 388–90; in 1980s, 266–67; paradox of, *xix–xx*; perturbations in external environment of, 388; as public trusts, 393; regulatory burdens of, 276–78, 468N56; social functions of, 388–89; subordination of academic mission of, 366–69, 371–83; as term, 457N16; and threatened financial viability, *xxiv*, 350–57. *See also* Academic medical centers

Academic health systems, 372, 379–81. *See also* Academic integrated delivery systems; Integrated delivery systems

Academic integrated delivery systems (Academic IDSs), 365, 488N49, 489N58. *See also* Integrated delivery systems

Academic integrity, lower sense of, 343

Academic medical centers: and charity care, 118–22, 264–67; growth of graduate medical education in, 183–84; and increased clinical competition, 181, 190, 235, 267–70, 352; and increased medical care, 163–68, 221–28, 231–36; role of, 123–24; and the public, 114–35; as term, 114. *See also* Academic health centers

Academic medicine: as career, 13–14, 15–16; growth of, 283; women in, 258–59

Academic Medicine, 311

Academic physicians, as dinosaurs, 373

Academic titles, standardization of, 41

Academic track, 294, 309

Academic values, persistence of, 168–73, 221

Accreditation, and licensing laws, 21

Accreditation Council for Graduate Medical Education, 314